FETAL AND EARLY POSTNATAL PROGRAMMING AND ITS INFLUENCE ON ADULT HEALTH

Oxidative Stress and Disease

Series Editors

Lester Packer, PhD
Enrique Cadenas, MD, PhD

University of Southern California School of Pharmacy Los Angeles, California

FETAL AND EARLY POSTNATAL PROGRAMMING AND ITS INFLUENCE ON ADULT HEALTH

EDITED BY

MULCHAND S. PATEL
JENS H. NIELSEN

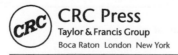

CRC Press
Taylor & Francis Group
Boca Raton London New York

CRC Press is an imprint of the
Taylor & Francis Group, an **informa** business

CRC Press
Taylor & Francis Group
6000 Broken Sound Parkway NW, Suite 300
Boca Raton, FL 33487-2742

First issued in paperback 2020

© 2017 by Taylor & Francis Group, LLC
CRC Press is an imprint of Taylor & Francis Group, an Informa business

No claim to original U.S. Government works

ISBN-13: 978-1-4987-7064-4 (hbk)
ISBN-13: 978-0-367-65789-5 (pbk)

Library of Congress Cataloging-in-Publication Data

Names: Patel, Mulchand S., editor. | Nielsen, Jens Høiriis, editor.
Title: Fetal and early postnatal programming and its influence on adult health / [edited by] Mulchand S. Patel and Jens H. Nielsen.
Other titles: Oxidative stress and disease.
Description: Boca Raton : Taylor & Francis, 2017. | Series: Oxidative stress and disease | Includes bibliographical references.
Identifiers: LCCN 2016055986 | ISBN 9781498770644 (hardback : alk. paper)
Subjects: | MESH: Prenatal Exposure Delayed Effects | Maternal Nutritional Physiological Phenomena | Maternal-Fetal Exchange–physiology | Maternal Exposure–adverse effects | Fetal Development
Classification: LCC RG559 | NLM WQ 210 | DDC 618.2/42–dc23
LC record available at https://lccn.loc.gov/2016055986

Visit the Taylor & Francis Web site at
http://www.taylorandfrancis.com

and the CRC Press Web site at
http://www.crcpress.com

Contents

SECTION I   Development of the Early Programming Concept

SECTION II   Maternal Malnutrition and Fetal Programming

SECTION III   Early Postnatal Programming

SECTION IV   Human Studies on Early Programming

SECTION V Epigenetic Mechanisms of Early Programming

SECTION VI Interventions

Series Preface

Oxidative stress is an underlying factor in health and disease. In this series, the importance of oxidative stress and disease associated with cell and organ systems of the body is highlighted by exploring the scientific evidence and the clinical applications of this knowledge. This series is intended for researchers in the biomedical sciences, clinicians, and all persons with an interest in the health sciences. The potential of such knowledge for healthy development, healthy aging, and disease prevention warrants further understanding on how oxidants and antioxidants modulate cell and tissue function.

Based on the concept of *Developmental Origins of Health and Disease*, the editors, Mulchand S. Patel and Jens H. Nielsen, organized a series of chapters with high relevance to acquired health problems ranging from insulin-resistance states to cancer to mental disorders and several more. The chapters discuss some of the molecular mechanisms that are implicated in the alteration of normal developmental programs and, moreover, provide some interventional programs aimed at lessening their adverse effects on health. Patel and Nielsen have edited an outstanding book with a collection of chapters that brings awareness to global health problems from different perspectives: maternal malnutrition and fetal programming, early postnatal programming, epigenetic mechanisms, and interventions.

Lester Packer
Enrique Cadenas
Series Editors
Oxidative Stress and Disease Series

Preface

A groundbreaking hypothesis on *Fetal Origins of Adult Disease* proposed by the late Sir Professor David Barker and his associates 25 years ago highlighted a possible link between fetal nutritional experience and development of disease risk later in adult life. Later, this hypothesis was revised to include the early postnatal period during which the newborn continues to grow rapidly and hence can be influenced by environmental factors, most notably modified nutrition, predisposing to an increased risk for adult-onset diseases. This concept is now recognized as the *Developmental Origins of Health and Disease* and is supported by outcomes of a large number of animal studies and a smaller number of observational studies in humans. A large segment of the world population today experiences one or more of the multitude of acquired health problems (such as obesity, type 2 diabetes, hypertension, cardiovascular disease, hyperlipidemia, insulin resistance, cancer, autoimmune diseases, mental disorders, etc.) due partly to abnormal nutritional experiences during the early period of life (fetal and/or early infancy). Maternal obesity and maternal malnutrition during gestation and lactation can contribute to developmental programming in the offspring. The beneficial effects of breastfeeding on reducing childhood obesity as well as the impact of early nutritional intervention on gut microbiomes are becoming increasingly recognized. Emerging evidence indicates that epigenetic modifications contribute to molecular and cellular changes in the offspring, predisposing to adverse health outcomes later in life. Epigenetic alterations may also, in part, be responsible for generational effects observed in animal studies. There is an urgent need for a better understanding of the molecular mechanisms responsible for altering normal developmental programs as well as exploring innovative interventional programs to lessen their adverse effects on health. Interventions to reduce maternal weight gain during prepregnancy and pregnancy periods and to decrease metabolic stress by dietary modification including nutraceutical supplementation are being evaluated for lessening the burden of early programming in the offspring. Some aspects of developmental programming are covered in recent reviews, but there is a paucity of books which are devoted to the various aspects of developmental programming. This book focuses on the current knowledge on several interrelated aspects of cellular programming as well as future research directions on this increasingly important global health problem.

Editors

Mulchand S. Patel earned a PhD in animal science (nutritional biochemistry) from the University of Illinois, Urbana–Champaign. He is a SUNY Distinguished Professor, UB Distinguished Professor, professor of biochemistry, and associate dean for Research and Biomedical Education at Jacobs School of Medicine and Biomedical Sciences, University at Buffalo, the State University of New York. Earlier he served as a chairman of the Department of Biochemistry at the same school. Professor Patel has been a member of the American Society for Biochemistry and Molecular Biology and the American Society for Nutrition for more than 40 years.

Professor Patel's research interests focus on the structure–function relationship of the human pyruvate dehydrogenase complex and genetic defects in this complex and developmental programming due to early life nutritional interventions. He has published nearly 250 original papers, invited reviews, and book chapters, and coedited six books. He has received several scientific achievement awards including a Fulbright Research Scholar Award to India. He has served as a co-organizer of several international conferences in the areas of his research interests and has presented his research at many international conferences.

Jens H. Nielsen earned an MSc and DSc in biochemistry and cell biology from the University of Copenhagen, Denmark. He was the head of the Department of Cell Biology at the Hagedorn Research Institute for several years before he became a professor at the Department of Biomedical Sciences, Faculty of Health and Medical Sciences, University of Copenhagen. He has been a visiting professor at the Hormone Research Institute, University of California, San Francisco. He has served as a board member and the chairman for the Danish Society for Biochemistry and Molecular Biology and a board member of the Danish Centre for Fetal Programming.

Professor Nielsen's research interests focus on the pathogenesis of type 1 and type 2 diabetes, in particular, the regulation of the development, growth, and function of the pancreatic β-cells. He has published 150 original papers and reviews. He has received several awards including the Arnold Lazarow Memorial Lecture from the University of Minnesota, Minneapolis and St. Paul. He has served as an organizer of several international meetings on diabetes and islet cell biology.

Contributors

Edward Archer
Enduring *FX*
Columbia, South Carolina

Francisco Bolaños-Jimenez
UMR Physiologie des Adaptations
  Nutritionnelles INRA Université
  de Nantes
Nantes, France

Charlotte Brøns
Department of Endocrinology (Diabetes
  and Metabolism)
Rigshospitalet
Copenhagen, Denmark

Tine Dalgaard Clausen
Department of Gynecology and Obstetrics
Nordsjaellands Hospital
Hilleroed, Denmark

and

Institute of Clinical Medicine
Faculty of Health and Medical Sciences
University of Copenhagen
Copenhagen, Denmark

Débora C. Damasceno
Department of Gynecology and Obstetrics
Botucatu Medical School, UNESP
São Paulo, Brazil

Peter Damm
Center for Pregnant Women with Diabetes
Department of Obstetrics
Rigshospitalet
Copenhagen, Denmark

and

Institute of Clinical Medicine
Faculty of Health and Medical Sciences
University of Copenhagen
Copenhagen, Denmark

Mina Desai
Department of Obstetrics and
  Gynecology
David Geffen School of Medicine at
  UCLA and LABioMed at Harbor–
  UCLA Medical Center
Los Angeles, California

Sherin U. Devaskar
Department of Pediatrics
Division of Neonatology and
  Developmental Biology

and

Neonatal Research Center of the UCLA
  Children's Discovery and Innovation
  Institute
David Geffen School of Medicine at
  UCLA
Los Angeles, California

Liesbeth Duijts
Department of Pediatrics and
  Department of Epidemiology
Erasmus University Medical Center
Rotterdam, the Netherlands

Jerad H. Dumolt
Department of Exercise and Nutrition
  Sciences
School of Public Health and Health
  Professions
University at Buffalo
The State University of New York
Buffalo, New York

Janine F. Felix
Department of Pediatrics and
  Department of Epidemiology
The Generation R Study Group
Erasmus University Medical Center
Rotterdam, the Netherlands

Cilius Esmann Fonvig
Department of Pediatrics
The Children's Obesity Clinic
Copenhagen University Hospital
    Holbæk
Holbæk, Denmark

and

The Novo Nordisk Foundation Center
    for Basic Metabolic Research
Section of Metabolic Genetics
The Faculty of Health and Medical
    Sciences
University of Copenhagen
Copenhagen, Denmark

Romy Gaillard
Department of Pediatrics and
    Department of Epidemiology
The Generation R Study Group
Erasmus University Medical Center
Rotterdam, the Netherlands

Louise Groth Grunnet
Department of Endocrinology (Diabetes
    and Metabolism)
Rigshospitalet
Copenhagen, Denmark

Torben Hansen
The Novo Nordisk Foundation Center
    for Basic Metabolic Research
Section of Metabolic Genetics
The Faculty of Health and Medical
    Sciences
University of Copenhagen
Copenhagen, Denmark

Jerrold J. Heindel
Division of Extramural Research and
    Training
National Institute of Environmental
    Health Sciences
Research Triangle Park, North Carolina

David J. Hill
Lawson Health Research Institute
St. Joseph's Health Care
London, Ontario, Canada

Jens-Christian Holm
Department of Pediatrics
The Children's Obesity Clinic
Copenhagen University Hospital
Holbæk, Denmark

and

The Novo Nordisk Foundation Center
    for Basic Metabolic Research
Section of Metabolic Genetics
The Faculty of Health and Medical
    Sciences
University of Copenhagen
Copenhagen, Denmark

Azadeh Houshmand-Oeregaard
Department of Obstetrics
Center for Pregnant Women with
    Diabetes
Rigshospitalet
Copenhagen, Denmark

Isabela Iessi
Department of Biomedical Sciences
University of Copenhagen
Copenhagen, Denmark

and

Department of Gynecology and
    Obstetrics
Botucatu Medical School
UNESP
São Paulo, Brazil

Vincent W.V. Jaddoe
Department of Pediatrics and
    Department of Epidemiology
The Generation R Study Group
Erasmus University Medical Center
Rotterdam, the Netherlands

Caroline Jaksch
Department of Biomedical Sciences
University of Copenhagen
Copenhagen, Denmark

and

Centre for Fetal Programming
Copenhagen, Denmark

Josep C. Jimenez-Chillaron
Institut de Recerca Pediàtrica
Hospital Sant Joan de Déu
Esplugues de Llobregat
Barcelona, Spain

Louise Kelstrup
Department of Obstetrics
Center for Pregnant Women with
    Diabetes
Rigshospitalet
Copenhagen, Denmark

Maria S. Landa
Department of Molecular Genetics and
    Biology of Complex Diseases
Institute of Medical Research
    A Lanari–IDIM
University of Buenos Aires
    National Council of Scientific and
    Technological Research (CONICET)
Ciudad Autónoma de Buenos Aires,
    Argentina

Lea H. Larsen
Department of Biomedical Sciences
Faculty of Health and Medical Sciences
University of Copenhagen
Copenhagen, Denmark

Suzanne G. Laychock
Department of Pharmacology and
    Toxicology
Jacobs School of Medicine and
    Biomedical Sciences
University at Buffalo
The State University of New York
Buffalo, New York

Tejas Limaye
Diabetes Unit
King Edward Memorial Hospital and
    Research Centre
Pune, India

Saleh Mahmood
Department of Biochemistry
Jacobs School of Medicine and
    Biomedical Sciences
University at Buffalo
The State University of New York
Buffalo, New York

Elisabeth R. Mathiesen
Department of Endocrinology
Center for Pregnant Women with
    Diabetes
Rigshospitalet
Copenhagen, Denmark

and

Institute of Clinical Medicine
Faculty of Health and Medical Sciences
University of Copenhagen
Copenhagen, Denmark

Samantha McDonald
Department of Exercise Science
University of South Carolina
Columbia, South Carolina

Michelle Mendez
Department of Nutrition–Gillings
    School of Public Health
Carolina Population Center and
    Lineberger Cancer Center
University of North Carolina
Chapel Hill, North Carolina

Rosalio Mercado-Camargo
Facultad de Químico–Farmacobiología
Universidad Michoacana de San
    Nicolás de Hidalgo
Morelia, Mexico

Ole H. Mortensen
Department of Biomedical Sciences
Faculty of Health and Medical Sciences
University of Copenhagen
Copenhagen, Denmark

L.M. Nicholas
University of Cambridge Metabolic
    Research Laboratories and MRC
    Metabolic Diseases Unit
Wellcome Trust–MRC Institute of
    Metabolic Science
Addenbrooke's Hospital
Cambridge, United Kingdom

Jens Høiriis Nielsen
Department of Biomedical Sciences
Faculty of Health and Medical Sciences
University of Copenhagen
Copenhagen, Denmark

S.E. Ozanne
University of Cambridge Metabolic
    Research Laboratories and MRC
    Metabolic Diseases Unit
Wellcome Trust–MRC Institute of
    Metabolic Science
Addenbrooke's Hospital
Cambridge, United Kingdom

Mulchand S. Patel
Department of Biochemistry
Jacobs School of Medicine and
    Biomedical Sciences
University at Buffalo
The State University of New York
Buffalo, New York

Oluf Pedersen
The Novo Nordisk Foundation Center
    for Basic Metabolic Research
Section of Metabolic Genetics
The Faculty of Health and Medical
    Sciences
University of Copenhagen
Copenhagen, Denmark

Andreas Friis Pihl
The Children's Obesity Clinic
Department of Pediatrics
Copenhagen University Hospital
    Holbæk

Sara Pinney
Children's Hospital of Philadelphia
Philadelphia, Pennsylvania

Carlos J. Pirola
Department of Molecular Genetics and
    Biology of Complex Diseases
Institute of Medical Research
    A Lanari–IDIM
University of Buenos Aires
    National Council of Scientific
    and Technological Research
    (CONICET)
Ciudad Autónoma de Buenos Aires,
    Argentina

Todd C. Rideout
Department of Exercise and Nutrition
    Sciences
School of Public Health and Health
    Professions
University at Buffalo
The State University of New York
Buffalo, New York

Guadalupe L. Rodríguez-González
Reproductive Biology Department
National Institute of Medical Sciences
    and Nutrition Salvador Zubirán
Mexico City, Mexico

Michael G. Ross
Department of Obstetrics and
    Gynecology
David Geffen School of Medicine at
    UCLA and LABioMed at Harbor–
    UCLA Medical Center
Los Angeles, California

Susana Santos
Department of Pediatrics and
    Department of Epidemiology
The Generation R Study Group
Erasmus University Medical Center
Rotterdam, the Netherlands

Kartik Shankar
Department of Pediatrics
Arkansas Children's Nutrition Center
University of Arkansas for Medical
    Sciences
Little Rock, Arkansas

Bo-Chul Shin
Department of Pediatrics
Division of Neonatology and
    Developmental Biology and the
    Neonatal Research Center of the
    UCLA Children's Discovery and
    Innovation Institute
David Geffen School of Medicine at
    UCLA
Los Angeles, California

Rebecca Simmons
Perelman School of Medicine
Children's Hospital of Philadelphia
University of Pennsylvania
Philadelphia, Pennsylvania

Silvia Sookoian
Department of Clinical and Molecular
    Hepatology
Institute of Medical Research
    A Lanari–IDIM
University of Buenos Aires
    National Council of Scientific
    and Technological Research
    (CONICET)
Ciudad Autónoma de Buenos Aires,
    Argentina

Mariana Tellechea
Department of Molecular Genetics and
    Biology of Complex Diseases
Institute of Medical Research
    A Lanari–IDIM
University of Buenos Aires
    National Council of Scientific and
    Technological Research (CONICET)
Ciudad Autónoma de Buenos Aires,
    Argentina

Keshari M. Thakali
Department of Pediatrics
Arkansas Children's Nutrition Center
University of Arkansas for Medical
    Sciences
Little Rock, Arkansas

Héctor Urquiza-Marín
Facultad de Químico–Farmacobiología
Universidad Michoacana de San
    Nicolás de Hidalgo
Morelia, Mexico

Umesh D. Wankhade
Department of Pediatrics
Arkansas Children's Nutrition Center
University of Arkansas for Medical
    Sciences
Little Rock, Arkansas

Chittaranjan Yajnik
Diabetes Unit
King Edward Memorial Hospital and
    Research Centre
Pune, India

Elena Zambrano
Reproductive Biology Department
National Institute of Medical Sciences
    and Nutrition
Salvador Zubirán
Mexico City, Mexico

Section I

Development of the Early Programming Concept

1 The Developmental Origins of Health and Disease—Where Did It All Begin?

L.M. Nicholas and S.E. Ozanne

CONTENTS

1.1 THE DEVELOPMENTAL ORIGINS OF ADULT DISEASE—ORIGINS OF THE HYPOTHESIS

One of the earliest proposals establishing the association between early life events and the risk for disease in adult life was more than 80 years ago by Kermack and colleagues. In 1934, in their investigation of specific death rates in England and Wales from 1845, Scotland from 1860, and Sweden from 1751, they found a fall in death rates from all causes, which could be attributed to improved conditions during the individual's childhood (Kermack et al. 1934). Some 40 years later, this association was supported by a Norwegian study by Forsdahl who found that infant mortality (a reliable index of standard of living in Norway) between birth and 9 years of age was positively correlated to later atherosclerotic heart disease mortality (Forsdahl 1977). Interestingly, he found that this was the case only for those who grew up in conditions of poverty and were then exposed to affluence in adult life (Forsdahl 1977) thus providing the first evidence that early programming effects are most pronounced when there is a mismatch in nutritional availability between early and later life.

It was only 10 years later, beginning in the early 1980s, that there was an increasing number of studies published, which investigated factors associated with the incidence of hypertension and death from cardiovascular disease and its relationship to those operating in early life. For example, Marmot et al. suggested that early life experiences could not be excluded when explaining their observation of an independent relationship between height and death from coronary disease (and other causes) (Marmot et al. 1984), especially when considering height as an indicator of early nutritional status. Another prospective study by Wadsworth et al. involving 5632 subjects born during one week in March 1946 in the United Kingdom found that birth weight was inversely associated with adult systolic (but not diastolic) blood pressure in both women and men (Wadsworth et al. 1985).

In 1986, in their effort to provide an explanation for the paradox that although the steep increase in ischemic heart disease during the earlier part of the 20th century in England and Wales had been associated with rising prosperity, the disease was now more common in poorer and lower income groups, Barker and Osmond explored the association between poor living standards and ischemic heart disease by a detailed geographical comparison of infant mortality between 1921 and 1925 and death in adults from ischemic heart disease and other leading causes between 1968 and 1978 (Barker and Osmond 1986). They found a positive correlation between mortality associated with ischemic heart disease and stroke and infant mortality rates, which was remarkably consistent in both males and females in all age groups and in the different geographical areas (Barker and Osmond 1986). Barker and colleagues concluded that the geographical distribution of ischemic heart disease in England and Wales was reflected by variations in nutrition in early life, which was expressed pathologically on exposure to later dietary influences (Barker and Osmond 1986).

1.2   THE RELATIONSHIP BETWEEN LOW BIRTH WEIGHT, HYPERTENSION, AND CARDIOVASCULAR DISEASE

Early in the 20th century, many infants were poorly nourished partly due to maternal malnutrition and ill health prompting Barker and Osmond to make the pioneering conclusion that it was likely nutrition during *prenatal* life that was a factor in determining risk for ischemic heart disease in adult life (Barker and Osmond 1986). Moreover, they suggested blood pressure as one link between the intrauterine environment and risk of cardiovascular disease (Barker and Osmond 1987). This prompted Barker and colleagues to carry out a number of epidemiological studies, this time using birth weight as a crude index of *in utero* experiences to investigate the impact of maternal undernutrition on the risk of hypertension and cardiovascular disease in adult life. Two studies, published in 1988, confirmed the earlier findings of Wadsworth et al. regarding the inverse relationship between systolic blood pressure and birth weight (Wadsworth et al. 1985), this time in a cohort of 9921 children at 10 years of age (Barker and Osmond 1988) and 3259 adults aged 36 (Barker et al. 1989). Soon after, Barker et al. proposed, for the first time, a possible mechanism by which this could occur. They found that the highest blood pressures occurred in men and women who had been *small* babies with *large* placentas (Barker et al. 1990). The authors postulated that discordance between fetal and placental weight may lead to circulatory adaptation in the fetus, altered arterial structure in the child, and consequently hypertension in the adult (Barker et al. 1990). Around the same time, a study investigating the association between birth weight and blood pressure in a cohort of Swedish male army conscripts found that being born small resulted in increased *diastolic* blood pressure in early adult life (Gennser et al. 1988). Interestingly, the authors disregarded systolic pressure in this study because they found that several men with a high diastolic blood pressure had normal systolic pressure (Gennser et al. 1988). Taken together, these studies suggested that being born small either due to prenatal undernutrition and/or uteroplacental insufficiency contributed to increased risk for hypertension that was identifiable in childhood and persisted in adult life.

Soon after the initial studies focusing on birth weight and blood pressure, Barker et al. carried out a study of over 5000 men born in Hertfordshire, England during 1911–1930 and found that men with the lowest weights at birth and at 1 year of age had the highest death rates from ischemic heart disease. As weight at birth and at 1 year was the only measure collected in this cohort, they concluded that the association between low birth weight and ischemic heart disease mortality was due to environmental influences producing poor fetal and infant growth (Barker et al. 1989). Furthermore, these findings led to the suggestion that promotion of infant growth in babies of below average birth weight (~3.5 kg) may be beneficial for reducing cardiovascular deaths since heavier weight at 1 year was accompanied by large reductions in death rates (Barker et al. 1989).

Studies published 10 years later by Eriksson et al. involving two separate cohorts of men born at the Helsinki University Hospital between 1924 and 1944 clearly showed, however, that not only is coronary heart disease associated with low birth weight but that rapid postnatal weight gain in these boys who were previously thin at birth was associated with *further* increased risk (Eriksson et al. 2001, 1999). The authors found that the adverse effects of rapid weight gain on later coronary heart disease were already apparent as early as 3 years of age (Eriksson et al. 2001) and was highest in boys who were thin at birth but whose weight caught up so that they had an average or above average body mass from age 7 (Eriksson et al. 1999). Similar findings were also observed in females but where coronary heart disease in men was associated more with *thinness* at birth followed by increased body mass, in women this was the case when they were born *short* in relation to placental size and were later tall in childhood (Forsen et al. 1999). Not surprisingly, this association was stronger in the daughters of taller mothers since this indicates that prenatal growth of these female infants was constrained (Forsen et al. 1999). These findings were the first since that of Forsdahl in 1977 to show the potential adverse effects on cardiovascular health when there is a mismatch between prenatal and postnatal nutrition.

Similar findings were also made in the context of increased blood pressure. Catch-up growth between birth and 7 years of age amplified the risk of hypertension associated with low birth weight (Eriksson et al. 2000) in a subset of the same cohort of Finnish men and women as previously published by Eriksson et al. (2001, 1999). Also, in the large Shanghai Women's Health Study, which involved more than 75,000 participants, women who were born with a low birth weight and became heavy or both heavy and tall at age 15 had a five- to sevenfold increased odds of developing early onset hypertension (Zhao et al. 2002).

In November 1990, David Barker summarized the findings hitherto regarding the association between low birth weight, hypertension, and cardiovascular disease in a publication titled "The fetal and infant origins of adult disease—the womb may be more important than the home." He argued that adult degenerative disease was not only based on the interaction between genes and an adverse environment in adult life (as previously thought) but also encompassed programming by the environment in fetal and infant life (Barker et al. 1990).

1.3 THE RELATIONSHIP BETWEEN LOW BIRTH WEIGHT, OBESITY, AND TYPE 2 DIABETES

Before the emergence of the fetal and infant origins of adult disease hypothesis, it was a widely accepted truth that type 2 diabetes mellitus (T2DM) was totally genetically determined (Hales and Barker 1992). In 1991, however, Hales and colleagues showed, in the same Hertfordshire cohort where associations between birth weight and cardiovascular disease had been made, that there was a continuous inverse relationship between birth weight and impaired glucose tolerance in men at 64 years of age (Hales et al. 1991). Those individuals with the lowest birth weight had a sixfold increased risk of developing T2DM when compared to the heaviest (Hales et al. 1991). A follow-up study to confirm and extend this association in a different population was published in 1993, this time involving both men and women aged 50 years born in Preston in the United Kingdom. The authors found that being born with a lower birth weight was associated with impaired glucose tolerance and T2DM in both male and female adults (Phipps et al. 1993). Moreover, these men and women also had a high ratio of placental weight to birth weight, which the authors concluded could be due to maternal undernutrition (Phipps et al. 1993). These findings have also been replicated in a cohort of young men (Robinson et al. 1992). Further support is offered by studies carried out on both men and women in the United States, which also found an inverse association between birth weight and the risk for T2DM in adulthood (Curhan et al. 1996; Rich-Edwards et al. 1999). Importantly, this association persisted even after adjusting for ethnicity, childhood socioeconomic status, and adult lifestyle factors (Rich-Edwards et al. 1999). Similar findings have subsequently been replicated in over 100 studies worldwide representing many ethnic groups.

Glucose induces insulin secretion in a biphasic pattern: an initial component (first phase) that develops rapidly but lasts only a few minutes, followed by a sustained component (second phase) (Seino et al. 2011). T2DM is characterized by loss of first-phase insulin secretion and reduced second-phase secretion. Before the development of frank T2DM, however, a decrease in the first phase of glucose stimulated insulin secretion is already present in people with impaired glucose tolerance (Cerasi and Luft 1967; Luzi and DeFronzo 1989). Thus, Hales and Barker put forth the suggestion that exposure to undernutrition during fetal life results in compromised development of the islets of Langerhans and/or β-cells and that this is a major factor in the etiology of T2DM (Hales and Barker 2001).

Despite the strong epidemiological evidence of a link between impaired fetal growth and future risk of T2DM, there were suggestions that the association between low birth weight and risk of T2DM in some studies could theoretically be explained by a genetically determined reduced fetal growth rate. Thus, in their study, Poulsen and colleagues specifically studied monozygotic twins discordant for T2DM, which allowed elimination of a putative influence of the genotype per se on the fetal growth rate (Poulsen et al. 1997). They found that within monozygotic twins, the diabetic twin had a lower birth weight compared to their genetically identical nondiabetic cotwin. These findings, therefore, argue against the possibility that the association between low birth weight and T2DM is solely due to having a genetic susceptibility to T2DM, which coincidentally also impairs fetal growth (Poulsen et al. 1997).

In addition to glucose intolerance, a study by Law et al. involving 1184 men in Hertfordshire and Preston in the United Kingdom found that adult men who experienced reduced growth during fetal life and infancy had a higher waist-to-hip ratio, which is an indicator of abdominal fatness (Law et al. 1992). Moreover, just like the risk for glucose intolerance and T2DM, the degree of adiposity tracked positively with placental weight-to-birth weight ratio (Law et al. 1992). This highlighted the potential twofold impact of impaired fetal and infant growth on T2DM risk since obesity increases the risk of insulin resistance and consequently T2DM and this would add to the risk resulting from poor early growth (Hales and Barker 1992). Indeed, in their study, Hales and colleagues found that the mean 2-hour glucose concentration ranged from 5.8 mmol/L in men who were in the highest tertile of weight at 1 year but the lowest tertile of current body mass index (BMI) (<25.4) to 7.7 mmol/L in men in the lowest tertile of weight at 1 year and the highest tertile of current BMI (>28) (Hales et al. 1991). Additionally, there was a similar additive effect of obesity and low weight at 1 year on fasting 32–33 split proinsulin concentration (Hales and Barker 2001); a partly processed form of insulin that in high concentrations may indicate insulin resistance and pancreatic islet dysfunction (Nagi et al. 1990).

In addition to pancreatic β-cell dysfunction, insulin resistance also contributes to the development of T2DM (Kahn et al. 2006). Thus, following the findings discussed earlier, Phillips et al. sought to determine whether insulin resistance could also be a consequence of reduced early growth. They found that both men and women who were thin at birth were more insulin resistant in later life (mean age of 52 years). Importantly, this association was independent of adult BMI and waist-to-hip ratio (Phillips et al. 1994). Obesity per se is also associated with an increased risk of insulin resistance. In obese individuals, adipose tissue releases increased amounts of nonesterified fatty acids, glycerol, hormones, proinflammatory cytokines, and other factors that are involved in the development of insulin resistance (Kahn et al. 2006). This study provided the earliest evidence that adults at the greatest risk of T2DM are those that experienced impaired growth during fetal life and that are obese in adult life; people who were thin at birth but obese as adults were the most resistant to insulin (Phillips et al. 1994). Furthermore, catch-up growth specifically between birth and 3 years of age was also found to contribute to the insulin resistance risk spectrum encompassing low birth weight with or without adult obesity (Ong et al. 2004).

1.4 THE RELATIONSHIP BETWEEN BIRTH WEIGHT AND THE METABOLIC SYNDROME

Epidemiological studies carried out across different countries and continents (some of which we have highlighted) have showed a clear association between low birth weight and the risk for hypertension, glucose intolerance, insulin resistance, and obesity. These comorbidities along with dyslipidemia are major components of the metabolic syndrome, which is associated with increased mortality from coronary heart disease (Fontbonne et al. 1991). In 1991, Hales and Barker first alluded to their hypothesis that the various components of the metabolic syndrome are the result of suboptimal development during intrauterine and early infant life (Hales and Barker 1992). This prompted Barker et al. to explore this possible association in a cohort of men in Hertfordshire. Indeed, men who were born small and had low weight at 1 year of age had impaired glucose tolerance or T2DM, together with hypertension as well as raised fasting serum triglyceride concentrations around age 64 (Barker et al. 1993). They also found that both men and women (in Preston) with the metabolic syndrome at around 50 years of age had low birth weight, a small head circumference, and low ponderal index at birth (Barker et al. 1993). Combining these findings and the intrauterine developmental trajectory, the authors postulated that the influences that program the metabolic syndrome may act early in gestation (Barker et al. 1993).

1.5 MECHANISMS UNDERLYING THE EARLY ORIGINS OF ADULT HEALTH AND DISEASE

In 1992, Hales and Barker coined the "thrifty phenotype" hypothesis in an attempt to explain the association between poor fetal and infant growth and the increased risk of developing impaired glucose tolerance and metabolic syndrome in adult life. The central element of this hypothesis is that if the growing fetus is malnourished during gestation due to suboptimal maternal nutrition, placental dysfunction, stress, and/or other factors there is an adaptive response to optimize the growth of key body organs, for example, heart and brain, to the detriment of others, for example, muscle and the endocrine pancreas (Hales and Barker 1992, 2001). In addition, the hypothesis proposed that metabolic programming would occur leading the fetus to maximize metabolic efficiency in terms of both the storage and usage of nutrients, which is designed to enhance postnatal survival under conditions of intermittent or poor nutrition. These adaptations, however, were proposed to become detrimental when nutrition is more abundant in the postnatal environment than it had been in the prenatal environment (Gluckman and Hanson 2004) (Figure 1.1). This is supported by studies in sub-Saharan Africa. For example, Motala showed that in rural Cameroon where there is chronic malnutrition, the rates of diabetes are only about 1% as there is a match between the pre- and postnatal environments (Motala 2002). Furthermore, in their studies of the Hertfordshire cohort, Hales and colleagues found that those who were born small and were obese as adults when the study was conducted had the worst glucose tolerance of all the groups (Hales et al. 1991).

Numerous studies have since been published that provide unequivocal support that fetal and/or infant malnutrition (which can be brought about by maternal malnutrition or other maternal/placental abnormalities) followed by catch-up growth programs a lifetime risk of hypertension and cardiovascular disease in the offspring. The implications of this are huge when considering the fact that around 70–90% of infants who are born small for their gestational age show some catch-up growth within the first years of life (Karlberg and Albertsson-Wikland 1995). Furthermore, in contemporary affluent societies, the biological predisposition to catch-up growth

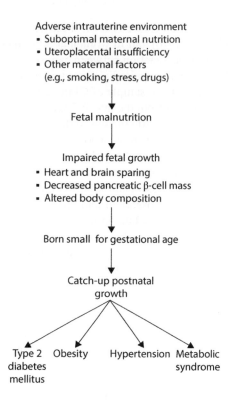

Adverse intrauterine environment
- Suboptimal maternal nutrition
- Uteroplacental insufficiency
- Other maternal factors
  (e.g., smoking, stress, drugs)

Fetal malnutrition

Impaired fetal growth
- Heart and brain sparing
- Decreased pancreatic β-cell mass
- Altered body composition

Born small for gestational age

Catch-up postnatal
growth

Type 2   Obesity   Hypertension Metabolic
diabetes   syndrome
mellitus

FIGURE 1.1 Exposure to suboptimal nutrition during fetal development results in an adaptive response to optimize the growth of key body organs to the detriment of others. This leads to an increased risk of metabolic and cardiovascular disease especially when fetal malnutrition is followed by catch-up growth in postnatal life.

in low birth weight babies results in accelerated postnatal growth, which overshoots their genetic target thus resulting in children with greater BMI, percentage body fat, total fat mass, and central fat distribution (Ong et al. 2000).

One of the pivotal elements of the "thrifty phenotype" hypothesis is the concept of a "critical" period during which specific nutritional perturbations may cause long-term changes in development and adverse outcomes in the offspring in later life. Historical events such as the Dutch famine of 1944–1945 during which rations were strictly imposed on all sections of the population including pregnant and nursing mothers, provided an opportunity to study associations between maternal under-nutrition during specific periods of gestation and the risk of chronic adult disease in babies born around the period. By comparing glucose and insulin responses to a standard oral glucose load in participants exposed to famine at any stage during gestation with those who were born in the year before or conceived in the year after, Ravelli and colleagues showed, for the first time, that exposure to famine during gestation decreased glucose tolerance in adults aged 50 years and that this effect was most pronounced when exposure occurred during mid- or late gestation (Ravelli et al. 1998). In contrast, exposure to maternal undernutrition during early gestation has a greater impact on future risk of obesity that was present in men at 19 years of age (Ravelli et al. 1976) and in women at 50 years of age (Ravelli et al. 1999). Further support for the association between exposure to maternal undernutrition during fetal development and impaired glucose tolerance in later life came from a study by Li et al. involving a large sample of Chinese adults that were exposed to the Chinese famine, which lasted from the late 1950s to the early 1960s. They found that exposure to famine during fetal life increased the risk of hyperglycemia in adult life. This association was strongest in adults who were more affluent and consumed a Western-style diet in adult life (Li et al. 2010). Moreover, these individuals were also at risk of developing the metabolic syndrome in adult life (Li et al. 2011).

Interestingly, in contrast to the association between famine exposure and subsequent risk for metabolic disease, Roseboom and colleagues found that exposure to the Dutch famine in early, mid-, and late gestation in a population that was previously well nourished had no impact on blood pressure on adult life (Roseboom et al. 1999). This led them to suggest that it is the composition rather than the quantity of a pregnant woman's diet that conferred these risks since the famine would have resulted in a proportionate reduction in caloric intake from protein, fat, and carbohydrate (Roseboom et al. 1999).

Bateson and Gluckman subsequently suggested that the "thrifty phenotype" concept may be too limited as an overarching hypothesis and that the adaptive responses of the embryo or fetus to a range of prenatal environments should be viewed in a broader, evolutionary context. They, therefore, proposed the "predictive adaptive response" hypothesis, the central tenet of which is that developing organisms receive information about the quality of their external environment and in response formulate predictions about future *extra*uterine conditions and prepare themselves adaptively for this environment. They proposed that for individuals whose early environment had predicted a high level of nutrition in adult life and who are consequently heavier at birth, the better their postnatal conditions, the better their adult health. Conversely, if an individual experienced conditions in fetal life, which predicted poor postnatal nutrition, this person was expected to be worse off if there is a relative excess of nutrition in postnatal life (Bateson et al. 1999; Gluckman et al. 2007). Regardless of whether the responses to poor fetal growth is an adaptation to preserve the growth of more important organs or predictive of future nutritional availability, the end result is still the programming of a lifetime of reduced functional capacity and disease risk. This is especially the case in the 21st century due to the increased likelihood of a nutritional mismatch between the fetal and postnatal environment; a majority of low birth weight babies are born in developing countries (de Onis et al. 1998) and it is these countries that are being affected most by the obesity epidemic, especially in urban areas (WHO and Consultation 2003).

1.6 THE DEVELOPMENTAL ORIGINS OF HEALTH AND DISEASE—FUTURE DIRECTIONS

The initial epidemiological studies of individuals born in the United Kingdom during the first half of the last century consistently demonstrated that having a low birth weight is associated with an increased risk of cardiovascular disease, T2DM, and other aspects of the metabolic syndrome in adult life and that this was linear across the birth weight spectrum (Hales et al. 1991). However, in more contemporary cohorts, and particularly those with a high prevalence of maternal obesity, the relationship has been shown to be U-shaped or reverse J-shaped with both high birth weight and low birth weight being associated with increased disease risk. This was first reported by McCance and colleagues who studied birth weight as a risk factor for diabetes among the Pima Indians in Arizona; they observed that there was a U-shaped, rather than a simple linear association present, that is, the rates of T2DM in those with low as well as high birth weights were almost twice as high when compared to those of normal birth weight (McCance et al. 1994). Furthermore, they found that the incidence of gestational diabetes mellitus (GDM) accounted for much of the diabetes in high birth weight individuals (McCance et al. 1994) and that these individuals were also more obese, had higher glucose concentrations, and an increased risk of being diagnosed as diabetic in childhood (Pettitt et al. 1993). Hence, both maternal under- and overnutrition appear to play an important role in fetal growth and development. Consequently, in recent years, there has been growing interest on the effects of maternal overweight/obesity on the health of the offspring in childhood and adult life especially in the context of the current global obesity epidemic, which has also recruited women of reproductive age with more women entering pregnancy with a BMI in the overweight or obese range (Kumanyika et al. 2008). Obese women are at an increased risk of developing insulin resistance and GDM (Catalano et al. 2003) and of giving birth to a large baby with increased fat mass (Pettitt et al. 1993; Catalano 2003; Catalano and Ehrenberg 2006; Silverman et al. 1998). Importantly, exposure to either maternal obesity or to impaired glucose tolerance during pregnancy is also associated with an increased risk of obesity and features of insulin resistance in childhood, adolescence, and adult life (Boney et al. 2005; Dorner and Plagemann 1994; Whitaker 2004). This suggests that exposure to maternal obesity may result in an "intergenerational cycle" of obesity and insulin resistance (Kumanyika et al. 2008; Zhang et al. 2011; Zhang et al. 2011).

The link between obesity in pregnancy and adverse maternal and infant outcomes has also resulted in a growing focus on the nutritional health of women and lifestyle interventions that can be safely introduced in the overweight/obese woman either before or during pregnancy. Current practice guidelines recommend that women should be counseled prior to conception and encouraged to make lifestyle changes both before and during pregnancy including following an exercise program (American College of Obstetricians and Gynecologists 2013). Indeed, two large-scale, multicenter randomized control trials, the LIMIT and UK Pregnancies Better Eating and Activity Trial (UPBEAT) study, have investigated the efficacy of a complex and comprehensive behavioral intervention, including a combination of dietary, exercise, and behavioral strategies versus standard antenatal care. These studies showed some favorable maternal weight-related outcomes (Dodd et al. 2014; Poston et al. 2015). Furthermore, the LIMIT trial reported that infants born to women allocated to lifestyle advice were less likely to be macrosomic, that is, to weigh more than 4 kg (Dodd et al. 2014). Importantly, these studies highlight the fact that women are able and willing to change their behavior during pregnancy.

In the 30 years since David Barker first proposed his hypothesis that different patterns of growth in early life lead to an increased risk of cardiovascular and

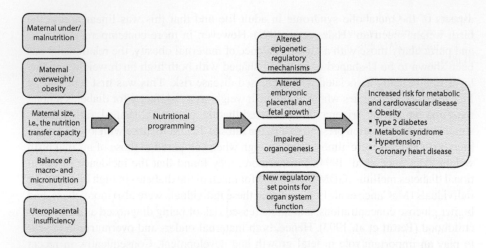

FIGURE 1.2 Various suboptimal maternal factors can program a lifetime of cardiometabolic vulnerability in the offspring through epigenetic changes, which are recruited within the developing embryo and/or fetus.

metabolic disease in adult life, there has been an accumulation of compelling epidemiological, clinical, and experimental evidence to support and extend this hypothesis (Figure 1.2). Investigations into the molecular mechanisms underlying the programming of obesity, T2DM, and cardiovascular disease have highlighted the sensitivity of the offspring epigenome to maternal obesity; epigenetic changes, which are recruited within the developing embryo and/or fetus, may be the conduit through which a life of metabolic vulnerability is programmed in tissues of metabolic importance (Figure 1.2). It is clear that this will set the trajectory of future studies thus leading to novel mechanistic hypotheses to strengthen our understanding of how the impact of an adverse intrauterine environment is transduced from mother to baby and to subsequent generations. This will then allow us to develop the robust interventions required to improve both maternal and infant health outcomes.

REFERENCES

American College of Obstetricians and Gynecologists (2013) ACOG Committee opinion no. 549: obesity in pregnancy. *Obstet Gynecol* 121, 213–217.

Barker, D. J., Bull, A. R., Osmond, C., and Simmonds, S. J. (1990) Fetal and placental size and risk of hypertension in adult life. *BMJ* 301, 259–262.

Barker, D. J., Hales, C. N., Fall, C. H., Osmond, C., Phipps, K., and Clark, P. M. (1993) Type 2 (non-insulin-dependent) diabetes mellitus, hypertension and hyperlipidaemia (syndrome X): Relation to reduced fetal growth. *Diabetologia* 36, 62–67.

Barker, D. J., and Osmond, C. (1986) Infant mortality, childhood nutrition, and ischaemic heart disease in England and Wales. *Lancet* 1, 1077–1081.

Barker, D. J., and Osmond, C. (1987) Death rates from stroke in England and Wales predicted from past maternal mortality. *Br Med J (Clin Res Ed)* 295, 83–86.

Barker, D. J., and Osmond, C. (1988) Low birth weight and hypertension. *BMJ* 297, 134–135.

Barker, D. J., Osmond, C., Golding, J., Kuh, D., and Wadsworth, M. E. (1989) Growth in utero, blood pressure in childhood and adult life, and mortality from cardiovascular disease. *BMJ* 298, 564–567.

Barker, D. J., Winter, P. D., Osmond, C., Margetts, B., and Simmonds, S. J. (1989) Weight in infancy and death from ischaemic heart disease. *Lancet* 2, 577–580.

Bateson, P., Bateson, P. P. G., and Martin, P. R. (1999) *Design for a life: How behaviour develops*, Vintage.

Boney, C. M., Verma, A., Tucker, R., and Vohr, B. R. (2005) Metabolic syndrome in childhood: Association with birth weight, maternal obesity, and gestational diabetes mellitus. *Pediatrics* 115, e290–e296.

Catalano, P. M. (2003) Obesity and pregnancy—The propagation of a viscous cycle? *J Clin Endocrinol Metab* 88, 3505–3506.

Catalano, P. M., and Ehrenberg, H. M. (2006) The short- and long-term implications of maternal obesity on the mother and her offspring. *BJOG* 113, 1126–1133.

Catalano, P. M., Kirwan, J. P., Haugel-de Mouzon, S., and King, J. (2003) Gestational diabetes and insulin resistance: Role in short- and long-term implications for mother and fetus. *J Nutr* 133, 1674S–1683S.

Cerasi, E., and Luft, R. (1967) The plasma insulin response to glucose infusion in healthy subjects and in diabetes mellitus. *Acta Endocrinol (Copenh)* 55, 278–304.

Curhan, G. C., Willett, W. C., Rimm, E. B., Spiegelman, D., Ascherio, A. L., and Stampfer, M. J. (1996) Birth weight and adult hypertension, diabetes mellitus, and obesity in US men. *Circulation* 94, 3246–3250.

de Onis, M., Blossner, M., and Villar, J. (1998) Levels and patterns of intrauterine growth retardation in developing countries. *Eur J Clin Nutr* 52(Suppl 1), S5–S15.

Dodd, J. M., Turnbull, D., McPhee, A. J., Deussen, A. R., Grivell, R. M., Yelland, L. N., Crowther, C. A., Wittert, G., Owens, J. A., and Robinson, J. S. (2014) Antenatal lifestyle advice for women who are overweight or obese: LIMIT randomised trial. *BMJ* 348.

Dorner, G., and Plagemann, A. (1994) Perinatal hyperinsulinism as possible predisposing factor for diabetes mellitus, obesity and enhanced cardiovascular risk in later life. *Horm Metab Res* 26, 213–221.

Eriksson, J. G., Forsén, T., Tuomilehto, J., Osmond, C., and Barker, D. J. P. (2001) Early growth and coronary heart disease in later life: Longitudinal study. *BMJ* 322, 949–953.

Eriksson, J. G., Forsén, T., Tuomilehto, J., Winter, P. D., Osmond, C., and Barker, D. J. P. (1999) Catch-up growth in childhood and death from coronary heart disease: Longitudinal study. *BMJ* 318, 427–431.

Eriksson, J., Forsen, T., Tuomilehto, J., Osmond, C., and Barker, D. (2000) Fetal and childhood growth and hypertension in adult life. *Hypertension* 36, 790–794.

Fontbonne, A., Charles, M. A., Thibult, N., Richard, J. L., Claude, J. R., Warnet, J. M., Rosselin, G. E., and Eschwege, E. (1991) Hyperinsulinaemia as a predictor of coronary heart disease mortality in a healthy population: The Paris Prospective Study, 15-year follow-up. *Diabetologia* 34, 356–361.

Forsdahl, A. (1977) Are poor living conditions in childhood and adolescence an important risk factor for arteriosclerotic heart disease? *Br J Prev Soc Med* 31, 91–95.

Forsen, T., Eriksson, J. G., Tuomilehto, J., Osmond, C., and Barker, D. J. (1999) Growth in utero and during childhood among women who develop coronary heart disease: Longitudinal study. *BMJ* 319, 1403–1407.

Gennser, G., Rymark, P., and Isberg, P. E. (1988) Low birth weight and risk of high blood pressure in adulthood. *Br Med J (Clin Res Ed)* 296, 1498–1500.

Gluckman, P. D., and Hanson, M. A. (2004) Living with the past: Evolution, development, and patterns of disease. *Science* 305, 1733–1736.

Gluckman, P. D., Hanson, M. A., and Beedle, A. S. (2007) Early life events and their consequences for later disease: A life history and evolutionary perspective. *Am J Hum Biol* 19, 1–19.

Hales, C. N., and Barker, D. J. P. (1992) Type 2 (non-insulin-dependent) diabetes mellitus: The thrifty phenotype hypothesis. *Diabetologia* 35, 595–601.

Hales, C. N., and Barker, D. J. P. (2001) The thrifty phenotype hypothesis. *Br Med Bull* 60, 5–20.

Hales, C. N., Barker, D. J., Clark, P. M., Cox, L. J., Fall, C., Osmond, C., and Winter, P. D. (1991) Fetal and infant growth and impaired glucose tolerance at age 64. *BMJ* 303, 1019–1022.

Kahn, S. E., Hull, R. L., and Utzschneider, K. M. (2006) Mechanisms linking obesity to insulin resistance and type 2 diabetes. *Nature* 444, 840–846.

Karlberg, J., and Albertsson-Wikland, K. (1995) Growth in full-term small-for-gestational-age infants: From birth to final height. *Pediatr Res* 38, 733–739.

Kermack, W. O., McKendrick, A. G., and McKinlay, P. L. (1934) Death-rates in Great Britain and Sweden. Some general regularities and their significance. *Lancet* 223, 698–703.

Kumanyika, S. K., Obarzanek, E., Stettler, N., Bell, R., Field, A. E., Fortmann, S. P., Franklin, B. A., Gillman, M. W., Lewis, C. E., Poston, W. C., 2nd, Stevens, J., and Hong, Y. (2008) Population-based prevention of obesity: The need for comprehensive promotion of healthful eating, physical activity, and energy balance: A scientific statement from American Heart Association Council on Epidemiology and Prevention, Interdisciplinary Committee for Prevention (formerly the expert panel on population and prevention science). *Circulation* 118, 428–464.

Law, C. M., Barker, D. J., Osmond, C., Fall, C. H., and Simmonds, S. J. (1992) Early growth and abdominal fatness in adult life. *J Epidemiol Community Health* 46, 184–186.

Li, Y., He, Y., Qi, L., Jaddoe, V. W., Feskens, E. J., Yang, X., Ma, G., and Hu, F. B. (2010) Exposure to the Chinese famine in early life and the risk of hyperglycemia and type 2 diabetes in adulthood. *Diabetes* 59, 2400–2406.

Li, Y., Jaddoe, V. W., Qi, L., He, Y., Wang, D., Lai, J., Zhang, J., Fu, P., Yang, X., and Hu, F. B. (2011) Exposure to the Chinese famine in early life and the risk of metabolic syndrome in adulthood. *Diabetes Care* 34, 1014–1018.

Luzi, L., and DeFronzo, R. A. (1989) Effect of loss of first-phase insulin secretion on hepatic glucose production and tissue glucose disposal in humans. *Am J Physiol* 257, E241–E246.

Marmot, M. G., Shipley, M. J., and Rose, G. (1984) Inequalities in death–Specific explanations of a general pattern? *Lancet* 1, 1003–1006.

McCance, D. R., Pettitt, D. J., Hanson, R. L., Jacobsson, L. T. H., Knowler, W. C., and Bennett, P. H. (1994) Birth weight and non-insulin dependent diabetes: Thrifty genotype, thrifty phenotype, or surviving small baby genotype? *BMJ* 308, 942–945.

Motala, A. A. (2002) Diabetes trends in Africa. *Diabetes Metab Res Rev* 18, S14–S20.

Nagi, D. K., Hendra, T. J., Ryle, A. J., Cooper, T. M., Temple, R. C., Clark, P. M., Schneider, A. E., Hales, C. N., and Yudkin, J. S. (1990) The relationships of concentrations of insulin, intact proinsulin and 32–33 split proinsulin with cardiovascular risk factors in type 2 (non-insulin-dependent) diabetic subjects. *Diabetologia* 33, 532–537.

Ong, K. K. L., Ahmed, M. L., Emmett, P. M., Preece, M. A., and Dunger, D. B. (2000) Association between postnatal catch-up growth and obesity in childhood: Prospective cohort study. *BMJ* 320, 967–971.

Ong, K. K., Petry, C. J., Emmett, P. M., Sandhu, M. S., Kiess, W., Hales, C. N., Ness, A. R., and Dunger, D. B. (2004) Insulin sensitivity and secretion in normal children related to size at birth, postnatal growth, and plasma insulin-like growth factor-I levels. *Diabetologia* 47, 1064–1070.

Pettitt, D. J., Nelson, R. G., Saad, M. F., Bennett, P. H., and Knowler, W. C. (1993) Diabetes and obesity in the offspring of Pima Indian women with diabetes during pregnancy. *Diabetes Care* 16, 310–314.

Phillips, D. I., Barker, D. J., Hales, C. N., Hirst, S., and Osmond, C. (1994) Thinness at birth and insulin resistance in adult life. *Diabetologia* 37, 150–154.

Phipps, K., Barker, D. J., Hales, C. N., Fall, C. H., Osmond, C., and Clark, P. M. (1993) Fetal growth and impaired glucose tolerance in men and women. *Diabetologia* 36, 225–228.

Poston, L., Bell, R., Croker, H., Flynn, A. C., Godfrey, K. M., Goff, L., Hayes, L., Khazaezadeh, N., Nelson, S. M., Oteng-Ntim, E., Pasupathy, D., Patel, N., Robson, S. C., Sandall, J., Sanders, T. A. B., Sattar, N., Seed, P. T., Wardle, J., Whitworth, M. K., and Briley, A. L. (2015) Effect of a behavioural intervention in obese pregnant women (the UPBEAT study): a multicentre, randomised controlled trial. *The Lancet Diabetes & Endocrinology* 3, 767–777.

Poulsen, P., Vaag, A. A., Kyvik, K. O., Moller Jensen, D., and Beck-Nielsen, H. (1997) Low birth weight is associated with NIDDM in discordant monozygotic and dizygotic twin pairs. *Diabetologia* 40, 439–446.

Ravelli, A. C., van der Meulen, J. H., Michels, R. P., Osmond, C., Barker, D. J., Hales, C. N., and Bleker, O. P. (1998) Glucose tolerance in adults after prenatal exposure to famine. *Lancet* 351, 173–177.

Ravelli, A. C., van Der Meulen, J. H., Osmond, C., Barker, D. J., and Bleker, O. P. (1999) Obesity at the age of 50 y in men and women exposed to famine prenatally. *Am J Clin Nutr* 70, 811–816.

Ravelli, G. P., Stein, Z. A., and Susser, M. W. (1976) Obesity in young men after famine exposure in utero and early infancy. *N Engl J Med* 295, 349–353.

Rich-Edwards, J. W., Colditz, G. A., Stampfer, M. J., Willett, W. C., Gillman, M. W., Hennekens, C. H., Speizer, F. E., and Manson, J. E. (1999) Birthweight and the risk for type 2 diabetes mellitus in adult women. *Ann Intern Med* 130, 278–284.

Robinson, S., Walton, R. J., Clark, P. M., Barker, D. J., Hales, C. N., and Osmond, C. (1992) The relation of fetal growth to plasma glucose in young men. *Diabetologia* 35, 444–446.

Roseboom, T. J., van der Meulen, J. H., Ravelli, A. C., van Montfrans, G. A., Osmond, C., Barker, D. J., and Bleker, O. P. (1999) Blood pressure in adults after prenatal exposure to famine. *J Hypertens* 17, 325–330.

Seino, S., Shibasaki, T., and Minami, K. (2011) Dynamics of insulin secretion and the clinical implications for obesity and diabetes. *J Clin Invest* 121, 2118–2125.

Silverman, B. L., Rizzo, T. A., Cho, N. H., and Metzger, B. E. (1998) Long-term effects of the intrauterine environment: The Northwestern University Diabetes in Pregnancy Center. *Diabetes Care* 21, B142–B149.

Wadsworth, M. E., Cripps, H. A., Midwinter, R. E., and Colley, J. R. (1985) Blood pressure in a national birth cohort at the age of 36 related to social and familial factors, smoking, and body mass. *Br Med J (Clin Res Ed)* 291, 1534–1538.

Whitaker, R. C. (2004) Predicting preschooler obesity at birth: The role of maternal obesity in early pregnancy. *Pediatrics* 114, e29–e36.

WHO, J., and Consultation, F. E. (2003) Diet, nutrition and the prevention of chronic diseases. *World Health Organ Tech Rep Ser* 916, i-viii, 1–149, backcover.

Zhang, S., Rattanatray, L., McMillen, I. C., Suter, C. M., and Morrison, J. L. (2011) Periconceptional nutrition and the early programming of a life of obesity or adversity. *Prog Biophys Mol Biol* 106, 307–314.

Zhang, S., Rattanatray, L., Morrison, J. L., Nicholas, L. M., Lie, S., and McMillen, I. C. (2011) Maternal obesity and the early origins of childhood obesity: Weighing up the benefits and costs of maternal weight loss in the periconceptional period for the offspring. *Exp Diabetes Res* 2011, 1–10.

Zhao, M., Shu, X. O., Jin, F., Yang, G., Li, H.-L., Liu, D.-K., Wen, W., Gao, Y.-T., and Zheng, W. (2002) Birthweight, childhood growth and hypertension in adulthood. *Int J Epidemiol* 31, 1043–1051.

2 The Maternal Resources Hypothesis and Childhood Obesity

Edward Archer and Samantha McDonald

CONTENTS

2.1 INTRODUCTION

This chapter presents the "maternal resources hypothesis" (MRH), a novel theory of nongenetic inheritance and evolution that explains the etiology of childhood obesity and metabolic diseases (Archer 2015a). The MRH posits that the recent increases in the global prevalence of obesity and type II diabetes are driven by nongenetic evolutionary processes known as maternal effects. The term "maternal effects" describes how a mother's phenotype (i.e., her traits or characteristics, e.g., body mass and behavior) alters prenatal and postnatal development, thereby influencing the survival and health trajectories of the offspring; these effects are independent of genotype. The MRH provides a comprehensive explanatory and predictive narrative of how progressive socioenvironmental changes over the past century have led to heritable alterations in the cellularity of the human body (i.e., relative number and function of muscle, fat, and insulin producing cells) with concomitant changes in appetite and nutrient partitioning (i.e., the digestion, utilization, and storage of consumed foods and beverages). These metabolic distortions disproportionately increased the amount of energy stored as lipid in adipocytes (i.e., fat in fat cells), thereby reducing the effective caloric intake of meals (i.e., the amount of energy available to metabolically active tissues in the postprandial period). Reductions in the effective caloric intake of a meal accelerated appetitive processes and led to positive energy balance via decreases in the intermeal period (e.g., snacking) and/or increases in the energy density of each meal (e.g., "supersizing").

Over the past century, these metabolic distortions snowballed from one generation to the next via accumulative maternal effects and led to the twin epidemics of obesity and type II diabetes in both humans and nonhuman animals such as dogs, cats, and horses. While the MRH is germane to all mammals, herein we focus our discussion on the intergenerational transmission and evolution of body mass, and metabolic and behavioral phenotypes via accumulative maternal effects in humans. The foundational assumptions of the MRH:

1. The human body is a complex, dynamical system in which all cells, tissues, and organs compete for nutrient energy.
2. The competition for nutrient energy and consequent nutrient partitioning (i.e., oxidation, anabolism, and/or storage of nutrient energy) is determined primarily by the cellularity of the body (i.e., relative number and type of cells) and physical activity (PA) behaviors.
3. *In utero* (prenatal) development determines the initial cellularity and behavioral trajectories of the human body.
4. Maternal phenotype (e.g., body cellularity, energy stores, and behavior) determines prenatal development and strongly influences postnatal development. Therefore, the initial body cellularity and behavioral trajectories of the next generation are engendered by the previous generation's phenotype via nongenetic inheritance (i.e., maternal effects).
5. The childhood obesity "epidemic" is the result of accumulative maternal effects that progressively altered matrilineal prenatal nutrient-energy metabolism and consequent fetal outcomes and health trajectories.

2.2 BACKGROUND

The increased global prevalence of obesity, increments in body mass, adiposity, and/or metabolic dysfunction have been documented in humans as well as many other mammalian species inclusive of pets (e.g., dogs, cats, horses), and laboratory and wild animals (e.g., rodents, monkeys, deer, elk) (Klimentidis et al. 2011; Flather et al. 2009). Given this fact, current anthropocentric theories positing the dominant influence of modern or Western diets, "thrifty genes," and/or obesogenic environments are biased and inadequate. Because valid scientific theories must provide a comprehensive explanatory and predictive narrative of the phenomena under investigation, any theory of human obesity and metabolic dysfunction must also explain the increased prevalence of these phenomena in other mammalian species. To date, the MRH (Archer 2015a) is the only theory that incorporates and explains the extant evidence inclusive of nonhuman animals.

2.3 OVERVIEW OF THE MRH

The human body is a complex, dynamical system that evolved in environments where survival necessitated significant levels of energy expenditure (EE) from physical exertion (e.g., evasion of predators, hunting). However, over the past few centuries, continuous socioenvironmental changes (e.g., sanitation, thermoneutrality, labor/time-saving technologies) induced considerable decrements in physical exertion and EE with concomitant improvements in the quantity of nutrient-energy availability (i.e., an enhanced food supply) (Archer and Blair 2011; Archer 2015a). As a result, maternal phenotype (e.g., body mass, behavior) evolved rapidly and led to progressive changes in matrilineal nutrient-energy metabolism and nutrient partitioning (Archer 2015a).

During the early part of the 20th century, these changes augmented maternal energy resources (e.g., body mass) and as a consequence, increased the nutrient energy available for fetal development in the intrauterine milieu. The enriched nutritive prenatal environment led to increasingly robust and larger infants with both greater lifespan and an increased resistance to disease (Cutler et al. 2006). With each passing generation, as female infants matured they progressively recapitulated their robustness and body size in their offspring via maternal effects (i.e., phenotype begetting phenotype, independent of genotype; e.g., see Wolf and Wade 2009). For example, over the last century there were progressive, accumulative maternal effects leading to both phenotypic remodeling and evolution such as increases in height (Kagawa et al. 2011), body stature and mass (Ogden et al. 2004), birth weight (Chike-Obi et al. 1996), organ mass (Thompson and Cohle 2004; Shepard et al. 1988), head circumference (Karvonen et al. 2012; Ounsted et al. 1985), and fat mass/adiposity (Olds 2009). Nevertheless, unremitting socioenvironmental evolution over multiple generations (e.g., the ubiquity of labor/time-saving devices and passive entertainment) eventually led to substantial declines in maternal PA (Church et al. 2011; Archer et al. 2013a,b), cardiorespiratory fitness (Gahche et al. 2014; de Moraes Ferrari et al. 2013), and subsequent prenatal metabolic (i.e., glycemic and lipidemic) control (Ioannou et al. 2007; Selvin et al. 2014).

The loss of maternal prenatal metabolic control perturbed maternal–fetal nutrient partitioning and overwhelmed placental compensatory mechanisms. This markedly increased the energy substrates in the intrauterine milieu thereby *permanently* and *irreversibly* altering fetal development and consequent metabolic and behavioral phenotypes of offspring. These phenotypic changes included the disproportionate and/or dysfunctional development of fetal pancreatic β-cells, adipocytes, and myocytes (Tong et al. 2009; Huang et al. 2012; Portha et al. 2011). Combined, these anatomic, metabolic, and behavioral disturbances increased appetite and biased tissue-specific competition for nutrient energy toward adipogenesis (i.e., adipogenic nutrient partitioning) via intensified insulin secretion, hyperplastic adiposity in confluence with reduced skeletal muscle (SM) force generation resulting in reductions in cardiorespiratory fitness and PA. Or stated simply, these prenatal maternal effects led to offspring being predisposed to positive energy balance due to "moving less and eating more."

In the postnatal period, social (i.e., vicarious) learning led to decrements in PA and increments in sedentary behaviors that further exacerbated the prenatally induced metabolic dysfunctions (i.e., reduced glycemic/lipidemic control). The consequence of this metabolic and behavioral phenotypic evolution was a progressive and enduring competitive advantage of adipocytes in the acquisition and sequestering of nutrient energy (i.e., adipogenic nutrient partitioning) that was progressively recapitulated in subsequent generations via maternal effects. As such, the current prevalence of obesity and metabolic diseases is simply the result of progressive alterations in the competitive milieu of the human body due to changes in cellularity and behavior.

The intergenerational transmission and evolution of dysfunctional matrilineal energy metabolism were accelerated via increments in the use of cesarean sections that led to the artificial selection for progressively larger, increasingly physically inactive, and metabolically compromised offspring. This medicalization of childbirth allowed both the metabolically compromised fetuses and the metabolically and behaviorally dysfunctional mothers who gestated them to survive and reproduce. Consequently, the frequency of obese, inactive, metabolically compromised phenotypes increased across the globe. This is evidenced by the rapid increases in the proportions of class II and III obesity among children and adolescents (Skelton et al. 2009). One hundred years ago, the majority of these individuals (and their mothers) would have died during childbirth due to cephalopelvic disproportion (i.e., incongruity of fetal head size and birth canal capacity) (Box 2.1).

By the late 20th century, an evolutionary tipping point in metabolically compromised maternal phenotypes and consequent matrilineal prenatal energy metabolism was reached in many populations (e.g., African Americans). Beyond this point, the intergenerational transmission of dysfunctional metabolic and behavioral phenotypes via accumulative, nonadaptive maternal effects ensured the competitive dominance of adipocytes over skeletal myocytes and other tissues in the acquisition and sequestering of nutrient energy. Consequently, obesity- and energy-contingent metabolic diseases such as type II diabetes mellitus became virtually inevitable in significant portions of these populations.

BOX 2.1   SUPPORTING EVIDENCE FOR THE MRH

The only irrefutable difference between an individual classified as obese (i.e., overfat) and an individual with "normal" adiposity is the relative number and/or size of their fat cells (Hirsch and Batchelor 1976; Salans et al. 1973)

Childhood obesity and maternal obesity are very strong predictors of adult obesity (Whitaker et al. 1997; Whitaker 2004)

Early development is a major determinant of the adipocyte number (Spalding et al. 2008)

The adipocyte number increases throughout early development (Hager et al. 1977)

The adipocyte number is a primary determinant of obesity (Spalding et al. 2008; Bjorntorp 1996)

Increments in fat mass are a function of adiposity (Forbes 2000)

Adipose tissue of young obese children differ both qualitatively and quantitatively from lean children (Knittle et al. 1979)

Monozygotic twins concordant for birth weight exhibit similar adipocyte numbers, while in those discordant for birth weight, the smaller twin displays both lower body weight and lower adipocyte number (Ginsberg-Fellner 1981)

2.4 MECHANISMS FOR PRENATAL MATERNAL EFFECTS

2.4.1 ROLE OF SM ACTIVATION

SM is the principal tissue for regulating the competitive milieu of the human body because its activation (i.e., contraction) plays a major role in metabolic control by maintaining insulin sensitivity via insulin-mediated glucose disposal (Baron et al. 1988) and fatty acid oxidation (Aas et al. 2005). As such, SM is an essential element in nutrient-energy partitioning (Bergouignan et al. 2011, 2009). PA is the primary determinant of SM activation, and marked reductions in PA result in substantial decrements in metabolic control resulting in transient hyperglycemia (i.e., glycemic excursions), hyperlipidemia, and subsequent increases in adipogenic nutrient partitioning. This inactivity-induced loss of metabolic control and insulin sensitivity is the result of reductions in total SM energy demands leading to decrements in fatty acid oxidation (Jensen 2003; Hamilton et al. 2007) and the repletion of SM glycogen stores and subsequent reductions in free 5' adenosine monophosphate-activated protein kinase (AMPK) and insulin sensitivity (Litherland et al. 2007; Jensen et al. 2011).

2.4.2 PREGNANCY AND INSULIN RESISTANCE

Pregnancy is a naturally insulin-resistant state characterized by numerous metabolic alterations that promote adipogenic nutrient partitioning (i.e., the accretion of adipose tissue) via impaired insulin sensitivity (Barbour et al. 2007). While pregnancy-induced reductions in insulin sensitivity are necessary for optimal fetal growth, progressive reductions in maternal PA and consequent reductions in SM activation and increments insulin resistance over the past half-century acted synergistically with the naturally occurring metabolic sequelae of pregnancy to exacerbate the negative metabolic consequences of inactivity (Krogh-Madsen et al. 2010; Olsen et al. 2008; Thyfault and Krogh-Madsen 2011; Friedrichsen et al. 2013). The confluence of the naturally occurring decrements in insulin sensitivity of pregnancy with inactivity-driven insulin resistance drove fetal developmental pathologies via the increased availability of energy substrates to the intrauterine environment.

Consistent evidence has demonstrated that fetal exposure to excess intrauterine energy stimulates the hypertrophy and hyperplasia of pancreatic β-cells leading to fetal hyperinsulinemia (Martens and Pipeleers 2009; Steinke and Driscoll 1965; Portha et al. 2011; Catalano et al. 1998) that precipitates adipocyte hyperplasia (Chandler-Laney et al. 2011; Herrera and Amusquivar 2000; Kalkhoff 1991; Long et al. 2012). Additionally, increased energy availability upregulates fetal fatty acid and glucose transporters (Long et al. 2012) thereby increasing the direct free fatty acid uptake and storage as triglyceride in fetal adipocytes (Shadid et al. 2007; Szabo and Szabo 1974), while altering fetal SM development via increases in collagen accumulation and crosslinking in fetal SM (Tong et al. 2009; Huang et al. 2012).

2.4.3 PROGRESSIVE MATERNAL EFFECTS VIA REDUCTIONS IN MATERNAL PA

Progressive reductions in maternal PA and increments in sedentary behaviors (e.g., television viewing) have been documented over the past half-century. From the

1960s to 2010, maternal household PA EE decreased (~1200–1500 kcals/week), with concomitant increases in time spent in sedentary behaviors (Archer et al. 2013a,b). By the 1990s, women and mothers allocated more time to screen-based media use than to all forms of PA combined (Archer et al. 2013a,b). In addition, a majority of pregnant women reported spending more than 50% of their day in sedentary behaviors (Evenson et al. 2011). In concert with the progressive increments in sedentarism, inactivity, and decrements in EE during PA were the progressive decrements in population level metabolic control (Ioannou et al. 2007) and substantial increases in maternal pregravid obesity (Heslehurst et al. 2007), gestational weight gain (Helms et al. 2006), and gestational diabetes (Dabelea et al. 2005).

The confluence of these mechanisms led to offspring with greater adipocyte cellularity (i.e., hyperplastic adiposity), altered insulin function, and dysfunctional SM development. And because cellularity (i.e., body mass at the cellular level) is a strong mediator of appetite, and reduced SM function decreases strength-to-weight ratio thereby increasing the requisite effort of PA and propensity to be sedentary, these fetal pathologies led to the predisposition to "eat more and move less." This is supported by the well-established low levels of PA, high levels of sedentary behaviors, and altered appetite regulation found among overweight and obese individuals (Troiano et al. 2008; Matthews et al. 2008; Shook et al. 2015).

2.5 MECHANISMS FOR POSTNATAL MATERNAL EFFECTS

Although prenatal development is the greatest determinant of the obese and/or metabolically compromised phenotype, the postnatal environment in which a child is reared can ameliorate or exacerbate the prenatally induced predispositions. For example, the intergenerational transmission of behavior has been consistently documented among social animals inclusive of humans (Broadhurst 1961; Jablonka and Lamb 2007). As such, the processes of postnatal maternal effects provide nongenetic mechanisms by which the behavioral phenotype of the mother or caregiver (e.g., physically inactive and highly sedentary) is recapitulated in the behavioral phenotype of infants, children, and adolescents. Mechanisms include social learning and modeling (i.e., observational, operant, and/or classical conditioning; Notten et al. 2012; Ricks 1985; Franks et al. 2005; Skinner 1953).

For example, it is well established that a mother's television (TV) viewing behaviors influence her children's TV behaviors (Notten et al. 2012), and over the past 50 years, screen-based media use has increased significantly. By the 21st century, mothers and children were spending the vast majority of their leisure time using screen-based media (Robinson 2011). Television is often used as a surrogate caregiver (i.e., "babysitter") (Taveras et al. 2009) for precisely the same reason that it is detrimental to infants and children: it captures their attention and keeps them relatively immobile. In a nonmedia-enhanced world, children and adolescents stimulate their neuromusculoskeletal systems via movement and "exploration" facilitated by PA and the activation of SM. Decrements in PA during critical periods of development, such as childhood, lead to reductions in the physiological resources (e.g., muscle force development and coordination) necessary for PA. And because osteocytes (i.e., bone cells), myocytes, and adipocytes share a common pool of stem cells, every kilocalorie of energy that is not used to build muscle and bone and optimize metabolic health will be used to further increase adipocyte size and/or number (Tong et al. 2009; Yan et al. 2012). As such, nonadaptive, prenatal maternal effects will be exacerbated by a poor maternal behavioral phenotype in the postnatal period. Stated more simply, children who grow up with an inactive, sedentary caregiver are more likely to be sedentary, inactive, and metabolically compromised as adults (Thompson et al. 2013; Franks et al. 2005).

2.6   NUTRIENT PARTITIONING AND ITS DETERMINANTS

Human EE is a continuous process but energy intake is discontinuous. Therefore, survival necessitates both the acquisition and storage of energy to meet EE demands (i.e., basal metabolism and PA) during intermeal periods. To meet the energy demands of basal metabolism and PA in the postabsorptive period (i.e., after the previous meal has been digested, oxidized, and/ stored), more energy must be consumed and stored at each meal than can be immediately oxidized. To accomplish this, each type of cell (or tissue) uses evolutionarily conserved strategies to partition energy for survival. For example, nutrient energy in the form of lipid or carbohydrate is stored in SM to facilitate PA. This storage is accomplished via insulin and/or contraction-mediated glucose disposal and fatty acid uptake (Litherland et al. 2007; Bergouignan et al. 2013). Lipid and carbohydrate are stored in the liver via a number of processes to ensure adequate levels of blood sugar to support the metabolic needs of the central nervous system and provide lipid for SM oxidation. Energy is stored in adipocytes to provide lipid substrates for both the liver and SM in the postabsorptive period or during periods of insufficient energy intake.

The partitioning of nutrient energy to specific tissues or organs is determined by the competitive milieu of the body and mediated by a number of factors. Cellularity and PA are the largest determinants of nutrient partitioning, but other determinants such as hormonal status play a major role during specific periods (e.g., puberty, pregnancy, and menopause). With respect to cellularity, there is clear evidence of a competitive advantage of adipocytes in the acquisition and storage of nutrient energy via the strong inverse relationship between the oxidation of dietary fat and obesity. In the postprandial period, obese individuals (i.e., people with a greater relative number of fat cells) store more fatty acids as lipid in adipocytes, while lean individuals oxidize a greater relative amount (Westerterp 2009). There is also evidence of the competitive advantage of adipocytes due to inactivity; individuals with low levels of SM activation due to physical inactivity partition more glucose to the production of saturated fatty acids via *de novo lipogenesis* (Petersen et al. 2007) and therefore partition more saturated fatty acids for storage in adipocytes (Binnert et al. 1998; Koutsari et al. 2011). As such, an excessive number of adipocytes (i.e., obesity) and physical inactivity act synergistically to create and exacerbate adipogenic nutrient-energy partitioning via the partitioning of energy (e.g., glucose and fatty acids) during the postprandial period (Westerterp 2009; Petersen et al. 2007; Bergouignan et al. 2006; Hamilton et al. 2007; Litherland et al. 2007). Given the impact of cellularity and PA on nutrient partitioning and the fact that prenatal development determines the initial trajectory of both cellularity and PA, accumulative maternal effects provide a powerful explanation for the inheritance and evolution of obesity and metabolic diseases.

2.7 THE FETAL DETERMINANTS OF EFFECTIVE ENERGY (CALORIC) INTAKE

There is an evolutionarily conserved relationship between energy intake and EE, and organisms can only survive if their effective energy intake meets or exceeds EE. In mammals, the evolutionarily conserved relationship between energy intake and expenditure is determined by allometric relationships established during *in utero* development (i.e., the physiologic scaling of various tissues and organs due to differential hyperplasia). Any perturbation of this relationship will lead to morphological alterations that may or may not be adaptive. Given that all tissues compete for energy, and that adipocytes evolved to store and sequester energy in the form of lipid, *caeteris paribus*, individuals with a greater relative number of adipocytes will store a disproportionate amount of energy from each meal as lipid in adipocytes. This adipogenic nutrient partitioning decreases the effective energy intake of the meal (i.e., the amount of energy available to metabolically active tissues in the postprandial period) and results in increases in appetite, a reduced intermeal period and/or greater energy density at the next meal, positive energy balance, and subsequent increases in adiposity.

The extant empirical evidence, as described, clearly suggests that poor prenatal metabolic control alters fetal development and that excessive intrauterine energy *permanently and irreversibly* alters body cellularity and consequent competitive milieu via a disproportionate increase in adipocytes and altered pancreatic β-cell function (Archer 2015a; Catalano and Hauguel-De Mouzon 2011; Pedersen 1967/1977; Reusens et al. 2007).

2.8 APPETITE, NUTRIENT PARTITIONING, AND POSITIVE ENERGY BALANCE

The greatest determinants of appetite are basal metabolic processes and PA (Blundell et al. 2012, 2003), whereas the primary determinants of nutrient partitioning are body cellularity (i.e., body composition on the cellular level) and PA. As such, when obese individuals partition more nutrient energy from each meal to storage, less energy is available for basal metabolic processes and PA. As a result, the metabolic stimuli that inhibit hunger and appetitive processes (e.g., adenosine triphosphate [ATP]/adenosine diphosphate [ADP] ratio, hepatic energy flux, glucose, and fatty acid oxidation) are reduced. Consequently, appetite will increase at an accelerated pace until more energy is consumed (Friedman 1995; Mayer 1957). Additionally, the relative energy deprivation of nonadipose tissues (e.g., the brain) may result in a perception of fatigue, potentially explaining why individuals struggling with obesity often suffer from fatigue (Wlodek and Gonzales 2003). Moreover, fatigue may also lead to inactivity and the associated decrements in metabolic control that drive appetite. To overcome the perception of fatigue and hunger, these individuals may reduce their intermeal interval by snacking and/or increasing the energy density of their next meal. This context leads to a positive feedback loop of excessive caloric intake and positive energy balance that exacerbates the vicious cycle of adipogenic nutrient-energy partitioning, decrements in PA with concomitant decreases in metabolic control, and increments in adiposity.

2.9 ACCUMULATIVE AND "CORRECTIVE" MATERNAL EFFECTS

The scientific literature on maternal effects and metabolic functioning in both humans and nonhuman animals is unequivocal (Brooks et al. 1995; Kurnianto et al. 1998; Patterson et al. 2008). Ovum transfer and cross-fostering studies have clearly demonstrated that the intrauterine milieu and early postnatal periods can induce, augment, or ameliorate metabolic dysfunction in a single generation, independent of genotype. Recently, an embryo transfer study by Garg et al. (2013) demonstrated that the inheritance of pathological metabolic phenotypes can be halted or ameliorated when the embryo is transferred and gestated in a "normal metabolic environment" (Garg et al. 2013). Brooks et al. (1995) examined ovum donations in humans and found that the "only discernible factor" influencing infant birth weight was the surrogate mother's body mass (Brooks et al. 1995). Combined, these results suggest that maternal phenotypes are transmissible to the next generation via maternal effects, and with respect to obesity and metabolic diseases, the intrauterine environment overwhelms any variation in genotype.

2.10 PRACTICAL IMPLICATIONS OF THE MRH

As posited in the MRH, accumulative, progressive maternal effects have significantly altered matrilineal energy metabolism such that obesity and metabolic diseases have reached epidemic proportions globally. Nevertheless, substantial changes in maternal prenatal behavior have the potential to productively impact the health of future generations. Given the potent effects of SM activation on metabolic health, PA throughout the life course, and especially in the preconception and prenatal periods, may serve as an effective strategy to prepare girls, adolescent females, and pregnant women to improve their metabolic control and ensure a healthy pregnancy. Given the current evolutionary context, PA and exercise during the prenatal period are essential to improve glycemic and lipidemic control and enable women to protect their fetuses from irreversible developmental overgrowth (e.g., increased adipocytes) and metabolic dysfunction.

As demonstrated by ovum transfer studies and a diverse body of literature, the predisposition to poor metabolic control due to the nongenetic inheritance of metabolically compromised phenotypes from previous generations (i.e., mother, grandmother) may be ameliorated if fetal development occurs in a "normal" metabolic intrauterine environment (Kurnianto et al. 1998; Patterson et al. 2008). This suggests that the inheritance of acquired characteristics (i.e., metabolically compromised phenotype) may be interrupted and potentially reversed with an adequate dose of maternal PA in the prenatal period and child PA in the postnatal period. Unfortunately, many existing prenatal exercise interventions are of an insufficient dose to positively influence perinatal outcomes (e.g., gestational weight gain, birth weight) and health trajectories (McDonald et al. 2015) (Box 2.2).

> ## BOX 2.2   GLOSSARY FOR THE MRH
>
> **Adipogenic Nutrient Partitioning:** Competitive advantage of adipocytes in the acquisition and sequestering of nutrient energy.
>
> **Effective Energy (Caloric) Intake:** The amount of nutrient energy available to metabolically active tissues in the postprandial and postabsorptive periods.
>
> **Maternal Effects:** A form of nongenetic inheritance in which a mother's phenotype is recapitulated in offspring independent of genotype. Also known as the Inheritance of Acquired Characteristics (Archer 2015b).
>
> **Nutrient Energy:** Energy derived from the consumption of food and beverages that is available for metabolic processes.
>
> **Nutrient Partitioning:** The metabolic fate of nutrient energy to oxidation, anabolism, and/or storage. Body composition on the cellular level and PA are the primary determinants (Krogh-Madsen et al. 2010; Thyfault and Krogh-Madsen 2011; Bergouignan et al. 2006).
>
> **Obesity:** The excessive storage of nutrient energy due to excessive adipose tissue cellularity.
>
> **Phenotype:** An individual's observable traits and characteristics, inclusive of metabolic, anthropometric, and metabolic characteristics.
>
> **Phenotypic Evolution:** The progressive or regressive remodeling of a characteristic over time (e.g., intergenerational changes in body size and/or mass).

2.11   SUMMARY OF THE MRH

Over the past century, the use of technology made life easier, simpler, and safer while improving nutritional status around the world. Initially, these changes led to increased robustness and better health. Yet, with each passing generation, the ubiquity of labor and time-saving devices decreased the amount of PA necessary in daily life while increasing sedentary behaviors such as watching TV. Because the contraction of SM via PA is essential for metabolic control, these reductions in PA and increments in sedentary behavior led to decrements in insulin sensitivity and increases in insulin resistance in many individuals, especially those who did not engage in daily leisure-time PA (e.g., exercise). The increasing trend of metabolic dysfunction had dire consequences for children born to inactive and larger mothers. The confluence of inactivity-induced insulin resistance with the naturally occurring insulin resistance of pregnancy led to infants born metabolically compromised as a result of a greater relative number of fat cells, altered insulin production, and less efficient SM. Consequently, these infants are predisposed to altered growth trajectories and a physically inactive lifestyle. And, because of their increased relative number of fat cells at birth (i.e., greater adipose tissue cellularity), they will store more of the calories consumed as fat, thereby lowering the effective caloric intake of each meal. This in turn increases appetite, the frequency of meals, and the energy density of each meal, thereby perpetuating the vicious cycle of adipogenic nutrient partitioning and physical inactivity.

For humans, the consequences of the MRH are profound: infants born with an excessive number of fat cells, altered insulin production, and decreased SM function are *permanently* and *irreversibly* predisposed to positive energy balance ("eating more and moving less"). As such, because willpower and volition cannot compete with evolution, interventions based on the energy balance conceptualization of obesity ("move more and eat less") will be entirely ineffective while contributing to the ever-present moralizing and demoralizing social discourse and stigma that individuals struggling with obesity face each day.

REFERENCES

Aas, V., M. Rokling-Andersen, A. J. Wensaas, G. H. Thoresen, E. T. Kase, and A. C. Rustan. 2005. Lipid metabolism in human skeletal muscle cells: Effects of palmitate and chronic hyperglycaemia. *Acta Physiol Scand* 183 (1):31–41. doi:10.1111/j.1365-201X.2004.01381.x.

Archer, E. 2015a. The childhood obesity epidemic as a result of nongenetic evolution: The maternal resources hypothesis. *Mayo Clin Proc* 90 (1):77–92. doi:10.1016/j.mayocp.2014.08.006.

Archer, E. 2015b. In reply—Maternal, paternal, and societal efforts are needed to "cure" childhood obesity. *Mayo Clin Proc* 90 (4):555–557. doi:10.1016/j.mayocp.2015.01.020.

Archer, E., and S. N. Blair. 2011. Physical activity and the prevention of cardiovascular disease: From evolution to epidemiology. *Prog Cardiovasc Dis* 53 (6):387–396.

Archer, E., C. J. Lavie, S. M. McDonald, D. M. Thomas, J. R. Hébert, S. E. Taverno Ross, K. L. McIver, R. M. Malina, and S. N. Blair. 2013a. Maternal inactivity: 45-year trends in mothers' use of time. *Mayo Clin Proc* 88 (12):1368–1377. doi:10.1016/j.mayocp.2013.09.009.

Archer, E., R. P. Shook, D. M. Thomas, T. S. Church, P. T. Katzmarzyk, J. R. Hebert, K. L. McIver, G. A. Hand, C. J. Lavie, and S. N. Blair. 2013b. 45-year trends in women's use of time and household management energy expenditure. *PLoS One* 8 (2):e56620. doi:10.1371/journal.pone.0056620.

Barbour, L. A., C. E. McCurdy, T. L. Hernandez, J. P. Kirwan, P. M. Catalano, and J. E. Friedman. 2007. Cellular mechanisms for insulin resistance in normal pregnancy and gestational diabetes. *Diabetes Care* 30 (Supplement 2):S112–S119. doi:10.2337/dc07-s202.

Baron, A. D., G. Brechtel, P. Wallace, and S. V. Edelman. 1988. Rates and tissue sites of non-insulin- and insulin-mediated glucose uptake in humans. *Am J Phys Endo Met* 255 (6):E769–E774.

Bergouignan, A., I. Momken, E. Lefai, E. Antoun, D. A. Schoeller, C. Platat, I. Chery, A. Zahariev, H. Vidal, L. Gabert, S. Normand, D. Freyssenet, M. Laville, C. Simon, and S. Blanc. 2013. Activity energy expenditure is a major determinant of dietary fat oxidation and trafficking, but the deleterious effect of detraining is more marked than the beneficial effect of training at current recommendations. *Am J Clin Nutr* 98 (3):648–658. doi:10.3945/ajcn.112.057075.

Bergouignan, A., D. A. Schoeller, S. Normand, G. Gauquelin-Koch, M. Laville, T. Shriver, M. Desage, Y. Le Maho, H. Ohshima, C. Gharib, and S. Blanc. 2006. Effect of physical inactivity on the oxidation of saturated and monounsaturated dietary fatty acids: Results of a randomized trial. *PLoS Clin Trials* 1 (5):e27.

Bergouignan, A., F. Rudwill, C. Simon, and S. Blanc. 2011. Physical inactivity as the culprit of metabolic inflexibility: Evidence from bed-rest studies. *J Appl Physiol* 111 (4):1201–1210. doi:10.1152/japplphysiol.00698.2011.

Bergouignan, A., G. Trudel, C. Simon, A. Chopard, D. A. Schoeller, I. Momken, S. B. Votruba, M. Desage, G. C. Burdge, G. Gauquelin-Koch, S. Normand, and S. Blanc. 2009. Physical inactivity differentially alters dietary oleate and palmitate trafficking. *Diabetes* 58 (2):367–376. doi:10.2337/db08-0263.

Binnert, C., C. Pachiaudi, M. Beylot, D. Hans, J. Vandermander, P. Chantre, J. P. Riou, and M. Laville. 1998. Influence of human obesity on the metabolic fate of dietary long- and medium-chain triacylglycerols. *Am J Clin Nutr* 67 (4):595–601.

Bjorntorp, P. 1996. The regulation of adipose tissue distribution in humans. *Int J Obes Relat Metab Disord* 20 (4):291–302.

Blundell, J. E., P. Caudwell, C. Gibbons, M. Hopkins, E. Naslund, N. King, and G. Finlayson. 2012. Role of resting metabolic rate and energy expenditure in hunger and appetite control: A new formulation. *Dis Model Mech* 5 (5):608–613. doi:10.1242/dmm.009837.

Blundell, J. E., R. J. Stubbs, D. A. Hughes, S. Whybrow, and N. A. King. 2003. Cross talk between physical activity and appetite control: Does physical activity stimulate appetite? *Proc Nutr Soc* 62 (3):651–661.

Broadhurst, P. L. 1961. Analysis of maternal effects in the inheritance of behaviour. *Anim Behav* 9 (3–4):129–141. doi:10.1016/0003-3472(61)90001-X.

Brooks, A. A., M. R. Johnson, P. J. Steer, M. E. Pawson, and H. I. Abdalla. 1995. Birth weight: Nature or nurture? *Early Hum Dev* 42 (1):29–35.

Catalano, P. M., N. M. Drago, and S. B. Amini. 1998. Longitudinal changes in pancreatic beta-cell function and metabolic clearance rate of insulin in pregnant women with normal and abnormal glucose tolerance. *Diabetes Care* 21 (3):403–408.

Catalano, P. M., and S. Hauguel-De Mouzon. 2011. Is it time to revisit the Pedersen hypothesis in the face of the obesity epidemic? *Am J Obstet Gynecol* 204 (6):479–487. doi:10.1016/j.ajog.2010.11.039.

Chandler-Laney, P. C., N. C. Bush, D. J. Rouse, M. S. Mancuso, and B. A. Gower. 2011. Maternal glucose concentration during pregnancy predicts fat and lean mass of prepubertal offspring. *Diabetes Care* 34 (3):741–5. doi:10.2337/dc10-1503.

Chike-Obi, U., R. J. David, R. Coutinho, and S. Y. Wu. 1996. Birth weight has increased over a generation. *Am J Epidemiol* 144 (6):563–569.

Church, T. S., D. M. Thomas, C. Tudor-Locke, P. T. Katzmarzyk, C. P. Earnest, R. Q. Rodarte, C. K. Martin, S. N. Blair, and C. Bouchard. 2011. Trends over 5 decades in U.S. occupation-related physical activity and their associations with obesity. *PLoS One* 6 (5):e19657. doi:10.1371/journal.pone.0019657.

Cutler, David, Angus Deaton, and Adriana Lleras-Muney. 2006. The determinants of mortality. *J Econ Perspect* 20 (3):97–120. doi:10.1257/jep.20.3.97.

Dabelea, D., J. K. Snell-Bergeon, C. L. Hartsfield, K. J. Bischoff, R. F. Hamman, and R. S. McDuffie. 2005. Increasing prevalence of gestational diabetes mellitus (GDM) over time and by birth cohort: Kaiser Permanente of Colorado GDM Screening Program. *Diabetes Care* 28 (3):579–584.

de Moraes Ferrari, G. Luis, M. Maia Bracco, V. K. Rodrigues Matsudo, and M. Fisberg. 2013. Cardiorespiratory fitness and nutritional status of schoolchildren: 30-year evolution. *J Pediatr* 89 (4):366–373. doi:10.1016/j.jped.2012.12.006.

Flather, C.H., M.S. Knowles, and S.J. Brady. 2009. *Population and Harvest Trends of Big Game and Small Game Species: A Technical Document Supporting the USDA Forest Service Interim Update of the 2000 RPA Assessment. Gen. Tech. Rep. RMRS-GTR-219.* Fort Collins, CO: U.S. Department of Agriculture, Forest Service, Rocky Mountain Research Station.

Forbes, G. B. 2000. Body fat content influences the body composition response to nutrition and exercise. *Ann N Y Acad Sci* 904:359–365.

Franks, P. W., E. Ravussin, R. L. Hanson, I. T. Harper, D. B. Allison, W. C. Knowler, P. A. Tataranni, and A. D. Salbe. 2005. Habitual physical activity in children: The role of genes and the environment. *Am J Clin Nutr* 82 (4):901–908.

Friedman, M. I. 1995. Control of energy intake by energy metabolism. *Am J Clin Nutr* 62 (5):1096S–1100S.

Friedrichsen, M., B. Mortensen, C. Pehmoller, J. B. Birk, and J. F. Wojtaszewski. 2013. Exercise-induced AMPK activity in skeletal muscle: Role in glucose uptake and insulin sensitivity. *Mol Cell Endocrinol* 366 (2):204–214. doi:10.1016/j.mce.2012.06.013.

Gahche, J., T. Fakhouri, D.D. Carroll, V.L. Burt, CY. Wang, and J.E. Fulton. 2014. *Cardiorespiratory Fitness Levels among U.S. Youth Aged 12–15 Years: United States, 1999–2004 and 2012; NCHS Data Brief No. 153*. Hyattsville, MD: CDC; National Center for Health Statistics.

Garg, M., M. Thamotharan, Y. Dai, P. W. Lee, and S. U. Devaskar. 2013. Embryo-transfer of the F2 postnatal calorie restricted female rat offspring into a control intra-uterine environment normalizes the metabolic phenotype. *Metabolism* 62 (3):432–441. doi:10.1016/j.metabol.2012.08.026.

Ginsberg-Fellner, F. 1981. Growth of adipose tissue in infants, children and adolescents: Variations in growth disorders. *Int J Obes* 5 (6):605–611.

Hager, A., L. Sjostrm, B. Arvidsson, P. Bjorntorp, and U. Smith. 1977. Body fat and adipose tissue cellularity in infants: A longitudinal study. *Metabolism* 26 (6):607–614.

Hamilton, M. T., D. G. Hamilton, and T. W. Zderic. 2007. Role of low energy expenditure and sitting in obesity, metabolic syndrome, type 2 diabetes, and cardiovascular disease. *Diabetes* 56 (11):2655–2667.

Helms, E., C. C. Coulson, and S. L. Galvin. 2006. Trends in weight gain during pregnancy: a population study across 16 years in North Carolina. *Am J Obstet Gynecol* 194 (5):e32-4. doi: 10.1016/j.ajog.2006.01.025.

Herrera, E., and E. Amusquivar. 2000. Lipid metabolism in the fetus and the newborn. *Diabetes Metab Res Rev* 16 (3):202–210. doi:10.1002/1520-7560(200005/06)16:3<202::AID-DMRR116>3.0.CO;2-#.

Heslehurst, N., L. J. Ells, H. Simpson, A. Batterham, J. Wilkinson, and C. D. Summerbell. 2007. Trends in maternal obesity incidence rates, demographic predictors, and health inequalities in 36,821 women over a 15-year period. *Bjog* 114 (2):187–194.

Hirsch, J., and B. Batchelor. 1976. Adipose tissue cellularity in human obesity. *Clin Endocrinol Metab* 5 (2):299–311.

Huang, Y., J. X. Zhao, X. Yan, M. J. Zhu, N. M. Long, R. J. McCormick, S. P. Ford, P. W. Nathanielsz, and M. Du. 2012. Maternal obesity enhances collagen accumulation and cross-linking in skeletal muscle of ovine offspring. *PLoS One* 7 (2):e31691. doi:10.1371/journal.pone.0031691.

Ioannou, G. N., C. L. Bryson, and E. J. Boyko. 2007. Prevalence and trends of insulin resistance, impaired fasting glucose, and diabetes. *J Diabetes Complications* 21 (6):363–370. doi:10.1016/j.jdiacomp.2006.07.005.

Jablonka, E., and M. J. Lamb. 2007. Precis of evolution in four dimensions. *Behav Brain Sci* 30 (4):353–365; discussion 365–389.

Jensen, J., P. I. Rustad, A. J. Kolnes, and Y. C. Lai. 2011. The role of skeletal muscle glycogen breakdown for regulation of insulin sensitivity by exercise. *Front Physiol* 2:112.

Jensen, M. D. 2003. Fate of fatty acids at rest and during exercise: Regulatory mechanisms. *Acta Physiol Scand* 178 (4):385–390.

Kagawa, M., Y. Tahara, K. Moji, R. Nakao, K. Aoyagi, and A. P. Hills. 2011. Secular changes in growth among Japanese children over 100 years (1900–2000). *Asia Pac J Clin Nutr* 20 (2):180–189.

Kalkhoff, R. K. 1991. Impact of maternal fuels and nutritional state on fetal growth. *Diabetes* 40 Suppl 2:61–65.

Karvonen, M., M. L. Hannila, A. Saari, and L. Dunkel. 2012. New Finnish reference for head circumference from birth to 7 years. *Ann Med* 44 (4):369–374. doi:10.3109/07853890.2011.558519.

Klimentidis, Y. C., T. M. Beasley, H. Y. Lin, G. Murati, G. E. Glass, M. Guyton, W. Newton, M. Jorgensen, S. B. Heymsfield, J. Kemnitz, L. Fairbanks, and D. B. Allison. 2011. Canaries in the coal mine: A cross-species analysis of the plurality of obesity epidemics. *Proc Biol Sci* 278 (1712):1626–1632.

Knittle, J. L., K. Timmers, F. Ginsberg-Fellner, R. E. Brown, and D. P. Katz. 1979. The growth of adipose tissue in children and adolescents. Cross-sectional and longitudinal studies of adipose cell number and size. *J Clin Invest* 63 (2):239–246. doi:10.1172/jci109295.

Koutsari, C., A. H. Ali, M. S. Mundi, and M. D. Jensen. 2011. Storage of circulating free fatty acid in adipose tissue of postabsorptive humans: Quantitative measures and implications for body fat distribution. *Diabetes* 60 (8):2032–2040.

Krogh-Madsen, R., J. P. Thyfault, C. Broholm, O. H. Mortensen, R. H. Olsen, R. Mounier, P. Plomgaard, G. van Hall, F. W. Booth, and B. K. Pedersen. 2010. A 2-wk reduction of ambulatory activity attenuates peripheral insulin sensitivity. *J Appl Physiol* 108 (5):1034–1040.

Kurnianto, E., A. Shinjo, and D. Suga. 1998. Prenatal and postnatal maternal effects on body weight in cross-fostering experiment on two subspecies of mice. *Exp Anim* 47 (2):97–103.

Litherland, G. J., N. J. Morris, M. Walker, and S. J. Yeaman. 2007. Role of glycogen content in insulin resistance in human muscle cells. *J Cell Physiol* 211 (2):344–352.

Long, N. M., D. C. Rule, M. J. Zhu, P. W. Nathanielsz, and S. P. Ford. 2012. Maternal obesity upregulates fatty acid and glucose transporters and increases expression of enzymes mediating fatty acid biosynthesis in fetal adipose tissue depots. *J Anim Sci* 90 (7):2201–2210. doi:10.2527/jas.2011-4343.

Martens, G. A., and D. Pipeleers. 2009. Glucose, regulator of survival and phenotype of pancreatic beta cells. *Vitam Horm* 80:507–539.

Matthews, C. E., K. Y. Chen, P. S. Freedson, M. S. Buchowski, B. M. Beech, R. R. Pate, and R. P. Troiano. 2008. Amount of time spent in sedentary behaviors in the United States, 2003–2004. *Am J Epidemiol* 167 (7):875–881. doi:10.1093/aje/kwm390.

Mayer, J. 1957. Correlation between metabolism and feeding behavior and multiple etiology of obesity. *Bull N Y Acad Med* 33 (11):744–761.

McDonald, S. M., J. Liu, S. Wilcox, E. Y. Lau, and E. Archer. 2015. Does dose matter in reducing gestational weight gain in exercise interventions? A systematic review of literature. *J Sci Med Sport* (0). doi:10.1016/j.jsams.2015.03.004.

Notten, N., G. Kraaykamp, and R.P. Konig. 2012. Family media matters: Unraveling the intergenerational transmission of reading and television tastes. *Sociol Perspect* 55 (4):683–706.

Ogden, C. L., C. D. Fryar, M. D. Carroll, and K. M. Flegal. 2004. Mean body weight, height, and body mass index, United States 1960–2002. *Adv Data* (347):1–17.

Olds, T. S. 2009. One million skinfolds: Secular trends in the fatness of young people 1951–2004. *Eur J Clin Nutr* 63 (8):934–946. doi:10.1038/ejcn.2009.7.

Olsen, R. H., R. Krogh-Madsen, C. Thomsen, F. W. Booth, and B. K. Pedersen. 2008. Metabolic responses to reduced daily steps in healthy nonexercising men. *JAMA* 299 (11):1261–1263. doi:10.1001/jama.299.11.1259.

Ounsted, M., V. A. Moar, and A. Scott. 1985. Head circumference charts updated. *Arch Dis Child* 60 (10):936–939.

Patterson, C. M., A. A. Dunn-Meynell, and B. E. Levin. 2008. Three weeks of early-onset exercise prolongs obesity resistance in DIO rats after exercise cessation. *Am J Physiol Regul Integr Comp Physiol* 294 (2):R290–R301. doi:10.1152/ajpregu.00661.2007.

Pedersen, J. 1967/1977. *The Pregnant Diabetic and Her Newborn: Problems and Management.* Copenhagen: Munksgaard.

Petersen, K. F., S. Dufour, D. B. Savage, S. Bilz, G. Solomon, S. Yonemitsu, G. W. Cline, D. Befroy, L. Zemany, B. B. Kahn, X. Papademetris, D. L. Rothman, and G. I. Shulman. 2007. The role of skeletal muscle insulin resistance in the pathogenesis of the metabolic syndrome. *Proc Natl Acad Sci USA* 104 (31):12587–12594.

Portha, B., A. Chavey, and J. Movassat. 2011. Early-life origins of type 2 diabetes: Fetal programming of the beta-cell mass. *Exp Diabetes Res* 2011:105076. doi:10.1155/2011/105076.

Reusens, B., S. E. Ozanne, and C. Remacle. 2007. Fetal determinants of type 2 diabetes. *Curr Drug Targets* 8 (8):935–941.

Ricks, M. H. 1985. The social transmission of parental behavior: Attachment across generations. *Monogr Soc Res Child Dev* 50 (1/2):211–227. doi:10.2307/3333834.

Robinson, J. 2011. IT, TV and time displacement: What Alexander Szalai anticipated but couldn't know. *Soc Indic Res* 101 (2):193–206.

Salans, L. B., S. W. Cushman, and R. E. Weismann. 1973. Studies of human adipose tissue. Adipose cell size and number in nonobese and obese patients. *J Clin Invest* 52 (4):929–41. doi:10.1172/jci107258.

Selvin, E., C. M. Parrinello, D. B. Sacks, and J. Coresh. 2014. Trends in prevalence and control of diabetes in the United States, 1988–1994 and 1999–2010. *Ann Intern Med* 160 (8):517–525. doi:10.7326/m13-2411.

Shadid, S., C. Koutsari, and M. D. Jensen. 2007. Direct free fatty acid uptake into human adipocytes in vivo: Relation to body fat distribution. *Diabetes* 56 (5):1369–1375. doi: 10.2337/db06-1680.

Shepard, T. H., M. Shi, G. W. Fellingham, M. Fujinaga, J. M. FitzSimmons, A. G. Fantel, and M. Barr. 1988. Organ weight standards for human fetuses. *Pediatr Pathol* 8 (5):513–524.

Shook, R. P., G. A Hand, C. Drenowatz, J. R Hebert, A. E Paluch, J. E Blundell, J. O Hill, P. T Katzmarzyk, T. S Church, and S. N Blair. 2015. Low levels of physical activity are associated with dysregulation of energy intake and fat mass gain over 1 year. *Am J Clin Nutr* 102 (6):1332–1338. doi:10.3945/ajcn.115.115360.

Skelton, J. A., S. R. Cook, P. Auinger, J. D. Klein, and S. E. Barlow. 2009. Prevalence and trends of severe obesity among U.S. children and adolescents. *Acad Pediatr* 9 (5):322–329. doi:10.1016/j.acap.2009.04.005.

Skinner, B.F. 1953. *Science and Human Behavior*. New York, NY: Macmillan.

Spalding, K. L., E. Arner, P. O. Westermark, S. Bernard, B. A. Buchholz, O. Bergmann, L. Blomqvist, J. Hoffstedt, E. Naslund, T. Britton, H. Concha, M. Hassan, M. Ryden, J. Frisen, and P. Arner. 2008. Dynamics of fat cell turnover in humans. *Nature* 453 (7196):783–787. doi:10.1038/nature06902.

Steinke, J., and S. G. Driscoll. 1965. The extractable insulin content of pancreas from fetuses and infants of diabetic and control mothers. *Diabetes* 14 (9):573–578.

Szabo, A. J., and O. Szabo. 1974. Placental free-fatty-acid transfer and fetal adipose-tissue development: An explantation of fetal adiposity in infants of diabetic mothers. *Lancet* 2 (7879):498–499.

Taveras, E. M., K. H. Hohman, S. Price, S. L. Gortmaker, and K. Sonneville. 2009. Televisions in the bedrooms of racial/ethnic minority children: How did they get there and how do we get them out? *Clin Pediatr (Phila)* 48 (7):715–719. doi:10.1177/0009922809335667.

Thompson, A. L., L. S. Adair, and M. E. Bentley. 2013. Maternal characteristics and perception of temperament associated with infant TV exposure. *Pediatrics* 131 (2):e390–e397. doi:10.1542/peds.2012-1224.

Thompson, W. S., and S. D. Cohle. 2004. Fifteen-year retrospective study of infant organ weights and revision of standard weight tables. *J Forensic Sci* 49 (3):575–585.

Thyfault, J. P., and R. Krogh-Madsen. 2011. Metabolic disruptions induced by reduced ambulatory activity in free living humans. *J Appl Physiol* 111 (4):1218–1224. doi: 10.1152/japplphysiol.00478.2011.

Tong, J. F., X. Yan, M. J. Zhu, S. P. Ford, P. W. Nathanielsz, and M. Du. 2009. Maternal obesity downregulates myogenesis and beta-catenin signaling in fetal skeletal muscle. *Am J Physiol Endocrinol Metab* 296 (4):E917–E924. doi:10.1152/ajpendo.90924.2008.

Troiano, R. P., D. Berrigan, K. W. Dodd, L. C. Masse, T. Tilert, and M. McDowell. 2008. Physical activity in the United States measured by accelerometer. *Med Sci Sports Exerc* 40 (1):181–188.

Westerterp, K. R. 2009. Dietary fat oxidation as a function of body fat. *Curr Opin Lipidol* 20 (1):45–49.

Whitaker, R. C. 2004. Predicting preschooler obesity at birth: The role of maternal obesity in early pregnancy. *Pediatrics* 114 (1):e29–e36.

Whitaker, R.C., J. A Wright, M. S Pepe, K. D Seidel, and W. H Dietz. 1997. Predicting obesity in young adulthood from childhood and parental obesity. *N Eng J Med* 337 (13):869–873.

Wlodek, D., and M. Gonzales. 2003. Decreased energy levels can cause and sustain obesity. *J Theor Biol* 225 (1):33–44.

Wolf, J. B, and M. J Wade. 2009. What are maternal effects (and what are they not)? *Phil Trans R S B: Biol Sci* 364 (1520):1107–1115. doi:10.1098/rstb.2008.0238.

Yan, X., M. J Zhu, M. V Dodson, and M. Du. 2012. Developmental programming of fetal skeletal muscle and adipose tissue development. *J Genomics* 1:29–38.

3 Developmental Programming by Environmental Chemicals and Their Influence on Health across the Lifespan

Jerrold J. Heindel and Michelle Mendez

CONTENTS

3.1 INTRODUCTION

Over the last several decades, there has been a major paradigm shift related in our understanding of the etiology of disease. It is now clear that diseases that appear across the lifespan often have their origins during development (*in utero* and early childhood): a concept called the Developmental Origins of Health and Disease (DOHaD). This concept posits that there are sensitive windows during development in which tissue development and function can be modified by environmental factors (e.g., poor maternal nutrition, stress, environmental chemicals, maternal disease/lifestyle), which can lead to increased susceptibility to disease/dysfunction across the life course (Gluckman et al. 2010; Barouki et al. 2012; Padmanabhan et al. 2016).

33

The DOHaD hypothesis of susceptibility to disease includes the following tenets (Barouki et al. 2012): (1) There are sensitive windows where exposures to environmental stressors can cause altered tissue programming leading to altered function and thus to increased susceptibility to disease/dysfunction across the lifespan. (2) Tissues are most sensitive to environmental stressors when they are developing which may include *in utero*, early postnatal, and late childhood or adolescence depending on the tissue/organ. (3) The increased susceptibility to disease can occur without any phenotype changes apparent at birth as the effects may involve subtle changes in gene expression, which lead to altered proteins, altered cell activity, number of cells, or cell locations. (4) Epigenetic modifications may underlie these changes in gene expression. (5) There is likely to be a latent period between the environmental stressor and onset of disease/dysfunction which can be from months to years to decades and even cross generations. (6) Some effects may be sexually dimorphic with effects only in males or females depending on the environmental stressor studied, and may also depend on genetic background (i.e., genetic polymorphisms), (7) The effects may only increase susceptibility to develop disease and the disease may not be apparent until a "second hit" occurs later in life. It is important to understand that these tenets underscore the DOHaD concept regardless of the environmental stressor (Heindel et al. 2015a).

The DOHaD concept originated from two separate scientific fields, nutrition and environmental health. The nutrition focus started with the finding that coronary heart disease is linked to impaired fetal growth due to severe malnutrition during fetal life (reviewed in Barker 2007). Over the years, there has been a focus on how poor nutrition can result in increased incidence of a variety of diseases later in life as noted in recent reviews (Gluckman et al. 2011; Lillycrop and Burdge 2012; Hanson and Gluckman 2015; Lane 2014). This focus on the importance of nutrition during development is now well known and accepted (Heindel et al. 2015a). However, the DOHaD paradigm as developed was never meant to be focused only on nutrition. The definition of DOHaD developed by the society with the same name is, "The Developmental Origins of Health and Disease is a multidisciplinary field that examines how environmental factors acting during the phase of developmental plasticity interact with genotypic variation to change the capacity of the organism to cope with its environment in later life." The words "environmental factors" thereby covers not only nutrition but also stress and environmental chemicals.

This review is focused on the DOHaD paradigm with the goal to highlight that "environment" in the DOHaD paradigm refers not just to nutrition but also environmental chemicals. We also show that the aspects of DOHaD that are applicable to nutrition are also applicable to environmental chemicals and highlight the DOHaD epidemiology literature with regard to environmental chemicals to show that the environmental chemical literature is as robust and focused on noncommunicable diseases as the nutritional literature.

Animal studies have long documented that the *in utero* developmental period is a sensitive window for perturbation by environmental chemicals. It has been clear since the 1950s that exposure to a wide variety of environmental chemicals *in utero* could be toxic to the developing fetus and lead to death, or birth defects. Indeed, governmental guidelines and long-standing study designs specifically examine chemicals for their *in utero* effects on death and birth defects (Chernoff et al. 1989). In a typical developmental toxicology study, the chemical is administered to the pregnant dam (mouse, rat, or rabbit), the offspring are examined just before birth for birth defects, and the uterus is examined for pregnancy loss. Thus, only death or birth defects like spina bifida or limb defects are detected. In this regard, just a few decades ago it was noted that between 2% and 5% of all live births have major developmental abnormalities (Beckman and Brent 1984). Up to 40% of these defects have been estimated to result from maternal exposures to harmful environmental agents that impact the intrauterine environment. The terrible limb defects caused when women took thalidomide during pregnancy is a human tragedy that proves the case (Finnell et al. 2002). While developmental toxicity protocols called for examination of the fetuses just prior to birth, other experimental designs expose the fetus to chemicals during development and allow live births and follow the pups throughout life. These studies have shown that depending on the agent, timing, and dose, environmental chemicals can cause not only death or malformations, but also premature birth or low birth weight and functional changes that could increase susceptibility to diseases that might not be apparent until later in life.

This discussion of developmental toxicology indicates that it is difficult to determine when the field of developmental origins of disease focusing on environmental chemical exposures actually started. However, one might consider that the work on dichlorodiphenyltrichloroethane (DDT), which was reviewed in the book, *Silent Spring*, by Rachel Carson in 1962 was a turning point for the field. She noted that DDT, a pesticide that was widely used to control mosquitoes, did not appear to have significant toxicity to adult birds but severely affected eggshells of the developing birds resulting in near extinction of the brown pelican and the bald eagle (Lundholm 1997).

A strong proof of principle in humans for the developmental origins of disease paradigm in the environmental health field came from studies that examined the use of an estrogenic drug, diethylstilbestrol (DES), during pregnancy that resulted in increased incidence of a rare vaginal cancer and reproductive abnormalities in both sons and daughters first published in 1971 (Newman et al. 1971; Tournaire et al. 2016). These effects in humans were shown to also occur in mice models (McLachlan and Newbold 1987; Newbold and McLachlan 1996).

A consensus statement from the Wingspread Conference in 1991 that brought together experts from a variety of environmental and endocrine fields first coined the term "endocrine disruptor" for chemicals that altered hormone action and focused attention on early development as a sensitive time for endocrine disruption, which helped to move the DOHaD field forward. Published results from the conference (Colborn et al. 1993) noted that "the chemicals of concern may have entirely different effects on the embryo, fetus, or perinatal organism than on the adult; the effects are most often manifested in offspring, not in the exposed parent; the timing of exposure in the developing organism is crucial in determining its character and future potential; and although critical exposure occurs during embryonic development, obvious manifestations may not occur until maturity." It also noted that "any perturbations of the endocrine system of a developing organism may alter the development of that organism: typically these effects are irreversible."

Several human tragedies provided further evidence for the increased sensitivity of developmental exposures to environmental chemicals including mercury contamination in Minamata Bay where exposure to mercury during pregnancy resulted in severe brain dysfunctions in the offspring (Yorifuji et al. 2015), and polychlorinated biphenyl (PCB) contamination of rice oil in Japan where the exposed mothers had only mild skin diseases and the offspring had serious brain problems including reduced intelligent quotient (IQ) (Hsu et al. 1985; Aoki 2001). While these effects of high-dose exposures to the mother were apparent in children in early life, maternal smoking during pregnancy, which is associated with increased postnatal weight gain and subsequent obesity in offspring (Ng et al. 2009; Ino 2010; Behl et al. 2013), provides proof of principle of adverse effects in later life of developmental exposures to common chemicals at environmentally relevant concentrations.

The first epidemiological studies that focused on developmental chemical exposures and later life disease outcomes were published in the mid-1970s and were focused on neurodevelopmental and behavioral effects (Weiss and Spyker 1974; Spyker 1975; Bellinger et al. 1984; Gladen et al. 1988), although the DOHaD hypothesis per se had not been developed at that time (Barker 1995). The hypothesis that exposure to an increasing number of chemicals may contribute to the global epidemic of obesity was further elaborated in Baillie-Hamilton (2002). The DOHaD field, with respect to chemical exposures, expanded starting around 2006 partly due to the publication of the obesogen hypothesis (Grun and Blumberg 2006) that focused on the developmental origins of obesity by environmental chemicals. This new focus under the DOHaD umbrella expanded the number and types of chemicals examined for developmental effects on disease susceptibility, as well as broadening the scope of the outcomes under study.

There has been an exponential increase in the number of publications in the field of environmental epidemiology through 2014 with 425 epidemiology publications that examined the association between exposure to environmental chemicals and a variety of health outcomes later in life (smoking and drugs excluded) (Heindel et al. 2017). Thus, the follow-up of the children studied in the birth cohorts that examined chemical-health outcome dyads is only now reaching 10–14 years of age, so there are few studies, which, taking advantage of stored samples or retrospective data, have long-term follow-up (Heindel et al. 2017; Karmaus et al. 2009; Halldorsson et al. 2012; Harris et al. 2013; La Merrill et al. 2013; Aschengrau et al. 2015). Thus, the majority of publications exploring long-term effects of early life chemical exposures focus on health effects that are apparent in childhood.

In this review, we provide an overview of the data linking developmental exposures to environmental chemicals to specific health outcomes with an emphasis on epidemiology studies and also incorporate animal studies where appropriate. We cannot cover the entire field of more than 400 publications but can give a short overview and then focus on specific chemical-health outcome dyads in neurodevelopmental and neurobehavioral studies, cancer, and cardiometabolic studies including obesity/diabetes to highlight specific examples. There have been numerous reviews focusing on both animal and human data that highlight the importance of chemical exposures in the DOHaD paradigm (Newbold 2011; Schug et al. 2013; Berghuis et al. 2015; Heindel et al. 2015a, b; Liu and Peterson 2015). The importance of the role of environmental chemicals in the DOHaD paradigm for disease has also been supported by society statements. These include the Endocrine Society (Diamanti-Kandarakis et al. 2009; Gore et al. 2015) and the recent Federation of Gynecology and Obstetrics (FOGO) opinion on reproductive health impacts of exposure to toxic environmental chemicals (Di Renzo et al. 2015).

3.2 OVERVIEW OF THE DOHaD EPIDEMIOLOGY LITERATURE FOCUSING ON ENVIRONMENTAL CHEMICALS

A recent review of the DOHaD epidemiology literature on chemical exposures (Heindel et al. 2017) found 425 publications through 2014. This review focused only on endpoints measured several months after birth, thus premature birth, birth weight, and any birth defects were not assessed. The large numbers of publications indicate not only a great interest but also a depth to the environmental chemical focus of DOHaD. The majority of these publications focused on neurological/neurobehavioral outcomes ($n = 211$) followed by cancer ($n = 59$), respiratory ($n = 50$), metabolic outcomes including obesity ($n = 35$), reproductive health ($n = 31$), immune disorders ($n = 29$), endocrine ($n = 22$), and cardiovascular dysfunctions ($n = 12$) with less than 10 publications each focusing on skin, musculoskeletal, thyroid, visual problems, gastrointestinal, liver (Heindel et al. 2017), and respiratory outcomes (Gascon et al. 2013, 2014, 2015). The number of publications with a specific health outcome is generally related to when publications in that discipline first appeared in the literature, with the earliest focus on neurodevelopmental/neurobehavioral outcomes and an emergence of obesity, immune, respiratory, and cardiovascular areas only in the last decade. Overall, 60 different chemicals have been examined in DOHaD publications (Heindel et al. 2017). The most studied environmental chemicals are PCBs (100 publications), organochlorine pesticides (60), mercury (61), lead (53), air pollutants/particulate matter (27), polycyclic aromatic hydrocarbons (PAHs) (23), nitrogen oxide/dioxides (20) and ozone (8), organophosphate pesticides (OPs) (22), and arsenic (16). In recent years, there has been a focus on chemicals with short half-lives including phthalates (plasticizers) (10), bisphenol A (BPA) (a component of polycarbonate) (9), and the newer chemicals polybrominated diphenyl ethers (PBDEs, flame retardants) (11), and the nonstick chemicals, perfluorooctanoic acids or sulfates (PFOA) (19) and PFOS (15). This overview (Heindel et al. 2017) and others (Fenton et al. 2012; Gascon et al. 2013; Yeung et al. 2014; Berghuis et al. 2015; Liu and Peterson 2015) indicate a large and growing body of evidence regarding the likely importance of developmental exposure to environmental chemicals and varied health outcomes in later life.

3.3 NEURODEVELOPMENTAL AND NEUROBEHAVIORAL STUDIES

The developing brain is extremely sensitive to environmental chemicals that can alter developmental programming leading to a myriad of neurodevelopmental and neurobehavioral problems that occur across the lifespan (Schug et al. 2015; Gore et al. 2015; Winneke 2011; Grandjean and Landrigan 2014; Tshala-Katumbay et al. 2015). Indeed, Grandjean noted that there is "strong evidence that industrial chemicals widely disseminated in the environment are important contributors to what we have called the global, silent pandemic of neurodevelopmental toxicity" (Grandjean and

Landrigan 2006). While 201 chemicals have the potential for neurodevelopmental toxicity (reviewed in Grandjean and Landrigan), only six—arsenic, lead, methylmercury, PCBs, OPs, and toluene—have been adequately shown to cause neurotoxicity in humans (Grandjean and Landrigan 2014).

Almost half of all the DOHaD epidemiology publications that focused on the role of environmental chemical exposures (211/425) examined some neurobehavioral and/or neurodevelopmental defect. This is to be expected because of the early focus on lead and mercury exposure *in utero* and early childhood and the subsequent increase in neurodevelopmental and neurobehavioral defects including loss of IQ. Both lead and methylmercury are well-established neurotoxicants that can have serious effects on the development and functioning of the human nervous system (Trasande et al. 2006; Grandjean and Landrigan 2014). Indeed, there are 26 publications examining the effects of developmental exposures to mercury and 20 publications examining the developmental effects of lead on just one measure of brain function: IQ (Heindel et al. 2017). It is clear that children exposed to lead even at levels thought to be safe, for example, <10 µg/dL, are at risk for reduced cognitive development including reduced IQ and poor academic performance (Bellinger 2008; Liu et al. 2013). There is no safe level of exposure to lead (Grandjean and Landrigan 2014).

Prenatal exposure to mercury, measured as mercury concentration in cord blood and maternal hair, due mainly to methylmercury contamination of meat from pilot whales, was examined in a birth cohort in the Faroe Islands (Debes et al. 2016). Total mercury in hair (reflecting long-term exposure) and in blood (a measure of short-term exposure) are both validated biomarkers of methyl mercury intake correlated with seafood consumption (Sheehan et al. 2014). Mercury exposure to the mother was shown to be associated with cognitive defects (most pronounced in language, attention, and memory) in the children measured at age 7 (Grandjean et al. 1997), 14, and 22 years, indicating that the effect of mercury toxicity is permanent and persists into adulthood (Debes et al. 2016) albeit at smaller effect sizes. Nonetheless, at 22 years major domains of brain functions as well as general intelligence were still affected (Debes et al. 2016). In addition, functional magnetic resonance imaging (MRI) scans showed abnormally expanded activation of brain regions in response to sensory stimulation and motor tasks in adolescents from the Faroe Island birth cohort (White et al. 2011), thus linking behavioral with structural and biochemical brain changes.

Although there are fewer studies, recent reviews show that developmental exposure to arsenic is associated with reduced intellectual development (Tyler and Allan 2014), but uncertainty remains regarding effects at very low doses (Rodriguez-Barranco et al. 2013; Tsuji et al. 2015; Rodrigues et al. 2016). Early life exposure to other metals, including cadmium and manganese, is also hypothesized to adversely affect neurodevelopment, but further research is needed as results to date are limited and mixed (Rodriguez-Barranco et al. 2013; Mora et al. 2015; Sanders et al. 2015).

Exposure to a variety of phthalates has also been associated with learning and memory problems. Phthalates are lipid soluble with a half-life of less than 24 hours in humans; they are not persistent and do not accumulate (Wittassek and Angerer 2008). Phthalate exposure is usually measured via their main metabolites in urine (Ejaredar et al. 2015). Low-molecular-weight phthalates such as dimethyl phthalate, diethyl phthalate, and dibutyl phthalate are used in cosmetics and lotions and as delivery agents in aerosols, while high-molecular-weight phthalates such as di(ethylhexyl) phthalate (DEHP) and butylbenzyl phthalate (BBZP) are mainly used as plasticizers and adhesives; they can leach over time (reviewed in Ejaredar et al. 2015). Developmental exposures to low-molecular-weight phthalates in general have been associated with attention problems, poorer overall executive functions in children aged 4–9 (Engel et al. 2010) and higher levels of aggression, problems in working memory and attention problems (Cho et al. 2010), and decreases in psychomotor development, increased odds of psychomotor delay, as well as decreases in mental development at 3 years of age (Whyatt et al. 2012). Developmental exposure to higher weight phthalates DEHP or dipentyl phthalate (DIPP) has been shown to result in decreased anogenital distance (AGD) in animal studies, which is an indication of decreased androgen production (Gray et al. 2016). Such androgenic effects may partly explain the influence of phthalates on behavioral outcomes. Swan has shown that first trimester phthalate exposure (DEHP) is associated with reduced AGD in newborn boys (Swan et al. 2015), which was associated with less masculine play behaviors as reported by parents (Swan et al. 2010). In addition to the variety of learning and behavioral problems associated with phthalate exposures, developmental exposure to low-molecular-weight phthalates has actually been associated with decreased IQ (Factor-Litvak et al. 2014). Full-scale IQ was inversely associated with prenatal exposure to dibutyl phthalate (DnBP) and diisobutyl phthalate (DiBP), measured as urinary metabolites. IQ was 6.7 and 7.6 points lower in children of mothers exposed to highest vs. lowest quartiles of DnBP and DiBP, respectively, when IQ was assessed at age 7.

Loss of IQ points has also been shown for exposure to OPs such as chlorpyrifos. Simultaneous publications from three separate laboratories showed that developmental exposure to organophosphates led to a loss of IQ points in the offspring that were similar to that found with lead exposure (Bouchard et al. 2011). Bouchard et al. (2011) measured urinary dialkyl phosphate (DAP) metabolites in urine to assess OP exposure in a birth cohort study (Center for the Health Assessment of Mothers and Children of Salinas [CHAMACOS]), in the Salinas Valley in California. Average maternal DAP concentrations were associated with poorer scores for working memory, processing speed, verbal comprehension, perceptual reasoning, and full scale IQ at age 7. Children in the highest DAP exposure had an average deficit of 7.0 IQ points compared with children in the lowest quintile (Bouchard et al. 2011). Engel et al. (2011) also measured total DAP metabolites as a measure of maternal OP exposure in the Mount Sinai Children's Health Study in New York City. Prenatal exposure was negatively associated with aspects of neurodevelopment at 12 and 24 months and also at 6–9 years of age (perceptual reasoning and working memory). Rauh et al. (2006) examined prenatal exposure to chlorpyrifos and effects through 3 years in an inner city minority population. They measured detectable levels of chlorpyrifos 99.7% in personal air samples and 64–70% umbilical cord blood samples collected at birth. Highly exposed children scored on average 6.5 points on the Bayley Psychomotor Development Index and 3.3 points lower on the Bayley Mental Development Index at age 3 years. Highly exposed children were defined as those in the highest tertile among subjects with detectable chlorpyrifos measured in cord blood (used as measure of exposures during pregnancy given evidence of limited variability over time in personal air measures; half-life of chlorpyrifos in blood is 27 hours). Though not apparent at 12 months, deficits in motor activity emerged by age 3 years, with exposed children more likely to show behavioral problems manifest as attention-deficit/hyperactivity disorder (ADHD) symptoms.

Recent reviews, including a systematic review, note that adverse effects of prenatal exposure to OPs may be stronger than those of postnatal exposure, although the data on postnatal exposures are limited (Berghuis et al. 2015; Hernandez et al. 2016). The effects of OPs on neurodevelopmental outcomes are thought to be influenced by genetics, with more severe effects in children with paraoxonase-1 (PON-1) polymorphisms, which impact the metabolism of the OPs (Engel et al. 2011). More research is needed to determine whether associations are causal, whether they persist or emerge over the longer term, and whether the mixed results reported in the studies conducted so far may be due in part to limited power to detect sex-specific effects, or effects in genetically susceptible subgroups. The inconsistent results may also relate to the heterogeneous outcomes analyzed across studies, as it remains uncertain whether the programmed effects of specific chemicals may be limited to particular neurodevelopmental or psychological domains (González-Alzaga et al. 2014).

PBDEs are a class of persistent chemicals widely used as flame retardants in furniture, carpets, and other consumer products (Lorber 2008). Three birth cohort studies identified consistent exposure–response relationships linking PBDE exposure with lower IQ (Herbstman et al. 2010; Eskenazi et al. 2013; Chen et al. 2014). For example, PBDEs measured in cord blood were associated with abnormal mental and physical development at ages 12–48 and 72 months. For every natural log-unit change in BDE 100, IQ scores were on average 3.4–4.0 point lower at 48 and 72 months (Herbstman et al. 2010). It has been proposed that thyroid disruption may be important in the action of these flame retardants to alter learning and memory (Dingemans et al. 2011). *In vitro* studies have shown that PBDEs can bind to not only thyroid hormone but also estrogen, androgen, progesterone, and glucocorticoid receptors indicating additional modes of action (Dingemans et al. 2011).

Along with cognitive and motor skills, other neurological endpoints associated with developmental exposures to environmental chemicals include ADHD and attention problems (Aguiar et al. 2010; Polanska et al. 2013; Berghuis et al. 2015) and autism/autism spectrum disorders (Rossignol et al. 2014; Fujiwara et al. 2016; Keil and Lein 2016), with fewer studies on depression and schizophrenia (Brown 2009). Toxicants implicated in autism spectrum disorder include pesticides, phthalates, PCBs, solvents, air pollutants, BPA, and heavy metals; however, the evidence is inconclusive at this time for a specific role for any environmental chemical. Though many aspects of brain development and behavioral outcomes have been linked to developmental exposures to a variety of environmental chemicals, as noted, many areas have limited publications. The literature to date has assessed a limited number of chemicals, and a limited number of endpoints, indicating a need for more studies.

3.4 CANCER

A nascent literature suggests that perinatal chemical exposures may increase the risk of adult onset as well as childhood cancers (Birnbaum and Fenton 2003; Fenton et al. 2012; Heindel et al. 2017). Leukemia/lymphoma is the most studied, followed by testicular, brain, and breast cancer (Heindel et al. 2017) with a few publications examining environmental exposures during development and ovarian, bone, liver, kidney, and skin cancers. Support for perinatal programming of adult-onset cancer stemmed from the now established increased risk of rare forms of vaginal cancer, as well as of breast cancer, in women exposed *in utero* to DES, a potent synthetic estrogen prescribed to their mothers during pregnancy (Palmer et al. 2006; Troisi et al. 2007, 2017; Newbold 2012; Hilakivi-Clarke 2014; Mahalingaiah et al. 2014).

Due to the challenge of estimating past prenatal exposures in research on adults, the epidemiological literature examining the relationship between prenatal chemical exposures and cancers in adulthood is very limited. However, several human studies with very long-term follow-up suggest that in addition to DES, there may be increases in adult cancers associated with prenatal and/or childhood exposure to DDT (Cohn et al. 2010, 2015), tetrachloroethylene (TCE) (Aschengrau et al. 2015), arsenic (Mohammed Abdul et al. 2015), and PAHs from air pollution (Bonner et al. 2005). Animal studies show that *in utero* exposure to dibenzo[*a*]pyrene produces lymphoma in the offspring, supporting the human data (Yu et al. 2006; Castro et al. 2008b).

Developmental and lifelong exposure to environmentally relevant exposures to arsenic in mice results in lung cancer (Waalkes et al. 2014) and developmental exposures increased the incidence of hepatic tumors in mice with a *ras* gene polymorphism (Nohara et al. 2014) and in C3H mice (Liu et al. 2004). Similarly, humans exposed to high levels of arsenic *in utero* and during childhood (<15 years) in Chile via water contamination had fourfold increases in lung and sevenfold increases in bladder cancer 35–40 years after the exposures ended (Steinmaus et al. 2013, 2014). Likewise, early life exposure to the organochlorine pesticide DDT has been associated with increases in mammary cancers in mice (Ho et al. 2012), consistent with findings in humans (Cohn et al. 2015). Prenatal exposure to PAHs has also been linked to cancers in animal studies (Yu et al. 2006; Castro et al. 2008b). Though developmental exposure has not been specifically examined, TCE has been associated with cancers in animal experiments (Guyton et al. 2014). Together, these data support the ability of developmental exposures that include not only drugs such as DES, but also solvents (e.g., TCE), organochlorine compounds (e.g., DDT), PAHs, and naturally occurring metals such as arsenic to result in increased susceptibility to a variety of cancers over the lifespan.

In addition to susceptibility to adult cancers after a long latency period, there are close to 30 publications that have examined the relationship between exposures to pesticides, organic solvents, and air pollutants on leukemia/lymphoma diagnosed in infancy and childhood (Heindel et al. 2017). Increased risks have been reported for diverse chemicals including maternal exposure to household cleaning products, pest control treatments, and paternal occupational chemical exposures. Additional research is critical to identify these risks and inform prevention efforts. Epidemiological studies are needed to provide further insight on the existence of genetically vulnerable subgroups or on postnatal lifestyle factors that may help to mitigate these risks.

Consistent with the data in humans, rodent studies also indicate that *in utero* exposure to other chemicals may also increase the risk of adult as well as childhood onset cancers, with postulated effects of endocrine disrupting chemicals that include BPA and phthalates along with PAHs and metals, among others (Birnbaum and Fenton 2003; Yu et al. 2006; Murray et al. 2007; Castro et al. 2008a; Tokar et al. 2011; Fenton et al. 2012; Steinmaus et al. 2013). Similar to other health outcomes, this literature suggests that the mechanisms involved may include epigenetic effects, altered tissue structure that may affect future development, and changes in sex hormone function. Further research is needed to better understand the links between early chemical exposures and subsequent risk of cancer and how to mitigate both harmful exposures and the resulting health risks.

3.5 OBESITY AND CARDIOMETABOLIC DISORDERS

There is growing evidence linking developmental exposure to a variety of environmental chemicals with excess weight gain and obesity in both animal models and human epidemiology studies of birth cohorts (La Merrill and Birnbaum 2011; Tang-Peronard et al. 2011; Thayer et al. 2012; Heindel et al. 2015b; Liu and Peterson 2015). Such effects may be mediated at least in part through effects manifested by reduced fetal growth: many of the chemicals hypothesized to promote obesity and cardiometabolic dysfunction have been associated with lower birth weight (Govarts et al. 2012; Bach et al. 2015). Smaller size at birth is strongly associated with both long-term obesity and cardiometabolic dysfunction, particularly when followed by rapid infant weight gain (Ong and Loos 2006; Gishti et al. 2014; Yeung et al. 2014). Mediation through impaired fetal growth provides a link between research on the programming of long-term health effects by prenatal chemical exposures and the earliest nutrition research on the DOHaD concept, which examined adult health outcomes associated with birth weights in the lower end of the normal range (Barker 1995). Indeed, there is strong and consistent evidence from meta-analyses of over 20 epidemiological studies that maternal smoking during pregnancy is associated with both smaller size at birth and subsequent obesity in the offspring in childhood (Behl et al. 2013). As noted, this literature on smoking provides proof of principle that chemical exposures during development may have lasting effects on impact weight gain and risk of obesity in later life.

Current epidemiological research on other chemicals most strongly supports a role in programming of obesity by early life exposure to dichlorodiphenyldichloroethylene (DDE), the major metabolite of the persistent organochlorine pesticide DDT (Liu and Peterson 2015). Exposure to moderate levels of $p'p'$-DDE during pregnancy is associated with rapid infant weight gain, overweight in childhood and adulthood, and measures of abdominal fatness such as the waist-to-height ratio (Karmaus et al. 2009; Mendez et al. 2011; Warner et al. 2013; Delvaux et al. 2014; Agay-Shay et al. 2015; Iszatt et al. 2015). However, null associations have been reported at higher exposures (Cupul-Uicab et al. 2010, 2013; Garced et al. 2012; Hoyer, Ramlau-Hansen et al. 2014). This is consistent with the hypothesis that effects of these chemicals may be nonmonotonic; while low doses of endocrine disrupting chemicals may be obesogenic, high levels may instead impair growth (Vandenberg et al. 2012). Additional research is needed to determine whether susceptibility to DDE-associated excess weight gain may vary not only with exposure level, but may also depend on factors including child sex and genetic polymorphisms.

Results are less consistent for the more limited research linking obesity with prenatal exposure to other persistent organic pollutants, including perfluorinated chemicals (PFOA/PFOS) (used to repel water and in nonstick pans), various PCBs, PBDEs (flame retardants), and hexachlorobenzene (HCB) (a pesticide) (Liu and Peterson 2015). As noted in a recent review (Liu and Peterson 2015), *in utero* and childhood exposures to PBDEs were shown to be associated with increased body mass index (BMI) at age 7 in a sexually dimorphic manner, with effects among boys but not girls in the only study on prenatal exposure to this chemical (Erkin-Cakmak et al. 2015). HCB has been associated with increased risk of overweight in Spanish birth cohorts (Valvi et al. 2012, 2013). Developmental exposure to PFOA resulted in increased BMI and waist circumference in females but not males at age 20 years (Halldorsson et al. 2012), indicating that some effects from prenatal exposures may remain into adulthood. Only two of seven studies found prenatal exposure to various PCBs to be associated with subsequent increased weight gain or obesity (Liu and Peterson 2015). However, as noted above for DDE, it is uncertain to what extent these mixed results may be explained in part by differential effects dependent on exposure dose, child sex, or genetic polymorphisms. These results, while not sufficient, indicate the possibility that chemicals in these classes are obesogens in humans as has been noted in some animal models (Hines et al. 2009; Suvorov et al. 2009). While data are still inconclusive, there are plausible mechanisms of action linking persistent organic pollutants to obesity, with evidence that these chemicals may affect adipocyte differentiation, peroxisome proliferator-activated receptor (PPAR) expression, estrogenic activity, and epigenetic modification, including associations seen in human cohorts where the same chemicals have been linked to obesity (Casals-Casas and Desvergne n.d.; Ho et al. 2012; Warner et al. 2013; Huen et al. 2014).

Along with persistent chemicals, several recent studies have examined whether, consistent with laboratory data, perinatal exposure to nonpersistent chemicals with short half-lives, such as BPA and phthalates, is associated with obesity in humans (Newbold et al. 2009; Heindel et al. 2015b; Janesick and Blumberg 2016). Results so far have been inconsistent (Kim and Park 2014; Buckley et al. 2015, 2016; Liu and Peterson 2015; Valvi et al. 2015; Maresca et al. 2016). Indeed, higher prenatal exposure to phthalates has been shown to be inversely associated with obesity (Buckley et al. 2015, 2016; Valvi et al. 2015; Maresca et al. 2016), as have some recent studies on prenatal exposure to BPA (Harley et al. 2013; Braun et al. 2014; Liu and Peterson 2015; Buckley et al. 2016b). Nonetheless, there are also human data suggesting that prenatal as well as ongoing postnatal exposure to phthalates and BPA is associated with weight gain and obesity, including central fatness (Valvi et al. 2013; Song et al. 2014; Ranciere et al. 2015; Deierlein et al. 2016). Further research examining whether early exposure to nonpersistent chemicals may increase risk of obesity must address key challenges that undermine the studies to date. These include the following: (1) determining whether associations are independent of higher intakes of packaged foods which are a major source of exposure to these chemicals (Serrano et al. 2014; Stacy et al. 2016); (2) improving characterization of exposure by using multiple rather than single biomarker measures, given the high within-person variability of these chemicals (Johns et al. 2015); (3) carefully evaluating not only the timing (i.e., pre- vs. postnatal) but also the range of exposure that may confer risk, particularly as there is evidence of nonmonotonic dose–response (Angle et al. 2013); and (4) exploring whether there are susceptible subgroups characterized by gender, genetic profile, or postnatal diet (Wei et al. 2011; Bautista et al. 2015). Failure to address these issues may lead to measurement error resulting in inaccurate characterization of chronic exposure to these chemicals, may fail to isolate any obesogenic effects these exposures from dietary patterns that may be correlated with these exposures, and may overlook effects that may be limited to susceptible population subgroups.

There is compelling evidence in laboratory animals that along with obesity, developmental chemical exposures are associated with increased cardiometabolic dysfunction (Maull et al. 2012; Nadal 2013; Gore et al. 2015; Sargis 2015). However, few human studies have directly examined the extent to which exposure to contaminants during early life may promote not only obesity, but also the cardiometabolic dysfunction that ultimately culminates in meaningful morbidity and mortality (Yeung et al. 2014). Like obesity, the human evidence that early chemical exposures may program cardiometabolic dysfunction is strongest for maternal smoking during pregnancy. Maternal smoking has been associated with diabetes, hypertension, and dyslipidemia in later life through relationships that may be largely mediated through obesity (Montgomery and Ekbom 2002; Cupul-Uicab et al. 2012a, b; de Jonge et al. 2013; Mattsson et al. 2013; Haynes et al. 2014; Jaddoe et al. 2014; Bao et al. 2016).

Thus far, only a handful of epidemiological studies have directly examined the cardiometabolic health effects of early life exposure to prenatal chemicals besides tobacco. These studies suggest that there may be associations between persistent organic pollutants such as DDT/DDE with blood pressure both at age 4 years and in adulthood (La Merrill et al. 2013; Vafeiadi et al. 2015) as well as with higher levels of insulin at age 5 years (Tang-Peronard et al. 2015); air pollution and increased carotid artery arterial stiffness in young adulthood (Breton et al. 2016); and arsenic exposure and subsequent increases in blood pressure and kidney dysfunction (Hawkesworth et al. 2013). As for obesity, BPA and phthalates, nonpersistent chemicals for which there are important methodological challenges and concerns, have not been strongly associated with cardiometabolic risk markers in children at age 4 years in the limited research so far (Vafeiadi et al. 2016).

Though evidence of adverse cardiometabolic effects is limited for prenatal chemical exposures, there is a growing literature in older children and adults suggesting that ongoing *postnatal* exposure to certain environmental chemicals may promote cardiometabolic disorders including diabetes and cardiovascular diseases (Lind et al. 2012b; Kelishadi et al. 2013; Taylor et al. 2013; Jensen et al. 2014; Poursafa et al. 2014; Song et al. 2016; Lee et al. 2016). These relationships may be independent of obesity, and in some cases may occur in the absence of obesity, as illustrated by associations between cardiometabolic outcomes and postnatal levels of some chemicals (e.g., PCBs, arsenic), which are not strongly associated with weight status (Lind et al. 2012a; Lee et al. 2014; Penell et al. 2014; Wiberg et al. 2014).

Given the limited and inconsistent results so far, further research is needed to establish the extent to which developmental exposure to environmental chemicals may cause obesity as well as cardiometabolic dysfunction in humans. To maximize the effectiveness of public health intervention, it will be important to determine whether any apparent effects are independent of ongoing postnatal exposure to these chemicals, which may correlate with prenatal levels of exposure. There is also a need for research to determine whether postnatal lifestyle factors, including post-natal nutrition patterns, may help to mitigate the risk of any lasting (DiVall 2013) adverse effects of early chemical exposures (Bautista et al. 2015). Prevailing patterns of postnatal nutrition, which vary from cohort to cohort, may be important determinants of whether researchers identify significant lasting effects of early life chemical exposures in a particular study.

3.6   EPIGENETIC REGULATION

Supported by evidence from animal studies (Baccarelli and Bollati 2009; Vaiserman 2014; van Dijk et al. 2015b; Waring et al. 2016), epigenetic modification has been proposed as a potential underlying mechanism through which early exposure to environmental chemicals may promote long-term health risks (Lee et al. 2009; Vaiserman 2015) as has been proposed for nutrition during development in humans (Lee 2015; Godfrey et al. 2016). Though limited, there is mounting evidence in human studies that chemical exposures modify the epigenome. Most research so far has been conducted in adults. As noted in recent reviews, diverse chemicals including arsenic, particulate matter, DDE, perfluorinated compounds, BPA, and PAHs have been associated with differential deoxyribonucleic acid (DNA) methylation (Baccarelli and Ghosh 2012; Bailey and Fry 2014; Argos 2015; Ruiz-Hernandez et al. 2015). Similarly, early life exposure to tobacco has been found to have an epigenetic signature (Green and Marsit 2015; Maccani and Maccani 2015; Ladd-Acosta et al. 2016). However, the nascent literature has not yet determined the biological or functional consequences of these changes in DNA methylation. It is also uncertain to what extent the mixed results of studies to date may be due to differences in technologies and assays, or to differences in epigenetic outcome measures (e.g., locus specific vs. global methylation, leukocytes vs. peripheral whole blood). Recent studies suggest functional consequences of epigenetic regulation may depend not only on locus-specific effects, but also on modifications, which may be apparent only in specific cell types, and effects that may be limited to specific target organs or tissues (e.g., liver, adipose). There is also evidence suggesting that mechanisms may involve epigenetic alterations besides DNA methylation, such as histone modifications or microRNAs (miRNAs) (Martinez et al. 2014; Vaiserman 2014; van Dijk et al. 2015a). Few human studies have examined these alternative epigenetic measures, particularly concurrently with DNA methylation (Baccarelli and Ghosh 2012; Nye et al. 2014). Moreover, much of the evidence so far comes from animal studies and it is uncertain to what these findings translate to humans (Waring et al. 2016).

Despite these limitations, the evidence to date supports a link between chemical exposures, epigenetic regulation, and health outcomes. For example, examination of locus-specific changes in DNA methylation associated with arsenic exposure identified effects in genes such as PLA2G2C, which encodes an enzyme relevant for skin carcinogens, inflammation, and lipid metabolism, consistent with the carcinogenic and cardiovascular effects of arsenic exposure (Argos et al. 2014). Studies have also identified epigenetic changes in cord blood associated specifically with prenatal exposure to arsenic (Cardenas et al. 2015b; Rojas et al. 2015). A recent study found effects specific to tissues (placenta and umbilical artery) not detected in cord blood (Cardenas et al. 2015a). These findings highlight the importance of continuing to increase the specificity of epigenetic measures in epidemiologic research. Several studies have suggested that differential DNA methylation at specific loci, such as retinoid X receptorα (RXRα) and hypoxia-inducible factor 3 alpha (HIF3A) measured in tissues at birth, is associated with subsequent adiposity (Godfrey et al. 2011; Pan et al. 2015), although it is uncertain whether these associations are causal (Richmond et al. 2016). Further research examining the extent to which adverse effects of environmental chemicals on health outcomes, including obesity and chronic disease risks, are epigenetically regulated is needed. It will be particularly important to gain insights on whether such effects may be modifiable by nutritional factors, providing a potential opportunity for public health intervention (Huang et al. 2015; Romagnolo et al. 2016).

3.7 METHODOLOGICAL CHALLENGES

Bolstered by evidence from the laboratory, a growing epidemiological literature suggests that chemical exposures in early life can influence a constellation of health outcomes in later life. However, results as noted above are both limited and heterogeneous. This may be in part due to methodological challenges specific to linking environmental chemical exposures during early development to health outcomes later in life. It is important that future research addresses a number of key issues to improve our ability to determine whether associations in epidemiological literature reflect causal relationships.

3.7.1 EXPOSURE ESTIMATION

Biomarkers are typically used to estimate aggregate exposure because contact with the same chemical may occur via multiple routes (e.g., inhalation, ingestion, dermal absorption) and sources (e.g., personal care and household products, air, soil, dust, and water) (Wilson et al. 2003; Morgan et al. 2005; Gehring et al. 2013; Botton et al. 2014; Hormann et al. 2014; Levallois et al. 2014; Rhie et al. 2014; Caspersen et al. 2016; Lang et al. 2016; Stacy et al. 2016). Though the use of biomarkers may be critical, misclassification of exposure based on biomarker measures is a concern, particularly for nonpersistent chemicals. Many short-lived chemicals are optimally measured in urine as they are rapidly metabolized and cleared from the circulation; the low concentrations measured in blood may be more susceptible to misclassification (Calafat et al. 2015). However, for some chemicals, notably BPA and also some phthalate metabolites, within-person variability in urine concentrations both throughout the day and from day to day can be so substantial that it may result in problematic misclassification if exposure estimates are based—as is typical—on a single spot urine, and even a single 24-hour urine sample (Preau et al. 2010; Ye et al. 2011; Fisher et al. 2015; Johns et al. 2015). Multiple samples collected at varied times over several days have been recommended to reduce such misclassification, through approaches such as averaging repeated measures, or using measures from pooled urine samples collected in each individual, as well as by developing measurement error models with a validation study subsample (Spiegelman 2010; Calafat et al. 2015; Perrier et al. 2016).

Sample contamination during collection, handling, and storage may also lead to considerable exposure measurement error particularly for phthalates and BPA, which are widely used in laboratory and medical equipment (Calafat et al. 2015). A final challenge is ensuring that measures of exposure reflect the vulnerable time windows of interest (e.g., pre- or early pregnancy, later pregnancy, infancy) (Engel and Wolff 2013). While many studies on the effects of early life exposure to chemicals have focused exclusively on samples collected in pregnancy, continued exposure in infancy may be considerable, and may have important health consequences, as is the case for childhood lead exposure (Engel and Wolff 2013; Lang et al. 2016). More research is needed to examine the effects of both cumulative exposure and exposure mixtures, as it has been hypothesized that there may be synergistic effects of exposure to multiple chemicals (Braun et al. 2016).

3.7.2 ANALYSIS CONSIDERATIONS

The potential for uncontrolled confounding in observational research exploring the health effects of early life exposure to chemicals is a major concern (Engel and Wolff 2013). It is far from certain that studies to date have adequately addressed possible confounding by factors such as socioeconomic status, home environments, and nutritional and dietary factors. Diet is a special concern as it may be a source of exposure to a number of chemicals (e.g., due to food packaging, contaminated soil, or marine environments) and may be an independent risk factor for a variety of outcomes such as obesity and neurodevelopment. Along with synergies, the potential for confounding by other chemical exposures poses another challenge, as multicollinearity may reduce statistical power in studies of small to moderate sample size (Braun et al. 2016). Effect modification as a result of varied susceptibility to adverse effects of certain exposures, for example, as a consequence of factors such as genetic polymorphisms (Engel et al. 2011; Duarte-Salles et al. 2012, 2013) is understudied, as unfortunately little is known about such susceptibility. Given evidence that associations between some chemical exposures and health outcomes may be nonmonotonic, it is important that future studies examine the shape of dose–response relationships rather than assuming linear relationships (Vandenberg et al. 2012). This and other challenges to statistical power issue make efforts to combine small studies, or to conduct larger studies with common exposure and outcome measures, particularly important (Gehring et al. 2013).

3.8 SUMMARY AND CONCLUSIONS

This review focused on an important but lesser known aspect of the DOHaD paradigm, the importance of exposure to environmental chemicals during development and health outcomes later in life. The DOHaD field has focused on the problems of over- and undernutrition during development as a major contributor to the increased susceptibility to disease across the lifespan without noting the perhaps equally important role for exposure to environmental chemicals. As noted above and shown in Figure 3.1, nutritional changes during development and exposure to environmental chemicals both share the same tenets and mechanisms. Indeed as noted in this review and reviewed in detail elsewhere (Heindel et al. 2017), there are over 60 chemical exposures during development that have been studied for their impact on diseases across the lifespan in human epidemiology studies. The majority of these chemicals are toxic at least in part due to the fact that they inter-fere with hormone action during development resulting in functional changes in gene expression that may persist and result in increased susceptibility to diseases across the lifespan. Furthermore, there is widespread exposure to these chemi-cals across the globe. These environmental chemicals have been associated with a wide variety of human health outcomes including neurodevelopmental and learn-ing problems, cancers, reproductive dysfunctions, respiratory problems, immune dysfunctions, obesity, diabetes, and other aspects of cardiometabolic diseases including metabolic syndrome. Altering nutrition during development has also been associated with a variety of diseases and in some cases the same diseases have been shown to be susceptible to both nutritional and chemical perturbations (Figure 3.2). Thus, it is now clear that developmental programming by both nutri-tional changes and environmental chemicals can result in increased susceptibil-ity to a variety of health outcomes across the lifespan with obesity being a good example (Figure 3.3). Therefore, it is critical that these two seemingly disparate research areas become more integrated as it likely that both chemicals and nutri-tion during development can alter programing leading to increased susceptibility to disease and thus they need to be examined together to determine their separate and integrative effects on health across the lifespan and generations. Improving nutrition and reducing exposure to environmental chemicals during development likely offer the best opportunity to actually prevent disease.

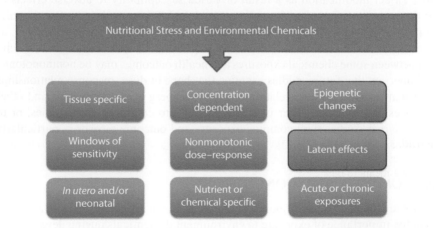

FIGURE 3.1 Nutritional stress or environmental chemical exposures cause similar effects during development.

Nutritional Stress	Environmental Chemicals
- Cardiovascular disease/ hypertension	- Cardiovascular disease/hypertension
- Obesity/diabetes	- Obesity/diabetes/metabolic syndrome
- Infertility	- Breast, prostate, and uterine cancers
- Dyslipidemia	- Early puberty
- Neurodevelopment	- Infertility
- Respiratory	- Susceptibility to infections
- Depression	- Neurodegenerative diseases
- Schizophrenia	- Autoimmune diseases
- Renal disease	- Endometriosis/uterine fibroids
- Cancer	- Learning and behavior/ADHD
	- Cancer

FIGURE 3.2 Nutritional stress or environmental chemical exposures during development lead to many of the same health outcomes. This is not an exhaustive listing but was developed to show health outcomes that are likely to be affected by both nutritional changes and exposure to environmental chemicals as well as health outcomes that are being examined in one area that could be examined in the other.

Developmental Nutrition	Environmental Chemicals	
- Maternal obesity	- Bisphenol A (BPA)	- Smoking/nicotine
	- Organotins	- Genistein
- Gestational diabetes	- Perflurooctanoic acids	- Monosodium glutamate
- Developmental high fat diet	- Phthalates	- Diethylstilbestrol
	- Polybrominated diphenyl ethers (PBDEs)	- Polychlorinated biphenyl ethers (PCBs)
- Developmental high sugar diet		
- Developmental altered protein diet	- Persistent organic pollutants (POPs)	- Organochlorine pesticides
	- Benzo[a] pyrene	- Arsenic
- High birth weight/low birth weight	- Air pollution	- Lead

FIGURE 3.3 Examples of perturbations in nutrition or exposure to environmental chemicals during development that can lead to obesity later in life. This listing shows some examples and is not meant to be a complete list. It is likely that both nutrition and chemical exposures play a role in the susceptibility to develop obesity; thus, more research is needed to examine their interaction. This model is likely to be useful for many of the other health outcomes.

REFERENCES

Agay-Shay, K., D. Martinez, D. Valvi, R. Garcia-Esteban, X. Basagana, O. Robinson, M. Casas, J. Sunyer and M. Vrijheid (2015). Exposure to endocrine-disrupting chemicals during pregnancy and weight at 7 years of age: A multi-pollutant approach. *Environ Health Perspect* 123(10): 1030–1037.

Aguiar, A., P. A. Eubig and S. L. Schantz (2010). Attention deficit/hyperactivity disorder: A focused overview for children's environmental health researchers. *Environ Health Perspect* 118(12): 1646–1653.

Angle, B. M., R. P. Do, D. Ponzi, R. W. Stahlhut, B. E. Drury, S. C. Nagel, W. V. Welshons, C. L. Besch-Williford, P. Palanza, S. Parmigiani, F. S. vom Saal and J. A. Taylor (2013). Metabolic disruption in male mice due to fetal exposure to low but not high doses of bisphenol A (BPA): Evidence for effects on body weight, food intake, adipocytes, leptin, adiponectin, insulin and glucose regulation. *Reprod Toxicol* 42: 256–268.

Aoki, Y. (2001). Polychlorinated biphenyls, polychlorinated dibenzo-p-dioxins, and polychlorinated dibenzofurans as endocrine disrupters—What we have learned from Yusho disease. *Environ Res* 86(1): 2–11.

Argos, M. (2015). Arsenic exposure and epigenetic alterations: Recent findings based on the illumina 450K DNA methylation array. *Curr Environ Health Rep* 2(2): 137–144.

Argos, M., L. Chen, F. Jasmine, L. Tong, B. L. Pierce, S. Roy, R. Paul-Brutus, M. V. Gamble, K. N. Harper, F. Parvez, M. Rahman, M. Rakibuz-Zaman, V. Slavkovich, J. A. Baron, J. H. Graziano, M. G. Kibriya and H. Ahsan, H (2014). Gene-specific differential DNA methylation and chronic arsenic exposure in an epigenome-wide association study of adults in Bangladesh. *Environ Health Perspect* 123(1): 64–71.

Aschengrau, A., M. R. Winter, V. M. Vieira, T. F. Webster, P. A. Janulewicz, L. G. Gallagher, J. Weinberg and D. M. Ozonoff (2015). Long-term health effects of early life exposure to tetrachloroethylene (PCE)-contaminated drinking water: A retrospective cohort study. *Environ Health* 14: 36.

Baccarelli, A. and V. Bollati (2009). Epigenetics and environmental chemicals. *Curr Opin Pediatr* 21(2): 243–251.

Baccarelli, A. and S. Ghosh (2012). Environmental exposures, epigenetics and cardiovascular disease. *Curr Opin Clin Nutr Metab Care* 15(4): 323–329.

Bach, C. C., B. H. Bech, N. Brix, E. A. Nohr, J. P. Bonde and T. B. Henriksen (2015). Perfluoroalkyl and polyfluoroalkyl substances and human fetal growth: A systematic review. *Crit Rev Toxicol* 45(1): 53–67.

Bailey, K. A. and R. C. Fry (2014). Arsenic-associated changes to the epigenome: What are the functional consequences? *Curr Environ Health Rep* 1: 22–34.

Baillie-Hamilton, P. F. (2002). Chemical toxins: A hypothesis to explain the global obesity epidemic. *J Altern Complement Med* 8(2): 185–192.

Bao, W., K. B. Michels, D. K. Tobias, S. Li, J. E. Chavarro, A. J. Gaskins, A. A. Vaag, F. B. Hu and C. Zhang (2016). Parental smoking during pregnancy and the risk of gestational diabetes in the daughter. *Int J Epidemiol* 45(1): 160–169.

Barker, D. J. (1995). Fetal origins of coronary heart disease. *BMJ* 311(6998): 171–174.

Barker, D. J. P. (2007). The origins of the developmental origins theory. *J Internl Med* 261(5): 412–417.

Barouki, R., P. D. Gluckman, P. Grandjean, M. Hanson and J. J. Heindel (2012). Developmental origins of non-communicable disease: Implications for research and public health. *Environ Health* 11: 42.

Bautista, C. J., C. Guzman, G. L. Rodriguez-Gonzalez and E. Zambrano (2015). Improvement in metabolic effects by dietary intervention is dependent on the precise nature of the developmental programming challenge. *J Dev Orig Health Dis* 6(4): 327–334.

Beckman, D. A. and R. L. Brent (1984). Mechanisms of teratogenesis. *Annu Rev Pharmacol Toxicol* 24: 483–500.

Behl, M., D. Rao, K. Aagaard, T. L. Davidson, E. D. Levin, T. A. Slotkin, S. Srinivasan, D. Wallinga, M. F. White, V. R. Walker, K. A. Thayer and A. C. Holloway (2013). Evaluation of the association between maternal smoking, childhood obesity, and metabolic disorders: A national toxicology program workshop review. *Environ Health Perspect* 121(2): 170–180.

Bellinger, D. C. (2008). Very low lead exposures and children's neurodevelopment. *Curr Opin Pediatr* 20(2): 172–177.

Bellinger, D. C., H. L. Needleman, A. Leviton, C. Waternaux, M. B. Rabinowitz and M. L. Nichols (1984). Early sensory-motor development and prenatal exposure to lead. *Neurobehav Toxicol Teratol* 6(5): 387–402.

Berghuis, S. A., A. F. Bos, P. J. Sauer and E. Roze (2015). Developmental neurotoxicity of persistent organic pollutants: An update on childhood outcome. *Arch Toxicol* 89(5): 687–709.

Birnbaum, L. S. and S. E. Fenton (2003). Cancer and developmental exposure to endocrine disruptors. *Environ Health Perspect* 111(4): 389–394.

Bonner, M. R., D. Han, J. Nie, P. Rogerson, J. E. Vena, P. Muti, M. Trevisan, S. B. Edge and J. L. Freudenheim (2005). Breast cancer risk and exposure in early life to polycyclic aromatic hydrocarbons using total suspended particulates as a proxy measure. *Cancer Epidemiol Biomarkers Prev* 14(1): 53–60.

Botton, J., M. Kogevinas, E. Gracia-Lavedan, E. Patelarou, T. Roumeliotaki, C. Iniguez, L. Santa Marina, J. Ibarluzea, F. Ballester, M. A. Mendez, L. Chatzi, J. Sunyer and C. M. Villanueva (2014). Postnatal weight growth and trihalomethane exposure during pregnancy. *Environ Res* 136c: 280–288.

Bouchard, M. F., J. Chevrier, K. G. Harley, K. Kogut, M. Vedar, N. Calderon, C. Trujillo, C. Johnson, A. Bradman, D. B. Barr and B. Eskenazi (2011). Prenatal exposure to organophosphate pesticides and IQ in 7-year-old children. *Environ Health Perspect* 119(8): 1189–1195.

Braun, J. M., C. Gennings, R. Hauser and T. F. Webster (2016). What can epidemiological studies tell us about the impact of chemical mixtures on human health? *Environ Health Perspect* 124(1): A6–A9.

Braun, J. M., B. P. Lanphear, A. M. Calafat, S. Deria, J. Khoury, C. J. Howe and S. A. Venners (2014). Early-life bisphenol a exposure and child body mass index: A prospective cohort study. *Environ Health Perspect* 122(11): 1239–1245.

Breton, C. V., W. J. Mack, J. Yao, K. Berhane, M. Amadeus, F. Lurmann, F. Gilliland, R. McConnell, H. N. Hodis, N. Kunzli and E. Avol (2016). Prenatal air pollution exposure and early cardiovascular phenotypes in young adults. *PLoS One* 11(3): e0150825.

Brown, J. S., Jr. (2009). Effects of bisphenol-A and other endocrine disruptors compared with abnormalities of schizophrenia: An endocrine-disruption theory of schizophrenia. *Schizophr Bull* 35(1): 256–278.

Buckley, J. P., S. M. Engel, J. M. Braun, R. M. Whyatt, J. L. Daniels, M. A. Mendez, D. B. Richardson, Y. Xu, A. M. Calafat, M. S. Wolff, B. P. Lanphear, A. H. Herring and A. G. Rundle (2016). Prenatal phthalate exposures and body mass index among 4 to 7-year-old children: A pooled analysis. *Epidemiology* 27(3): 449–458.

Buckley, J. P., S. M. Engel, M. A. Mendez, D. B. Richardson, J. L. Daniels, A. M. Calafat, M. S. Wolff and A. H. Herring (2015). Prenatal phthalate exposures and childhood fat mass in a New York City cohort. *Environ Health Perspect* 124: 507–513.

Buckley, J. P., A. H. Herring, M. S. Wolff, A. M. Calafat and S. M. Engel (2016). Prenatal exposure to environmental phenols and childhood fat mass in the Mount Sinai Children's Environmental Health Study. *Environ Int* 91: 350–356.

Calafat, A. M., M. P. Longnecker, H. M. Koch, S. H. Swan, R. Hauser, L. R. Goldman, B. P. Lanphear, R. A. Rudel, S. M. Engel, S. L. Teitelbaum, R. M. Whyatt and M. S. Wolff (2015). Optimal exposure biomarkers for nonpersistent chemicals in environmental epidemiology. *Environ Health Perspect* 123(7): A166–A168.

Cardenas, A., E. A. Houseman, A. A. Baccarelli, Q. Quamruzzaman, M. Rahman, G. Mostofa, R. O. Wright, D. C. Christiani and M. L. Kile (2015a). In utero arsenic exposure and epigenome-wide associations in placenta, umbilical artery, and human umbilical vein endothelial cells. *Epigenetics* 10(11): 1054–1063.

Cardenas, A., D. C. Koestler, E. A. Houseman, B. P. Jackson, M. L. Kile, M. R. Karagas and C. J. Marsit (2015b). Differential DNA methylation in umbilical cord blood of infants exposed to mercury and arsenic in utero. *Epigenetics* 10(6): 508–515.

Casals-Casas, C. and B. Desvergne (n.d.) Endocrine disruptors: From endocrine to metabolic disruption. *Annu Rev Physiol* 73: 135–162.

Caspersen, I. H., H. E. Kvalem, M. Haugen, A. L. Brantsaeter, H. M. Meltzer, J. Alexander, C. Thomsen, M. Froshaug, N. M. Bremnes, S. L. Broadwell, B. Granum, M. Kogevinas and H. K. Knutsen (2016). Determinants of plasma PCB, brominated flame retardants, and organochlorine pesticides in pregnant women and 3 year old children in the Norwegian Mother and Child Cohort Study. *Environ Res* 146: 136–144.

Castro, D. J., W. M. Baird, C. B. Pereira, J. Giovanini, C. V. Lohr, K. A. Fischer, Z. Yu, F. J. Gonzalez, S. K. Krueger and D. E. Williams (2008a). Fetal mouse Cyp1b1 and transplacental carcinogenesis from maternal exposure to dibenzo(a, l)pyrene. *Cancer Prev Res (Phila)* 1(2): 128–134.

Castro, D. J., C. V. Lohr, K. A. Fischer, C. B. Pereira and D. E. Williams (2008b). Lymphoma and lung cancer in offspring born to pregnant mice dosed with dibenzo[a, L]pyrene: The importance of in utero vs. lactational exposure. *Toxicol Appl Pharmacol* 233(3): 454–458.

Chen, A., K. Yolton, S. A. Rauch, G. M. Webster, R. Hornung, A. Sjodin, K. N. Dietrich and B. P. Lanphear (2014). Prenatal polybrominated diphenyl ether exposures and neurodevelopment in U.S. children through 5 years of age: The HOME study. *Environ Health Perspect* 122(8): 856–862.

Chernoff, N., J. M. Rogers and R. J. Kavlock (1989). An overview of maternal toxicity and prenatal development: Considerations for developmental toxicity hazard assessments. *Toxicology* 59(2): 111–125.

Cho, S. C., S. Y. Bhang, Y. C. Hong, M. S. Shin, B. N. Kim, J. W. Kim, H. J. Yoo, I. H. Cho and H. W. Kim (2010). Relationship between environmental phthalate exposure and the intelligence of school-age children. *Environ Health Perspect* 118(7): 1027–1032.

Cohn, B. A., P. M. Cirillo and R. E. Christianson (2010). Prenatal DDT exposure and testicular cancer: A nested case-control study. *Arch Environ Occup Health* 65(3): 127–134.

Cohn, B. A., M. La Merrill, N. Y. Krigbaum, G. Yeh, J. S. Park, L. Zimmermann and P. M. Cirillo (2015). DDT exposure in utero and breast cancer. *J Clin Endocrinol Metab* 100(8): 2865–2872.

Colborn, T., F. S. vom Saal and A. M. Soto (1993). Developmental effects of endocrine-disrupting chemicals in wildlife and humans. *Environ Health Perspect* 101(5): 378–384.

Cupul-Uicab, L. A., M. Hernandez-Avila, E. A. Terrazas-Medina, M. L. Pennell and M. P. Longnecker (2010). Prenatal exposure to the major DDT metabolite 1,1-dichloro-2,2-bis(p-chlorophenyl)ethylene (DDE) and growth in boys from Mexico. *Environ Res* 110(6): 595–603.

Cupul-Uicab, L. A., M. A. Klebanoff, J. W. Brock and M. P. Longnecker (2013). Prenatal exposure to persistent organochlorines and childhood obesity in the U.S. collaborative perinatal project. *Environ Health Perspect* 121(9): 1103–1109.

Cupul-Uicab, L. A., R. Skjaerven, K. Haug, K. K. Melve, S. M. Engel and M. P. Longnecker (2012a). In utero exposure to maternal tobacco smoke and subsequent obesity, hypertension, and gestational diabetes among women in the MoBa cohort. *Environ Health Perspect* 120(3): 355–360.

Cupul-Uicab, L. A., R. Skjaerven, K. Haug, G. S. Travlos, R. E. Wilson, M. Eggesbo, J. A. Hoppin, K. W. Whitworth and M. P. Longnecker (2012b). Exposure to tobacco smoke in utero and subsequent plasma lipids, ApoB, and CRP among adult women in the MoBa cohort. *Environ Health Perspect* 120(11): 1532–1537.

de Jonge, L. L., H. R. Harris, J. W. Rich-Edwards, W. C. Willett, M. R. Forman, V. W. Jaddoe and K. B. Michels (2013). Parental smoking in pregnancy and the risks of adult-onset hypertension. *Hypertension* 61(2): 494–500.

Debes, F., P. Weihe and P. Grandjean (2016). Cognitive deficits at age 22 years associated with prenatal exposure to methylmercury. *Cortex* 74: 358–369.

Deierlein, A. L., M. S. Wolff, A. Pajak, S. M. Pinney, G. C. Windham, M. P. Galvez, M. J. Silva, A. M. Calafat, L. H. Kushi, F. M. Biro and S. L. Teitelbaum (2016). Longitudinal associations of phthalate exposures during childhood and body size measurements in young girls. *Epidemiology* 27: 492–499.

Delvaux, I., J. Van Cauwenberghe, E. Den Hond, G. Schoeters, E. Govarts, V. Nelen, W. Baeyens, N. Van Larebeke and I. Sioen (2014). Prenatal exposure to environmental contaminants and body composition at age 7–9 years. *Environ Res* 132: 24–32.

Di Renzo, G. C., J. A. Conry, J. Blake, M. S. DeFrancesco, N. DeNicola, J. N. Martin Jr, K. A. McCue, D. Richmond, A. Shah, P. Sutton, T. J. Woodruff, S. Z. van der Poel and L. C. Giudice (2015). International Federation of Gynecology and Obstetrics opinion on reproductive health impacts of exposure to toxic environmental chemicals. *Int J Gynecol Obstet* 131(3): 219–225.

Diamanti-Kandarakis, E., J. P. Bourguignon, L. C. Giudice, R. Hauser, G. S. Prins, A. M. Soto, R. T. Zoeller and A. C. Gore (2009). Endocrine-disrupting chemicals: An Endocrine Society scientific statement. *Endocr Rev* 30(4): 293–342.

Dingemans, M. M., M. van den Berg and R. H. Westerink (2011). Neurotoxicity of brominated flame retardants: (In)direct effects of parent and hydroxylated polybrominated diphenyl ethers on the (developing) nervous system. *Environ Health Perspect* 119(7): 900–907.

DiVall, S. A. (2013). The influence of endocrine disruptors on growth and development of children. *Curr Opin Endocrinol Diabetes Obes* 20(1): 50–55.

Duarte-Salles, T., M. A. Mendez, H. M. Meltzer, J. Alexander and M. Haugen (2013). Dietary benzo(a)pyrene intake during pregnancy and birth weight: Associations modified by vitamin C intakes in the Norwegian Mother and Child Cohort Study (MoBa). *Environ Int* 60: 217–223.

Duarte-Salles, T., M. A. Mendez, E. Morales, M. Bustamante, A. Rodriguez-Vicente, M. Kogevinas and J. Sunyer (2012). Dietary benzo(a)pyrene and fetal growth: Effect modification by vitamin C intake and glutathione S-transferase P1 polymorphism. *Environ Int* 45: 1–8.

Ejaredar, M., E. C. Nyanza, K. Ten Eycke and D. Dewey (2015). Phthalate exposure and childrens neurodevelopment: A systematic review. *Environ Res* 142: 51–60.

Engel, S. M., A. Miodovnik, R. L. Canfield, C. Zhu, M. J. Silva, A. M. Calafat and M. S. Wolff (2010). Prenatal phthalate exposure is associated with childhood behavior and executive functioning. *Environ Health Perspect* 118(4): 565–571.

Engel, S. M., J. Wetmur, J. Chen, C. Zhu, D. B. Barr, R. L. Canfield and M. S. Wolff (2011). Prenatal exposure to organophosphates, paraoxonase 1, and cognitive development in childhood. *Environ Health Perspect* 119(8): 1182–1188.

Engel, S. M. and M. S. Wolff (2013). Causal inference considerations for endocrine disruptor research in children's health. *Annu Rev Public Health* 34: 139–158.

Erkin-Cakmak, A., K. G. Harley, J. Chevrier, A. Bradman, K. Kogut, K. Huen and B. Eskenazi (2015). In utero and childhood polybrominated diphenyl ether exposures and body mass at age 7 years: The CHAMACOS study. *Environ Health Perspect* **123**(6): 636–642.

Eskenazi, B., J. Chevrier, S. A. Rauch, K. Kogut, K. G. Harley, C. Johnson, C. Trujillo, A. Sjodin and A. Bradman (2013). In utero and childhood polybrominated diphenyl ether (PBDE) exposures and neurodevelopment in the CHAMACOS study. *Environ Health Perspect* 121(2): 257–262.

Factor-Litvak, P., B. Insel, A. M. Calafat, X. Liu, F. Perera, V. A. Rauh and R. M. Whyatt (2014). Persistent associations between maternal prenatal exposure to phthalates on child IQ at age 7 years. *PLoS One* 9(12): e114003.

Fenton, S. E., C. Reed and R. R. Newbold (2012). Perinatal environmental exposures affect mammary development, function, and cancer risk in adulthood. *Annu Rev Pharmacol Toxicol* 52: 455–479.

Finnell, R. H., J. G. Waes, J. D. Eudy and T. H. Rosenquist (2002). Molecular basis of environmentally induced birth defects. *Annu Rev Pharmacol Toxicol* 42: 181–208.

Fisher, M., T. E. Arbuckle, R. Mallick, A. LeBlanc, R. Hauser, M. Feeley, D. Koniecki, T. Ramsay, G. Provencher, R. Berube and M. Walker (2015). Bisphenol A and phthalate metabolite urinary concentrations: Daily and across pregnancy variability. *J Expo Sci Environ Epidemiol* 25(3): 231–239.

Fujiwara, T., N. Morisaki, Y. Honda, M. Sampei and Y. Tani (2016). Chemicals, nutrition, and autism spectrum disorder: A mini-review. *Front Neurosci* 10: 174.

Garced, S., L. Torres-Sanchez, M. E. Cebrian, L. Claudio and L. Lopez-Carrillo (2012). Prenatal dichlorodiphenyldichloroethylene (DDE) exposure and child growth during the first year of life. *Environ Res* 113: 58–62.

Gascon, M., M. Casas, E. Morales, D. Valvi, A. Ballesteros-Gomez, N. Luque, S. Rubio, N. Monfort, R. Ventura, D. Martinez, J. Sunyer and M. Vrijheid (2015). Prenatal exposure to bisphenol A and phthalates and childhood respiratory tract infections and allergy. *J Allergy Clin Immunol* 135(2): 370–378.

Gascon, M., E. Morales, J. Sunyer and M. Vrijheid (2013). Effects of persistent organic pollutants on the developing respiratory and immune systems: A systematic review. *Environ Int* 52: 51–65.

Gascon, M., J. Sunyer, M. Casas, D. Martinez, F. Ballester, M. Basterrechea, J. P. Bonde, L. Chatzi, C. Chevrier, M. Eggesbo, A. Esplugues, E. Govarts, K. Hannu, J. Ibarluzea, M. Kasper-Sonnenberg, C. Klumper, G. Koppen, M. J. Nieuwenhuijsen, L. Palkovicova, F. Pele, A. Polder, G. Schoeters, M. Torrent, T. Trnovec, M. Vassilaki and M. Vrijheid (2014). Prenatal exposure to DDE and PCB 153 and respiratory health in early childhood: A meta-analysis. *Epidemiology* 25(4): 544–553.

Gehring, U., M. Casas, B. Brunekreef, A. Bergstrom, J. P. Bonde, J. Botton, C. Chevrier, S. Cordier, J. Heinrich, C. Hohmann, T. Keil, J. Sunyer, C. G. Tischer, G. Toft, M. Wickman, M. Vrijheid and M. Nieuwenhuijsen (2013). Environmental exposure assessment in European birth cohorts: Results from the ENRIECO project. *Environ Health* 12: 8.

Gishti, O., R. Gaillard, R. Manniesing, M. Abrahamse-Berkeveld, E. M. van der Beek, D. H. Heppe, E. A. Steegers, A. Hofman, L. Duijts, B. Durmus and V. W. Jaddoe (2014). Fetal and infant growth patterns associated with total and abdominal fat distribution in school-age children. *J Clin Endocrinol Metab* **99**(7): 2557–2566.

Gladen, B. C., W. J. Rogan, P. Hardy, J. Thullen, J. Tingelstad and M. Tully (1988). Development after exposure to polychlorinated biphenyls and dichlorodiphenyl dichloroethene transplacentally and through human milk. *J Pediatr* 113(6): 991–995.

Gluckman, P. D., M. A. Hanson and F. M. Low (2011). The role of developmental plasticity and epigenetics in human health. *Birth Defects Res C Embryo Today* 93(1): 12–18.

Gluckman, P. D., M. A. Hanson and M. D. Mitchell (2010). developmental origins of health and disease: Reducing the burden of chronic disease in the next generation. *Genome Med* **2**(2): 14.

Godfrey, K. M., P. M. Costello and K. A. Lillycrop (2016). Development, epigenetics and metabolic programming. *Nestle Nutr Inst Workshop Ser* 85: 71–80.

Godfrey, K. M., A. Sheppard, P. D. Gluckman, K. A. Lillycrop, G. C. Burdge, C. McLean, J. Rodford, J. L. Slater-Jefferies, E. Garratt, S. R. Crozier, B. S. Emerald, C. R. Gale, H. M. Inskip, C. Cooper and M. A. Hanson (2011). Epigenetic gene promoter methylation at birth is associated with child's later adiposity. *Diabetes* 60: 1528–1534.

González-Alzaga, B., M. Lacasaña, C. Aguilar-Garduño, M. Rodríguez-Barranco, F. Ballester, M. Rebagliato and A. F. Hernández (2014). A systematic review of neurodevelopmental effects of prenatal and postnatal organophosphate pesticide exposure. *Toxicol Lett* **230** (2): 104–121.

Gore, A. C., V. A. Chappell, S. E. Fenton, J. A. Flaws, A. Nadal, G. S. Prins, J. Toppari and R. T. Zoeller (2015). EDC-2: The Endocrine Society's Second Scientific Statement on Endocrine-Disrupting Chemicals. *Endocr Rev* 36(6): E1–E150.

Govarts, E., M. Nieuwenhuijsen, G. Schoeters, F. Ballester, K. Bloemen, M. de Boer, C. Chevrier, M. Eggesbo, M. Guxens, U. Kramer, J. Legler, D. Martinez, L. Palkovicova, E. Patelarou, U. Ranft, A. Rautio, M. S. Petersen, R. Slama, H. Stigum, G. Toft, T. Trnovec, S. Vandentorren, P. Weihe, N. W. Kuperus, M. Wilhelm, J. Wittsiepe and J. P. Bonde (2012). Birth weight and prenatal exposure to polychlorinated biphenyls (PCBs) and dichlorodiphenyldichloroethylene (DDE): A meta-analysis within 12 European Birth Cohorts. *Environ Health Perspect* 120(2): 162–170.

Grandjean, P. and P. J. Landrigan (2006).Developmental neurotoxicity of industrial chemicals. *Lancet* 368(9553): 2167–2178.

Grandjean, P. and P. J. Landrigan (2014). Neurobehavioural effects of developmental toxicity. *Lancet Neurol* 13(3): 330–338.

Grandjean, P., P. Weihe, R. F. White, F. Debes, S. Araki, K. Yokoyama, K. Murata, N. Sorensen, R. Dahl and P. J. Jorgensen (1997). Cognitive deficit in 7-year-old children with prenatal exposure to methylmercury. *Neurotoxicol Teratol* 19(6): 417–428.

Gray, L. E., Jr., J. Furr, K. R. Tatum-Gibbs, C. Lambright, H. Sampson, B. R. Hannas, V. S. Wilson, A. Hotchkiss and P. M. Foster (2016). Establishing the "Biological relevance" of dipentyl phthalate reductions in fetal rat testosterone production and plasma and testis testosterone levels. *Toxicol Sci* 149(1): 178–191.

Green, B. B. and C. J. Marsit (2015). Select prenatal environmental exposures and subsequent alterations of gene-specific and repetitive element DNA methylation in fetal tissues. *Curr Environ Health Rep* 2(2): 126–136.

Grun, F. and B. Blumberg (2006). Environmental obesogens: Organotins and endocrine disruption via nuclear receptor signaling. *Endocrinology* 147(6 Suppl): S50–S55.

Guyton, K. Z., K. A. Hogan, C. S. Scott, G. S. Cooper, A. S. Bale, L. Kopylev, S. Barone, S. L. Makris, B. Glenn, R. P. Subramaniam, M. R. Gwinn, R. C. Dzubow and W. A. Chiu (2014). Human health effects of tetrachloroethylene: Key findings and scientific issues. *Environ Health Perspect* 122(4): 325–334.

Halldorsson, T. I., D. Rytter, L. S. Haug, B. H. Bech, I. Danielsen, G. Becher, T. B. Henriksen and S. F. Olsen (2012). Prenatal exposure to perfluorooctanoate and risk of overweight at 20 years of age: A prospective cohort study. *Environ Health Perspect* 120 (5): 668–673.

Hanson, M. A. and P. D. Gluckman (2015). developmental origins of health and disease—Global public health implications. *Best Pract Res Clin Obstet Gynaecol* 29(1): 24–31.

Harley, K. G., R. Aguilar Schall, J. Chevrier, K. Tyler, H. Aguirre, A. Bradman, N. T. Holland, R. H. Lustig, A. M. Calafat and B. Eskenazi (2013). Prenatal and postnatal bisphenol A exposure and body mass index in childhood in the CHAMACOS cohort. *Environ Health Perspect* 121(4): 514–520, 520e511–516.

Harris, H. R., W. C. Willett and K. B. Michels (2013). Parental smoking during pregnancy and risk of overweight and obesity in the daughter. *Int J Obes* 37(10): 1356–1363.

Hawkesworth, S., Y. Wagatsuma, M. Kippler, A. J. Fulford, S. E. Arifeen, L. A. Persson, S. E. Moore and M. Vahter (2013). Early exposure to toxic metals has a limited effect on blood pressure or kidney function in later childhood, rural Bangladesh. *Int J Epidemiol* 42(1): 176–185.

Haynes, A., M. N. Cooper, C. Bower, T. W. Jones and E. A. Davis (2014). Maternal smoking during pregnancy and the risk of childhood type 1 diabetes in Western Australia. *Diabetologia* 57(3): 469–472.

Heindel, J. J., J. Balbus, L. Birnbaum, M. N. Brune-Drisse, P. Grandjean, K. Gray, P. J. Landrigan, P. D. Sly, W. Suk, D. Cory Slechta, C. Thompson and M. Hanson (2015a). developmental origins of health and disease: Integrating environmental influences. *Endocrinology* 156(10): 3416–3421.

Heindel, J. J., R. Newbold and T. T. Schug (2015b). Endocrine disruptors and obesity. *Nat Rev Endocrinol* 11(11): 653–661.

Heindel, J. J., L. A. Skalla, B. R. Joubert, C. H. Dilworth, and K.A. Gray, (2017). Review of developmental origins of health and disease research in environmental epidemiology. *Reproductive Toxicology* 68:34–48.

Herbstman, J. B., A. Sjodin, M. Kurzon, S. A. Lederman, R. S. Jones, V. Rauh, L. L. Needham, D. Tang, M. Niedzwiecki, R. Y. Wang and F. Perera (2010). Prenatal exposure to PBDEs and neurodevelopment. *Environ Health Perspect* 118(5): 712–719.

Hernandez, A. F., B. Gonzalez-Alzaga, I. Lopez-Flores and M. Lacasana (2016). Systematic reviews on neurodevelopmental and neurodegenerative disorders linked to pesticide exposure: Methodological features and impact on risk assessment. *Environ Int* 92–93: 657–679.

Hilakivi-Clarke, L. (2014). Maternal exposure to diethylstilbestrol during pregnancy and increased breast cancer risk in daughters. *Breast Cancer Res* 16(2): 208.

Hines, E. P., S. S. White, J. P. Stanko, E. A. Gibbs-Flournoy, C. Lau and S. E. Fenton (2009). Phenotypic dichotomy following developmental exposure to perfluorooctanoic acid (PFOA) in female CD-1 mice: Low doses induce elevated serum leptin and insulin, and overweight in mid-life. *Mol Cell Endocrinol* 304(1–2): 97–105.

Ho, S. M., A. Johnson, P. Tarapore, V. Janakiram, X. Zhang and Y. K. Leung (2012). Environmental epigenetics and its implication on disease risk and health outcomes. *Ilar J* 53(3–4): 289–305.

Hormann, A. M., F. S. Vom Saal, S. C. Nagel, R. W. Stahlhut, C. L. Moyer, M. R. Ellersieck, W. V. Welshons, P. L. Toutain and J. A. Taylor (2014). Holding thermal receipt paper and eating food after using hand sanitizer results in high serum bioactive and urine total levels of bisphenol A (BPA). *PLoS One* 9(10): e110509.

Hoyer, B. B., C. H. Ramlau-Hansen, T. B. Henriksen, H. S. Pedersen, K. Goralczyk, V. Zviezdai, B. A. Jonsson, D. Heederik, V. Lenters, R. Vermeulen, J. P. Bonde and G. Toft (2014). Body mass index in young school-age children in relation to organochlorine compounds in early life: A prospective study. *Int J Obes* 38(7): 919–925.

Hsu, S. T., C. I. Ma, S. K. Hsu, S. S. Wu, N. H. Hsu, C. C. Yeh and S. B. Wu (1985). Discovery and epidemiology of PCB poisoning in Taiwan: A four-year follow up. *Environ Health Perspect* 59: 5–10.

Huang, T., Y. Zheng, Q. Qi, M. Xu, S. H. Ley, Y. Li, J. H. Kang, J. Wiggs, L. R. Pasquale, A. T. Chan, E. B. Rimm, D. J. Hunter, J. E. Manson, W. C. Willett, F. B. Hu and L. Qi (2015). DNA methylation variants at HIF3A locus, B-vitamin intake, and long-term weight change: Gene-diet interactions in two U.S. cohorts *Diabetes* 64(9): 3146–3154.

Huen, K., P. Yousefi, A. Bradman, L. Yan, K. G. Harley, K. Kogut, B. Eskenazi and N. Holland (2014). Effects of age, sex, and persistent organic pollutants on DNA methylation in children. *Environ Mol Mutagen* 55(3): 209–222.

Ino, T. (2010). Maternal smoking during pregnancy and offspring obesity: Meta-analysis. *Pediatr Int* 52(1): 94–99.

Iszatt, N., H. Stigum, M. A. Verner, R. A. White, E. Govarts, L. P. Murinova, G. Schoeters, T. Trnovec, J. Legler, F. Pele, J. Botton, C. Chevrier, J. Wittsiepe, U. Ranft, S. Vandentorren, M. Kasper-Sonnenberg, C. Klumper, N. Weisglas-Kuperus, A. Polder and M. Eggesbo (2015). Prenatal and postnatal exposure to persistent organic pollutants and infant growth: A pooled analysis of seven European birth cohorts. *Environ Health Perspect* 123(7): 730–736.

Jaddoe, V. W., L. L. de Jonge, R. M. van Dam, W. C. Willett, H. Harris, M. J. Stampfer, F. B. Hu and K. B. Michels (2014). Fetal exposure to parental smoking and the risk of type 2 diabetes in adult women. *Diabetes Care* 37(11): 2966–2973.

Janesick, A. S. and B. Blumberg (2016). Obesogens: An emerging threat to public health. *Am J Obstet Gynecol* 214(5): 559–565.

Jensen, T. K., A. G. Timmermann, L. I. Rossing, M. Ried-Larsen, A. Grontved, L. B. Andersen, C. Dalgaard, O. H. Hansen, T. Scheike, F. Nielsen and P. Grandjean (2014). Polychlorinated biphenyl exposure and glucose metabolism in 9-year-old Danish children. *J Clin Endocrinol Metab* 99(12): E2643–E2651.

Johns, L. E., G. S. Cooper, A. Galizia and J. D. Meeker (2015). Exposure assessment issues in epidemiology studies of phthalates. *Environ Int* 85: 27–39.

Johnson, N. A., A. Ho, J. M. Cline, C. L. Hughes, W. G. Foster and V. L. Davis (2012). Accelerated mammary tumor onset in a HER2/Neu mouse model exposed to DDT metabolites locally delivered to the mammary gland. *Environ Health Perspect* 120(8): 1170–1176.

Karmaus, W., J. R. Osuch, I. Eneli, L. M. Mudd, J. Zhang, D. Mikucki, P. Haan and S. Davis (2009). Maternal levels of dichlorodiphenyl-dichloroethylene (DDE) may increase weight and body mass index in adult female offspring. *Occup Environ Med* 66(3): 143–149.

Keil, K. P. and P. J. Lein (2016). DNA methylation: A mechanism linking environmental chemical exposures to risk of autism spectrum disorders? *Environ Epigenet* 2(1):pii: dvv012.

Kelishadi, R., A. Askarieh, M. E. Motlagh, M. Tajadini, R. Heshmat, G. Ardalan, S. Fallahi and P. Poursafa (2013). Association of blood cadmium level with cardiometabolic risk factors and liver enzymes in a nationally representative sample of adolescents: The CASPIAN-III study. *J Environ Public Health* 2013: 142856.

Kim, S. H. and M. J. Park (2014). Phthalate exposure and childhood obesity. *Ann Pediatr Endocrinol Metab* 19(2): 69–75.

La Merrill, M. and L. S. Birnbaum (2011). Childhood obesity and environmental chemicals. *Mt Sinai J Med* 78(1): 22–48.

La Merrill, M., P. M. Cirillo, M. B. Terry, N. Y. Krigbaum, J. D. Flom and B. A. Cohn (2013). Prenatal exposure to the pesticide DDT and hypertension diagnosed in women before age 50: A longitudinal birth cohort study. *Environ Health Perspect* 121(5): 594–599.

Ladd-Acosta, C., C. Shu, B. K. Lee, N. Gidaya, A. Singer, L. A. Schieve, D. E. Schendel, N. Jones, J. L. Daniels, G. C. Windham, C. J. Newschaffer, L. A. Croen, A. P. Feinberg and M. Daniele Fallin (2016). Presence of an epigenetic signature of prenatal cigarette smoke exposure in childhood. *Environ Res* 144(Pt A): 139–148.

Lane, R. H. (2014). Fetal programming, epigenetics, and adult onset disease. *Clin Perinatol* 41(4): 815–831.

Lang, C., M. Fisher, A. Neisa, L. MacKinnon, S. Kuchta, S. MacPherson, A. Probert and T. E. Arbuckle (2016). Personal care product use in pregnancy and the postpartum period: Implications for exposure assessment. *Int J Environ Res Public Health* 13(1): pii: E105.

Lee, D. H., D. R. Jacobs, Jr. and M. Porta (2009). Hypothesis: A unifying mechanism for nutrition and chemicals as lifelong modulators of DNA hypomethylation. *Environ Health Perspect* 117(12): 1799–1802.

Lee, D. H., M. Porta, D. R. Jacobs, Jr. and L. N. Vandenberg (2014). Chlorinated persistent organic pollutants, obesity, and type 2 diabetes. *Endocr Rev* 35(4): 557–601.

Lee, H. A., S. H. Park, Y. S. Hong, E. H. Ha and H. Park (2016). The effect of exposure to persistent organic pollutants on metabolic health among KOREAN children during a 1-year follow-up. *Int J Environ Res Public Health* 13(3): pii: E270.

Lee, H. S. (2015). Impact of maternal diet on the epigenome during In utero life and the developmental programming of diseases in childhood and adulthood. *Nutrients* 7(11): 9492–9507.

Levallois, P., J. St-Laurent, D. Gauvin, M. Courteau, M. Prevost, C. Campagna, F. Lemieux, S. Nour, M. D'Amour and P. E. Rasmussen (2014). The impact of drinking water, indoor dust and paint on blood lead levels of children aged 1–5 years in Montreal (Quebec, Canada). *J Expo Sci Environ Epidemiol* 24(2): 185–191.

Lillycrop, K. A. and G. C. Burdge (2012). Epigenetic mechanisms linking early nutrition to long term health. *Best Prac Res Clin Endocrinol Metab* 26(5): 667–676.

Lind, P. M., L. Olsen and L. Lind (2012a). Circulating levels of metals are related to carotid atherosclerosis in elderly. *Sci Total Environ* 416: 80–88.

Lind, P. M., B. Zethelius and L. Lind (2012b). Circulating levels of phthalate metabolites are associated with prevalent diabetes in the elderly. *Diabetes Care* 35(7): 1519–1524.

Liu, J., L. Li, Y. Wang, C. Yan and X. Liu (2013). Impact of low blood lead concentrations on IQ and school performance in Chinese children. *PLoS One* 8(5): e65230.

Liu, J., Y. Xie, J. M. Ward, B. A. Diwan and M. P. Waalkes (2004). Toxicogenomic analysis of aberrant gene expression in liver tumors and nontumorous livers of adult mice exposed in utero to inorganic arsenic. *Toxicol Sci* 77(2): 249–257.

Liu, Y. and K. E. Peterson (2015). Maternal exposure to synthetic chemicals and obesity in the offspring: Recent findings. *Curr Environ Health Rep* 2(4): 339–347.

Lorber, M. (2008). Exposure of Americans to polybrominated diphenyl ethers. *J Expo Sci Environ Epidemiol* 18(1): 2–19.

Lundholm, C. D. (1997). DDE-induced eggshell thinning in birds: Effects of p, p'-DDE on the calcium and prostaglandin metabolism of the eggshell gland. *Comp Biochem Physiol C Pharmacol Toxicol Endocrinol* 118(2): 113–128.

Maccani, J. Z. and M. A. Maccani (2015). Altered placental DNA methylation patterns associated with maternal smoking: Current perspectives. *Adv Genomics Genet* 2015(5): 205–214.

Mahalingaiah, S., J. E. Hart, L. A. Wise, K. L. Terry, R. Boynton-Jarrett and S. A. Missmer (2014). Prenatal diethylstilbestrol exposure and risk of uterine leiomyomata in the Nurses' Health Study II. *Am J Epidemiol* 179(2): 186–191.

Maresca, M. M., L. A. Hoepner, A. Hassoun, S. E. Oberfield, S. J. Mooney, A. M. Calafat, J. Ramirez, G. Freyer, F. P. Perera, R. M. Whyatt and A. G. Rundle (2016). Prenatal exposure to phthalates and childhood body size in an urban cohort. *Environ Health Perspect* 124(4): 514–520.

Martinez, J. A., F. I. Milagro, K. J. Claycombe and K. L. Schalinske (2014). Epigenetics in adipose tissue, obesity, weight loss, and diabetes. *Adv Nutr* 5(1): 71–81.

Mattsson, K., K. Kallen, M. P. Longnecker, A. Rignell-Hydbom and L. Rylander (2013). Maternal smoking during pregnancy and daughters' risk of gestational diabetes and obesity. *Diabetologia* 56(8): 1689–1695.

Maull, E. A., H. Ahsan, J. Edwards, M. P. Longnecker, A. Navas-Acien, J. Pi, E. K. Silbergeld, M. Styblo, C.-H. Tseng, K. A. Thayer and D. Loomis (2012). Evaluation of the association between arsenic and diabetes: A National Toxicology Program workshop review. *Environ Health Perspect* 120(12): 1658–1670.

McLachlan, J. A. and R. R. Newbold (1987). Estrogens and development. *Environ Health Perspect* 75: 25–27.

Mendez, M. A., R. Garcia-Esteban, M. Guxens, M. Vrijheid, M. Kogevinas, F. Goni, S. Fochs and J. Sunyer (2011). Prenatal organochlorine compound exposure, rapid weight gain, and overweight in infancy. *Environ Health Perspect* 119(2): 272–278.

Mohammed Abdul, K. S., S. S. Jayasinghe, E. P. S. Chandana, C. Jayasumana and P. M. C. S. De Silva (2015). Arsenic and human health effects: A review. *Environ Toxicol Pharmacol* 40(3): 828–846.

Montgomery, S. M. and A. Ekbom (2002). Smoking during pregnancy and diabetes mellitus in a British longitudinal birth cohort. *BMJ* 324(7328): 26–27.

Mora, A. M., M. Arora, K. G. Harley, K. Kogut, K. Parra, D. Hernandez-Bonilla, R. B. Gunier, A. Bradman, D. R. Smith and B. Eskenazi (2015). Prenatal and postnatal manganese teeth levels and neurodevelopment at 7, 9, and 10.5 years in the CHAMACOS cohort. *Environ Int* 84: 39–54.

Morgan, M. K., L. S. Sheldon, C. W. Croghan, P. A. Jones, G. L. Robertson, J. C. Chuang, N. K. Wilson and C. W. Lyu (2005). Exposures of preschool children to chlorpyrifos and its degradation product 3,5,6–trichloro-2-pyridinol in their everyday environments. *J Expo Anal Environ Epidemiol* 15(4): 297–309.

Murray, T. J., M. V. Maffini, A. A. Ucci, C. Sonnenschein and A. M. Soto (2007). Induction of mammary gland ductal hyperplasias and carcinoma in situ following fetal bisphenol A exposure. *Reprod Toxicol* 23(3): 383–390.

Nadal, A. (2013). Obesity: Fat from plastics? Linking bisphenol A exposure and obesity. *Nat Rev Endocrinol* 9(1): 9-10.

Newbold, R. R. (2011). Developmental exposure to endocrine-disrupting chemicals programs for reproductive tract alterations and obesity later in life. *Am J Clin Nutr* 94: 1939S–1942S.

Newbold, R. R. (2012). Prenatal exposure to diethylstilbestrol and long-term impact on the breast and reproductive tract in humans and mice. *J Dev Orig Health Dis* 3(2): 73–82.

Newbold, R. R. and J. A. McLachlan (1996). Transplacental hormonal carcinogenesis: Diethylstilbestrol as an example. *Prog Clin Biol Res* 394: 131–147.

Newbold, R. R., E. Padilla-Banks and W. N. Jefferson (2009). Environmental estrogens and obesity. *Mol Cell Endocrinol* 304(1–2): 84–89.

Newman, W. J., A. L. Herbst, H. Ulfelder and D. C. Poskanzer (1971). Registry of clear-cell carcinoma of genital tract in young women. *N Engl J Med* 285(7): 407.

Ng, S. P., D. J. Conklin, A. Bhatnagar, D. D. Bolanowski, J. Lyon and J. T. Zelikoff (2009). Prenatal exposure to cigarette smoke induces diet- and sex-dependent dyslipidemia and weight gain in adult murine offspring. *Environ Health Perspect* 117(7): 1042–1048.

Nohara, K., T. Suzuki, S. Takumi and K. Okamura (2014). Increase in incidence of hepatic tumors caused by oncogenic somatic mutation in mice maternally exposed to inorganic arsenic and the multigenerational and transgenerational effects of inorganic arsenic. *Nihon Eiseigaku Zasshi* 69(2): 92–96.

Nye, M. D., R. C. Fry, C. Hoyo and S. K. Murphy (2014). Investigating epigenetic effects of prenatal exposure to toxic metals in newborns: Challenges and benefits. *Med Epigenet* 2(1): 53–59.

Ong, K. K. and R. J. Loos (2006). Rapid infancy weight gain and subsequent obesity: Systematic reviews and hopeful suggestions. *Acta Paediatr* 95(8): 904–908.

Padmanabhan, V., R. C. Cardoso and M. Puttabyatappa (2016). Developmental programming, a pathway to disease. *Endocrinology* 157(4): 1328–1340.

Palmer, J. R., L. A. Wise, E. E. Hatch, R. Troisi, L. Titus-Ernstoff, W. Strohsnitter, R. Kaufman, A. L. Herbst, K. L. Noller, M. Hyer and R. N. Hoover (2006). Prenatal diethylstilbestrol exposure and risk of breast cancer. *Cancer Epidemiol Biomarkers Prev* 15(8): 1509–1514.

Pan, H., X. Lin, Y. Wu, L. Chen, A. L. Teh, S. E. Soh, Y. S. Lee, M. T. Tint, J. L. MacIsaac, A. M. Morin, K. H. Tan, F. Yap, S. M. Saw, M. S. Kobor, M. J. Meaney, K. M. Godfrey, Y. S. Chong, P. D. Gluckman, N. Karnani and J. D. Holbrook (2015). HIF3A association with adiposity: The story begins before birth. *Epigenomics* 7(6): 937–950.

Penell, J., L. Lind, S. Salihovic, B. van Bavel and P. M. Lind (2014). Persistent organic pollutants are related to the change in circulating lipid levels during a 5 year follow-up. *Environ Res* 134: 190–197.

Perrier, F., L. Giorgis-Allemand, R. Slama and C. Philippat (2016). Within-subject pooling of biological samples to reduce exposure misclassification in biomarker-based studies. *Epidemiology* 27(3): 378–388.

Polanska, K., J. Jurewicz and W. Hanke (2013). Review of current evidence on the impact of pesticides, polychlorinated biphenyls and selected metals on attention deficit/hyperactivity disorder in children. *Int J Occup Med Environ Health* 26(1): 16–38.

Poursafa, P., E. Ataee, M. E. Motlagh, G. Ardalan, M. H. Tajadini, M. Yazdi and R. Kelishadi (2014). Association of serum lead and mercury level with cardiometabolic risk factors and liver enzymes in a nationally representative sample of adolescents: The CASPIAN-III study. *Environ Sci Pollut Res Int* 21(23): 13496–13502.

Preau, J. L., Jr., L. Y. Wong, M. J. Silva, L. L. Needham and A. M. Calafat (2010). Variability over 1 week in the urinary concentrations of metabolites of diethyl phthalate and di(2-ethylhexyl) phthalate among eight adults: An observational study. *Environ Health Perspect* 118(12): 1748–1754.

Ranciere, F., J. G. Lyons, V. H. Loh, J. Botton, T. Galloway, T. Wang, J. E. Shaw and D. J. Magliano (2015). Bisphenol A and the risk of cardiometabolic disorders: A systematic review with meta-analysis of the epidemiological evidence. *Environ Health* 14: 46.

Rauh, V. A., R. Garfinkel, F. P. Perera, H. F. Andrews, L. Hoepner, D. B. Barr, R. Whitehead, D. Tang and R. W. Whyatt (2006). Impact of prenatal chlorpyrifos exposure on neurodevelopment in the first 3 years of life among inner-city children. *Pediatrics* 118(6): e1845–e1859.

Rhie, Y. J., H. K. Nam, Y. J. Oh, H. S. Kim and K. H. Lee (2014). Influence of bottle-feeding on serum bisphenol a levels in infants. *J Korean Med Sci* 29(2): 261–264.

Richmond, R. C., G. C. Sharp, M. E. Ward, A. Fraser, O. Lyttleton, W. L. McArdle, S. M. Ring, T. R. Gaunt, D. A. Lawlor, G. Davey Smith and C. L. Relton (2016). DNA methylation and BMI: Investigating identified methylation sites at HIF3A in a causal framework. *Diabetes* 65(5): 1231–1244.

Rodrigues, E. G., D. C. Bellinger, L. Valeri, M. O. Hasan, Q. Quamruzzaman, M. Golam, M. L. Kile, D. C. Christiani, R. O. Wright and M. Mazumdar (2016). Neurodevelopmental outcomes among 2 to 3-year-old children in Bangladesh with elevated blood lead and exposure to arsenic and manganese in drinking water. *Environ Health* 15: 44.

Rodriguez-Barranco, M., M. Lacasana, C. Aguilar-Garduno, J. Alguacil, F. Gil, B. Gonzalez-Alzaga and A. Rojas-Garcia (2013). Association of arsenic, cadmium and manganese exposure with neurodevelopment and behavioural disorders in children: A systematic review and meta-analysis. *Sci Total Environ* 454–455: 562–577.

Rojas, D., J. E. Rager, L. Smeester, K. A. Bailey, Z. Drobna, M. Rubio-Andrade, M. Styblo, G. Garcia-Vargas and R. C. Fry (2015). Prenatal arsenic exposure and the epigenome: Identifying sites of 5-methylcytosine alterations that predict functional changes in gene expression in newborn cord blood and subsequent birth outcomes. *Toxicol Sci* 143(1): 97–106.

Romagnolo, D. F., K. D. Daniels, J. T. Grunwald, S. A. Ramos, C. R. Propper and O. I. Selmin (2016). Epigenetics of breast cancer: Modifying role of environmental and bioactive food compounds. *Mol Nutr Food Res*.60(6): 1310-1329.

Rossignol, D. A., S. J. Genuis and R. E. Frye (2014). Environmental toxicants and autism spectrum disorders: A systematic review. *Transl Psychiatry* 4: e360.

Ruiz-Hernandez, A., C. C. Kuo, P. Rentero-Garrido, W. Y. Tang, J. Redon, J. M. Ordovas, A. Navas-Acien and M. Tellez-Plaza (2015). Environmental chemicals and DNA methylation in adults: A systematic review of the epidemiologic evidence. *Clin Epigenetics* 7(1): 55.

Sanders, A. P., B. Claus Henn and R. O. Wright (2015). Perinatal and childhood exposure to cadmium, manganese, and metal mixtures and effects on cognition and behavior: A review of recent literature. *Curr Environ Health Rep* 2(3): 284–294.

Sargis, R. M. (2015). Metabolic disruption in context: Clinical avenues for synergistic perturbations in energy homeostasis by endocrine disrupting chemicals. *Endocr Disruptors* 3(1): e1080788.

Schug, T. T., R. Barouki, P. Gluckman, P. Grandjean, M. Hanson and J. J. Heindel (2013). PPTOX III: Environmental stressors in the developmental origins of disease: Evidence and mechanisms. *Toxicol Sci* 131(2): 343–350.

Schug, T. T., A. M. Blawas, K. Gray, J. J. Heindel and C. P. Lawler (2015). Elucidating the links between endocrine disruptors and neurodevelopment. *Endocrinology* 156(6): 1941–1951.

Serrano, S. E., J. Braun, L. Trasande, R. Dills and S. Sathyanarayana (2014). Phthalates and diet: A review of the food monitoring and epidemiology data. *Environ Health* 13(1): 43.

Sheehan, M. C., T. A. Burke, A. Navas-Acien, P. N. Breysse, J. McGready and M. A. Fox (2014). Global methylmercury exposure from seafood consumption and risk of developmental neurotoxicity: A systematic review. *Bull World Health Organ* 92(4): 254F–269F.

Song, Y., E. L. Chou, A. Baecker, N. Y. You, Y. Song, Q. Sun and S. Liu (2016). Endocrine-disrupting chemicals, risk of type 2 diabetes, and diabetes-related metabolic traits: A systematic review and meta-analysis. *J Diabetes* 8(4): 516–532.

Song, Y., R. Hauser, F. B. Hu, A. A. Franke, S. Liu and Q. Sun (2014). Urinary concentrations of bisphenol A and phthalate metabolites and weight change: A prospective investigation in U.S. women. *Int J Obes* 38(12): 1532–1537.

Spiegelman, D. (2010). Approaches to uncertainty in exposure assessment in environmental epidemiology. *Annu Rev Public Health* 31: 149–163.

Spyker, J. M. (1975). Assessing the impact of low level chemicals on development: Behavioral and latent effects. *Fed Proc* 34(9): 1835–1844.

Stacy, S. L., M. Eliot, A. M. Calafat, A. Chen, B. P. Lanphear, R. Hauser, G. D. Papandonatos, S. Sathyanarayana, X. Ye, K. Yolton and J. M. Braun (2016). Patterns, variability, and predictors of urinary bisphenol A concentrations during childhood. *Environ Sci Technol.* 50(11): 5981–5990.

Steinmaus, C., C. Ferreccio, J. Acevedo, Y. Yuan, J. Liaw, V. Duran, S. Cuevas, J. Garcia, R. Meza, R. Valdes, G. Valdes, H. Benitez, V. VanderLinde, V. Villagra, K. P. Cantor, L. E. Moore, S. G. Perez, S. Steinmaus and A. H. Smith (2014). Increased lung and bladder cancer incidence in adults after in utero and early-life arsenic exposure. *Cancer Epidemiol Biomarkers Prev* 23(8): 1529–1538.

Steinmaus, C. M., C. Ferreccio, J. A. Romo, Y. Yuan, S. Cortes, G. Marshall, L. E. Moore, J. R. Balmes, J. Liaw, T. Golden and A. H. Smith (2013). Drinking water arsenic in northern chile: High cancer risks 40 years after exposure cessation. *Cancer Epidemiol Biomarkers Prev* 22(4): 623–630.

Suvorov, A., M. C. Battista and L. Takser (2009). Perinatal exposure to low-dose 2,2′,4,4′-tetrabromodiphenyl ether affects growth in rat offspring: What is the role of IGF-1? *Toxicology* 260(1–3): 126–131.

Swan, S. H., F. Liu, M. Hines, R. L. Kruse, C. Wang, J. B. Redmon, A. Sparks and B. Weiss (2010). Prenatal phthalate exposure and reduced masculine play in boys. *Int J Androl* 33(2): 259–269.

Swan, S. H., S. Sathyanarayana, E. S. Barrett, S. Janssen, F. Liu, R. H. Nguyen and J. B. Redmon (2015). First trimester phthalate exposure and anogenital distance in newborns. *Hum Reprod* 30(4): 963–972.

Tang-Peronard, J. L., H. R. Andersen, T. K. Jensen and B. L. Heitmann (2011). Endocrine-disrupting chemicals and obesity development in humans: A review. *Obes Rev* 12(8): 622–636.

Tang-Peronard, J. L., B. L. Heitmann, T. K. Jensen, A. M. Vinggaard, S. Madsbad, U. Steuerwald, P. Grandjean, P. Weihe, F. Nielsen and H. R. Andersen (2015). Prenatal exposure to persistent organochlorine pollutants is associated with high insulin levels in 5-year-old girls. *Environ Res* 142: 407–413.

Taylor, K. W., R. F. Novak, H. A. Anderson, L. S. Birnbaum, C. Blystone, M. Devito, D. Jacobs, J. Kohrle, D. H. Lee, L. Rylander, A. Rignell-Hydbom, R. Tornero-Velez, M. E. Turyk, A. L. Boyles, K. A. Thayer and L. Lind (2013). Evaluation of the association between persistent organic pollutants (POPs) and diabetes in epidemiological studies: A national toxicology program workshop review. *Environ Health Perspect* 121(7): 774–783.

Thayer, K. A., J. J. Heindel, J. R. Bucher and M. A. Gallo (2012). Role of environmental chemicals in diabetes and obesity: A National Toxicology Program workshop review. *Environ Health Perspect* 120(6): 779–789.

Tokar, E. J., W. Qu and M. P. Waalkes (2011). Arsenic, stem cells, and the developmental basis of adult cancer. *Toxicol Sci* 120 (Suppl 1): S192–S203.

Tournaire, M., S. Epelboin, E. Devouche, G. Viot, J. Le Bidois, A. Cabau, A. Dunbavand and A. Levadou (2016). Adverse health effects in children of women exposed in utero to diethylstilbestrol (DES). *Therapie* 71: 395–404.

Trasande, L., C. B. Schechter, K. A. Haynes and P. J. Landrigan (2006). Mental retardation and prenatal methylmercury toxicity. *Am J Ind Med* 49(3): 153–158.

Troisi, R., E. E. Hatch, J. R. Palmer, L. Titus, S. J. Robboy, W. C. Strohsnitter, A. L. Herbst, E. Adam, M. Hyer and R. N. Hoover (2016). Prenatal diethylstilbestrol exposure and high-grade squamous cell neoplasia of the lower genital tract. *Am J Obstet Gynecol* 215(3): 322.e1-322.e8.

Troisi, R., E. E. Hatch, L. Titus-Ernstoff, M. Hyer, J. R. Palmer, S. J. Robboy, W. C. Strohsnitter, R. Kaufman, A. L. Herbst and R. N. Hoover (2007). Cancer risk in women prenatally exposed to diethylstilbestrol. *Int J Cancer* 121(2): 356–360.

Tshala-Katumbay, D., J. C. Mwanza, D. S. Rohlman, G. Maestre and R. B. Oria (2015). A global perspective on the influence of environmental exposures on the nervous system. *Nature* 527(7578): S187–S192.

Tsuji, J. S., M. R. Garry, V. Perez and E. T. Chang (2015). Low-level arsenic exposure and developmental neurotoxicity in children: A systematic review and risk assessment. *Toxicology* 337: 91–107.

Tyler, C. R. and A. M. Allan (2014). The effects of arsenic exposure on neurological and cognitive dysfunction in human and rodent studies: A review. *Curr Environ Health Rep* 1: 132–147.

Vafeiadi, M., V. Georgiou, G. Chalkiadaki, P. Rantakokko, H. Kiviranta, M. Karachaliou, E. Fthenou, M. Venihaki, K. Sarri, M. Vassilaki, S. A. Kyrtopoulos, E. Oken, M. Kogevinas and L. Chatzi (2015). Association of prenatal exposure to persistent organic pollutants with obesity and cardiometabolic traits in early childhood: The rhea mother-child cohort (Crete, Greece). *Environ Health Perspect* 123(10): 1015–1021.

Vafeiadi, M., T. Roumeliotaki, A. Myridakis, G. Chalkiadaki, E. Fthenou, E. Dermitzaki, M. Karachaliou, K. Sarri, M. Vassilaki, E. G. Stephanou, M. Kogevinas and L. Chatzi (2016). Association of early life exposure to bisphenol A with obesity and cardiometabolic traits in childhood. *Environ Res* 146: 379–387.

Vaiserman, A. (2014). Early-life exposure to endocrine disrupting chemicals and later-life health outcomes: An epigenetic bridge? *Aging Dis* 5(6): 419–429.

Vaiserman, A. (2015). Epidemiologic evidence for association between adverse environmental exposures in early life and epigenetic variation: A potential link to disease susceptibility? *Clin Epigenetics* 7(1): 96.

Valvi, D., M. Casas, M. A. Mendez, A. Ballesteros-Gomez, N. Luque, S. Rubio, J. Sunyer and M. Vrijheid (2013). Prenatal bisphenol a urine concentrations and early rapid growth and overweight risk in the offspring. *Epidemiology* 24(6): 791–799.

Valvi, D., M. Casas, D. Romaguera, N. Monfort, R. Ventura, D. Martinez, J. Sunyer and M. Vrijheid (2015). Prenatal phthalate exposure and childhood growth and blood pressure: Evidence from the Spanish INMA-Sabadell birth cohort study. *Environ Health Perspect* 123(10): 1022–1029.

Valvi, D., M. A. Mendez, D. Martinez, J. O. Grimalt, M. Torrent, J. Sunyer and M. Vrijheid (2012). Prenatal concentrations of polychlorinated biphenyls, DDE, and DDT and overweight in children: A prospective birth cohort study. *Environ Health Perspect* 120(3): 451–457.

van Dijk, S. J., P. L. Molloy, H. Varinli, J. L. Morrison and B. S. Muhlhausler (2015a). Epigenetics and human obesity. *Int J Obes* 39(1): 85–97.

van Dijk, S. J., R. L. Tellam, J. L. Morrison, B. S. Muhlhausler and P. L. Molloy (2015b). Recent developments on the role of epigenetics in obesity and metabolic disease. *Clin Epigenetics* 7(1): 1–13.

Vandenberg, L. N., T. Colborn, T. B. Hayes, J. J. Heindel, D. R. Jacobs, Jr., D. H. Lee, T. Shioda, A. M. Soto, F. S. vom Saal, W. V. Welshons, R. T. Zoeller and J. P. Myers (2012). Hormones and endocrine-disrupting chemicals: Low-dose effects and nonmonotonic dose responses. *Endocr Rev* 33(3): 378–455.

Waalkes, M. P., W. Qu, E. J. Tokar, G. E. Kissling and D. Dixon (2014). Lung tumors in mice induced by "whole-life" inorganic arsenic exposure at human-relevant doses. *Arch Toxicol* 88(8): 1619–1629.

Waring, R. H., R. M. Harris and S. C. Mitchell (2016). In utero exposure to carcinogens: Epigenetics, developmental disruption and consequences in later life. *Maturitas* 86: 59–63.

Warner, M., R. Aguilar Schall, K. G. Harley, A. Bradman, D. Barr and B. Eskenazi (2013). In utero DDT and DDE exposure and obesity status of 7-year-old Mexican-American children in the CHAMACOS cohort. *Environ Health Perspect* 121(5): 631–636.

Wei, J., Y. Lin, Y. Li, C. Ying, J. Chen, L. Song, Z. Zhou, Z. Lv, W. Xia, X. Chen and S. Xu (2011). Perinatal exposure to bisphenol A at reference dose predisposes offspring to metabolic syndrome in adult rats on a high-fat diet. *Endocrinology* 152(8): 3049–3061.

Weiss, B. and J. M. Spyker (1974). The susceptibility of the fetus and child to chemical pollutants. Behavioral implications of prenatal and early postnatal exposure to chemical pollutants. *Pediatrics* 53(5): 851–859.

White, R. F., C. L. Palumbo, D. A. Yurgelun-Todd, K. J. Heaton, P. Weihe, F. Debes and P. Grandjean (2011). Functional MRI approach to developmental methylmercury and polychlorinated biphenyl neurotoxicity. *Neurotoxicology* 32(6): 975–980.

Whyatt, R. M., X. Liu, V. A. Rauh, A. M. Calafat, A. C. Just, L. Hoepner, D. Diaz, J. Quinn, J. Adibi, F. P. Perera and P. Factor-Litvak (2012). Maternal prenatal urinary phthalate metabolite concentrations and child mental, psychomotor, and behavioral development at 3 years of age. *Environ Health Perspect* 120(2): 290–295.

Wiberg, B., P. M. Lind and L. Lind (2014). Serum levels of monobenzylphthalate (MBzP) is related to carotid atherosclerosis in the elderly. *Environ Res* 133: 348–352.

Wilson, N. K., J. C. Chuang, C. Lyu, R. Menton and M. K. Morgan (2003). Aggregate exposures of nine preschool children to persistent organic pollutants at day care and at home. *J Expo Anal Environ Epidemiol* 13(3): 187–202.

Winneke, G. (2011). Developmental aspects of environmental neurotoxicology: Lessons from lead and polychlorinated biphenyls. *J Neurol Sci* 308(1–2): 9–15.

Wittassek, M. and J. Angerer (2008). Phthalates: Metabolism and exposure *Int J Androl* 31(2): 131–138.

Ye, X., L. Y. Wong, A. M. Bishop and A. M. Calafat (2011). Variability of urinary concentrations of bisphenol A in spot samples, first morning voids, and 24-hour collections. *Environ Health Perspect* 119(7): 983–988.

Yeung, E. H., C. Robledo, N. Boghossian, C. Zhang and P. Mendola (2014). Developmental origins of cardiovascular disease. *Curr Epidemiol Rep* 1(1): 9–16.

Yorifuji, T., T. Kato, Y. Kado, A. Tokinobu, M. Yamakawa, T. Tsuda and S. Sanada (2015). Intrauterine exposure to methylmercury and neurocognitive functions: Minamata disease. *Arch Environ Occup Health* 70(5): 297–302.

Yu, Z., C. V. Loehr, K. A. Fischer, M. A. Louderback, S. K. Krueger, R. H. Dashwood, N. I. Kerkvliet, C. B. Pereira, J. E. Jennings-Gee, S. T. Dance, M. S. Miller, G. S. Bailey and D. E. Williams (2006). In utero exposure of mice to dibenzo[a, l]pyrene produces lymphoma in the offspring: Role of the aryl hydrocarbon receptor. *Cancer Res* 66(2): 755–762.

Section II

Maternal Malnutrition and Fetal Programming

4 Protein Deficiency and Pancreatic Development

David J. Hill

CONTENTS

4.1   INTRODUCTION

Intrauterine growth restriction (IUGR) is a proxy for a number of developmental deficiencies, including fetal genetic mutations, placental dysfunction, maternal uterine vessel abnormalities, and the adequacy of maternal nutrition. Infants born small for gestational age (SGA) were shown in numerous cohort studies to carry increased risks for the development of chronic diseases such as type 2 diabetes, hypertension, cardiovascular disorders, and osteoporosis in adult life (Barker 1994). A direct link between maternal nutritional sufficiency and the development of adult metabolic diseases was shown through a study of individuals who experienced the Dutch famine of 1944/1945 (Painter et al. 2005). Calorie restriction in third trimester during the famine increased the risk of subsequent glucose intolerance and type 2 diabetes in the offspring, whereas exposure earlier in gestation resulted in a higher body mass index (BMI) and waist circumference at age 50 years, particularly in women (Ravelli et al. 1999).

More specifically, the birth morphometry of infants with SGA is related to an increased risk of metabolic diseases in adulthood (Bernstein et al. 1997). Infants born with a low ponderal index and who were also thin, but with normal body length, were more prone to develop insulin resistance as adults and demonstrated impaired glucose tolerance, accompanied by a reduced muscle lipid content and lower rates of muscle glycolysis (Ravelli et al. 1998, 1999; Garofano et al. 1997). This phenotype suggests that the fetal insult occurred subsequent to 36 weeks gestation, which is when the fetus accumulates subcutaneous and visceral fat, and tissue glycogen stores (Alvarez et al. 1997). Infants who were proportionally small at birth with lower body length tended to became hypertensive as adults with increased risk of cardiovascular diseases (Reusens et al. 1995). The reduction in body length suggests that in these infants the fetal insult occurred earlier in gestation. Thus, critical windows may exist during embryonic and fetal life, and perhaps in the neonatal period, where relative nutritional deficiencies may program the risk for particular adult disease profiles. These windows are likely to reflect critical periods or organ development, and one organ central to metabolic disease is the pancreas. Phenotypic changes to the pancreatic islets of Langerhans cannot be studied in the human neonate given the present limitations of resolution of noninvasive molecular imaging methodologies. Animal models of maternal nutritional restriction during pregnancy have therefore been essential to determine both short-term changes in pancreatic structure and function in the offspring, and their long-term implications for metabolism.

4.2   THE LOW PROTEIN DIET MODEL OF MATERNAL DIETARY RESTRICTION

Several rodent models have been utilized to study the direct effects of maternal nutritional availability on fetal tissues or indirect effects through changes in uteroplacental function. These include a reduction in overall calorie availability in the pregnant rat or mouse (Martin et al. 1997; Manuel-Apolinar et al. 2014), a reduction in uteroplacental blood flow by uterine vessel occlusion (Simmons et al. 2001), or nicotine administration to the dam to constrict the uterine blood vessels (Somm et al. 2008). A widely utilized model has been the administration of a protein-reduced but isocalorific diet, either throughout pregnancy, during distinct windows representing the first, second, or third weeks of pregnancy or extending until weaning around 21 days of postnatal life (Chamson-Reig et al. 2006). Such low protein (LP) diets typically provide protein in the form of casein with a reduction to 6–9% weight per total weight compared to 17–24% protein in the control chow. The LP diet is made isocalorific by additional supplementation with carbohydrate. Some studies have adjusted the methionine content of LP diets back to control dietary values to separate the effects of general protein deficiency from the specific importance of methionine for deoxyribonucleic acid (DNA) methylation, contributing to epigenetic patterning of gene expression (Rees et al. 2006). A human equivalent of these long-term metabolic implications following deficient protein availability during pregnancy would be the reduced birth weight associated with restricted maternal protein intake in vegetarian women in rural India, as characterized by the Pune Maternal Nutrition Study (Roa et al. 2001; Fall 2009).

Provision of an LP diet to pregnant rats resulted in a reduction in maternal levels of branched and nonbranched chain amino acids including leucine, isoleucine, and phenylalanine (Bhasin et al. 2009). Additionally, transfer of amino acids across the placenta to the fetus of the LP-fed dam is reduced as a result of a decreased expression of amino acid transporters such as the neutral amino acid transporter-2 (Snat2)

(Rosario et al. 2011). This was shown to be linked to a downregulation of placental mammalian target of rapamycin (mTOR) and insulin receptor signaling, mTOR being an integrative signal between nutrient uptake and tissue growth. However, in the above study, the LP diet contained only 4% protein. In a study using the same strain of rat subjected to a 9% protein diet, the expression of Snat2 and other genes in the amino acid response pathway, such as activating transcription factor-3 (Atf3) and asparagine synthetase (Asns), were increased compared to dams receiving an 18% protein diet (Strakovsky et al. 2010). The increase in the expression levels of these genes correlated with the extent of IUGR in the offspring. Consequently, it was suggested that the placental changes might provide a signal to the fetus for an adaptive response that predisposed to metabolic disease in later life. In the presence of a very LP diet, this adaptive mechanism may fail and IUGR will result. Human IUGR, which may have a number of causes other than nutritional imbalance, is associated with a reduced presence of placental amino acid transporters in addition to a reduction in iron and lipid transport (Glazier et al. 1997; Johansson et al. 2003, Magnusson et al. 2004).

The effects of a maternal LP diet on the metabolism of the offspring may also be influenced through an increased exposure to maternal glucocorticoids *in utero*. The placental expression of 11 β-hydroxysteroid dehydrogenase type 2, an enzyme that metabolizes glucocorticoids to inactive derivatives, was reduced in offspring of a LP-fed dams (Bertram et al. 2001; Ostreicher et al. 2010). Cortisol has also been shown to downregulate the expression of the important transcription factor Pdx1 in the embryonic pancreas, which may subsequently limit insulin release and β-cell differentiation.

4.3 METABOLIC AND PANCREATIC PHENOTYPE AT BIRTH

The feeding of an LP diet to rats throughout gestation results is an approximate 10% reduction in mean litter birth weight at term (Petrik et al. 1999). However, birth weight is not reproducibly lowered if the model is applied to the mouse (Cox et al. 2010). The offspring of LP-fed rats exhibited an altered circulating amino acid profile, with the greatest reduction being in circulating taurine. Corticosterone levels are increased in such animals, and circulating levels of insulin-like growth factor-I (IGF-I) are reduced (Herbert and Carillo 1982). In both mice and rats, maternal exposure to LP throughout gestation caused a significant reduction in the weight of the pancreas and liver of the offspring at birth, but not brain. Within the pancreas, the β-cell mass and mean islet size were both significantly lower than for control diet-fed dams (Petrik et al. 1999). Once islets of Langerhans were isolated in late fetal life, those from LP-fed rats had a lower basal insulin release than control islets, with less insulin release when challenged with glucose, arginine, or leucine (Cherif et al. 1998).

Mechanistically, exposure to a maternal LP diet until weaning in rats altered both the cell-cycle kinetics of β-cells in the offspring and the local presence of growth factors within the pancreatic environment. Offspring experiencing an LP diet had a decreased rate of β-cell replication and a higher rate of β-cell apoptosis (Petrik et al. 1999). Based on the presence of cell cycle–specific proteins *in situ*, detected by immunocytochemistry, the β-cell cycle length was longer in offspring of LP-fed rats because of an extended G1 phase. This appears to be linked to a reduced activation of key mitogenic signaling pathways within β-cells such as the phosphorylation of forkhead-O1 (FoxO1) and extracellular signal-related kinase 1/2 (Erk1/2) (Rafacho et al. 2009). The pancreatic expression of IGF-II within the pancreas was also reduced, as was the key transcription factor for β-cell differentiation, Pdx1 (Petrik et al. 1999). IGF-II can function as both a mitogen and prevent apoptosis of β-cells within the pancreas in early life (Hill 2011). In the Goto Kahizaki (GK) rat model of type 2 diabetes, the production of IGF-II in the fetus is defective (Serradas et al. 2002). These animals exhibit an impaired regeneration of β-cell following partial pancreatectomy, demonstrating the importance of IGF-II for the maintenance of β-cell mass (Plachot et al. 2001). It has been suggested that the phenotypic changes to the β-cell following exposure to an LP diet in early life are not simply a blunting of growth and survival but a premature switch from proliferation to differentiation (Rodriguez-Trejo et al. 2012). This was based on the higher expression of mRNAs following birth for 13 key genes required for β-cell maturation, including hepatocyte nuclear factor α (*Hnf1a*), hepatocyte nuclear factor 4α (*Hnf4a*), Rfx6, and solute carrier family 2, member 2 (*Slc2a2*).

We found in the rat that intraislet vascular density was lower in the offspring of LP-fed mothers at birth (Nicholson et al. 2010) and remained lower than in control-fed animals in adulthood. This is relevant to islet functional capacity as signaling occurs across the basement membrane separating the β-cell from capillary endothelial cells. Such signaling is mediated by both integrins and the paracrine actions of locally produced growth factors that include vascular endothelial growth factor (VEGF) and hepatocyte growth factor (HGF) (Johannson et al. 2006; Nikolova et al. 2006). VEGF-A is required to maintain a fenestrated endothelium within the islet that allows for rapid glucose sensing from the circulation and the excretion of insulin into the hepatic portal vein (Johannson et al. 2006). In offspring from LP-fed rats, the number of β-cells exhibiting both VEGF and the VEGF receptors was reduced compared to those receiving control diet (Nicholson et al. 2010). Changes to the microvascular density were not specific to the pancreas, but also observed in the endometrium, ovaries, and skeletal muscle (Ferreira et al. 2010), and the changes extended to function with a reduction in endothelial dilatation (Sathishkumar et al. 2009). LP diet-related deficiencies in islet vascular density may reflect underlying changes in the presence of endothelial progenitor cells (EPCs). We and others have demonstrated that such cells, when delivered exogenously, were capable of increasing β-cell mass through the promotion of islet angiogenesis, and by enhanced proliferation of existing β-cells or by the differentiation of progenitors (Hess et al. 2003; Hasegawa et al. 2007). The pancreatic population of EPCs was quantified by immunostaining for nestin, CD34, and c-kit and was shown to be decreased in parallel with β-cell mass in the offspring of LP-fed rats (Joanette et al. 2004).

Exposure to an LP diet during gestational weeks 1 and 2 of pregnancy alone resulted in a significant decrease in the mean islet area in the offspring on the day of birth with a particular deficiency in the number of large islets (Chamson-Reig et al. 2006). This again suggests that the effects of the LP diet on islet phenotype were exerted as early as pancreatic organogenesis. Exposure of rats to the LP diet during either weeks 2 or 3 of gestation also resulted in a significant decrease in β-cell mass and reduced pancreatic Pdx1 expression at birth. Some gender-specific differences were observed with week 2 being the most critical period for β-cell mass in females, while week 3 was more relevant for male offspring (Thyssen et al. 2003). Thus, a number of critical windows may exist for altered endocrine pancreatic development in response to an LP insult, extending from implantation of the embryo through to maturation of differentiated β-cells in the neonate.

The changes in the phenotype or abundance of resident stem or progenitor populations within pancreas may be determined very early in life. When pregnant rats were given the LP diet in the preimplantation period only, from conception to 4 days, both the birth weight and postnatal growth rate of offspring were impaired compared to control-fed animals (Kwong et al. 2000). When blastocysts were harvested at the time of implantation they already exhibited a reduced cell number within the inner cell mass, which is the source of all embryonic stem cells, and at a slightly later stage of development within the trophectoderm, which gives rise to the placenta (Kwong et al. 2000).

The pancreatic phenotype in the offspring following exposure to the LP diet could be linked to changes in resident progenitor β-cells within the pancreas, with origins during pancreatic organogenesis. We and others have recently described such a resident precursor population within both the islets and the small but abundant endocrine cell clusters of the pancreas (Smukler et al. 2011; Beamish et al. 2016). These cells express low levels of insulin but are functionally inactive as they lack adequate levels of the Glut2 glucose transporter. In contrast to differentiated β-cells, the precursor cells are highly proliferative and have multilineage capacity, being able to give rise to all pancreatic endocrine cell types as well as neural lineages (Beamish et al. 2016). Further evidence that dietary restriction in early life alters a β-cell progenitor phenotype was obtained *in vitro*. Islets were isolated from neonatal mice exposed *in utero* to a control or LP diet and were dedifferentiated during culture over 4 weeks to yield ductal epithelial cell-like cells that expressed cytokeratin 19 but no longer expressed insulin (Beamish et al. 2007). Duct-like cells could be redifferentiated to form pseudoislets in the presence of IGF-II and fibroblast growth factor-7 (FGF7). The proliferation rate of cell cultures from LP-fed offspring was significantly lower compared to those from control-fed animals and their ability to form pseudoislets and reexpress insulin was virtually abolished. In line with the morphological findings, the relative expression of transcription factors required for the differentiation of functional β-cells within the pseudoislets such as Pdx1, Pax6, and Ngn3 was significantly reduced for cells from LP-exposed mice (Beamish et al. 2007).

4.4 LONG-TERM CHANGES IN PANCREATIC AND METABOLIC FUNCTION AND PLASTICITY

If a maternal LP diet is replaced by control diet in rodent models at birth then the islet morphology and β-cell mass in the offspring will partially recover, but if extended until weaning the changes are irreversible and will lead to glucose intolerance in later life (Boujendar et al. 2002). This can be partly explained by the importance of the neonatal period for β-cell maturation in rodents, and the associated turnover of endocrine cells from progenitors that occurs to yield β-cell populations that are glucose responsive (Trudeau et al. 2000). These processes are essential for setting a plasticity for both islet function and number for lifelong glucose homeostasis. When LP feeding was extended to weaning, islets from offspring possessed a lower β-cell mass with impaired glucose-stimulated insulin release (Petrik et al. 1999). In addition to direct long-term programming of β-cell function by an LP diet, there are also likely to be indirect effects, including changes to insulin secretion in response to stimulation by the autonomic nervous system. Perinatal protein restriction was shown to alter vagus nerve electrophysiology to reduce the insulinotrophic effects of acetylcholine within parasympathetic pathways (de Oliveira et al. 2011).

The window of fetal exposure to an LP diet did not appear to change the trajectory toward glucose intolerance as adults, nor did gender; however, the pancreatic phenotype did alter with gender. When rats were exposed to an LP diet for the first 2 weeks of gestation only, or weeks 2 or 3 alone, all became glucose intolerant by 130 days of age (Chamson-Reig et al. 2009). Pancreatic morphology was examined in the offspring on postnatal day 21 compared to the day of birth. Although the mean islet area and the number of β-cells were reduced at birth regardless of the period of LP, the deficit was greatest in those given LP in gestational week 2 in females and in week 3 in males, and this was greater than for animals exposed to LP continuously. As adults, the glucose intolerance seen in male offspring that received an LP diet in early life was predominantly due to peripheral insulin resistance, while for females the primary defect was a decreased β-cell mass. Also, islets from either gender were more prone to cytokine-induced apoptosis following exposure *in vitro* (Reusens et al. 2011). These deficiencies could be transmitted to the F2 generation when F1 pregnant females born from LP-fed mothers were maintained on normal protein diet through gestation.

While glucose-stimulated insulin release remains impaired throughout life in offspring from rodents receiving an LP diet during pregnancy, there is also evidence that the turnover and generation of new β-cells are compromised. Several laboratories have examined the impact of a gestational LP diet in the mouse on the plasticity of β-cells in the offspring to recover from experimental depletion using streptozotocin (STZ) (Cox et al. 2010; Goosse et al. 2014). Mice subject to an LP diet during gestation and neonatal life were unable to recover β-cell mass following a subtotal depletion of these cells by treatment with STZ (Cox et al. 2010). It cannot be concluded if the failure of islet plasticity is primarily due to an intrinsic change in the regenerative mechanisms within β-cells or their progenitors or is due to a failure of angiogenesis within the supporting islet microvasculature, which was also impaired. There was a paradoxical increase in the number of Pdx1[+]/insulin[-] putative β-cell progenitors (Cox et al. 2010) in the offspring of LP-fed mice following STZ, suggesting that their differentiation into mature β-cells might have been impaired. A specific block on β-cell maturation during regeneration following exposure to an LP diet is supported by a failure to increase the number of insulin-positive cell clusters, or individual insulin-positive cells adjacent to the pancreatic ducts as was seen on control-fed animals. This would suggest a failure of endocrine cell neogenesis as a legacy of LP exposure. The longer term implication of LP exposure was a permanent reduction in the numbers of islets relative to animals receiving STZ that were control-fed in early life, especially in females. The failure of islet plasticity is consistent with changes in other tissues following exposure to LP in early life, such as an impaired recovery of male adult rats following ischemia reperfusion (Ryan et al. 2012).

The deficits in pancreatic β-cell mass occurring in the F1 generation where rats or mice were exposed to an LP diet *in utero* can be transmitted through subsequent generations. A reduced mean birth weight was found in F1 offspring. However, when F1 females gave birth while receiving control diet throughout gestation, the F2 generation newborns were of slightly increased birth weight and the F3 offspring were of normal size at birth (Frantz et al. 2011). However, the islet density and size continued to be reduced relative to controls in the F2 and F3 offspring. While this was associated with glucose intolerance in adulthood for F1 and F2 offspring, in the F3 generation the lower β-cell mass was compensated for by an increased insulin sensitivity. However, others have noted that F2 generation females born to F1 animals that were exposed to an LP diet *in utero* demonstrate glucose intolerance during pregnancy (Benyshek et al. 2006; Ignacio-Souza et al. 2013). It is, therefore, possible that F3 females might show a continued legacy of impaired glucose metabolism when they subsequently become pregnant. This would imply a transmission across at least three generations.

4.5 EARLY DIETARY INSULT AND THE MAMMALIAN TARGET OF RAPAMYCIN AXIS

mTOR is a serine/threonine kinase that represents a major crossroads in intracellular signaling that connects the sensing of nutritional availability with growth and maturation signals transmitted by peptide growth factors and hormones. The result is a well-tuned integration of cell proliferation and protein translation to suit the cellular external environment (Peng et al. 2002; Jacinto and Hall 2003; Hay and Soneneberg 2004; Martin and Hall 2005; Tee and Blenis 2005). There are two functional complexes of mTOR, mTOR complex 1 (mTORC1) that incorporates the protein regulatory-associated protein of mTOR (Raptor) and mTORC2 that includes rapamycin-insensitive companion of mammalian target of rapamycin (RICTOR). When mTORC1 is activated by growth factors or amino acids, there is a downstream phosphorylation (activation) of ribosomal S6 kinase1 (S6K1) and eukaryote initiation factor 4E-binding protein 1 (4E-BP1), which upregulates cellular protein translation. However, activation of mTORC2 is more closely linked to entry of cells into the proliferative cycle through the phosphorylation of PKCα (Balcazar et al. 2009; Jacinto et al. 2004), such that cell proliferation and function can be balanced. Rapamycin is a specific inhibitor of mTORC1 and mTORC2 at high doses (Sarbassov et al. 2006; Rosner and Hengstschlager 2008). The tuberous sclerosis complex (*TSC*) genes function as specific inhibitors of mTOR.

The regulation of β-cell mass and insulin secretion is integrated with nutritional availability through the mTOR pathway, and rapamycin inhibits β-cell proliferation *in vitro* through predominantly the inhibition of mTORC1 (Nir et al. 2007; Niclauss et al. 2011). The increase in pancreatic β-cell mass that occurs in response to persistent hyperglycemia is prevented by rapamycin treatment *in vivo* (Fraenkel et al. 2008). As would therefore be expected, a deletion of the *TSC2* gene resulted in an increase in mTOR signaling and greater cell proliferation and hypertrophy (Rachdi et al. 2008; Bartolome et al. 2010). The survival of β-cells is also linked to mTOR signaling because the ability of IGF-I or II to prevent apoptosis is mediated by mTOR acting downstream of Akt signaling (Cai et al. 2008). Similar survival effects are seen with glucagon-like peptide-1 (GLP-1), but in that case through the activation of cyclic adenosine monophosphate (AMP) (Kwon et al. 2004).

Young offspring from rats given an LP diet during gestation had a decrease in the amounts of mTOR protein and activated p70 S6K1 within the pancreatic islets, associated with the expected impairment of glucose and amino acid-stimulated insulin release (Filiputti et al. 2008, 2010). Neonatal mice from dams receiving control diet during gestation were able to regenerate their β-cell mass over 4 weeks if this was previously reduced by approximately 70% by administration of STZ (Cox et al. 2013). However, mice from dams given an LP diet could not replace their β-cell mass, suggesting that exposure to an LP diet had severely impaired β-cell plasticity. Male offspring subsequently became severely diabetic. Changes in the expression of genes in the mTOR pathway were examined within whole pancreas or isolated islets within this model. Messenger RNAs encoding mTOR and cell cycle genes such as cdk2 were much reduced following STZ and recovered in mice from control diet-fed mothers but not those receiving an LP diet (Cox et al. 2013; Alejandro et al. 2014). Conversely, the expression of *TSC2* was significantly increased in the LP + STZ animals, but expression of *Raptor* or *Rictor* was not changed. Isolated islets exposed to rapamycin from offspring of control-fed mice exhibited a decrease in the rate of DNA synthesis to the low levels seen in islets from LP-exposed offspring and had an increased rate of apoptosis. A prevention of mTOR signaling within islets, as seen in the LP diet model, therefore has prolonged detrimental effects on islet plasticity and survival.

Recently, the mTOR pathway in pancreatic β-cells has been shown to integrate with the Hippo-Yes-associated protein (Yap) pathway during cell proliferation and its relationship to the retention of β-cell function. Yap is a transcriptional coactivator, which, in the absence of negative regulation, interacts with the TEA domain (TEAD) family of transcription factors that promote the expression of genes controlling cell proliferation and survival (Hansen et al. 2015). Yap is highly expressed early in pancreas development in the mouse embryo but expression decreases as β-cells differentiate and becomes undetectable in adult islets (George et al. 2012). Experimental reactivation of Yap signaling in β-cells results in renewed cell proliferation (George et al. 2015). Signaling through the mTOR pathway was shown to be directly linked to Yap activation allowing for a continued basal mitogenesis of β-cells while these cells can simultaneously remain functionally active (Hansen et al. 2015). However, a permanent suppression of mTOR signaling as seen in offspring of LP-fed mice will likely reduce the physiological turnover of β-cells and result in a progressive loss of β-cell mass through the suppression of the Yap pathway.

4.6   EPIGENETIC MODIFICATION OF GENE EXPRESSION FOLLOWING EXPOSURE TO A LOW PROTEIN DIET

Epigenetic biochemical modifications to genomic DNA or the supporting chromatin in response to environmental changes *in utero*, including nutritional metabolites, can alter the metabolic axis in the offspring for life and may be transmittable to future generations. The most common modifications in terms of metabolic imprinting are differential DNA methylation and changes in acetylation or methylation of lysine in the histone regions of chromatin (Fuks 2005; Simmons 2007). The ability to alter DNA methylation on cytosine is due to the actions of methyltransferase enzymes, with cytosine residues occurring frequently in guanine-cytosine (GC)-rich sequences within gene promoter regions. An absence or a limited methylation of promoter regions typically results in a greater expression of the associated proteins, whereas increased methylation results in a decrease expression. Histone proteins can be modified at the amino terminus by acetylation, methylation, and other modifications, which change the compactness of the DNA–chromatin complex and alter the ability of transcription factors to bind to gene promoter regions. Dietary manipulation during gestation can alter gene promoter DNA methylation (Cooney et al. 2002). Adult humans malnourished *in utero* during the Dutch hunger winter of 1944 and who subsequently developed type 2 diabetes showed a decreased methylation of the IGF-II gene promoter (Heijmans et al. 2008). Conversely, maternal diabetes was associated with altered methylation of genes involved with glucose metabolism and cell replication in cord blood cells from the newborns (El Hajj et al. 2013).

During pancreas organogenesis nutritional insults can cause epigenetic changes in the expression of the transcription factor Pdx1, which is necessary for the differentiation of β-cells from progenitors and for insulin biosynthesis. IUGR in the rat was accompanied by a reduced expression of *Pdx1* mRNA in the fetal pancreas, which was subsequently suppressed throughout life with animals becoming glucose intolerant (Pinney and Simmons 2012). This occurred no matter whether animals were restored to normal protein diet at birth or at weaning (Abuzgaia et al. 2015). When islets were isolated from IUGR fetuses, there was a reduced level of acetylation on H3 and H4 histones within the *Pdx1* promoter, preventing transcriptional activation by Upstream stimulatory factor 1 (USF1) (Park et al. 2008). Following birth the histone compaction continued around the *Pdx1* gene with a reduction in H3 acetylation but increased methylation of H3K9, and an age-related reduction in *Pdx1* expression resulting in a smaller β-cell mass with impaired glucose-stimulated insulin secretion. A second gene that can be epigenetically modified in β-cells is *HNF4α*, which is required for β-cell development from progenitor populations. Rats born to mothers fed an LP diet during gestation showed a reduced expression of HNF4α in pancreas with a decreased acetylation of the P2 promoter at the H3 region and enhanced methylation at H3K9 (Sandovici et al. 2011). These changes are normally age related but occurred prematurely in offspring exposed to an LP diet. It is likely that long-lived epigenetic modifications to the expression of genes controlling β-cell mass and function occur as a result of early exposure to an LP diet, but the phenotype of poor glucose tolerance may well involve epigenetic changes to genes controlling tissue insulin sensitivity also. Such changes to the expression of the glucose transporter, Glut4, in peripheral tissues have been reported (Raychaudhuri et al. 2008).

Programming of a transgenerational transmission of impaired β-cell function as a result of LP exposure could also be mediated through mitochondrial DNA, which is exclusively inherited from the mother. Because mitochondria in β-cells directly regulate glucose-stimulated insulin secretion by providing adenosine triphosphate (ATP) for energy-dependent ion channel activation, permanent changes to mitochondrial gene expression associated with altered function may be transmittable across generations. β-Cells have much higher ATP requirements than many other cell types but are equipped with lower endogenous levels of antioxidants (Rashidi et al. 2009). Exposure of the F1 generation to an LP diet *in utero* resulted in an increased generation of reactive oxidant species and a reduced expression of mitochondrial gene cytochrome c oxidase 1 (COX1) (Lee et al. 2011), resulting in permanent damage to mitochondrial function (Theys et al. 2011; Simmons et al. 2005). These changes were restored by taurine supplementation to the LP diet (Lee et al. 2011).

4.7   PREMATURITY OF CELLULAR AGING

The lifelong changes in the phenotype and function of the pancreas in offspring exposed to a maternal LP diet may also represent a premature aging of tissues and the associated cellular oxidative stress and decreased cellular plasticity. Cellular aging and the onset of senescence are controlled by telomerase, which shortens the telomere length within chromosomes each time a cell undergoes mitosis. In humans, the telomere length reduction starts during embryogenesis with a rapid decline after week 6 of gestation and a more gradual decline until birth and thereafter (Cheng et al. 2013). The telomerase enzymes include telomerase reverse transcriptase (TERT) and the RNA template (TERC). Cellular and physiological stress causes an increased rate of telomere shortening throughout life (Shalev et al. 2013). Thus, a reduced copy number of the *Terc* gene was reported in placenta from infants with IUGR leading to decreased telomerase and enhanced telomere shortening (Biron-Shental et al. 2011). TERT is present in the mitochondria as well as the nucleus and mitochondrial levels are increased in response to cellular oxidative stress as occurs in offspring of diabetic mothers as measured in cord blood mononuclear cells (Li et al. 2014). The altered ratio of TERT within mitochondria compared to nuclei could result in cellular aging with a reduction in β-cell survival and plasticity, coupled with premature insulin resistance in peripheral tissues such as muscle, adipose, and liver. The numbers of shortened telomeres increased more rapidly with aging in rat tissues for animals exposed to an LP diet *in utero*, including the pancreatic islets (Cherif et al. 2003). This was associated with an increased expression of p16[INK], which is an inhibitor of β-cell proliferation (tarry-Adkins et al. 2013). Consequently, the lifespan of the offspring from mothers who received an LP diet was shortened compared to those from control-fed mothers (Jennings et al. 1999), and the normal age-related reduction in responsiveness of β-cells to glucose occurred prematurely (Morimoto et al. 2012).

4.8   REVERSAL OF PANCREATIC DYSFUNCTION BY DIETARY SUPPLEMENTATION WITH TAURINE

Taurine is an abundant sulfur-containing amino acid with tissue levels being greatest in brain, proinflammatory cells, and pancreas (Briel et al. 1972). It is localized to both α- and β-cells within the islets (Bustamante et al. 2001). Adult humans can maintain adequate endogenous taurine levels by metabolism from dietary methionine and cysteine, but the synthetic capacity is much lower in the neonate and reduced yet further in infants with IUGR (Zelikovic et al. 1990). There are widespread cellular actions of taurine including a regulation of cell volume, extracellular and intracellular calcium mobilization, and an antiapoptotic action in hepatocytes, endothelial cells, macrophages, and renal tubules (Huxtable 1992; Palmi et al. 1999; Wu et al. 1999; Barua et al. 2001; Takikawa et al. 2001; Verzola et al. 2001). The ability of taurine to prevent apoptosis is mediated by the Fas pathway. Animals born to LP diet-fed rats have an increased presence of immunoreactive Fas and Fas ligand within islets, which contributes toward a higher rate of β-cell apoptosis, especially at the time of neonatal developmental apoptosis around postnatal day 14. Similarly, nutritional supplementation of mothers with methyl donors such as folic acid, or micronutrient-rich vegetables may also improve newborn outcome (Potdar et al. 2014).

Taurine levels are reduced in the blood of pregnant rats given an LP diet compared to controls, and taurine levels in the fetus are depleted more than any other amino acid (Reusens et al. 1995; Cherif et al. 1998). Taurine supplementation of an LP diet alone was also able to reverse all of the changes in β-cell physiology in the offspring that resulted from feeding an LP diet. These included a normalization of β-cell mass and proliferative rate, the islet microvascular density, glucose and amino acid-stimulated insulin release, and the local abundance of IGF-II and VEGF (Cherif et al. 1998; Boujendar et al. 2002, 2003). The ability of taurine to enhance glucose-stimulated insulin secretion involves an increased flux of both extracellular and intracellular Ca^{2+} through activation or both the phosphokinase A (PKA) and PKC pathways (Batista et al. 2012; Carneiro et al. 2009; Ribeiro et al. 2010). The cross talk between these pathways is disrupted following exposure to LP resulting in a decreased efficiency of insulin exocytosis, which is restored by taurine (Lippo et al. 2015). In addition, taurine has been shown to increase levels of the ATP-sensitive K^+ATP channels on β-cells (Vettorazzi et al. 2014). Both Fas and Fas ligand presence were reduced by taurine supplementation resulting in less β-cell apoptosis. Additionally, supplementing the tissue culture medium of isolated rat islets with taurine, or adding taurine to an LP diet, prevented interleukin-1 (IL-1) and transforming growth factor α (TGF-α) induced apoptosis within β-cells and restored insulin secretion (Merezak et al. 2001). This suggests that selective nutritional supplementation can alter endocrine pancreatic development and functional trajectory and can offset the damage in early life caused by an LP diet.

4.9 REVERSAL OF PANCREATIC DYSFUNCTION WITH STATIN TREATMENT

In addition to their cholesterol lowering actions, statins also exert pleiotropic actions. These include increased nitric oxide (NO) synthesis and antioxidant effects leading to improved endothelial cell function (Wang et al. 2008), a reduction of atherosclerotic plaque (Ikeda et al. 2000; Dulak et al. 2006; Wang et al. 2008), and anti-inflammatory actions with a reduction in circulating C-reactive protein and inflammatory cytokines. Offspring from rats given an LP diet during gestation showed improved blood vessel dilation following treatment with atorvastatin (Torrens et al. 2009). This is likely to be associated with microvascular angiogenesis also as statin treatment increased the numbers of circulating EPCs in a pig model (Mohler et al. 2009), increased proliferation of EPCs *in vitro* (Assmus et al. 2003), and delayed diabetes onset in two different mouse models of T1D, including STZ treatment (Rydgren et al. 2007). These actions are independent of the ability of statins to inhibit hydroxymethylglutaryl-CoA synthase (HMG-CoA) reductase activity (Rydgren and Sandler 2009). Following experimental reduction in β-cell mass with STZ in neonatal rats, subsequent treatment with atorvastatin improved the recovery in β-cell mass and of glucose tolerance (Marchand et al. 2010). This was accompanied by an increase in the number of proliferating intraislet endothelial cells and the proliferation of adjacent β-cells. Therefore, it is not clear if the ability of statins to rescue β-cell mass is a direct action on the proliferation of remaining β-cells or indirect through an enhanced presence of EPCs from bone marrow leading to islet vasculogenesis.

4.10   CONCLUSIONS

Some of the effects of maternal protein deprivation on fetal β-cell mass and function involve changes to placental function but many are direct. Mechanisms involve changes to progenitor cell number and differentiation capacity and long-term changes in β-cell proliferation, survival, and plasticity (Figure 4.1). These involve a resetting of key integrative intracellular pathways such as mTOR and Hippo-Yes, but may have a root cause in an advancement in the rate of cellular aging. Certain amino acids, such as taurine, appear to be particularly important for determining a normal trajectory for β-cell development. If the nutritional insult is reversed at birth a limited recovery is possible, but if extended to weaning then the effects are long lasting and impair the ability of β-cells to recover from metabolic stress, resulting in diabetes. This suggests that a reversal of risk in the context of the low birth weight human infant may require nutritional supplementation or pharmacological intervention either *in utero* or in early postnatal life.

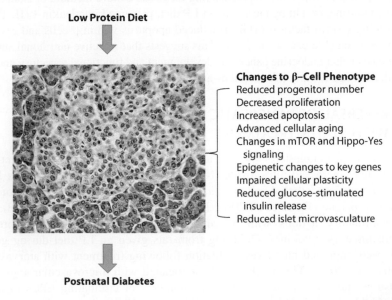

Low Protein Diet

Changes to β–Cell Phenotype
Reduced progenitor number
Decreased proliferation
Increased apoptosis
Advanced cellular aging
Changes in mTOR and Hippo-Yes signaling
Epigenetic changes to key genes
Impaired cellular plasticity
Reduced glucose-stimulated insulin release
Reduced islet microvasculature

Postnatal Diabetes

FIGURE 4.1   Mechanisms implicated in the long-lasting reduction of β-cell mass and function in the offspring of animals exposed to a maternal low protein diet during gestation and neonatal life.

ACKNOWLEDGMENTS

For cited studies, the author is grateful to research funding from the Alan Thicke Centre for Juvenile Diabetes Research, the Program of Experimental Medicine, Department of Medicine, Western University, and the European Commission Framework 7 Program.

REFERENCES

Abuzgaia, A.M., Hardy, D.B. and Arany, E. 2015. Regulation of postnatal pancreatic Pdx1 and downstream target genes after gestational exposure to protein restriction in rats. *Reproduction* 149:293–303.

Alejandro, E.U., Gregg, B., Wallen, T. et al. 2014. Maternal diet-induced microRNAs and mTOR underlie β cell dysfunction in offspring. *J Clin Invest* 124:4395–4410.

Alvarez, C., Martin, M.A., Goya, L. et al. 1997. Contrasted impact of maternal rat food restriction on fetal endocrine pancreas. *Endocrinology* 138:2267–2273.

Assmus, B., Urbich, C., Aicher, A. et al. 2003. HMG-CoA reductase inhibitors reduce senescence and increase proliferation of endothelial progenitor cells via regulation of cell cycle regulatory genes. *Circ Res* 92:1049–1055.

Balcazar, N., Sathyamurthy, A. Elghazi, L. et al. 2009. mTORC1 activation regulates β-cell mass and proliferation by modulation of cyclin D2 synthesis and stability. *J Biol Chem* 284:7832–7842.

Barker, D.J. 1994. *Programming the Baby. Mothers, Babies, Disease in Later Life*. London: Br Med J Publishing Group, pp. 14–36.

Bartolome, A., Guillen, C. and Benito, M. 2010. Role of TSC1-TSC2 complex in the integration of insulin and glucose signaling involved in pancreatic β-cell proliferation. *Endocrinology* 151:3084–3094.

Barua, M., Liu, Y. and Quinn, M.R. 2001. Taurine chloramine inhibits inducible nitric oxide synthase and TNF-alpha gene expression in activated alveolar macrophages: Decreased NF-kappaB activation and IkappaB kinase activity. *J Immunol* 167:2275–2281.

Batista, T.M., Ribeiro, R.A., Amaral, A.G. et al. 2012. Taurine supplementation restores glucose and carbachol-induced insulin secretion in islets from low-protein diet rats: Involvement of Ach-M3R, Synt 1 and SNAP-25 proteins. *J Nutr Biochem* 23:306–312.

Beamish, C.A., Strutt, B., Arany, E.J. et al. 2007. Imaging of re-differentiated islet like clusters using a novel immunocytochemical method. *Diabetes* 56 (Suppl 1):1678P.

Beamish, C.A., Strutt, B.J., Arany, E.J. et al. 2016. Insulin-positive, Glut2-low cells present within mouse pancreas exhibit lineage plasticity and are enriched within extra-islet endocrine cell clusters. *Islets* 8:65–82.

Benyshek, D.C., Johnston, C.S. and Martin, J.F. 2006. Glucose metabolism is altered in the adequately-nourished grand-offspring (F3 generation) of rats malnourished during gestation and perinatal life. *Diabetologia* 49:1117–1119.

Bernstein, J.M., Goran, M.I., Amini, S.B. et al. 1997. Differential growth of fetal tissues during the second half of pregnancy. *Am J Obstet Gynecol* 176:28–32.

Bertram, C., Trowern, A.R., Copin, N. et al. 2001. The maternal diet during pregnancy programs altered expression of the glucocorticoid receptor and type 2 11β-hydroxysteroid dehydrogenase: Potential molecular mechanisms underlying the programming of hypertension in utero. *Endocrinology* 142:2841–2853.

Bhasin, K.K., van Nas, A., Martin, L.J. et al. 2009. Maternal low-protein diet or hypercholesterolemia reduces circulating essential amino acids and leads to intrauterine growth retardation. *Diabetes* 58:559–566.

Biron-Shental, T., Kidron, D., Sukenik-Halevy, R. et al. 2011. TERC telomerase subunit gene copy number in placentas from pregnancies complicated with intrauterine growth restriction. *Early Hum Dev* 87:73–75.

Boujendar, S., Arany, E., Hill, D.J. et al. 2003. Taurine supplementation during fetal life reverses the vascular impairment caused to the endocrine pancreas by a low protein diet. *J Nutr* 133:2820–2825.

Boujendar, S., Reusens, B., Merezak, S. et al. 2002. Taurine supplementation to a low protein diet during foetal and early postnatal life restores normal proliferation and apoptosis of rat pancreatic islets. *Diabetologia* 45:856–866.

Briel, G., Gylfe, E., Hellman, B. et al. 1972. Microdetermination of free amino acids in pancreatic islets isolated from obese-hyperglycemic mice. *Acta Physiol Scand* 84:247–253.

Bustamante, J., Lobo, M.V., Alonso, F.J. et al. 2001. An osmotic-sensitive taurine pool is localized in rat pancreatic islet cells containing glucagon and somatostatin. *Am J Physiol Endocrinol Metab* 281:E1275–E1285.

Cai, Y., Wang, Q., Ling, Z. et al. 2008. Akt activation protects pancreatic beta cells from AMPK-mediated death through stimulation of mTOR. *Biochem Pharmacol* 75:1981–1993.

Carneiro, E.M., Latorraca, M.Q., Araujo, E. et al. 2009. Taurine supplementation modulates glucose homeostasis and islet function. *J Nutr Biochem* 20:503–511.

Chamson-Reig, A., Thyssen, S., Arany, E. et al. 2006. Altered pancreatic morphology in the offspring of pregnant rats given reduced dietary protein is time and gender specific. *J Endocrinol* 191:83–92.

Chamson-Reig, A., Thyssen, S.M., Hill, D.J. et al. 2009. Exposure of the pregnant rat to low protein diet causes impaired glucose homeostasis in the young adult offspring by different mechanisms in males and females. *Exp Biol Med* 234:1425–1436.

Cheng, G., Kong, F., Luan, Y. et al. 2013. Differential shortening rate of telomere length in the development of human fetus. *Biochem Biophys Res Commun* 442:112–115.

Cherif, H., Reusens, B., Ahn, M-T. et al. 1998. Effects of taurine on the insulin secretion of rat fetal islets from dams fed a low protein diet. *J Endocrinol* 159:341–348.

Cherif, H., Tarry, J.L., Ozanne, S.E. et al. 2003. Ageing and telomeres: A study into organ- and gender-specific telomere shortening. *Nucleic Acids Res* 31:1576–1583.

Cooney, C.A., Dave, A.A. and Wolff, G.L. 2002. Maternal methyl supplements in mice affect epigenetic variation and DNA methylation of offspring. *J Nutr* 132:2393S–2400S.

Cox, A.R., Arany, E.J. and Hill, D.J. 2010. The effects of low protein during gestation on mouse pancreatic development and β-cell regeneration. *Pediatr Res* 68:16–22.

Cox, A.R., Beamish, C.A., Carter, D.E. et al. 2013. Cellular mechanisms underlying failed beta cell regeneration in offspring of protein-restricted pregnant mice. *Exp Biol Med* 238:1147–1159.

De Oliveira, J.C., Scomparin, D.X., Andreazzi, A.E. et al. 2011. Metabolic imprinting by maternal protein malnourishment impairs vagal activity in adult rats. *J Neuroendocrinol* 23:148–157.

Dulak, J., Loboda, A., Jazwa, A. et al. 2006. Atorvastatin affects several angiogenic mediators in endothelial cells. *Endothelium* 12:233–241.

El Hajj, N., Pliushch, G., Schneider, E. et al. 2013. Metabolic programming of MEST DNA methylation by intrauterine exposure to gestational diabetes mellitus. *Diabetes* 62:1320–1328.

Fall, C. 2009. Maternal nutrition: Effects on health in the next generation. *Indian J Med Res* 130:593–599.

Ferreira, R.V., Gombar, F.M., da Silva Faria, T. et al. 2010. Metabolic programming of ovarian angiogenesis and folliculogenesis by maternal malnutrition during lactation. *Fertil Steril* 93:2572–2580.

Filiputti, E., Ferreira, F., Souza, K.L. et al. 2008. Impaired insulin secretion and decreased expression of the nutritionally responsive ribosomal kinase protein S6K-1 in pancreatic islets from malnourished rats. *Life Sci* 82:542–48.

Filiputti, E., Rafacho, A., Araujo, E.P. et al. 2010. Augmentation of insulin secretion by leucine supplementation in malnourished rats: Possible involvement of the phosphatidylinositol 3-phosphate kinase/mammalian target protein of rapamycin pathway. *Metabolism* 59:635–644.

Fraenkel, M., Ketzinel-Gilad, M., Ariav, Y. et al. 2008. mTOR inhibition by rapamycin prevents beta-cell adaptation to hyperglycemia and exacerbates the metabolic state in type 2 diabetes. *Diabetes* 57:945–957.

Frantz, E.D., Barbosa Aquila, M., da Rocha Pinheiro-Mulder, A. et al. 2011. Transgenerational endocrine pancreatic adaptation in mice from maternal protein restriction in utero. *Mech Ageing Dev* 132:110–116.

Fuks, S. 2005. DNA methylation and histone modifications: teaming up to silence genes. *Curr Opin Genet Dev* 15:490–495.

Garofano, A., Czernichow, P., and Breant, B. 1997. In utero undernutrition impairs rat beta-cell development. *Diabetologia* 40:1231–1234.

George, N.M., Boerner, B.P., Mir, S.U. et al. 2015. Exploiting expression of Hippo effector, Yap, for expansion of functional islet mass. *Mol Endocrinol* 29:1594–1607.

George, N.M., Day, C.E., Boerner, B.P. et al. 2012. Hippo signaling regulates pancreas development through inactivation of Yap. *Mol Cell Biol* 32:5116–5128.

Glazier, J.D., Cetin, I., Perugino, G. et al. 1997. Association between the activity of the system A amino acid transporter in the microvillous plasma membrane of the human placenta and severity of fetal compromise in intrauterine growth restriction. *Pediatr Res* 42:514–519.

Goosse, K., Bouckenooghe, T., Sisino, G. et al. 2014. Increased susceptibility to streptozotocin and impeded regeneration capacity of beta-cells in adult offspring of malnourished rats. *Acta Physiol* 210:99–109.

Hansen, C.G., Ng, Y.L., Lam, W-L.M. et al. 2015. The Hippo pathway effectors YAP and TAZ promote cell growth by modulating amino acid signaling to mTORC1. *Cell Res* 25:1299–1313.

Hasegawa, Y., Ogihara, T., Yamada, T. et al. 2007. Bone marrow (BM) transplantation promotes β-cell regeneration after acute injury through BM cell mobilization. *Endocrinology* 148:2006–2015.

Hay, N. and Soneneberg, N. 2004. Upstream and downstream of mTOR. *Genes Dev* 18:1926–1945.

Heijmans, B.T., Tobi, E.W. et al. 2008. Persistent epigenetic differences associated with prenatal exposure to famine in humans. *Proc Natl Acad Sci USA* 105:17046–17049.

Herbert, D.C. and Carillo, A.J. 1982. The hypophyseal-adrenal axis in the protein-calorie malnourished rat. *Horm Metab Res* 14:205–207.

Hess, D., Li, L., Sakano, S. et al. 2003. Bone marrow derived stem cells rescue hyperglycemia by regeneration of recipient islets. *Nature Biotech* 21:763–770.

Hill, D.J. 2011. Nutritional programming of pancreatic β-cell plasticity. *World J Diabetes* 2:119–132.

Huxtable, R.J. 1992. Physiological actions of taurine. *Physiol Rev* 72:101–163.

Ignacio-Souza, L.M., Reis, S.R., Arantes, V.C. et al. 2013. Protein restriction in early life is associated with changes in insulin sensitivity and pancreatic β-cell function during pregnancy. *Br J Nutr* 109:236–247.

Ikeda, U., Shimpo, M., Ohki, P. et al. 2000. Fluvastatin inhibits matrix metalloproteinase-1 expression in human vascular endothelial cells. *Hypertension* 36:325–329.

Jacinto, E. and Hall M.N. 2003. TOR signalling in bugs, brain and brawn. *Nature Rev Mol Cell Biol* 4:117–126.

Jacinto, E., Loewith, R., Schmidt, A. et al. 2004. Mammalian TOR complex 2 controls the actin cytoskeleton and is rapamycin insensitive. *Nat Cell Biol* 6:1122–1228.

Jennings, B.J., Ozanne, S.E. and Hales, C.N. 1999. Early growth determines longevity in male rats and may be related to telomere shortening. *FEBS Lett* 488:4–8.

Joanette, E., Reusens, B., Arany, E. et al. 2004. Low protein diet during early life causes a reduction in the frequency of cells immunopositive for nestin and CD34 in both pancreatic ducts and islets in the rat. *Endocrinology* 145:3004–3013.

Johansson, M., Karlsson, L., Wennergren, M. et al. 2003. Activity and protein expression of Na+/K+ ATPase are reduced in microvillous syncytiotrophoblast plasma membranes isolated from pregnancies complicated by intrauterine growth restriction. *J Clin Endocrinol Metab* 88:2831–2837.

Johannson, M., Mattsson, G., Andersson, A. et al. 2006. Islet endothelial cells and pancreatic β-cell proliferation: Studies in vitro and during pregnancy in adult rats. *Endocrinology* 147:2314–2324.

Kwon, G., Marshall, C.A., Pappan, K.L. et al. 2004. Signaling elements involved in the metabolic regulation of mTOR by nutrients, incretins and growth factors in islets. *Diabetes* 53 (Suppl 3):S225–S232.

Kwong, W.Y., Wild, A.E., Roberts, P. et al. 2000. Maternal undernutrition during the preimplantation period of rat development causes blastocyst abnormalities and programming of postnatal hypertension. *Development* 127:4195–4202.

Lee, Y.Y., Lee, H-J., Lee, S-S. et al. 2011. Taurine supplementation restored the changes in pancreatic islet mitochondria in the fetal protein malnourished rat. *Br J Nutr* 106:1198–1206.

Li, P., Tong, Y., Yang, H. et al. 2014. Mitochondrial translocation of human telomerase reverse transcriptase in cord blood mononuclear cells of newborns with gestational diabetes mellitus mothers. *Diabetes Res Clin Pract* 103:310–318.

Lippo, B.R., Batista, T.M., de Rezende, L.F. et al. 2015. Low-protein diet disrupts the crosstalk between the PKA and PKC signaling pathways in isolated pancreatic islets. *J Nutr Biochem* 26:556–562.

Magnusson, A.L., Powell, T., Wennergren, M. et al. 2004. Glucose metabolism in the human preterm and term placenta of IUGR fetuses. *Placenta* 25:337–346.

Manuel-Apolinar, L., Rocha, L., Damasio, L. et al. 2014. Role of prenatal undernutrition in the expression of serotonin, dopamine and leptin receptors in adult mice: Implications of food intake. *Mol Med Rep* 9:407–412.

Marchand, K.C., Arany, E.J. and Hill, D.J. 2010. The effects of atorvastatin on the regeneration of pancreatic beta cells after streptozotocin treatment in the neonatal rodent. *Am J Physiol Endocrinol Metab* 299:E92–E100.

Martın, M.A., Alvarez, C., Goya, L. et al. 1997. Insulin secretion in adult rats that had experienced different underfeeding patterns during their development. *Am J Physiol* 272:E634–E640.

Martin, D.E. and Hall, M.N. 2005. The expanding TOR network. *Curr Opin Cell Biol* 17:158–166.

Merezak, S., Hardikar, A.A., Yajnik, C.S. et al. 2001. Intrauterine low protein diet increases fetal β cell sensitivity to NO and IL-1β: The protective role of taurine. *J Endocrinol* 171:299–308.

Mohler, E.R., Shi, Y., Moore, J. et al. 2009. Diabetes reduces bone marrow and circulating porcine endothelial progenitor cells, an effect ameliorated by atorvastatin and independent of cholesterol. *Cytometry Part A* 75A:75–82.

Morimoto, S., Calzada, L., Sosa, T.C. et al. 2012. Emergence of ageing-related changes in insulin secretion by pancreatic islets of male rat offspring of mothers fed a low protein diet. *Br J Nutr* 107:1562–1565.

Nicholson, M.J., Arany, E.J. and Hill, D.J. 2010. Changes in islet micro-vasculature following streptozotocin-induced β-cell loss and subsequent replacement in the neonatal rat. *Exp Biol Med* 235:189–198.

Niclauss, N., Bosco, D., Morel, P. et al. 2011. Rapamycin impairs proliferation of transplanted islet β cells. *Transplantation* 91:714–722.

Nikolova, G., Jabs, N., Konstantinova, I. et al. 2006. The vascular basement membrane: A 'niche' for insulin gene expression and β cell proliferation. *Dev Cell* 10:397–405.

Nir, T., Melton, D.A. and Dor, Y. 2007. Recovery from diabetes in mice by beta cell regeneration. *J Clin Invest* 117:2553–2561.

Ostreicher, I., Almeida, J.R., Campean, V. et al. 2010. Changes in 11beta-hydroxysteroid dehydrogenase type 2 expression in a low-protein rat model of intrauterine growth restriction. *Nephrol Dial Transplant* 25:3195–3203.

Painter, R.C., Roseboom, T.J. and Bleker, O.P. 2005. Prenatal exposure to the Dutch famine and disease in later life: An overview. *Reprod Toxicol* 20:345–352.

Palmi, M., Youmbi, G.T., Fusi, F. et al. 1999. Potentiation of mitochondrial $Ca2+$ sequestration by taurine. *Biochem Pharmacol* 58:1123–1131.

Park, J.H., Stoffers, D.A., Nicholls, R.D. et al. 2008. Development of type 2 diabetes following intrauterine growth retardation in rats is associated with progressive epigenetic silencing of Pdx1. *J Clin Invest* 118:2316–2324.

Peng, T., Golub, T.R. and Sabatini, D.M. 2002. The immunosuppressant rapamycin mimics a starvation-like signal distinct from amino acid and glucose deprivation. *Mol Cell Biol* 22:5575–5584.

Petrik, J., Reusens, B., Arany, E. et al. 1999. A low protein diet alters the balance of islet cell replication and apoptosis in the fetal and neonatal rat, and is associated with a reduced pancreatic expression of insulin-like growth factor-II. *Endocrinology* 140:4861–4873.

Pinney, S.E. and Simmons, R.A. 2012. Metabolic programming, epigenetics, and gestational diabetes mellitus. *Curr Diab Rep* 12:67–74.

Plachot, C., Movassat, J. and Portha, B. 2001. Impaired beta-cell regeneration after partial pancreatectomy in the adult Goto-Kahizaki rat, a spontaneous model of type II diabetes. *Histochem Cell Biol* 116:131–139.

Potdar, R.D., Sahariah, S.A., Gandhi, M. et al. 2014. Improving women's diet quality preconceptionally and during gestation: Effects on birth weight and prevalence of low birth weight—A randomized controlled efficacy trial in India (Mumbai Maternal Nutrition Project). *Am J Clin Nutr* 100:1257–1268.

Rachdi, L., Balcazar, N., Osorio-Duque, F. et al. 2008. Disruption of Tsc2 in pancreatic β cells induces β cell mass expansion and improved glucose tolerance in a TORC1-dependent manner. *Proc Natl Acad Sci USA* 105:9250–9255.

Rafacho, A., Giozzet, V.A., Boschero, A.C. et al. 2009. Reduced pancreatic beta-cell mass is associated with decreased FoxO1 and Erk1/2 protein phosphorylation in low protein malnourished rats. *Braz J Med Biol Res* 42:935–941.

Rashidi, A., Kirkwood, T.B. and Shanley, D.P. 2009. Metabolic evolution suggests an explanation for the weakness of antioxidant defences in beta-cells. *Mech Ageing Dev* 130:216–221.

Ravelli, A.C., van der Meulen, J.H. and Michels, R.P. 1998. Glucose tolerance in adults after prenatal exposure to the Dutch famine. *Lancet* 351:173–177.

Ravelli, A.C., van der Meulen, F.H., Osmond, C. et al. 1999. Obesity at the age of 50 y in men and women exposed to famine prenatally. *Am J Clin Nutr* 70:811–816.

Raychaudhuri, N., Raychaudhuri, S., Thamotharan, M. et al. 2008. Histone code modifications repress glucose transporter 4 expression in the intrauterine growth-restricted offspring. *J Biol Chem* 283:13611–13626.

Rees, W.D., Hay, S.M. and Cruikshank, M. 2006. An imbalance in the methionine content of the maternal diet reduces postnatal growth in the rat. *Metab Clin Exp* 55:763–770.

Reusens, B., Dahri, S., Snoeck, A. et al. 1995. Long-term consequences of diabetes and its complications may have a fetal origin: Experimental and epidemiological evidence. In Cowett, R.M., Ed., *Diabetes Nestle' Nutrition Workshop Series*. New York, NY: Raven Press, vol 35: pp. 187–198.

Reusens, B., Theys, N., Dumortier, O. et al. 2011. Maternal malnutrition programs the endocrine pancreas in progeny. *Am J Clin Nutr 94* (Suppl 6):1824S–1829S.

Ribeiro, R.A., Vanzela, E.C., Oliveira, C.A. et al. 2010. Taurine supplementation: Involvement of cholinergic phospholipase C and PKA pathways in potentiation of insulin secretion and Ca2+ handling in mouse pancreatic islets. *Br J Nutr* 104:1148–1155.

Roa, S., Yajnik, C.S., Kanade, A. et al. 2001. Intake of micronutrient-rich foods in rural Indian mothers is associated with the size of their babies at birth: Pune maternal nutrition study. *J Nutr* 131:1217–1224.

Rodriguez-Trejo, A., Guadalupe Ortiz-Lopez, M., Zambrano, E. et al. 2012. Developmental programming of neonatal pancreatic β-cells by a maternal low-protein diet in rats involves a switch from proliferation to differentiation. *Am J Physiol Endocrinol Metab* 302:E1431–E1439.

Rosario, F.J., Jansson, N., Kanai, Y. et al. 2011. Maternal protein restriction in the rat inhibits placental insulin, mTOR, and STAT3 signaling and down-regulates placental amino acid transporters. *Endocrinology* 152:1119–1129.

Rosner, M. and Hengstschläger, M. 2008. Cytoplasmic and nuclear distribution of the protein complexes mTORC1 and mTORC2: Rapamycin triggers dephosphorylation and delocalization of the mTORC2 components rictor and sin1. *Hum Mol Genet* 17:2934–2948.

Ryan, K.J., Elmes, M.J. and Langley-Evans, S.C. 2012. The effects of prenatal protein restriction on β-adrenergic signalling of the adult rat heart during ischaemia reperfusion. *J Nutr Metab* 2012:397389.

Rydgren, T. and Sandler, S. 2009. The protective effect of simvastatin against low dose streptozotocin induced type 1 diabetes in mice is independent of inhibition of HMG-CoA reductase. *Biochem Biophys Res Commun* 379:1076–1079.

Rydgren, T., Vaarala, O. and Sandler, S. 2007. Simvastatin protects against multiple low-dose streptozotocin-induced type 1 diabetes in CD-1 mice and recurrence of disease in nonobese diabetic mice. *J Pharmacol Exp Therapeutics* 323:180–185.

Sandovici, I., Smith, N.H., Nitert, M.D. et al. 2011. Maternal diet and aging alter the epigenetic control of a promoter-enhancer interaction at the Hnf4a gene in rat pancreatic islets. *Proc Natl Acad Sci USA.* 108:5449–5454.

Sarbassov, D.D., Ali, S.M., Sengupta, S. et al. 2006. Prolonged rapamycin treatment inhibits mTORC2 assembly and Akt/PKB. *Mol Cell* 22:159–168.

Sathishkumar, K., Elkins, R., Yallampalli, U. et al. 2009. Protein restriction during pregnancy induces hypertension and impairs endothelium-dependent vascular function in adult female offspring. *J Vasc Res* 46:229–239.

Serradas, P., Goya, L., Lacorne, M. et al. 2002. Fetal insulin and insulin-like growth factor-2 production is impaired in the GK rat model of type 2 diabetes. *Diabetes* 51:392–397.

Shalev, I., Entringer, S., Wadhwa, P.D. et al. 2013. Stress and telomere biology: A lifespan perspective. *Psychoneuroendocrinology* 38:1835–1842.

Simmons, R.A. 2007. Developmental origins of diabetes: The role of epigenetic mechanisms. *Curr Opin Endocrinol Diabetes Obes* 14:13–16.

Simmons, R.A., Suponitsky-Kroyter, I. and Selak, M.A. 2005. Progressive accumulation of mitochondrial DNA mutations and decline in mitochondrial function lead to beta-cell failure. *J Biol Chem* 280:28785–28791.

Simmons, R.A., Templeton, L.J. and Gertz, S.J. 2001. Intrauterine growth retardation leads to the development of type 2 diabetes in the rat. *Diabetes* 50:2279–2286.

Smukler, S.R., Arntfield, M.E., Razavi, R. et al. 2011. The adult mouse and human pancreas contain rare multipotent stem cells that express insulin. *Cell Stem Cell* 8:281–293.

Somm, E., Schwitzgebel, V.M., Vauthay, D.M. et al. 2008. Prenatal nicotine exposure alters early pancreatic islet and adipose tissue development with consequences on the control of body weight and glucose metabolism later in life. *Endocrinology* 149:6289–6299.

Strakovsky, R.S., Zhou, D. and Pan Y-X. 2010. A low-protein diet during gestation in rats activates the placental mammalian amino acid response pathway and programs the growth capacity of offspring. *J Nutr* 140:2116–2120.

Takikawa, Y., Miyoshi, H., Rust, C. et al. 2001. The bile acid-activated phosphatidylinositol 3-kinase pathway inhibits Fas apoptosis upstream of bid in rodent hepatocytes. *Gastroenterology* 120:1810–1817.

Tarry-Adkins, J.L., Martin-Gronert, M.S., Fernandez-Twinn, D.S. et al. 2013. Poor maternal nutrition followed by accelerated postnatal growth leads to alterations in DNA damage and repair, oxidative and nitrosative stress, and oxidative defense capacity in rat heart. *FASEB J* 27:379–390.

Tee, A.R. and Blenis, J. 2005. mTor, translational control and human disease. *Semin Cell Dev Biol* 16:29–37.

Theys, N., Ahn, M.T., Bouckenooghe, T. et al. 2011. Maternal malnutrition programs pancreatic islet mitochondrial dysfunction in the adult offspring. *J Nutr Biochem* 22:985–994.

Thyssen, S., Arany, E., Chamson-Reig, A. et al. 2003. Sexual differences impacts glucose homeostasis in protein restricted rats. *Can Diabet Assoc*, Ottawa Abstract 277.

Torrens, C., Kelsall, C.J., Hopkins, L.A. et al. 2009. Atorvastatin restores endothelial function in offspring of protein-restricted rats in a cholesterol-independent manner. *Hypertension* 53:661–667.

Trudeau, J.D., Dutz, J.P., Arany, E. et al. 2000. Neonatal β-cell apoptosis: A trigger for autoimmune diabetes? *Diabetes* 49:1–7.

Verzola, D., Bertoletto, M.B., Villaggio, B. et al. 2001. Taurine prevents apoptosis induced by high ambient glucose in human tubule renal cells. *J Invest Med* 50:443–451.

Vettorazzi, J.F., Ribeiro, R.A., Santos-Silva, J.C. et al. 2014. Taurine supplementation increases K_{ATP} channel protein content, improving Ca^{2+} handling and insulin secretion in islets from malnourished mice fed on a high fat diet. *Amino Acids* 46:2123–2136.

Wang, C.Y., Liu, P.Y. and Liao, J.K. 2008. Pleiotropic effects of statin therapy: Molecular mechanisms and clinical results. *Trends Mol Med* 14:37–44.

Wu, Q.D., Wang, J.H., Fennessy, F. et al. 1999. Taurine prevents high-glucose-induced human vascular endothelial cell apoptosis. *Am J Physiol* 277:C1229–C1238.

Zelikovic, I., Chesney, R.W., Friedman, A.L. et al. 1990. Taurine depletion in very low birth weight infants receiving prolonged total parenteral nutrition: Role of renal immaturity. *J Paediatr* 116:301–306.

5 Placental Insufficiency, Pancreatic Development, and Function

Sara Pinney and Rebecca Simmons

CONTENTS

5.1 INTRODUCTION

The development of disease later in life has been linked to exposure to an adverse intrauterine environment, as observed in offspring of pregnancies complicated by intrauterine growth restriction (IUGR), obesity, or diabetes (Hales and Barker 1992, 2001; Kermack et al. 1934; Ravelli et al. 1976, 1998; Valdez et al. 1994). The period from conception to birth is a time of rapid growth, cellular replication and differentiation, and functional maturation of organ systems. These processes are very sensitive to alterations in nutrient availability and an abnormal intrauterine metabolic milieu can have long-lasting effects on the offspring. Perhaps the best example of how nutrient availability during pregnancy affects long-term health and disease in the offspring is exemplified by the Dutch Hunger Winter. This period of famine occurred in the western part of the Netherlands during the winter of 1944–1945; the period of famine was clearly defined, and official food rations were documented. Extensive health care and birth weight registries still exist for this population, which have allowed numerous studies to be performed, which have clearly shown that prenatal exposure to famine is associated with the later development of diseases such as obesity, diabetes, and cardiovascular disease (Lumey et al. 2007).

5.2 INTRAUTERINE GROWTH RESTRICTION AND INSULIN SECRETION IN HUMANS

Glucose-stimulated insulin secretion and glucose removal are impaired severely in the IUGR human fetus (Nicolini et al. 1990). This may in part reflect decreased β-cell mass, which was severely reduced in IUGR fetuses (<1.5 kg) in one study (Van Assche et al. 1977). Béringue and colleagues did not find altered β-cell mass in less severely restricted human fetuses (<10th percentile for birth weight), although this lack of effect may also reflect the variety of causes of IUGR and range of gestational ages within the cohort (Béringue et al. 2002).

Insulin secretion relative to insulin sensitivity and hence demand is substantially impaired in children and adults who grow poorly before birth in most (Jensen et al. 2002; Veening et al. 2003; Mericq et al. 2005) but not all studies (Jaquet et al. 2000). Jensen et al. (2002) measured insulin secretion and insulin sensitivity in a well-matched Caucasian population of 19-year-old glucose tolerant men with birth weights of either below the 10th percentile (small for gestational age [SGA]) or between the 50th and 75th percentile (controls). To eliminate the major confounders such as "diabetes genes," none of the participants had a family history of diabetes, hypertension, or ischemic heart disease. There was no difference between the groups with regard to current weight, body mass index (BMI), body composition, and lipid profile. When controlled for insulin sensitivity, insulin secretion was reduced by 30%. However, insulin sensitivity was normal in the SGA subjects. The investigators hypothesized that defects in insulin secretion may precede defects in insulin action and that once SGA individuals accumulate body fat, they will develop insulin resistance (Jensen et al. 2002).

5.3 RESTRICTED FETAL GROWTH AND INSULIN SECRETION IN OTHER ANIMAL SPECIES

Animal models have a normal genetic background upon which environmental effects during gestation or early postnatal life can be tested for their role in inducing an abnormal metabolic phenotype. The most commonly used animal models for IUGR are caloric or protein restriction, induction of uteroplacental insufficiency (UPI), or glucocorticoid administration in the pregnant rodent, sheep, guinea pig, and nonhuman primate. Remarkably, results from many of these investigations seem to suggest a common offspring phenotype of impaired β-cell function consistent with what has been observed in humans after IUGR.

5.3.1 UTEROPLACENTAL INSUFFICIENCY

UPI is one of the most common causes of IUGR, as only in the face of severe malnutrition is fetal growth adversely affected by maternal diet, while in contrast UPI significantly reduces nutrient availability to the fetus even in the context of adequate maternal diet. Bilateral uterine artery ligation at day 18 of gestation in the rat (where term is 22 days) restricts fetal growth, and similar to the human IUGR condition, levels of glucose, insulin, insulin-like growth factor I (IGF-I), amino acids, and oxygen are reduced (Ogata et al. 1986; Simmons et al. 1992, 2001; Unterman et al. 1993 Boloker et al. 2002). At birth, IUGR newborns have decreased weight but normal β-cell mass. However, despite having normal numbers of β-cells, β-cell function is markedly impaired as demonstrated by blunted first phase insulin secretion. Glucose- and leucine-stimulated insulin release from isolated islets is markedly impaired, but insulin release in response to arginine is normal, suggesting that the secretory apparatus is intact (Simmons et al. 2001, 2005). As the animals age, β-cell mass progressively declines and by 6–9 months of age, β-cell mass in UPI offspring is only about 10% of control values (Simmons et al. 2001; Stoffers et al. 2003).

Placental restriction (PR) in the sheep, either through carunclectomy or maternal hyperthermia (Bell et al. 1987; Thureen et al. 1992; Ross et al. 1996; Anderson et al. 1997; Galan et al. 1999), limits placental delivery of substrates including oxygen and glucose to the PR fetus, which also exhibits the endocrine adaptations and reduced growth characteristic of human IUGR, including reduced circulating and tissue levels of IGF and other anabolic hormones and an early and amplified prenatal surge of cortisol (Robinson et al. 1979; Harding et al. 1985; Owens et al. 1987, 1989, 1994; Kind et al. 1995; Phillips et al. 1996). Before birth, the PR ovine fetus induced by surgical restriction of placental growth has reduced overall insulin secretion *in vivo*, although this is normal when corrected for insulin sensitivity (Owens et al. 2007). Similarly, the more severe hyperthermia-induced growth restriction in sheep also reduces basal- and glucose-stimulated insulin secretion in absolute terms (Limesand et al. 2005, 2006). After birth, the young growth-restricted adult sheep, particularly the male, has reduced basal- and glucose-stimulated insulin secretion, which is even more marked when adjusted for the reduced insulin sensitivity (Owens et al. 2007).

5.3.2 MATERNAL MALNUTRITION

In the rat, maternal dietary protein restriction (isocaloric 8% versus 20% protein) throughout gestation and lactation retards fetal growth, and the structure and function of the endocrine pancreas are altered in the offspring (Snoeck et al. 1990; Dahri et al. 1991; Petrik et al. 1999). Islet cell proliferation, size, and vascularization are reduced, and both pulsatile and peak insulin secretory capacity *in vivo* and *in vitro* are impaired in the newborn (Snoeck et al. 1990; Dahri et al. 1991; Petrik et al. 1999). Many of these defects persist into adulthood (Heywood et al. 2004; Dahri et al. 1991; Snoeck et al. 1990, Berney et al. 1997; Wilson and Hughes 1997; Bertin et al. 1999; Boujendar et al. 2003; Petrik et al. 1999; Petry et al. 2001). Of importance, there does not appear to be a gender-specific effect as the adult offspring female rats also exhibit reduced pancreatic insulin content and β-cell mass (Bertin et al. 1999).

Restricting the diet to 50% of total calories (termed total caloric restriction) during the last week of pregnancy also has significant effects on the pancreas. In male rats, β-cell mass is decreased at birth and at 21 days of age (Garofano et al. 1997). The effect is even more pronounced when caloric restriction is given throughout pregnancy (Dumortier et al. 2007). Likewise, extending caloric restriction after birth until weaning further impairs β-cell development, causing a reduction of 66% of the β-cell mass at 21 days (Garofano et al. 1998). In adulthood, these animals develop insulinopenia (Garofano et al. 1999). However, it is not known whether the insulin secretory defect is solely due to reduced β-cell mass or whether a restricted maternal diet induces a functional deficit independent of mass. In contrast to the studies by Garofano et al., studies by Bertin et al. did not observe any changes in β-cell mass or insulin content in the total caloric restriction group in adult male or female offspring. These studies only demonstrated an effect on the pancreas in adult offspring of dams fed a protein-restricted diet during the last week in pregnancy (Bertin et al. 1999).

5.4 MECHANISMS OF IMPAIRED INSULIN SECRETION

5.4.1 Regulation of β-Cell Mass

Intriguingly, offspring of all of the rodent models described above display marked reductions in β-cell mass indicating that the β-cell plays a primary role in the development of the metabolic phenotype. Several transcription factors have been shown to be essential for the development of the pancreas (reviewed in Habener et al. 2005). The embryonic development of β-cells is critically dependent on the function of the basic helix–loop–helix transcription factor neurogenin 3 (Ngn3). PDX-1 (also known as IDX1, IPF1, STF1, XlhBox8, GSF, and IUF) is a homeodomain-containing transcription factor that plays two critical roles, first in the early development of both endocrine and exocrine pancreas, and then in the later differentiation and function of the β-cell. Targeted homozygous disruption of PDX-1 in mice results in pancreatic agenesis (Jonsson et al. 1994; Offield et al. 1996); homozygous mutations yield a similar phenotype in humans (Stoffers et al. 1997a) and heterozygous mutations cause MODY in the human (Stoffers et al. 1997b; Bernardo et al. 2008).

During embryonic development, fewer Ngn3 (–20%) and Pdx1 (–47%) positive cells are present in the pancreas of calorically restricted as well as in UPI fetuses in comparison to controls, consistent with a decrease in the β-cell precursor pool (Stoffers et al. 2003; Dumortier et al. 2007). The loss of Pdx1 expression persists into adulthood contributing further to the progressive decline in β-cell mass and function (Stoffers et al. 2003). The molecular mechanisms relating to loss of Pdx1 expression are discussed below.

5.4.2 Islet Vascularity

The endocrine pancreas is a richly vascularized tissue. In rodents, each islet of Langerhans receives its blood supply from one to five afferent arterioles that branch into a glomerular-like network of microvessels and form a local intraislet portal system (Bonner-Weir 2000) through which blood flows from the central core of β-cells to the non-β-cell mantle. Endocrine microvessels are wider and thinner walled than the exocrine capillaries and possess 10 times as many fenestrations (Henderson and Moss 1985). Vascular endothelial growth factor (VEGF) is a dimeric glycosylated protein with structural homology to platelet-derived growth factor. VEGF is a strong mitogenic factor for endothelial cells (ECs) in various *in vitro* and *in vivo* systems (Leung et al. 1989; Thieme et al. 1995) and has been shown to increase the permeability of microvessels (Ferrara 2004; Ferrara et al. 1992).

In islets, strong VEGF staining has been demonstrated in β-cells and non-β-cells (Rooman et al. 1997). These observations suggest that continued low-level secretion of VEGF by islet cells may play a major role in the homeostasis of the rich intrainsular vasculature, in particular, in the maintenance of the fenestrated endothelium (Vasir et al. 2001). VEGF was also found to be weakly expressed by acinar cells in the exocrine pancreas. The two high-affinity receptors for VEGF, Flt-1 and Flk-1, are also expressed in adult and fetal islets of Langerhans and in the exocrine pancreas. VEGF receptor Flk-1 is expressed by the ECs (Christofori et al. 1995) and by the pancreatic ductal cells during fetal development. This suggests that VEGF and its receptor might also play a role in both endocrine pancreatic organogenesis and the population dynamics of pancreatic ducts (Oberg et al. 1994), especially because VEGF was shown to be mitogenic for the pancreatic ductal epithelium (Rooman et al. 1997). Recently, blood vessels were shown to provide not only metabolic sustenance but also inductive signals for endocrine pancreas development, and VEGF would be a major factor in this endothelium–endocrine cell interaction (Ranjan et al. 2009).

In previous studies, we observed reduced islet vascular density in fetal and neonatal UPI rats compared with controls (Ham et al. 2009; Jaeckle Santos et al. 2014). These changes in islet vascularity precede reductions in β-cell mass and are associated with changes in VEGF expression during the perinatal period. Caloric restriction during pregnancy also significantly reduces islet vascularity in the fetus (Boujendar et al. 2003). Studies performed by Rozance et al. (2015) and Rozance and Hay (2016) provide some insight into mechanisms that may be responsible for this phenotype. In their model of fetal growth restriction induced by maternal hyperthermia in the sheep, they also observed decreased islet vascularity in the fetus (Rozance et al. 2015; Rozance and Hay 2016). Pancreatic and islet ECs provide signals responsible for the normal formation, maturation, and function of the pancreatic β-cells. Hepatocyte growth factor (HGF) and VEGFA are paracrine hormones that mediate communication between pancreatic islet ECs and β-cells. They show that paracrine actions from ECs increase islet insulin content, and in ECs from growth-restricted animals, secretion of HGF is diminished. Given the potential feed-forward regulation of β-cell VEGFA and islet EC HGF, these two growth factors are highly integrated in normal pancreatic islet development and this regulation is decreased in IUGR fetuses, resulting in lower pancreatic islet insulin concentrations and insulin secretion (Rozance et al. 2015; Rozance and Hay 2016).

5.4.3 Mitochondrial Dysfunction

Multiple studies have shown that IUGR is associated with increased oxidative stress in the human fetus (Myatt et al. 1997; Karowicz-Bilinska et al. 2002; Ejima et al. 1999; Kato et al. 1997; Bowen et al. 2001; Wang and Walsh 1998, 2001). A major consequence of limited nutrient availability is an alteration in the redox state in susceptible fetal tissues leading to oxidative stress. In particular, low levels of oxygen, evident in growth-retarded fetuses, will decrease the activity of complexes of the electron transport chain, which will generate increased levels of reactive oxygen species (ROS) (Esposti and McLennan 1998; Chandel et al. 1996; Gorgias et al. 1996). Overproduction of ROS initiates many oxidative reactions that lead to oxidative damage not only in the mitochondria but also in cellular proteins, lipids, and nucleic acids. Increased ROS levels inactivate the iron–sulfur centers of the electron transport chain complexes and tricarboxylic acid cycle aconitase, resulting in shutdown of mitochondrial energy production.

A key adaptation enabling the fetus to survive in a limited energy environment may be the reprogramming of mitochondrial function (Gorgias et al. 1996; Peterside et al. 2003, Selak et al. 2003). However, these alterations in mitochondrial function can have deleterious effects, especially in cells that have a high-energy requirement, such as the β-cell. The β-cell depends upon the normal production of adenosine triphosphate (ATP) for nutrient-induced insulin secretion (Panten et al. 1984; Newgard and McGarry 1995; Schuit 1997; Mertz et al. 1996; Ortsater et al. 2002; Antinozzi et al. 2002; Malaisse et al. 1980; Lenzen et al. 1986) and proliferation (Noda et al. 2002). Thus, an interruption of mitochondrial function can have profound consequences for the β-cell.

Mitochondrial dysfunction can also lead to increased production of ROS, which will lead to oxidative stress if the defense mechanisms of the cell are overwhelmed. β-cells are especially vulnerable to attacks by ROS because expression of antioxidant enzymes in pancreatic islets is very low (Lenzen et al. 1996; Tiedge et al. 1997), and β-cells have a high oxidative energy requirement. Increased ROS impair glucose-stimulated insulin secretion (Noda et al. 2002; Maechler et al. 1999; Sakai et al. 2003), decrease gene expression of key β-cell genes (Kaneto et al. 1999, 2001, 2002a, b; Jonas et al. 1999, 2001; Efanova et al. 1998), and induce cell death (Moran et al. 2000; Donath et al. 1999; Silva et al. 2000).

We have found that UPI induces oxidative stress and marked mitochondrial dysfunction in the fetal β-cell (Simmons et al. 2005). ATP production is impaired and continues to deteriorate with age. The activities of complexes I and III of the electron transport chain progressively decline in IUGR islets. Mitochondrial DNA (mtDNA) point mutations accumulate with age and are associated with decreased mtDNA content and reduced expression of mitochondrial-encoded genes in IUGR islets. Mitochondrial dysfunction results in impaired insulin secretion. These results demonstrate that UPI induces mitochondrial dysfunction in the fetal β-cell leading to increased production of ROS, which in turn damage mtDNA (Simmons et al. 2005). A self-reinforcing cycle of progressive deterioration in mitochondrial function leads to a corresponding decline in β-cell function. Finally, a threshold in mitochondrial dysfunction and ROS production is reached and diabetes ensues (Figure 5.1).

A maternal low protein (LP) diet also seems to program an increased vulnerability of the endocrine pancreas to oxidative stress (Merezak et al. 2001, 2004, Goosse et al. 2009). Antioxidant enzymatic activities are diminished in islets of the progeny and at 3 months, superoxide dismutase activity was increased in LP islets; however, there was no activation of catalase or glutathione peroxidase. This unbalance could lead to oxidative stress. Furthermore, islets from fetal and adult LP progeny showed a higher rate of apoptosis after cytokines or oxidative stress aggression in *in vitro* experiments (Merezak et al. 2001, 2004). Higher nitric oxide (NO) production by islets from adult LP offspring may be an important factor to explain this subsequent cell death (Goosse et al. 2009).

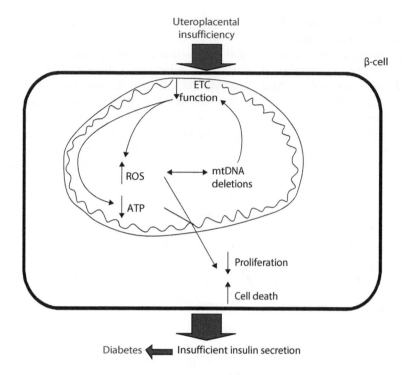

FIGURE 5.1   Decreased nutrient and oxygen availability to the fetus result in mitochondrial dysfunction which in turn results in increased production of reactive oxygen species (ROS) and decreased production of adenosine triphosphate (ATP). Mitochondrial dysfunction in key cells such as the β-cell in the pancreas decreases cell proliferation and increases cell death culminating in the development of type 2 diabetes.

5.4.4   MOLECULAR MECHANISMS: EPIGENETIC REGULATION

The metabolic or nutritional state of the organism directly influences epigenetic modifications, as essentially all known epigenetic modifications rely upon substrates derived from intermediary metabolism such as S-adenosyl methionine (SAM), acetyl CoA, α-ketoglutarate, and nicotinamide adenine dinucleotide (NAD⁺) (Kaelin and McKnight 2013). Studies in the IUGR rat demonstrate that fetal growth restriction induces epigenetic modifications of key genes regulating β-cell development (Park et al. 2008). Most notably, levels of *Pdx1* mRNA are reduced by more than 50% in UPI fetal rats as early as 24 hours after the onset of growth retardation and altered *Pdx1* expression persists after birth and progressively declines in the UPI animal. PDX1 is a homeodomain-containing transcription factor that plays a critical role in the early development of both endocrine and exocrine pancreas, and then in the later differentiation and function of the β-cell, making regulation of this target a key focus for understanding the pathological outcomes of UPI. Repression of *Pdx1* occurs in two waves, as early repression of this gene involves recruitment of the mSin3A histone deacetylase complex, followed later by Histone 3 lysine 9 (H3K9) dimethylation and eventual recruitment of dna methyltransferase 3A (DNMT3A) and cytosine methylation. Prior to cytosine methylation—at the neonatal stage—this epigenetic process is reversible and may define an important developmental window for therapeutic approaches. Indeed, early reversal of *Pdx1* deacetylation can prevent the onset of diabetes (Pinney et al. 2011), demonstrating that UPI-induced epigenetic modifications are responsible for the development of diabetes in this animal model (Figure 5.2).

Pdx1 represents one of the several key targets of epigenetic regulation that suffer long-term epigenetic reprogramming in response to maternal dietary conditions. For example, the pancreatic transcription factor *Hnf4α* is also epigenetically regulated

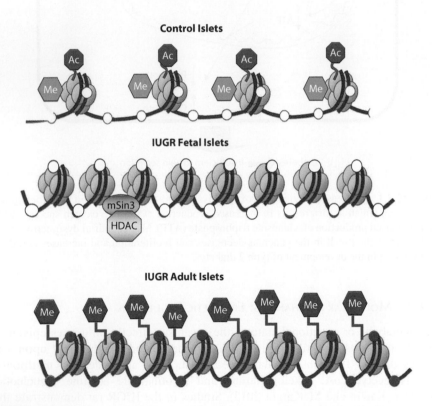

FIGURE 5.2 Summary of epigenetic changes at *Pdx1* in intrauterine growth restriction (IUGR) rats during the development of type 2 diabetes. In pancreatic β-cells (top), the *Pdx1* proximal promoter is normally found in an unmethylated (white circles) open chromatin state allowing access to transcription factors such as upstream stimulatory factor (USF)-1 and associated with nucleosomes characterized by acetylated (Ac) histones H3 and H4 and with trimethylated H3K4 (Me). In IUGR fetal and 2-week islets (middle), histone acetylation is progressively lost through association with an mSin3A–histone deacetylase (HDAC)1–DNA methyl transferase (DMT)1 repressor complex, with trimethylated H3K4 disappearing and dimethylated H3K9 appearing after birth. IUGR adult islets (bottom) are characterized by inactive chromatin with dimethylated H3K9 (Me) and extensive DNA methylation (dark gray circles) locking in the transcriptionally silent state of *Pdx1*.

by maternal diet and aging in rat islets from offspring of protein-restricted dams (Sandovici et al. 2011). Here, increased DNA methylation and repressive histone modifications at the P2 promoter of *Hnf4α* were linked to a significant reduction in expression, while reversal of DNA methylation and histone modifications could reactivate transcription of *Hnf4α* via the P2 promoter.

UPI also induces genome-wide changes in DNA methylation. In a previous study, using a novel method of assessment of genome-wide DNA methylation, *HpaII* tiny fragment enrichment by ligation-mediated polymerase chain reaction (PCR) (HELP) assay, we found that UPI in the rat causes consistent and nonrandom changes in cytosine methylation, affecting <1% of *HpaII* sites in the genome (Thompson et al. 2010). The majority of these changes take place not at promoters but at intergenic sequences, many of which are evolutionarily conserved. Furthermore, some of these loci are in proximity to genes manifesting concordant changes in gene expression and are enriched near genes that regulate processes that are markedly impaired in UPI islets (e.g., vascularization, proliferation, insulin secretion, and cell death). This epigenomic dysregulation precedes the development of diabetes and is therefore a potential mediator of the pathogenesis of the disease, preserving cellular memory of the long antecedent intrauterine event. Finally, our identification of differential methylation at conserved intergenic and potentially *cis*-regulatory sites emphasizes the limitations of study designs that focus solely on promoters and/or CpG islands. We showed that changes in methylation, even when not located at promoters, are correlated with transcriptional changes at adjacent genes, consistent with suggestions from previous studies (Irizarry et al. 2009).

There are numerous studies in humans examining the relationship between fetal nutrient availability and epigenetic modifications in the offspring (Rakyan et al. 2011). Many of these are confounded by small sample size, cellular heterogeneity of tissues examined, and lack of validation. Moreover, most DNA methylation assays are performed in total peripheral blood monocytes, where the unique methylation profiles of the various cellular lineages complicate interpretation of the data. Despite these issues, multiple studies in diverse populations repeatedly show changes in DNA methylation associated with low birth weight and/or altered nutrient availability. Thus, it is likely that an adverse *in utero* milieu does indeed induce epigenetic modifications in the offspring, but whether these modifications have biological relevance remains to be determined. The field of "epigenetic epidemiology" remains an active and a growing field of investigation.

5.5   CONCLUSIONS

The combined epidemiological, clinical, and animal studies clearly demonstrate that the intrauterine environment influences both growth and development of the fetus and the subsequent development of adult diseases. There are specific critical windows during development, often coincident with periods of rapid cell division, during which a stimulus or insult may have long-lasting consequences on tissue or organ function postnatally. Studies using animal models suggest that mitochondrial dysfunction and oxidative stress are linked to epigenetic modifications, which in turn play a pivotal role in the pathogenesis of the fetal origins of adult disease.

The near future promises advances on at least three fronts. First, the burgeoning field of epigenetic epidemiology is in its early days, but surveys of epigenetic marks in children who experience adverse placental environments promise to yield a wealth of knowledge regarding the mechanisms responsible for long-term metabolic reprogramming. A number of potential issues with extant studies exist, as for example, birth weight is only one marker of an adverse fetal environment and confining studies to this population only may lead to erroneous conclusions regarding etiology. But this approach has great promise, particularly as it grows in scope and sophistication. Second, advances in epigenomics and in epigenetic "editing" in model organisms should continue to provide mechanistic insights regarding the molecular basis for Developmental Origins of Health and Disease (DOHaD) and to offer fundamental insights into early development. Finally, correction of metabolic abnormalities will of course be one of the key goals for future efforts, as mitochondrial function and even epigenetic marks remain more promising candidates for therapeutic intervention than one's genomic sequence, at least for the foreseeable future.

REFERENCES

Anderson AH, Fennessey PV, Meschia G et al. Placental transport of threonine and its utilization in the normal and growth-restricted fetus. *Am J Physiol*. 1997;272:E892–E900.

Antinozzi PA, Ishihara H, Newgard CB et al. Mitochondrial metabolism sets the maximal limit of fuel-stimulated insulin secretion in a model pancreatic beta cell. A survey of four fuel secretagogues. *J Biol Chem*. 2002;277:11746–11755.

Bell AW, Wilkening RB, Meschia G. Some aspects of placental function in chronically heat-stressed ewes. *J Dev Physiol*. 1987;9:17–29.

Béringue F, Blondeau B, Castellotti MC et al. Endocrine pancreas development in growth-retarded human fetuses. *Diabetes*. 2002;51:385–391.

Bernardo AS, Hay CW, Docherty K. Pancreatic transcription factors and their role in the birth, life and survival of the pancreatic beta cell. *Mol Cell Endocrinol*. 2008;294:1–9.

Berney DM, Desai M, Palmer DJ et al. The effects of maternal protein deprivation on the fetal rat pancreas: Major structural changes and their recuperation. *J Pathol*. 1997;183:109–115.

Bertin E, Gangnerau MN, Bailbe D et al. Glucose metabolism and β-cell mass in adult offspring of rats protein and/or energy restricted during the last week of pregnancy. *Am J Physiol*. 1999;277:E11–E17.

Boloker J, Gertz SJ, Simmons RA. Gestational diabetes leads to the development of diabetes in adulthood in the rat. *Diabetes*. 2002;51:1499–1506.

Bonner-Weir S. Perspective: Postnatal pancreatic β-cell growth. *Endocrinology*. 2000;141:1926–1929.

Boujendar S, Arany E, Hill D et al. Taurine supplementation of a low protein diet fed to rat dams normalizes the vascularization of the fetal endocrine pancreas. *J Nutr*. 2003;133:2820–2825.

Bowen RS, Moodley J, Dutton MF et al. Oxidative stress in pre-eclampsia. *Acta Obstet Gynecol Scand*. 2001;80:719–725.

Chandel NS, Budinger GRS, Schumacker PT. Molecular oxygen modulates cytochrome c oxidase function. *J Biol Chem*. 1996;271:8672–18677.

Christofori G, Naik P, Hanahan D. Vascular endothelial growth factor and its receptors, flt-1 and flk-1, are expressed in normal pancreatic islets and throughout islet cell tumorigenesis. *Mol Endocrinol*. 1995;9:1760–1770.

Dahri S, Snoeck A, Reusens-Billen B et al. Islet function in off-spring of mothers on low protein diet during gestation. *Diabetes*. 1991;40:115–120.

Donath MY, Gross DJ, Cerasi E et al. Hyperglycemia-induced β-cell apoptosis in pancreatic islets of Psammomys obesus during development of diabetes. *Diabetes*. 1999;48:738–744.

Dumortier O, Blondeau B, Duvillié B et al. Different mechanisms operating during different critical time-windows reduce rat fetal beta cell mass due to a maternal low protein or low-energy diet. *Diabetologia*. 2007;50:2495–2503.

Efanova IB, Zaitsev SV, Zhivotovsky B et al. Glucose and tolbutamide induce apoptosis in pancreatic β-cells. *J Biol Chem*. 1998;273:22501–22507.

Ejima K, Nanri H, Toki N et al. Localization of thioredoxin reductase and thioredoxin in normal human placenta and their protective effect against oxidative stress. *Placenta*. 1999;20:95–101.

Esposti MD, McLennan, H. Mitochondria and cells produce reactive oxygen species in virtual anaerobiosis: Relevance to ceramide-induced apoptosis. *FEBS Lett*. 1998;430:338–342.

Ferrara N. Vascular endothelial growth factor: Basic science and clinical progress. *Endocr Rev*. 2004;25:581–611.

Ferrara N, Houck K, Jakeman L et al. Molecular and biological properties of the vascular endothelial growth factor family of proteins. *Endocr Rev*. 1992;13:18–32.

Galan HL, Hussey MJ, Barbera A et al. Relationship of fetal growth to duration of heat stress in an ovine model of placental insufficiency. *Am J Obstet Gynecol*.1999;180:1278–1282.

Garofano A, Czernichow P, Bréant B. In utero undernutrition impairs rat beta-cell development. *Diabetologia*. 1997;40:1231–1234.

Garofano A, Czernichow P, Bréant B. Beta-cell mass and proliferation following late fetal and early postnatal malnutrition in the rat. *Diabetologia*. 1998;41:1114–1120.

Garofano A, Czernichow P, Bréant B. Effect of ageing on beta-cell mass and function in rats malnourished during the perinatal period. *Diabetologia*. 1999;42:711–718.

Goosse K, Bouckenooghe T, Balteau M et al. Implication of nitric oxide in the increased islet-cells vulnerability of adult progeny from protein-restricted mothers and its prevention by taurine. *J Endocrinol*. 2009;200:177–187.

Gorgias N, Maidatsi P, Tsolaki M et al. Hypoxic pretreatment protects against neuronal damage of the rat hippocampus induced by severe hypoxia. *Brain Res*. 1996;714:215–225.

Habener JF, Kemp DM, Thomas MK. Minireview: Transcriptional regulation in pancreatic development. *Endocrinology*. 2005;146:1025–1034.

Hales CN, Barker DJ. Type 2 (non-insulin-dependent) diabetes mellitus: The thrifty phenotype hypothesis. *Diabetologia*. 1992;35:595–601.

Hales CN, Barker DJ. The thrifty phenotype hypothesis. *Br Med Bull*. 2001;60:5–20.

Ham JN, Crutchlow MF, Desai BM et al. Exendin-4 normalizes islet vascularity in intrauterine growth restricted rats: Potential role of VEGF. *Pediatr Res*. 2009;66:42–46.

Harding JE, Jones CT, Robinson JS. Studies on experimental growth retardation in sheep. The effects of a small placenta in restricting transport to and growth of the fetus. *J Dev Physiol*. 1985;7:427–442.

Henderson JR, Moss MC. A morphometric study of the endocrine and exocrine capillaries of the pancreas. *Q J Exp Physiol*. 1985 Jul;70(3):347–356.

Heywood WE, Mian N, Milla PJ et al. Programming of defective rat pancreatic beta-cell function in offspring from mothers fed a low protein diet during gestation and the suckling periods. *Clin Sci*. 2004;07:37–45.

Irizarry RA, Ladd-Acosta C, Wen B et al. The human colon cancer methylome shows similar hypo and hypermethylation at conserved tissue-specific CpG island shores. *Nat Genet*. 2009 Feb;41(2):178–186.

Jaeckle Santos LJ, Li C, Doulias PT et al. Neutralizing Th2 inflammation in neonatal islets prevents β-cell failure in adult IUGR rats. *Diabetes.* 2014;63:1672–1684.

Jaquet D, Gaboriau A, Czernichow P et al. Insulin resistance early in adulthood in subjects born with intrauterine growth retardation. *J Clin Endocrinol Metab.* 2000;85:1401–1406.

Jensen CB, Storgaard H, Dela F et al. Early differential defects of insulin secretion and action in 19-year-old Caucasian men who had low birth weight. *Diabetes.* 2002;51:1271–1280.

Jonas JC, Laybutt DR, Steil GM et al. High glucose stimulates early response gene c-Myc expression in rat pancreatic beta cells. *J Biol Chem.* 2001;276:35375–35381.

Jonas JC, Sharma A, Hasenkamp W et al. Chronic hyperglycemia triggers loss of pancreatic beta cell differentiation in an animal model of diabetes. *J Biol Chem.* 1999;274:14112–14121.

Jonsson J, Carlsson L, Edlund T et al. Insulin-promoter-factor 1 is required for pancreas development in mice. *Nature.* 1994;371:606–609.

Kaelin WG, Jr, McKnight SL. Influence of metabolism on epigenetics and disease. *Cell.* 2013;153:56–69.

Kaneto H, Kajimoto Y, Fujitani Y et al. Oxidative stress iwnduces p21 expression in pancreatic islet cells: Possible implication in beta-cell dysfunction. *Diabetologia.* 1999;42:1093–1097.

Kaneto H, Xu G, Fujii N et al. Involvement of c-Jun N-terminal kinase in oxidative stress-mediated suppression of insulin gene expression. *J Biol Chem.* 2002a;277:30010–30018.

Kaneto HH, Xu G, Fujii N et al. Involvement of protein kinase C beta 2 in c-myc induction by high glucose in pancreatic beta-cells. *J Biol Chem.* 2002b;277:3680–3685.

Kaneto H, Xu G, Song KH et al. Activation of the hexosamine pathway leads to deterioration of pancreatic beta-cell function through the induction of oxidative stress. *J Biol Chem.* 2001;276:31099–31104.

Karowicz-Bilinska A, Suzin J, Sieroszewski, P. Evaluation of oxidative stress indices during treatment in pregnant women with intrauterine growth retardation. *Med Sci Monit.* 2002;8:CR211–CR216.

Kato H, Yoneyama Y, Araki T. Fetal plasma lipid peroxide levels in pregnancies complicated by preeclampsia. *Gynecol Obstet Invest.* 1997;43:158–161.

Kermack WO, McKendrick AG, McKinlay PL. Death-rates in Great Britain and Sweden: Expression of specific mortality rates as products of two factors, and some consequences thereof. *J Hyg.* 1934;34:433–457.

Kind KL, Owens JA, Robinson JS et al. Effect of restriction of placental growth on expression of IGFs in fetal sheep: Relationship to fetal growth, circulating IGFs and binding proteins. *J Endocrinol.* 1995;146:23–34.

Lenzen S, Drinkgern J, Tiedge M. Low antioxidant enzyme gene expression in pancreatic islets compared with various other mouse tissues. *Free Radic Biol Med.* 1996;20:463–466.

Lenzen S, Schmidt W, Rustenbeck I et al. 2-Ketoglutarate generation in pancreatic β-cell mitochondria regulates insulin secretory action of amino acids and 2-keto acids. *Biosci Rep.* 1986;6:163–169.

Leung DW, Cachianes G, Kuang WJ et al. Vascular endothelial growth factor is a secreted angiogenic mitogen. *Science.* 1989 Dec 8;246(4935):1306–1309.

Limesand SW, Jensen J, Hutton JC et al. Diminished β-cell replication contributes to reduced β-cell mass in fetal sheep with intrauterine growth restriction. *Am J Physiol.* 2005;288:R1297–R1305.

Limesand SW, Rozance PJ, Zerbe GO et al. Attenuated insulin release and storage in fetal sheep pancreatic islets with intrauterine growth restriction. *Endocrinology.* 2006;147:1488–1497.

Lumey L, Stein AD, Kahn HS et al. Cohort profile: The Dutch Hunger winter families study. *Int J Epidemiol.* 2007;36:1196–1204.

Maechler P, Jornot L, Wollheim CB. Hydrogen peroxide alters mitochondrial activation and insulin secretion in pancreatic beta cells. *J Biol Chem.* 1999;274:27905–27913.

Malaisse WJ, Hutton JC, Carpinelli AR et al. The stimulus-secretion coupling of amino acid-induced insulin release. Metabolism and cationic effects of leucine. *Diabetes.* 1980;29:431–437.

Merezak S, Hardikar AA, Yajnik CS et al. Intrauterine low protein diet increases fetal beta-cell sensitivity to NO and IL-1 beta: The protective role of taurine. *J Endocrinol.* 2001;171:299–308.

Merezak S, Reusens B, Renard A et al. Effect of maternal low protein diet and taurine on the vulnerability of adult Wistar rat islets to cytokines. *Diabetologia.* 2004;47:669–675.

Mericq V, Ong KK, Bazaes R et al. Longitudinal changes in insulin sensitivity and secretion from birth to age three years in small-and appropriate-for-gestational-age children. *Diabetologia.* 2005;48:2609–2614.

Mertz RJ, Worley JF, III, Spencer B et al. Activation of stimulus-secretion coupling in pancreatic β-cells by specific products of glucose metabolism. *J Biol Chem.* 1996;271:4838–4845.

Moran A, Zhang HJ, Olsonm LK et al. Differentiation of glucose toxicity from β-cell exhaustion during the evolution of defective insulin gene expression in the pancreatic islet cell line, HIT-T15. *J Clin Invest.* 2000;99:534–539.

Myatt L, Eis ALW, Brockman DE et al. Differential localization of superoxide dismutase isoforms in placental villous tissue of normotensive, pre-eclamptic, and intrauterine growth-restricted pregnancies. *J Histochem Cytochem.* 1997;45:1433–1438.

Newgard CB, McGarry JD. Metabolic coupling factors in pancreatic β-cell signal transduction. *Annu Rev Biochem.* 1995;64:689–719.

Nicolini U, Hubinot C, Santolaya J et al. Effects of fetal intravenous glucose challenge in normal and growth retarded fetuses. *Hormone Metab Res.* 1990;22:426–430.

Noda M, Yamashita S, Takahashi N et al. Switch to anaerobic glucose metabolism with NADH accumulation in the beta-cell model of mitochondrial diabetes. Characteristics of betaHC9 cells deficient in mitochondrial DNA transcription. *J Biol Chem.* 2002;277:41817–41826.

Oberg C, Waltenberger J, Claesson-Welsh L et al. Expression of protein tyrosine kinases in islet cells: Possible role of the Flk-1 receptor for beta-cell maturation from duct cells. *Growth Factors.* 1994;10(2):115–126.

Offield MF, Jetton TL, Labosky PA et al. PDX-1 is required for pancreatic outgrowth and differentiation of the rostral duodenum. *Development.* 1996;122:983–995.

Ogata ES, Bussey ME, Finley S. Altered gas exchange, limited glucose and branched chain amino acids, and hypoinsulinism retard fetal growth in the rat. *Metabolism.* 1986;35:970–977.

Ortsater H, Liss P, Akerman KEO. Contribution of glycolytic and mitochondrial pathways in glucose-induced changes in islet respiration and insulin secretion. *Pflugers Arch Eur J Physiol.* 2002;444:506–512.

Owens JA, Falconer J, Robinson JS. Effect of restriction of placental growth on fetal and utero-placental metabolism. *J Dev Physiol.* 1987;9:225–238.

Owens JA, Falconer J, Robinson JS. Glucose metabolism in pregnant sheep when placental growth is restricted. *Am J Physiol.* 1989;257:R350–R357.

Owens JA, Kind KL, Carbone F et al. Circulating insulin-like growth factors-I and -II and substrates in fetal sheep following restriction of placental growth. *J Endocrinol.* 1994;140:5–13.

Owens JA, Gatford KL, De Blasio MJ et al. Restriction of placental growth in sheep impairs insulin secretion but not sensitivity before birth. *J Physiol.* 2007;584:935–949.

Panten U, Zielman S, Langer J et al. Regulation of insulin secretion by energy metabolism in pancreatic β-cell mitochondria. *Biochem J*. 1984;219:189–196.

Park JH, Stoffers DA, Nicholls RD et al. Development of type 2 diabetes following intrauterine growth retardation in rats is associated with progressive epigenetic silencing of Pdx1. *J Clin Invest*. 2008;118:2316–2324.

Peterside IE, Selak MA, Simmons RA. Impaired oxidative phosphorylation in hepatic mitochondria of growth retarded rats alters glucose metabolism. *Am J Physiol*. 2003;285:E1258–E1264.

Petrik J, Reusens B, Arany E et al. A low protein diet alters the balance of islet cell replication and apoptosis in the fetal and neonatal rat and is associated with a reduced pancreatic expression of insulin-like growth factor-II. *Endocrinology*. 1999 Oct;140(10):4861–4873.

Petry CJ, Dorling MW, Pawlak DB et al. Diabetes in old male offspring of rat dams fed a reduced protein diet. *Int J Exp Diabetes Res*. 2001;2:139–143.

Phillips ID, Simonetta G, Owens JA et al. Placental restriction alters the functional development of the pituitary-adrenal axis in the sheep fetus during late gestation. *Pediatr Res*. 1996 Dec;40(6):861–866.

Pinney SE, Jaeckle Santos LJ, Han Y et al. Exendin-4 increases histone acetylase activity and reverses epigenetic modifications that silence Pdx1 in the intrauterine growth retarded rat. *Diabetologia*. 2011;54:2606–2614.

Rakyan VK, Down TA, Balding DJ et al. Epigenome-wide association studies for common human diseases. *Nat Rev Genet*. 2011;12:529–541.

Ranjan AK, Joglekar MV, Hardikar AA. Endothelial cells in pancreatic islet development and function. *Islets*. 2009 Jul-Aug;1(1):2–9.

Ravelli AC, van der Meulen JH, Michels RP et al. Glucose tolerance in adults after prenatal exposure to famine. *Lancet* 1998; 17;351(9097):173–177.

Ravelli GP, Stein ZA, Susser MW. Obesity in young men after famine exposure in utero and early infancy. *New Engl J Med*. 1976;295, 349–353.

Robinson JS, Kingston EJ, Jones CT et al. Studies on experimental growth retardation in sheep. The effect of removal of endometrial caruncles on fetal size and metabolism. *J Dev Physiol*.1979;1:379–398.

Rooman I, Schuit F, Bouwens L. Effect of vascular endothelial growth factor on growth and differentiation of pancreatic ductal epithelium. *Lab Invest*. 1997;76:225–232.

Ross JC, Fennessey PV, Wilkening RB et al. Placental transport and fetal utilization of leucine in a model of fetal growth retardation. *Am J Physiol*.1996;270:E491–E503.

Rozance PJ, Anderson M, Martinez M et al. Placental insufficiency decreases pancreatic vascularity and disrupts hepatocyte growth factor signaling in the pancreatic islet endothelial cell in fetal sheep. *Diabetes*. 2015;64:555–564.

Rozance PJ, Hay WW Jr. Pancreatic islet hepatocyte growth factor and vascular endothelial growth factor A signaling in growth restricted fetuses. *Mol Cell Endocrinol*. 2016 Nov 5;435:78–84.

Sakai K, Matsumoto K, Nishikawa T et al. Mitochondrial reactive oxygen species reduce insulin secretion by pancreatic β-cells. *Biochem Biophys Res Comm*. 2003;300:216–222.

Sandovici I, Smith NH, Nitert MD et al. Maternal diet and aging alter the epigenetic control of a promoter-enhancer interaction at the Hnf4a gene in rat pancreatic islets. *Proc Natl Acad Sci USA*. 2011;108:5449–5454.

Schuit, F. Metabolic fate of glucose in purified islet cells. Glucose regulated anaplerosis in β-cells. *J Biol Chem*. 1997;272:18572–18579.

Selak MA, Storey BT, Peterside IE et al. Impaired oxidative phosphorylation in skeletal muscle contributes to insulin resistance and hyperglycemia. *Am J Physiol*. 2003;285:E130–E137.

Silva JP, Kohler M, Graff C et al. Impaired insulin secretion and β-cell loss in tissue specific knockout mice with mitochondrial diabetes. *Nat Genet*. 2000;26:336–340.

Simmons RA, Gounis AS, Bangalore SA, Ogata ES. Intrauterine growth retardation: Fetal glucose transport is diminished in lung but spared in brain. *Pediatr Res* 1992 31:59-63.

Simmons RA, Suponitsky-Kroyter I, Selak MA. Progressive accumulation of mitochondrial DNA mutations and decline in mitochondrial function lead to β-cell failure. *J Biol Chem*. 2005;280:28785–28791.

Simmons RA, Templeton LJ, Gertz SJ. Intrauterine growth retardation leads to the development of type 2 diabetes in the rat. *Diabetes*. 2001;50:2279–2286.

Snoeck A, Remacle C, Reusens B et al. Effect of a low protein diet during pregnancy on the fetal rat endocrine pancreas. *Biol Neonate*. 1990;57:107–118.

Stoffers DA, Desai BM, DeLeon DD et al. Neonatal exendin-4 prevents the development of diabetes in the intrauterine growth retarded rat. *Diabetes*. 2003;52:734–740.

Stoffers DA, Ferrer J, Clarke WL et al. Early-onset type-II diabetes mellitus (MODY4) linked to IPF1. *Nat Genet*. 1997a;17:138–139.

Stoffers DA, Zinkin NT, Stanojevic V et al. Pancreatic agenesis attributable to a single nucleotide deletion in the human IPF1 gene coding sequence. *Nat Genet*. 1997b 15:106–110.

Thieme H, Aiello LP, Takagi H et al. Comparative analysis of vascular endothelial growth factor receptors on retinal and aortic vascular endothelial cells. *Diabetes*. 1995 Jan;44(1):98–103.

Thompson RF, Fazzari MJ, Niu H et al. Experimental intrauterine growth restriction induces alterations in DNA methylation and gene expression in pancreatic islets of rats. *J Biol Chem*. 2010;285:15111–15118.

Thureen PJ, Trembler KA, Meschia G et al. Placental glucose transport in heat-induced fetal growth retardation. *Am J Physiol*.1992;263:R578–R585.

Tiedge M, Lortz S, Drinkgern J et al. Relationship between antioxidant enzyme gene expression and antioxidant defense status of insulin-producing cells. *Diabetes*. 1997;46:1733–1742.

Unterman TG, Simmons RA, Glick RP et al. Circulating levels of insulin, insulin-like growth factor-I (IGF-I), IGF-II, and IGF-binding proteins in the small for gestational age fetal rat. *Endocrinology*. 1993;132:327–336.

Valdez R, Athens MA, Thompson GH et al. Birthweight and adult health outcomes in a biethnic population in the USA. *Diabetologia*. 1994;37:624–631.

Van Assche FA, De Prins F, Aerts L et al. The endocrine pancreas in small-for-dates infants. *Br J Obstet Gynaecol*.1977;84:751–753.

Vasir B, Jonas JC, Steil GM et al. Gene expression of VEGF and its receptors Flk-1/KDR and Flt-1 in cultured and transplanted rat islets. *Transplantation*. 2001;71:924–935.

Veening MA, van Weissenbruch MM, Heine RJ et al. β-cell capacity and insulin sensitivity in prepubertal children born small for gestational age. Influence of body size during childhood. *Diabetes*. 2003;52:1756–1760.

Wang Y, Walsh SW. Placental mitochondria as a source of oxidative stress in pre-eclampsia. *Placenta*. 1998;19:581–586.

Wang Y, Walsh SW. Increased superoxide generation is associated with decreased superoxide dismutase activity and mRNA expression in placental trophoblast cells in pre-eclampsia. *Placenta*. 2001;22:206–212.

Wilson MR, Hughes SJ. The effect of maternal protein deficiency during pregnancy and lactation on glucose tolerance and pancreatic islet function in adult rat offspring. *J Endocrinol*. 1997;154:177–185.

6 Regulation of Skeletal Muscle GLUT4 in Intrauterine Growth Restriction Offspring

Bo-Chul Shin and Sherin U. Devaskar

CONTENTS

6.1 INTRODUCTION

Glucose is the major energy source for mammalian cells as well as an important substrate for protein and lipid synthesis. Mammalian cells take up glucose from extracellular fluid into the cell through glucose transporters (Zhao and Keating 2007). The mammalian genome contains 14 isoforms of the glut family exhibiting tissue-specific expression (Scheepers et al. 2004; Wu and Freeze 2002; Joost and Thorens 2001; Takata et al. 1997). In healthy individuals, despite alternating periods of fasting and feeding, plasma glucose levels are primarily well maintained within a narrow range under the hormonal action of insulin and glucagon and other counterregulatory hormones that regulate concentrations of blood glucose in living organisms (Govers 2014). A specific insulin-responsive isoform of the facilitative glucose transporter protein family, glucose transporter protein 4 (GLUT4), is mainly expressed in fat and skeletal muscle cells and is essential in maintaining glucose homeostasis (Cushman and Wardzala 1980; Suzuki and Kono 1980).

Insulin is a hormone that plays a key role in the regulation of blood glucose concentrations. In the absence of insulin, the basal membrane permeability for glucose is low because GLUT4 is excluded from the plasma membrane and is localized in vesicles inside the cell. In this case, most GLUT4 is localized in GLUT4 storage compartments, early endosomes, and tubulovesicular structures within cells (Holman and Cushman 1994). Under insulin stimulation, insulin activates the intracellular signaling cascades, with a fraction of intracellular GLUT4-containing tubulovesicular membranes fusing with the plasma membrane, thus delivering GLUT4 to the surface of the cells (Thoidis and Kandror 2001; Cushman and Wardzala 1980; Suzuki and Kono 1980). This leads to a dramatic increase in glucose uptake by translocation of GLUT4 from the intracellular tubulovesicular elements into the plasma membrane (Slot et al. 1991; Ozanne et al. 2003). In healthy normal conditions, this process is readily reversible such that when insulin concentrations decline, GLUT4 transporters are separated from the plasma membrane by endocytosis and are recycled back to their intracellular storage compartments. In this way, the primary mechanism of insulin action in GLUT4 translocation is to stimulate tethering and fusion of trafficking vesicles to specific fusion sites in the plasma membrane (Ozanne et al. 2003; Koumanov et al. 2005). However, under a lack of insulin, or an inability to adequately respond to insulin at the target sites of action, symptoms of diabetes mellitus ensue.

In the case of reduced systemic insulin concentrations, exogenous insulin administration brings about recovery from abnormal to normal glucose homeostasis affected by normalizing the physiological GLUT4 translocation process, as is seen in type 1 diabetes mellitus. On the other hand, when a lack of response to exogenous insulin is encountered due to insulin resistance, an ineffective GLUT4 translocation contributes toward this metabolic outcome of type 2 diabetes mellitus. In response to oxidative stress, GLUT4 also translocates from intracellular vesicles to the plasma membrane (Horie et al. 2008). In addition to insulin, exercise also causes translocation of GLUT4 from an intracellular location to the plasma membrane in skeletal muscle via activation of adenosine monophosphate (AMP) kinase (Sherman et al. 1996).

GLUT4 can also be regulated at the messenger RNA (mRNA) level. Glut4 mRNA was reduced by fasting (40%) in the skeletal muscle of 2-month-old rats under 48 hours of fasting, and increased by *in vitro* incubation with insulin (25%) or insulin plus glucose (Silva et al. 2005). Interestingly, a decline in skeletal muscle GLUT4 expression and protein concentrations was noted in intrauterine growth-restricted (IUGR) rats as well in response to maternal calorie restriction (CR) (Thamotharan et al. 2005). Therefore, glut4 gene expression or transcriptional activity has a profound impact on insulin-mediated glucose disposal making it essential to understand the underlying mechanisms toward creating future therapies. In this chapter, we focus on the transcriptional and posttranscriptional aspects of GLUT4 and the impact of such regulation on its function mainly in the IUGR offspring.

6.2   INTRAUTERINE GROWTH RESTRICTION (IUGR) OFFSPRING

The placenta is a major organ that interfaces between the mother and fetus, carrying oxygen and nutrients into the developing baby. Intrauterine environment exposed to placental insufficiency or poor maternal energy intake such as hypoxia, malnutrition, and high blood pressure during pregnancy affects fetal growth resulting in low birth weight. Other causes of IUGR may include congenital anomalies, infections, or drug and substance misuse (Figueras and Gardosi 2010; Wu et al. 2006; Jang et al. 2015; Dunlop et al. 2015; Neitzke et al. 2011). IUGR is distinctly different from small for gestational age (SGA). Newborn infants whose estimated body weight is below the 10th percentile for gestational age constitute the definition of SGA (Battaglia and Lubchenco 1967; Tuuli et al. 2011). The birth weight of an infant is a critical anticipatory factor that preempts survival, postnatal growth, and further development (Figueras and Gardosi 2010; Jang et al. 2015; Hay et al. 2016; Tuuli et al. 2011). On the other hand, IUGR, which signifies intrauterine deceleration of growth, is a main factor that may result in late fetal loss, morbidity, and mortality (Battaglia and Lubchenco 1967; Hay et al. 2016; Froen et al. 2004; McIntire et al. 1999). Specifically, morbidity and mortality are significantly high among term infants who are below the third percentile for weight at gestational age (McIntire et al. 1999). In addition, IUGR lends itself toward a predisposition for developing metabolic disorders in later life by aberrations in metabolic activity that may be permanent or programmed (Hales and Barker 2001; Barker 1997). An IUGR offspring is susceptible for developing cardiovascular disease (Barker 1997; Barker et al. 1993; Holemans et al. 2003; Barker and Osmond 1986), hypertension, insulin resistance, and obesity with type 2 diabetes mellitus (Barker et al. 1993; Simmons et al. 2001; Ozanne and Hales 2002; Berends and Ozanne 2012; Stocker et al. 2005; Wolf 2003; Morrison et al. 2010). Diabetes mellitus is one of the leading chronic diseases in almost every country. By studies designed to determine global diabetes prevalence among adults (20–79 years) for 216 countries between 2010 and 2030, it was estimated that the percentage of the population with diabetes mellitus will increase from 6.4% in 2010 to 7.7% by 2030. Specially, the number of diabetic adults will increase to 69% in developing countries, in comparison with 20% in developed countries (Shaw et al. 2010).

Given these staggering numbers, we embarked on establishing a cause-and-effect paradigm between IUGR and long-term effects. To this end, we adapted an IUGR rat model as a surrogate for the IUGR human infant to enable study of long-term and transgenerational consequences. The model employed was a maternal malnutrition model consisting of 50% caloric restriction beginning in midgestation through late gestation. This dietary manipulation resulted in IUGR with low birth weights of pups (Garg et al. 2012; Thamotharan et al. 2005). The postnatal and adult IUGR and postnatal growth-restricted offspring demonstrated changes in hepatic circadian genes (Freije et al. 2015), histone code modifications, subcellular localization, and translocation of skeletal muscle GLUT4 (Thamotharan et al. 2005; Tsirka et al. 2001; Raychaudhuri et al. 2008) due to maladaptation of postreceptor signaling molecules (Thamotharan et al. 2003; Abbasi et al. 2012; Oak et al. 2006). Glucose intolerance and lipid metabolic maladaptation (Dai et al. 2012; Tomi et al. 2013; Garg et al. 2006, 2012, 2013a) due to hepatopancreatic aberrations were observed along with deranged leptin signaling affecting hypothalamic neuropeptides that control appetite and energy expenditure thereby ultimately culminating in obesity (Gibson et al. 2015; Shin et al. 2014; Garg et al. 2013a).

6.3   GLUT4 GENE MANIPULATION

The normal plasma glucose concentration varies between 4 and 7 mM in normal individuals despite periods of feeding and fasting (Saltiel and Kahn 2001). Insulin resistance as related to type 2 diabetes resulting later in life due to IUGR consists of failure to stimulate trafficking of GLUT4 in fat and muscle. This aberration in GLUT4 translocation results in hyperglycemia and vascular and cardiovascular problems with abnormalities in insulin-dependent glucose utilization (James et al. 1988; Mueckler and Holman 1995). Lessons for this condition can be learned from genetically manipulated mouse models. Glut4-deficient mice without mediators of glucose transport in muscle and adipose tissue showed impaired insulin tolerance and glucose metabolism more so in females than in males. These mice displayed characteristics of a shortened lifespan, cardiac hypertrophy with increased glut1 expression in heart, and enhanced susceptibility to fatigue with reduced muscle carbohydrate stores (Katz et al. 1996; Gorselink et al. 2002; Wallberg-Henriksson and Zierath 2001). In contrast, transgenic mice overexpressing glut4 in skeletal muscle demonstrated improved glucose homeostasis in streptozotocin-induced diabetic mice, but failed to reverse the diabetic phenotype caused by insulinopenia with high blood glucose concentrations (Wallberg-Henriksson and Zierath 2001; Ikemoto et al. 1995). Interestingly, male glut4+/– mice with decreased glut4 expression in adipose tissue and skeletal muscle do not develop obesity or reduced muscle glucose uptake and hypertension as seen in humans with noninsulin-dependent diabetes mellitus, although increased circulating glucose and insulin concentrations exist (Stenbit et al. 1997; Tsao et al. 1999). Thus, in these glut4 heterozygous null mice, a 50% reduction in glut4 expression is noted. In our IUGR rat model (Thamotharan et al. 2005) decreased glut4 expression is seen on a physiological basis. This may be a useful model for characterizing the development of insulin resistance due to an IUGR beginning. IUGR offspring born to mothers exposed to prenatal nutrient restriction, regardless of postnatal nutritional alteration, showed a metabolic maladaptation related to skeletal muscle GLUT4 reduction, glucose intolerance, and the insulin resistance of GLUT4 translocation predisposing toward adult-onset chronic diseases (Thamotharan et al. 2005; Garg et al. 2013a). In this review, we focus on skeletal muscle GLUT4 aberrations and remedies as observed specifically in the IUGR offspring.

6.4   SIGNALING NECESSARY FOR INDUCING GLUT4 TRANSLOCATION IN IUGR

Skeletal muscle is composed of ~30–39% of an adult human body mass, although aging is associated with a preferential decrease (Janssen et al. 2000), and represents 85% of the total body glucose utilization, forming a primary location for insulin-stimulated glucose uptake (DeFronzo et al. 1981). In IUGR fetus, reduction of muscle mass or change of fiber composition may especially contribute to the increased risk of obesity or related metabolic complications seen as insulin resistance in aging IUGR individuals (Yates et al. 2014; Wells et al. 2007; Jensen et al. 2007). In addition, skeletal muscle plays a critical role in the regulation of metabolic homeostasis because it expresses an insulin responsive protein, GLUT4.

As a major hormone of metabolic regulation, insulin maintains a glucose homeostatic balance through translocation of GLUT4 containing intracellular vesicles in skeletal muscle to the sarcolemma. Insulin activates a number of intracellular signaling proteins such as insulin receptor substrate (IRS), phosphatidylinositol-3-kinases (PI3-kinases), pyruvate dehydrogenase kinase 1 (PDK1), protein kinase C (PKC), and protein kinase B (PKB or AKT) that ultimately facilitate GLUT4 translocation.

Under normal physiological conditions, when insulin binds to the insulin receptor (IR), GLUT4 translocates from intracellular pools to the cell surface, and fuses with the cell membrane, resulting in facilitating glucose transport into cells. In general, in insulin responsive tissues such as the skeletal muscle, insulin binds to the IR on the cell membrane and activates the tyrosine kinase domain of the receptor. The receptor then phosphorylates and afterward recruits IRS1/IRS2. Consequently, the phosphatidylinositol-3-kinase (PI3 kinase) enzyme with the Src homology 2 (SH2) domain binds to the Tyr phosphorylated IRS. PI3 kinase, AKT, and PDK1 regulate GLUT4 translocation to the plasma membrane (Alam et al. 2016; Alvim et al. 2015; Oak et al. 2006).

However, under the physiological state in an IUGR offspring exposed to low circulating insulin concentrations, a relative insulin resistance is observed, where translocation of GLUT4 is disrupted due to impaired insulin signaling in skeletal and other related tissues such as cardiac muscle and adipose tissue (Alam et al. 2016; Sadler et al. 2013). This impairment is related to maximal basal elevation of GLUT4 in skeletal muscle sarcolemma even before exogenous insulin is provided (Thamotharan et al. 2005; Oak et al. 2006).

Recently, small guanosine triphosphatase (GTPase) Rac1 has been classified as a downregulated signal component of Akt2 for GLUT4 translocation in skeletal muscle glucose uptake in response to insulin stimulation (Takenaka et al. 2014; Satoh 2014; Chiu et al. 2011). Interestingly, Rac1 is also involved in actin rearrangement that supports the movement of GLUT4 vesicles along the rapid reorganization of actin under insulin stimulation. This involvement of actin filament in Rac1 activity is being supported by results that demonstrate that in the presence of *an actin filament depolarizing agent, Latrunculin B*, Akt inhibitor blocks insulin-induced glucose uptake; however, the Rac1 inhibitor alone does not block insulin-induced glucose uptake, implying that actin filament is important for Rac1's function in this regard (Khayat et al. 2000; Sylow et al. 2014). In addition to the decrease in murine Akt2 and Rac1 expression seen with insulin resistance, a diminution in insulin-stimulated p-Akt occurs, dramatically reducing glucose uptake by 70% compared to control muscle (Sylow et al. 2014). Furthermore, the Rac1 expression pattern detected by Rac1 immunostaining in the transverse tubuli of skeletal muscle indicates less Rac1 redistribution in insulin-resistant mice (Sylow et al. 2013, 2014). Therefore, the increased expression of Rac1/Akt and insulin-responsive Rac1 redistribution in transverse tubuli may be required for enhancing function of dysregulated Rac1 and Akt signaling encountered with severe insulin resistance.

Considering the Rac1-related pathway, analysis of Rac1 redistribution under insulin treatment provides an explanation about enhanced insulin activities that may be extrapolated to the IUGR offspring exposed to moderate nutritional restriction during the adult phase of life.

In the IUGR offspring, although the adult male is more prone than the female in developing subsequent aberrancy in metabolic consequences (Owens et al. 2007), both sexes show diversity in the perturbed signaling molecules necessary for GLUT4 translocation.

In male rats with early protein restriction, the adult offspring expresses less PKCζ in skeletal muscle compared to control. This change impairs insulin action, which is not responsive to exogenous insulin stimulation in the IUGR skeletal muscle. This change is also noted in the face of no change in IR expression, although glut4 expression is reduced as seen soon after birth. In addition, the expression of insulin-induced signaling proteins, PKCζ p85α, and p110β, including GLUT4, decreases in the skeletal muscle biopsies of low birth weight humans similar to the reduction in PKCζ p85α, and GLUT4 observed in the IUGR male rat offspring. This implies that the rat model is a valuable surrogate for long-term human studies as similar aberrations are encountered in both species (Ozanne et al. 2005). Interestingly, the expression of skeletal muscle IR and Akt substrate of 160 kDa (AS160) increases in the male IUGR offspring; however, phosphorylation of IR, IRS-1, and AS160 fails to respond to insulin stimulation. These results are associated with increased plasma glucose and insulin concentrations reflecting insulin resistance initiated by impaired GLUT4 translocation due to impaired phosphorylation of insulin-induced AS160 (Blesson et al. 2014; Karlsson et al. 2005).

In contrast, in the female IUGR offspring, the basal expression of GLUT4, p-Akt, Akt2, and p-PDK1 increases in skeletal muscle, which may reflect a prosurvival adaptation in response to an *in utero* environment of restricted nutrition. Under such conditions *in utero*, increased p-Akt, Akt2, and p-PDK1 may be responsible for enhanced GLUT4 at the sarcolemma, thereby maximally capturing glucose in a situation of reduced transplacental glucose supply to the developing fetus. However, after birth during the postnatal and adult stages, when nutrition is restored to normalcy, this maximal increase in sarcolemmal GLUT4 cannot be further enhanced in response to exogenous insulin bringing about insulin resistance of further translocation of GLUT4 to the sarcolemma (Thamotharan et al. 2005; Oak et al. 2006). In our IUGR female adult rat offspring the block in translocating skeletal muscle GLUT4 lies especially in the absence of insulin-induced increase in total PKCζ expression causing insulin resistance (Oak et al. 2006). In addition, skeletal muscle Akt2 also decreases in both male and female IUGR fetus and young sheep fetus, besides showing reduced expression of various other insulin-signaling molecules (De Blasio et al. 2012; Thorn et al. 2009). Cumulatively, these studies support a prediabetic state related to insulin resistance exhibited by the skeletal muscle GLUT4 translocation machinery (Figure 6.1).

6.5   STRATEGIES FOR ENHANCING GLUT4 TRANSLOCATION AND THEREBY INSULIN SENSITIVITY IN IUGR OFFSPRING

6.5.1   Physical Exercise

Current lifestyle involving excessive calorie intake and a reduction in physical activity is detrimental to health. Physical exercise through muscle contraction increases

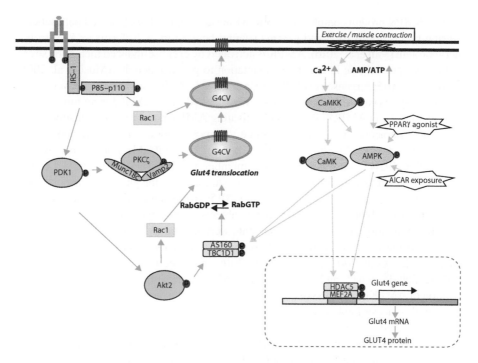

FIGURE 6.1 Schematic representation. Translocation of glucose transporter 4 by insulin or muscle contraction/exercise in skeletal muscle. Autophosphorylation of receptor by insulin activates diverse intracellular signaling proteins through the following signaling pathways. Exercise/muscle contraction including AMP-activated protein kinase (AMPK) activators, peroxisome proliferator-activated receptor type gamma (PPARγ) agonist, or 5′-aminoimidazole-4-carboxamide-1-β-D-ribofuranoside (AICAR) exposure induce glucose transporter protein 4 (glut4) gene expression or GLUT4 translocation. The impairment of phosphatidylinositol-3-kinases (PI3 kinase), pyruvate dehydrogenase kinase 1 (PDK1), protein kinase C (PKC)ζ, protein kinase B (PKB or AKT2), and AMPK activities results in metabolic disorders with insulin resistance due to defective GLUT4 translocation in the intrauterine growth restriction (IUGR) rat offspring.

skeletal muscle glucose uptake and insulin sensitivity by improving GLUT4 translocation (Mul et al. 2016; Lauritzen et al. 2010; Pate et al. 1995). Exercise improves skeletal muscle GLUT4 translocation by activating alternate pathways that do not require the IR or the postreceptor signaling molecules (Treadway et al. 1989; Grimditch et al. 1986; Wojtaszewski et al. 1999). Skeletal muscle contraction activates AMP-activated protein kinase (AMPK), Rac1, peroxisome proliferator-activated receptor-γ coactivator (PGC), and related molecules that in turn translocate GLUT4 to the sarcolemma thereby restoring insulin sensitivity of this process. This alternate pathway is exemplified in the muscle-specific IR knockout (KO) mice that present with severe insulin resistance. Physical exercise in these mice normalizes resting glucose uptake in soleus muscle due to enhanced GLUT4 translocation but these mice do not respond to exogenous insulin (Gannon et al. 2015a; Dos Santos et al. 2015; Richter and Hargreaves 2013; Mul et al. 2016; Sylow et al. 2016).

The AMPK protein complex is a protein kinase composed of alpha and beta subunit bearing two isoforms each and gamma subunit bearing three isoforms as a heterotrimeric protein (Mul et al. 2016). AMPK is activated by exercise-induced metabolic stress and plays a crucial role in metabolic adaptation to physical activity (Musi et al. 2001; Alvim et al. 2015; Jorgensen et al. 2006; Hardie 2013). AMPK activation is governed by two pathways: (1) an AMP-sensitive pathway that hydrolyzes ATP during muscle contraction increasing AMP/ATP ratio and activating AMPK and (2) a Ca^{2+}-sensitive pathway where intracellular Ca^{2+} increases due to depolarization with muscle contraction that activates Ca2+/calmodulin-dependent protein kinase (CaMK) or AMPK, AS160 (tre-2/USP6, BUB2, cdc16 domain family member 4 or TBC1D4), and TBC1D1 bringing about GLUT4-containing vesicles to the sarcolemma for glucose transport (Mul et al. 2016; Dos Santos et al. 2015; Cartee 2015; Jorgensen et al. 2006; Jessen et al. 2011). In muscle biopsies of human, male subjects with or without insulin resistance, AMPK expression and activity in basal state were similar (Musi et al. 2001; Kjobsted et al. 2016). Following an acute bout of exercise, a significant increase in AMPK alpha2 activity (Musi et al. 2001; Kjobsted et al. 2016; Jessen et al. 2011) with no change in AMPK alpha1, alpha2, and beta1 isoforms (Musi et al. 2001) was seen. In addition, ablation of AMPK alpha2 in skeletal muscle provokes the development of insulin resistance with glucose intolerance (Fujii et al. 2008). Recently, insulin-resistant subjects when compared to control subjects reflected an increase in AMPK $\alpha2\beta2\gamma3$ activity after an acute bout of exercise, while AMPK $\alpha1\beta2\gamma1$ and $\alpha2\beta2\gamma1$ increased during the 3-hour exercise recovery period (Kjobsted et al. 2016; Zhang et al. 2013a). This differential activation of the AMPK heterotrimeric enzyme plays a key role in regulating skeletal muscle metabolism in response to physical exercise. In addition, euglycemic–hyperinsulinemic clamp studies have confirmed that insulin fails to regulate AMPK activity supporting exercise-induced AMPK signaling as an alternate path of intervention particularly in the presence of insulin resistance (Kjobsted et al. 2016).

A similar approach is feasible in the IUGR adult offspring that expresses insulin resistance of skeletal muscle GLUT4 translocation. Addressing this specific issue, our studies demonstrated improved insulin sensitivity in the adult rat IUGR offspring that exercised on a treadmill at a speed of 11 m/min for 15 min/day from d21 to d60. Exercised IUGR offspring demonstrated increased skeletal muscle AMPK enzyme activity with decreased hepatic glucose production. In addition, these exercised IUGR rat offspring expressed lower glucose-stimulated insulin release and reduced plasma glucose concentrations in insulin tolerance tests. These changes were seen despite the absence of changes in insulin-induced glut4 expression or GLUT4 redistribution; however, exercise improved the overall insulin sensitivity in these rats (Garg et al. 2009).

In addition, after aerobic exercise training for 6 months in older humans at 50–80 years of age with no previous chronic diseases such as diabetes or cardiovascular disease, muscle biopsies revealed enhanced insulin sensitivity under increased AMPK expression, capillary density, glut4 expression, and glycogen synthetase activity with factors returning to the preexercise state except for capillary density following 2 months of detraining (Prior et al. 2015). More recently, studies in mice on a treadmill running at 20 m/min speed for 90 minutes increased serum interleukin 6 (IL-6) activating signal transducer and activator of transcription 3 (STAT3), which in turn increased glut4 expression and improved insulin sensitivity (Ikeda et al. 2016). However, transgenic glut4 KO mice with severe reduction to approximately 10% of normal glut4 expression fail to increase glucose uptake after exercise, unlike transgenic glut4 KO mice with only ~30–60% reduction (Howlett et al. 2013). Therefore, a threshold amount of glut4 expression is necessary for facilitating muscle glucose uptake by exercise-induced GLUT4 translocation (Howlett et al. 2013). In fact, physical exercise increases skeletal muscle glut4 expression while immobilization decreases glut4 expression (Ren et al. 1994; Op 't Eijnde et al. 2001). Glut4 gene expression may be epigenetically regulated under physical activity, thereby bringing about skeletal muscle adaptation.

Exercise increases histone 3 acetylation at lysine 36, a site associated with transcriptional elongation in human skeletal muscle, which releases histone deacetylases (HDACs) into cytoplasm and removes a transcriptional repressor (McGee et al. 2009). Notably, after exercise, HDAC5 is seen to dissociate from myocyte enhancer factor 2 (MEF2). Additionally, increased PGC1 and MEF2 expression was noted post-exercise, which further contributed to the increased expression of glut4. AMPK and CaMK phosphorylation also increased post-exercise contributing to the overall increase in glut4 expression (McGee and Hargreaves 2004; Smith et al. 2008; Dos Santos et al. 2015; Santos et al. 2014).

Furthermore, Rac1 signaling being AMPK independent as seen with no response to the AMPK-activating agent 5′-aminoimidazole-4-carboxamide-1-β-D-ribofuranoside (AICAR) in skeletal myotubes C2C12 (Sylow et al. 2013) demonstrates enhanced guanosine triphosphate (GTP) binding in response to exercise in both mice and human skeletal muscle. Increased Rac1 activity is known to regulate glucose uptake in skeletal muscle (Sylow et al. 2013, 2016), providing an additional target of manipulation in the IUGR adult offspring.

6.5.2 NUTRITIONAL INTERVENTION

Fisher-344 rats at 22–23 months of age were either accessing food ad libitum (AL) or subjected to *moderate* CR consuming only ~60–65% of AL intake. The CR group demonstrated a decrease in body mass and the isolated CR muscle cells inhibited increased glucose uptake with elevated phosphorylation of Akt2 or AS160 in response to insulin (Wang et al. 2016a, b). Thus, nutritional restriction may be an alternative intervention for improving insulin sensitivity. Hence, we exposed calorie restricted IUGR rat offspring to postnatal CR that led to protection in the adult against obesity and glucose intolerance. This protection was evident despite introduction of a high-fat diet in later life. However, while postnatal CR proved protective against metabolic derangements even after the food restriction was lifted postweaning, the concern is always the negative impact on the developing brain. Thus, it is important to consider other pharmacological interventions that are protective long term despite early introduction but balance this protection against ensuring normal neurodevelopment (Tomi et al. 2013; Dai et al. 2012; Garg et al. 2012).

6.5.3 PHARMACOLOGICAL INTERVENTIONS

Thiazolidinediones (TZDs) on the other hand are a class of antidiabetic drugs that enhance insulin sensitivity by specifically binding the peroxisome proliferator-activated receptors (PPAR)γ (Rangwala and Lazar 2004; Trobec et al. 2011). One such TZD, rosiglitazone, is used for glycemic control through improved insulin sensitivity (Mayerson et al. 2002; Raji et al. 2003; Bennett et al. 2004; Aronoff et al. 2000; Saltiel and Olefsky 1996). PPARγ is mainly expressed in adipose tissue, and plays an important role in adipocyte differentiation and the expression of adipocytic genes related to metabolism (Tontonoz et al. 1994; Vidal-Puig et al. 1996; Berger and Moller 2002; Oak et al. 2009). PPARγ is also expressed in skeletal muscle (Loviscach et al. 2000; Vidal-Puig et al. 1997; Park et al. 1997), the activation of which involves the regulation of signaling molecules such as fatty acid transport protein (FATP)-1, IRS-2, PDK4, PI3K, and Akt (Berger and Moller 2002; Trobec et al. 2011). We previously employed a PPARγ agonist, rosiglitazone, as an intervention in the IUGR rat offspring (Oak et al. 2009). Rosiglitazone treatment increased the insulin-induced plasma membrane association of GLUT4 and PKCζ. In addition, pAMPK/AMPK ratio also increased in the basal state. The regulation of these signaling molecules resulted in improving insulin sensitivity (Oak et al. 2009).

Insulin-like growth factor I (IGF-I) is an endocrine regulator during fetal development, while growth hormone (GH) is a postnatal endocrine regulator. GH and IGF-I effect PI3K/Akt and mitogen-activated protein kinase (MAPK) pathways by sharing tyrosine kinases on their specific receptors, which can serve as pharmacological targets (Trobec et al. 2011; Wali et al. 2012). In IUGR, the fetal circulating IGF-I or GH concentrations are significantly lower compared to the age-matched controls, while IGF-II concentrations are similar (Lassarre et al. 1991; Mirlesse et al. 1993). In addition, at birth IGF-I concentrations are lower in an IUGR infant, subsequently increasing toward normal during the first month of life (Leger et al. 1996). Thus, the lowered IGF-I concentrations at birth may serve as a biomarker of fetal growth restriction. Therefore, IGF-I or GH treatment can possibly ameliorate the adult maladaptive metabolic phenotype in the adult IUGR offspring (Leger et al. 1996; Chatelain 2000). GH treatment in an IUGR child is known to increase growth velocity dramatically, while discontinuation of GH decreases growth velocity (Kamp et al. 2001; Czernichow 2001). In addition, IGF-I administered into the amniotic fluid of sheep was seen to cross the fetal gut epithelium and circulate in the fetus, thereby increasing the growth rate in an IUGR offspring (Bloomfield et al. 2002a, b; Eremia et al. 2007). Recently, Reynold et al. reported on GH treatment from postnatal days 3 to 21 leading to an increase in insulin-stimulated glucose uptake with upregulation of genes related to GLUT4 translocation, such as Tyrp-IRS-1, p-AKT, and PPARγ, and also including GLUT4 itself. In addition, fat mass decreases after GH treatment (Reynolds et al. 2013). These results support the possible effects on reversing metabolic dysfunction through GH treatment during the suckling phase in the IUGR offspring.

6.6 TRANSGENERATIONAL EFFECT ON GLUT4 EXPRESSION IN THE IUGR OFFSPRING

Events that affect the *in utero* environment such as alterations in the nutritional supply are known to have long-term implications and induce chronic diseases including metabolic disorders. Offspring of a diabetic pregnancy develop aberrant glucose homeostasis (Thamotharan et al. 2007; Boloker et al. 2002). Similarly, a protein-restricted diet exposure of the F0 generation during gestation results in the inheritance of a phenotype with altered glucose and insulin metabolism with reduced skeletal muscle glut4 expression seen in the F2 offspring (Zambrano et al. 2005). Given this transgenerational influence of a gestational nutritional disruptor, it is imperative to introduce interventions early in life to reverse the metabolic derangements encountered in an IUGR offspring. However, the IUGR female offspring during pregnancy expresses gestational diabetes (Garg et al. 2010), hence it is not known whether gestational diabetes is responsible for an *in utero* environmental effect or if there is transgenerational transmission of this phenotype independent of the maternal IUGR offspring's *in utero* environment. Hence, we undertook embryo transfer experiments to tease out the effect of these two situations. Our embryo transfer experiments in rats determined that gestational nutritional restriction can also transmit metabolic aberrations to the F2 generation. Female F2 rats, procreated by F1 perinatal growth-restricted mothers but transferred as embryos to gestate in control mothers, were compared with the control F2 progeny (Thamotharan et al. 2007).

This F2 progeny was not growth restricted at birth but demonstrated fasting hyperglycemia, hyperinsulinemia, increased hepatic glucose production, and increased hepatic weight with no differences in postnatal growth patterns compared to the F2 control. In addition, skeletal muscle total GLUT4 and pAkt concentrations increased but plasma membrane-associated GLUT4 and total pPKCζ, and PKCζ enzyme activity necessary for insulin-induced GLUT4 translocation, decreased. Based on these observations, malprogramming due to gestational nutritional deficiency is evident and has far-reaching implications to many generations of progeny. Given this assumption, it stands to reason that epigenetic mechanisms should be explored as the basis for this transgenerational inheritance in an IUGR pregnant mother (Thamotharan et al. 2007; Garg et al. 2013b).

6.7 EPIGENETIC MODIFICATIONS OF GLUT4 EXPRESSION IN IUGR MUSCLE

The adult IUGR offspring demonstrates decreased GLUT4 in skeletal muscle, indicating the development of insulin resistance in later life (Thamotharan et al. 2005). Thus, intrauterine milieu of reduced nutrition permanently modifies glut4 expression in the offspring. Thus, besides defective skeletal muscle, GLUT4 translocation impairment of glut4 expression also exists (Pinney and Simmons 2009). Furthermore, this reduction is transmitted transgenerationally; therefore, exploration of epigenetic mechanisms seems reasonable.

Epigenetic mechanisms cause heritable silencing or activation of genes without a change in coding sequences. There are three processes that epigenetically can regulate gene expression: DNA methylation/demethylation and histone modifications that regulate gene transcription, and small noncoding RNAs (miRNAs) that dictate mRNA half-life and translational efficiency (Egger et al. 2004; Pinney and Simmons 2009; Dos Santos et al. 2015).

DNA methylation occurs in the C5 position of cytosine residues and may contribute to epigenetic silencing if imposed on gene promoters. DNA methylation of gene bodies has varied effects on gene expression depending on where it occurs. The maintenance of such CpG methylation is due to functional cooperation by DNA methyltransferases (DNMT) and catalyzed by ten-eleven translocation proteins (TETs). Histone modifications as epigenetic modifiers are the posttranslational modifications of histones (backbone of the DNA helices) by acetylation/deacetylation and methylation/demethylation of conserved lysine residues, thereby modifying gene expression by influencing the DNA and protein binding of transcription factors (transactivators, repressors). In general, histone acetylation activates transcriptionally competent DNA regions, whereas histone methylation can either activate or deactivate transcription based on the lysine residue involved. For example, methylation of histone 3 lysine 4 methylation (H3K4me) activates, while histone 3 lysine 9 methylation (H3K9me) represses gene transcription. Histone deacetylation is catalyzed by a class of HDACs, while acetylation is catalyzed by HATs. miRNAs on the other hand are small noncoding RNA molecules that regulate target gene expression through posttranscriptional gene regulation. This occurs by the miRNA binding to complementary 3′ untranslated region (UTR) of a target gene mRNA, thereby repressing or degrading specific target mRNAs (Cho 2011). More recently, long noncoding RNAs (lncRNAs) have also been determined to play a role in transcription. Although the biological functions of most miRNAs and lncRNAs have not been understood completely, an increasing number of studies reveal miRNAs and lncRNAs playing significant roles in human diseases (Egger et al. 2004; Dos Santos et al. 2015; Gupta et al. 2010; Cao 2014). Hence, it stands to reason that we explore the role of certain epigenetic mechanisms governing skeletal muscle glut4 expression in the adult IUGR offspring.

Analysis of the glut4 promotor region was carried out in transgenic mice that carried a mutation of a glut4 transactivating protein, namely MEF2. In transgenic mice created by replacing the MEF2 core consensus (CT*AAAAAT*AG) with a mutated sequence of CT*GGGCCC*AG, glut4 mRNA expression was ablated, supporting a critical role for MEF2 in glut4 gene expression (Thai et al. 1998). MyoD, another transcription factor, also enhances glut4 expression by binding with MEF2 and thyroid hormone receptor alpha 1 (TRα1). The association of these three nuclear factors has the most pronounced positive effect on glut4 transcription (Moreno et al. 2003; Santalucia et al. 2001).

Our studies focused on the skeletal muscle of the IUGR postnatal and adult offspring and demonstrated that MEF2D, an inhibitor of MEF2A (an activator), is increased while both MEF2A and MyoD are decreased when compared to age-matched controls. In addition, DNMTs demonstrate enhanced glut4 promoter binding in an age-specific manner, DNMT1 in the postnatal period, while both DNMT3a and DNMT3b in the adult IUGR offspring. These DNMTs in turn recruit increased amounts of methyl CpG binding protein 2 (MeCP2) to bind the glut4 promotor region. In addition, the covalent modifications of the histone code, namely histone 3 lysine 14 (H3K14) deacetylation, are governed by increased HDAC1 and enhanced association of HDAC4 with HDAC1. Further H3.K9 methylation by Suv39H1 methylase increased the recruitment of heterochromatin protein 1α, collectively inactivating postnatal and adult IUGR skeletal muscle glut4 gene transcription (Raychaudhuri et al. 2008).

In skeletal muscle, PGC-1α enhanced glut4 expression by coactivating MEF2 (Lin et al. 2005; Michael et al. 2001). In the IUGR rat offspring, CpG island methylation significantly increases in the PGC-1α promotor, which was associated with a reduction in PGC-1α gene expression with a reduction of PGC-1α transcription activity, thereby reducing glut4 expression (Zeng et al. 2013; Xie et al. 2015). In contrast to these two studies, low protein maternal diet in the female IUGR offspring upregulated MEF2 binding of the glut4 gene, mediated by enhanced H3Ac, H4Ac, and H3K4Me2 (Zheng et al. 2012), suggesting differences in the conditions resulting in IUGR. Notwithstanding this last study, trans-cinnamaldehyde, a component of the cinnamon extract, when applied to C2C12 murine myotubes augmented differentiation into myocytes by increasing MEF2 and PGC-1α expression, which in turn enhanced glut4 expression (Gannon et al. 2015b). Interestingly, novel small molecules, such as ZIN005, also increased PGC-1α mRNA in skeletal muscle of diabetic db/db mice unlike the decrease in hepatic PGC-1α expression and resultant reduction in gluconeogenesis, thereby enhancing insulin sensitivity overall (Zhang et al. 2013b). Altered expression of miRNAs as shown by miRNA microarray of the skeletal muscle of the IUGR rat offspring yielded the upregulation of miR-29, let-7a-2–30, and miR-140-5p, while miR-126a and miR-222-3p were downregulated. miR-29a when overexpressed in C2C12 cells downregulated both PPARδ and PGC-1α because PPARδ regulates PGC-1α expression. Similarly, increased miRNA-29a decreased both PPARδ and PGC-1α in the skeletal muscle of the IUGR rat offspring (Zhou et al. 2016). Furthermore after exercise, expression of *miR-23* decreases causing the upregulation of skeletal muscle *PGC-1α*, thereby mediating improved insulin sensitivity (Safdar et al. 2009).

6.8 SUMMARY

The IUGR offspring is prone toward developing glucose intolerance and skeletal muscle-specific insulin resistance as witnessed by a reduction in glut4 expression and the inability to translocate to the plasma membrane in response to insulin. Both these processes are regulated by differing molecular machinery providing targets for resolution. The importance for early intervention lies in the fact that this IUGR metabolic phenotype is transgenerationally transmitted evoking epigenetics, providing a contributing factor toward the worldwide epidemic of metabolic disorders, which include diabetes and obesity and their various complications.

REFERENCES

Abbasi, A., M. Thamotharan, B. C. Shin, M. C. Jordan, K. P. Roos, A. Stahl, and S. U. Devaskar. 2012. Myocardial macronutrient transporter adaptations in the adult pregestational female intrauterine and postnatal growth-restricted offspring. *Am J Physiol Endocrinol Metab* 302 (11):E1352–E1362.

Alam, F., A. Islam, I. Khalil, and S. H. Gan 2016. Metabolic control of type 2 diabetes by targeting the GLUT4 glucose transporter: Intervention approaches. *Curr Pharm Des* 22:3034–3049.

Alvim, R. O., M. R. Cheuhen, S. R. Machado, A. G. Sousa, and P. C. Santos. 2015. General aspects of muscle glucose uptake. *An Acad Bras Cienc* 87 (1):351–368.

Aronoff, S., S. Rosenblatt, S. Braithwaite, J. W. Egan, A. L. Mathisen, and R. L. Schneider. 2000. Pioglitazone hydrochloride monotherapy improves glycemic control in the treatment of patients with type 2 diabetes: A 6-month randomized placebo-controlled dose-response study. The Pioglitazone 001 Study Group. *Diabetes Care* 23 (11):1605–1611.

Barker, D. J. 1997. Fetal nutrition and cardiovascular disease in later life. *Br Med Bull* 53 (1):96–108.

Barker, D. J., C. N. Hales, C. H. Fall, C. Osmond, K. Phipps, and P. M. Clark. 1993. Type 2 (non-insulin-dependent) diabetes mellitus, hypertension and hyperlipidaemia (syndrome X): Relation to reduced fetal growth. *Diabetologia* 36 (1):62–67.

Barker, D. J., and C. Osmond. 1986. Infant mortality, childhood nutrition, and ischaemic heart disease in England and Wales. *Lancet* 1 (8489):1077–1081.

Battaglia, F. C., and L. O. Lubchenco. 1967. A practical classification of newborn infants by weight and gestational age. *J Pediatr* 71 (2):159–163.

Bennett, S. M., A. Agrawal, H. Elasha, M. Heise, N. P. Jones, M. Walker, and J. P. Wilding. 2004. Rosiglitazone improves insulin sensitivity, glucose tolerance and ambulatory blood pressure in subjects with impaired glucose tolerance. *Diabet Med* 21 (5):415–422.

Berends, L. M., and S. E. Ozanne. 2012. Early determinants of type-2 diabetes. *Best Pract Res Clin Endocrinol Metab* 26 (5):569–580.

Berger, J., and D. E. Moller. 2002. The mechanisms of action of PPARs. *Annu Rev Med* 53:409–435.

Blesson, C. S., K. Sathishkumar, V. Chinnathambi, and C. Yallampalli. 2014. Gestational protein restriction impairs insulin-regulated glucose transport mechanisms in gastrocnemius muscles of adult male offspring. *Endocrinology* 155 (8):3036–3046.

Bloomfield, F. H., M. K. Bauer, P. L. van Zijl, P. D. Gluckman, and J. E. Harding. 2002a. Amniotic IGF-I supplements improve gut growth but reduce circulating IGF-I in growth-restricted fetal sheep. *Am J Physiol Endocrinol Metab* 282 (2):E259–E269.

Bloomfield, F. H., B. H. Breier, and J. E. Harding. 2002b. Fate of (125)I-IGF-I administered into the amniotic fluid of late-gestation fetal sheep. *Pediatr Res* 51 (3):361–369.

Boloker, J., S. J. Gertz, and R. A. Simmons. 2002. Gestational diabetes leads to the development of diabetes in adulthood in the rat. *Diabetes* 51 (5):1499–1506.

Cao, J. 2014. The functional role of long non-coding RNAs and epigenetics. *Biol Proced Online* 16:11.

Cartee, G. D. 2015. Mechanisms for greater insulin-stimulated glucose uptake in normal and insulin-resistant skeletal muscle after acute exercise. *Am J Physiol Endocrinol Metab* 309 (12):E949–E959.

Chatelain, P. 2000. Children born with intra-uterine growth retardation (IUGR) or small for gestational age (SGA): Long-term growth and metabolic consequences. *Endocr Regul* 34 (1):33–36.

Chiu, T. T., T. E. Jensen, L. Sylow, E. A. Richter, and A. Klip. 2011. Rac1 signalling toward GLUT4/glucose uptake in skeletal muscle. *Cell Signal* 23 (10):1546–1554.

Cho, W. C. 2011. Grand challenges and opportunities in deciphering the role of non-coding RNAs in human diseases. *Front Genet* 2:1.

Cushman, S. W., and L. J. Wardzala. 1980. Potential mechanism of insulin action on glucose transport in the isolated rat adipose cell. Apparent translocation of intracellular transport systems to the plasma membrane. *J Biol Chem* 255 (10):4758–4762.

Czernichow, P. 2001. Treatment with growth hormone in short children born with intrauterine growth retardation. *Endocrine* 15 (1):39–42.

Dai, Y., S. Thamotharan, M. Garg, B. C. Shin, and S. U. Devaskar. 2012. Superimposition of postnatal calorie restriction protects the aging male intrauterine growth—Restricted offspring from metabolic maladaptations. *Endocrinology* 153 (9):4216–4226.

De Blasio, M. J., K. L. Gatford, M. L. Harland, J. S. Robinson, and J. A. Owens. 2012. Placental restriction reduces insulin sensitivity and expression of insulin signaling and glucose transporter genes in skeletal muscle, but not liver, in young sheep. *Endocrinology* 153 (5):2142–2151.

DeFronzo, R. A., E. Jacot, E. Jequier, E. Maeder, J. Wahren, and J. P. Felber. 1981. The effect of insulin on the disposal of intravenous glucose. Results from indirect calorimetry and hepatic and femoral venous catheterization. *Diabetes* 30 (12):1000–1007.

Dos Santos, J. M., M. L. Moreli, S. Tewari, and S. A. Benite-Ribeiro. 2015. The effect of exercise on skeletal muscle glucose uptake in type 2 diabetes: An epigenetic perspective. *Metabolism* 64 (12):1619–1628.

Dunlop, K., M. Cedrone, J. F. Staples, and T. R. Regnault. 2015. Altered fetal skeletal muscle nutrient metabolism following an adverse in utero environment and the modulation of later life insulin sensitivity. *Nutrients* 7 (2):1202–1216.

Egger, G., G. Liang, A. Aparicio, and P. A. Jones. 2004. Epigenetics in human disease and prospects for epigenetic therapy. *Nature* 429 (6990):457–463.

Eremia, S. C., H. A. de Boo, F. H. Bloomfield, M. H. Oliver, and J. E. Harding. 2007. Fetal and amniotic insulin-like growth factor-I supplements improve growth rate in intrauterine growth restriction fetal sheep. *Endocrinology* 148 (6):2963–2972.

Figueras, F., and J. Gardosi. 2010. Intrauterine growth restriction: New concepts in antenatal surveillance, diagnosis, and management. *Am J Obstet Gynecol* 204 (4):288–300.

Freije, W. A., S. Thamotharan, R. Lee, B. C. Shin, and S. U. Devaskar. 2015. The hepatic transcriptome of young suckling and aging intrauterine growth restricted male rats. *J Cell Biochem* 116 (4):566–579.

Froen, J. F., J. O. Gardosi, A. Thurmann, A. Francis, and B. Stray-Pedersen. 2004. Restricted fetal growth in sudden intrauterine unexplained death. *Acta Obstet Gynecol Scand* 83 (9):801–807.

Fujii, N., R. C. Ho, Y. Manabe, N. Jessen, T. Toyoda, W. L. Holland, S. A. Summers, M. F. Hirshman, and L. J. Goodyear. 2008. Ablation of AMP-activated protein kinase alpha2 activity exacerbates insulin resistance induced by high-fat feeding of mice. *Diabetes* 57 (11):2958–2966.

Gannon, N. P., C. A. Conn, and R. A. Vaughan. 2015a. Dietary stimulators of GLUT4 expression and translocation in skeletal muscle: A mini-review. *Mol Nutr Food Res* 59 (1):48–64.

Gannon, N. P., J. K. Schnuck, C. M. Mermier, C. A. Conn, and R. A. Vaughan. 2015b. Trans-cinnamaldehyde stimulates mitochondrial biogenesis through PGC-1alpha and PPARbeta/delta leading to enhanced GLUT4 expression. *Biochimie* 119:45–51.

Garg, M., M. Thamotharan, Y. Dai, V. Lagishetty, A. V. Matveyenko, W. N. Lee, and S. U. Devaskar. 2013a. Glucose intolerance and lipid metabolic adaptations in response to intrauterine and postnatal calorie restriction in male adult rats. *Endocrinology* 154 (1):102–113.

Garg, M., M. Thamotharan, Y. Dai, P. W. Lee, and S. U. Devaskar. 2013b. Embryo-transfer of the F2 postnatal calorie restricted female rat offspring into a control intra-uterine environment normalizes the metabolic phenotype. *Metabolism* 62 (3):432–441.

Garg, M., M. Thamotharan, Y. Dai, S. Thamotharan, B. C. Shin, D. Stout, and S. U. Devaskar. 2012. Early postnatal caloric restriction protects adult male intrauterine growth-restricted offspring from obesity. *Diabetes* 61 (6):1391–1398.

Garg, M., M. Thamotharan, S. A. Oak, G. Pan, D. C. Maclaren, P. W. Lee, and S. U. Devaskar. 2009. Early exercise regimen improves insulin sensitivity in the intrauterine growth-restricted adult female rat offspring. *Am J Physiol Endocrinol Metab* 296 (2):E272–E281.

Garg, M., M. Thamotharan, G. Pan, P. W. Lee, and S. U. Devaskar. 2010. Early exposure of the pregestational intrauterine and postnatal growth-restricted female offspring to a peroxisome proliferator-activated receptor-{gamma} agonist. *Am J Physiol Endocrinol Metab* 298 (3):E489–E498.

Garg, M., M. Thamotharan, L. Rogers, S. Bassilian, W. N. Lee, and S. U. Devaskar. 2006. Glucose metabolic adaptations in the intrauterine growth-restricted adult female rat offspring. *Am J Physiol Endocrinol Metab* 290 (6):E1218–E1226.

Gibson, L. C., B. C. Shin, Y. Dai, W. Freije, S. Kositamongkol, J. Cho, and S. U. Devaskar. 2015. Early leptin intervention reverses perturbed energy balance regulating hypothalamic neuropeptides in the pre- and postnatal calorie-restricted female rat offspring. *J Neurosci Res* 93 (6):902–912.

Gorselink, M., M. R. Drost, K. F. de Brouwer, G. Schaart, G. P. van Kranenburg, T. H. Roemen, M. van Bilsen, M. J. Charron, and G. J. van der Vusse. 2002. Increased muscle fatigability in GLUT-4-deficient mice. *Am J Physiol Endocrinol Metab* 282 (2):E348–E354.

Govers, R. 2014. Molecular mechanisms of GLUT4 regulation in adipocytes. *Diabetes Metab* 40 (6):400–410.

Grimditch, G. K., R. J. Barnard, S. A. Kaplan, and E. Sternlicht. 1986. Effect of training on insulin binding to rat skeletal muscle sarcolemmal vesicles. *Am J Physiol* 250 (5 Pt 1):E570–575.

Gupta, R. A., N. Shah, K. C. Wang, J. Kim, H. M. Horlings, D. J. Wong, M. C. Tsai, T. Hung, P. Argani, J. L. Rinn, Y. Wang, P. Brzoska, B. Kong, R. Li, R. B. West, M. J. van de Vijver, S. Sukumar, and H. Y. Chang. 2010. Long non-coding RNA HOTAIR reprograms chromatin state to promote cancer metastasis. *Nature* 464 (7291):1071–1076.

Hales, C. N., and D. J. Barker. 2001. The thrifty phenotype hypothesis. *Br Med Bull* 60:5–20.

Hardie, D. G. 2013. AMPK: A target for drugs and natural products with effects on both diabetes and cancer. *Diabetes* 62 (7):2164–2172.

Hay, W. W., Jr., L. D. Brown, P. J. Rozance, S. R. Wesolowski, and S. W. Limesand. 2016. Challenges in nourishing the IUGR fetus-Lessons learned from studies in the IUGR fetal sheep. *Acta Paediatr* 105:881–889.

Holemans, K., L. Aerts, and F. A. Van Assche. 2003. Fetal growth restriction and consequences for the offspring in animal models. *J Soc Gynecol Investig* 10 (7):392–399.

Holman, G. D., and S. W. Cushman. 1994. Subcellular localization and trafficking of the GLUT4 glucose transporter isoform in insulin-responsive cells. *Bioessays* 16 (10):753–759.

Horie, T., K. Ono, K. Nagao, H. Nishi, M. Kinoshita, T. Kawamura, H. Wada, A. Shimatsu, T. Kita, and K. Hasegawa. 2008. Oxidative stress induces GLUT4 translocation by activation of PI3-K/Akt and dual AMPK kinase in cardiac myocytes. *J Cell Physiol* 215 (3):733–742.

Howlett, K. F., S. Andrikopoulos, J. Proietto, and M. Hargreaves. 2013. Exercise-induced muscle glucose uptake in mice with graded, muscle-specific GLUT-4 deletion. *Physiol Rep* 1 (3):e00065.

Ikeda, S. I., Y. Tamura, S. Kakehi, H. Sanada, R. Kawamori, and H. Watada. 2016. Exercise-induced increase in IL-6 level enhances GLUT4 expression and insulin sensitivity in mouse skeletal muscle. *Biochem Biophys Res Commun* 473:947–952.

Ikemoto, S., K. S. Thompson, M. Takahashi, H. Itakura, M. D. Lane, and O. Ezaki. 1995. High fat diet-induced hyperglycemia: Prevention by low level expression of a glucose transporter (GLUT4) minigene in transgenic mice. *Proc Natl Acad Sci USA* 92 (8):3096–3099.

James, D. E., R. Brown, J. Navarro, and P. F. Pilch. 1988. Insulin-regulatable tissues express a unique insulin-sensitive glucose transport protein. *Nature* 333 (6169):183–185.

Jang, E. A., L. D. Longo, and R. Goyal. 2015. Antenatal maternal hypoxia: Criterion for fetal growth restriction in rodents. *Front Physiol* 6:176.

Janssen, I., S. B. Heymsfield, Z. M. Wang, and R. Ross. 2000. Skeletal muscle mass and distribution in 468 men and women aged 18–88 yr. *J Appl Physiol (1985)* 89 (1):81–88.

Jensen, C. B., H. Storgaard, S. Madsbad, E. A. Richter, and A. A. Vaag. 2007. Altered skeletal muscle fiber composition and size precede whole-body insulin resistance in young men with low birth weight. *J Clin Endocrinol Metab* 92 (4):1530–1534.

Jessen, N., D. An, A. S. Lihn, J. Nygren, M. F. Hirshman, A. Thorell, and L. J. Goodyear. 2011. Exercise increases TBC1D1 phosphorylation in human skeletal muscle. *Am J Physiol Endocrinol Metab* 301 (1):E164–E171.

Joost, H. G., and B. Thorens. 2001. The extended GLUT-family of sugar/polyol transport facilitators: Nomenclature, sequence characteristics, and potential function of its novel members (review). *Mol Membr Biol* 18 (4):247–256.

Jorgensen, S. B., E. A. Richter, and J. F. Wojtaszewski. 2006. Role of AMPK in skeletal muscle metabolic regulation and adaptation in relation to exercise. *J Physiol* 574 (Pt 1):17–31.

Kamp, G. A., D. Mul, J. J. Waelkens, M. Jansen, H. A. Delemarre-van de Waal, L. Verhoeven-Wind, M. Frolich, W. Oostdijk, and J. M. Wit. 2001. A randomized controlled trial of three years growth hormone and gonadotropin-releasing hormone agonist treatment in children with idiopathic short stature and intrauterine growth retardation. *J Clin Endocrinol Metab* 86 (7):2969–2975.

Karlsson, H. K., J. R. Zierath, S. Kane, A. Krook, G. E. Lienhard, and H. Wallberg-Henriksson. 2005. Insulin-stimulated phosphorylation of the Akt substrate AS160 is impaired in skeletal muscle of type 2 diabetic subjects. *Diabetes* 54 (6):1692–1697.

Katz, E. B., R. Burcelin, T. S. Tsao, A. E. Stenbit, and M. J. Charron. 1996. The metabolic consequences of altered glucose transporter expression in transgenic mice. *J Mol Med* 74 (11):639–652.

Khayat, Z. A., P. Tong, K. Yaworsky, R. J. Bloch, and A. Klip. 2000. Insulin-induced actin filament remodeling colocalizes actin with phosphatidylinositol 3-kinase and GLUT4 in L6 myotubes. *J Cell Sci* 113 (Pt 2):279–290.

Kjobsted, R., A. J. Pedersen, J. R. Hingst, R. Sabaratnam, J. B. Birk, J. M. Kristensen, K. Hojlund, and J. F. Wojtaszewski. 2016. Intact regulation of the AMPK signaling network in response to exercise and insulin in skeletal muscle of male patients with type 2 diabetes: Illumination of AMPK activation in recovery from exercise. *Diabetes* 65 (5):1219–1230.

Koumanov, F., B. Jin, J. Yang, and G. D. Holman. 2005. Insulin signaling meets vesicle traffic of GLUT4 at a plasma-membrane-activated fusion step. *Cell Metab* 2 (3):179–189.

Lassarre, C., S. Hardouin, F. Daffos, F. Forestier, F. Frankenne, and M. Binoux. 1991. Serum insulin-like growth factors and insulin-like growth factor binding proteins in the human fetus. Relationships with growth in normal subjects and in subjects with intrauterine growth retardation. *Pediatr Res* 29 (3):219–225.

Lauritzen, H. P., H. Galbo, T. Toyoda, and L. J. Goodyear. 2010. Kinetics of contraction-induced GLUT4 translocation in skeletal muscle fibers from living mice. *Diabetes* 59 (9):2134–2144.

Leger, J., M. Noel, J. M. Limal, and P. Czernichow. 1996. Growth factors and intrauterine growth retardation. II. Serum growth hormone, insulin-like growth factor (IGF) I, and IGF-binding protein 3 levels in children with intrauterine growth retardation compared with normal control subjects: Prospective study from birth to two years of age. Study Group of IUGR. *Pediatr Res* 40 (1):101–107.

Lin, J., C. Handschin, and B. M. Spiegelman. 2005. Metabolic control through the PGC-1 family of transcription coactivators. *Cell Metab* 1 (6):361–370.

Loviscach, M., N. Rehman, L. Carter, S. Mudaliar, P. Mohadeen, T. P. Ciaraldi, J. H. Veerkamp, and R. R. Henry. 2000. Distribution of peroxisome proliferator-activated receptors (PPARs) in human skeletal muscle and adipose tissue: Relation to insulin action. *Diabetologia* 43 (3):304–311.

Mayerson, A. B., R. S. Hundal, S. Dufour, V. Lebon, D. Befroy, G. W. Cline, S. Enocksson, S. E. Inzucchi, G. I. Shulman, and K. F. Petersen. 2002. The effects of rosiglitazone on insulin sensitivity, lipolysis, and hepatic and skeletal muscle triglyceride content in patients with type 2 diabetes. *Diabetes* 51 (3):797–802.

McGee, S. L., E. Fairlie, A. P. Garnham, and M. Hargreaves. 2009. Exercise-induced histone modifications in human skeletal muscle. *J Physiol* 587 (Pt 24):5951–5958.

McGee, S. L., and M. Hargreaves. 2004. Exercise and myocyte enhancer factor 2 regulation in human skeletal muscle. *Diabetes* 53 (5):1208–1214.

McIntire, D. D., S. L. Bloom, B. M. Casey, and K. J. Leveno. 1999. Birth weight in relation to morbidity and mortality among newborn infants. *N Engl J Med* 340 (16):1234–1238.

Michael, L. F., Z. Wu, R. B. Cheatham, P. Puigserver, G. Adelmant, J. J. Lehman, D. P. Kelly, and B. M. Spiegelman. 2001. Restoration of insulin-sensitive glucose transporter (GLUT4) gene expression in muscle cells by the transcriptional coactivator PGC-1. *Proc Natl Acad Sci USA* 98 (7):3820–3825.

Mirlesse, V., F. Frankenne, E. Alsat, M. Poncelet, G. Hennen, and D. Evain-Brion. 1993. Placental growth hormone levels in normal pregnancy and in pregnancies with intrauterine growth retardation. *Pediatr Res* 34 (4):439–442.

Moreno, H., A. L. Serrano, T. Santalucia, A. Guma, C. Canto, N. J. Brand, M. Palacin, S. Schiaffino, and A. Zorzano. 2003. Differential regulation of the muscle-specific GLUT4 enhancer in regenerating and adult skeletal muscle. *J Biol Chem* 278 (42):40557–40564.

Morrison, J. L., J. A. Duffield, B. S. Muhlhausler, S. Gentili, and I. C. McMillen. 2010. Fetal growth restriction, catch-up growth and the early origins of insulin resistance and visceral obesity. *Pediatr Nephrol* 25 (4):669–677.

Mueckler, M., and G. Holman. 1995. Homeostasis without a GLUT. *Nature* 377 (6545):100–101.

Mul, J. D., K. I. Stanford, M. F. Hirshman, and L. J. Goodyear. 2016. Exercise and regulation of carbohydrate metabolism. *Prog Mol Biol Transl Sci* 135:17–37.

Musi, N., N. Fujii, M. F. Hirshman, I. Ekberg, S. Froberg, O. Ljungqvist, A. Thorell, and L. J. Goodyear. 2001. AMP-activated protein kinase (AMPK) is activated in muscle of subjects with type 2 diabetes during exercise. *Diabetes* 50 (5):921–927.

Neitzke, U., T. Harder, and A. Plagemann. 2011. Intrauterine growth restriction and developmental programming of the metabolic syndrome: A critical appraisal. *Microcirculation* 18 (4):304–311.

Oak, S., C. Tran, M. O. Castillo, S. Thamotharan, M. Thamotharan, and S. U. Devaskar. 2009. Peroxisome proliferator-activated receptor-gamma agonist improves skeletal muscle insulin signaling in the pregestational intrauterine growth-restricted rat offspring. *Am J Physiol Endocrinol Metab* 297 (2):E514–E524.

Oak, S. A., C. Tran, G. Pan, M. Thamotharan, and S. U. Devaskar. 2006. Perturbed skeletal muscle insulin signaling in the adult female intrauterine growth-restricted rat. *Am J Physiol Endocrinol Metab* 290 (6):E1321–E1330.

Op 't Eijnde, B., B. Urso, E. A. Richter, P. L. Greenhaff, and P. Hespel. 2001. Effect of oral creatine supplementation on human muscle GLUT4 protein content after immobilization. *Diabetes* 50 (1):18–23.

Owens, J. A., P. Thavaneswaran, M. J. De Blasio, I. C. McMillen, J. S. Robinson, and K. L. Gatford. 2007. Sex-specific effects of placental restriction on components of the metabolic syndrome in young adult sheep. *Am J Physiol Endocrinol Metab* 292 (6):E1879–E1889.

Ozanne, S. E., and C. N. Hales. 2002. Early programming of glucose-insulin metabolism. *Trends Endocrinol Metab* 13 (9):368–373.

Ozanne, S. E., C. B. Jensen, K. J. Tingey, H. Storgaard, S. Madsbad, and A. A. Vaag. 2005. Low birthweight is associated with specific changes in muscle insulin-signalling protein expression. *Diabetologia* 48 (3):547–552.

Ozanne, S. E., G. S. Olsen, L. L. Hansen, K. J. Tingey, B. T. Nave, C. L. Wang, K. Hartil, C. J. Petry, A. J. Buckley, and L. Mosthaf-Seedorf. 2003. Early growth restriction leads to down regulation of protein kinase C zeta and insulin resistance in skeletal muscle. *J Endocrinol* 177 (2):235–241.

Park, K. S., T. P. Ciaraldi, L. Abrams-Carter, S. Mudaliar, S. E. Nikoulina, and R. R. Henry. 1997. PPAR-gamma gene expression is elevated in skeletal muscle of obese and type II diabetic subjects. *Diabetes* 46 (7):1230–1234.

Pate, R. R., M. Pratt, S. N. Blair, W. L. Haskell, C. A. Macera, C. Bouchard, D. Buchner, W. Ettinger, G. W. Heath, A. C. King et al. 1995. Physical activity and public health. A recommendation from the Centers for Disease Control and Prevention and the American College of Sports Medicine. *JAMA* 273 (5):402–407.

Pinney, S. E., and R. A. Simmons. 2009. Epigenetic mechanisms in the development of type 2 diabetes. *Trends Endocrinol Metab* 21 (4):223–229.

Prior, S. J., A. P. Goldberg, H. K. Ortmeyer, E. R. Chin, D. Chen, J. B. Blumenthal, and A. S. Ryan. 2015. Increased skeletal muscle capillarization independently enhances insulin sensitivity in older adults after exercise training and detraining. *Diabetes* 64 (10):3386–3395.

Raji, A., E. W. Seely, S. A. Bekins, G. H. Williams, and D. C. Simonson. 2003. Rosiglitazone improves insulin sensitivity and lowers blood pressure in hypertensive patients. *Diabetes Care* 26 (1):172–178.

Rangwala, S. M., and M. A. Lazar. 2004. Peroxisome proliferator-activated receptor gamma in diabetes and metabolism. *Trends Pharmacol Sci* 25 (6):331–336.

Raychaudhuri, N., S. Raychaudhuri, M. Thamotharan, and S. U. Devaskar. 2008. Histone code modifications repress glucose transporter 4 expression in the intrauterine growth-restricted offspring. *J Biol Chem* 283 (20):13611–13626.

Ren, J. M., C. F. Semenkovich, E. A. Gulve, J. Gao, and J. O. Holloszy. 1994. Exercise induces rapid increases in GLUT4 expression, glucose transport capacity, and insulin-stimulated glycogen storage in muscle. *J Biol Chem* 269 (20):14396–14401.

Reynolds, C. M., M. Li, C. Gray, and M. H. Vickers. 2013. Preweaning growth hormone treatment ameliorates adipose tissue insulin resistance and inflammation in adult male offspring following maternal undernutrition. *Endocrinology* 154 (8):2676–2686.

Richter, E. A., and M. Hargreaves. 2013. Exercise, GLUT4, and skeletal muscle glucose uptake. *Physiol Rev* (93) 3:993–1017.

Sadler, J. B., N. J. Bryant, G. W. Gould, and C. R. Welburn. 2013. Posttranslational modifications of GLUT4 affect its subcellular localization and translocation. *Int J Mol Sci* 14 (5):9963–9978.

Safdar, A., A. Abadi, M. Akhtar, B. P. Hettinga, and M. A. Tarnopolsky. 2009. miRNA in the regulation of skeletal muscle adaptation to acute endurance exercise in C57Bl/6J male mice. *PLoS One* 4 (5):e5610.

Saltiel, A. R., and C. R. Kahn. 2001. Insulin signalling and the regulation of glucose and lipid metabolism. *Nature* 414 (6865):799–806.

Saltiel, A. R., and J. M. Olefsky. 1996. Thiazolidinediones in the treatment of insulin resistance and type II diabetes. *Diabetes* 45 (12):1661–1669.

Santalucia, T., H. Moreno, M. Palacin, M. H. Yacoub, N. J. Brand, and A. Zorzano. 2001. A novel functional co-operation between MyoD, MEF2 and TRalpha1 is sufficient for the induction of GLUT4 gene transcription. *J Mol Biol* 314 (2):195–204.

Santos, J. M., S. Tewari, and S. A. Benite-Ribeiro. 2014. The effect of exercise on epigenetic modifications of PGC1: The impact on type 2 diabetes. *Med Hypotheses* 82 (6):748–753.

Satoh, T. 2014. Rho GTPases in insulin-stimulated glucose uptake. *Small GTPases* 5:e28102.

Scheepers, A., H. G. Joost, and A. Schurmann. 2004. The glucose transporter families SGLT and GLUT: Molecular basis of normal and aberrant function. *JPEN J Parenter Enteral Nutr* 28 (5):364–371.

Shaw, J. E., R. A. Sicree, and P. Z. Zimmet. 2010. Global estimates of the prevalence of diabetes for 2010 and 2030. *Diabetes Res Clin Pract* 87 (1):4–14.

Sherman, L. A., M. F. Hirshman, M. Cormont, Y. Le Marchand-Brustel, and L. J. Goodyear. 1996. Differential effects of insulin and exercise on Rab4 distribution in rat skeletal muscle. *Endocrinology* 137 (1):266–273.

Shin, B. C., Y. Dai, M. Thamotharan, L. C. Gibson, and S. U. Devaskar. 2014. Pre—And postnatal calorie restriction perturbs early hypothalamic neuropeptide and energy balance. *J Neurosci Res* 90 (6):1169–1182.

Silva, J. L., G. Giannocco, D. T. Furuya, G. A. Lima, P. A. Moraes, S. Nachef, S. Bordin, L. R. Britto, M. T. Nunes, and U. F. Machado. 2005. NF-kappaB, MEF2A, MEF2D and HIF1-a involvement on insulin- and contraction-induced regulation of GLUT4 gene expression in soleus muscle. *Mol Cell Endocrinol* 240 (1–2):82–93.

Simmons, R. A., L. J. Templeton, and S. J. Gertz. 2001. Intrauterine growth retardation leads to the development of type 2 diabetes in the rat. *Diabetes* 50 (10):2279–2286.

Slot, J. W., H. J. Geuze, S. Gigengack, D. E. James, and G. E. Lienhard. 1991. Translocation of the glucose transporter GLUT4 in cardiac myocytes of the rat. *Proc Natl Acad Sci USA* 88 (17):7815–7819.

Smith, J. A., T. A. Kohn, A. K. Chetty, and E. O. Ojuka. 2008. CaMK activation during exercise is required for histone hyperacetylation and MEF2A binding at the MEF2 site on the Glut4 gene. *Am J Physiol Endocrinol Metab* 295 (3):E698–E704.

Stenbit, A. E., T. S. Tsao, J. Li, R. Burcelin, D. L. Geenen, S. M. Factor, K. Houseknecht, E. B. Katz, and M. J. Charron. 1997. GLUT4 heterozygous knockout mice develop muscle insulin resistance and diabetes. *Nat Med* 3 (10):1096–1101.

Stocker, C. J., J. R. Arch, and M. A. Cawthorne. 2005. Fetal origins of insulin resistance and obesity. *Proc Nutr Soc* 64 (2):143–151.

Suzuki, K., and T. Kono. 1980. Evidence that insulin causes translocation of glucose transport activity to the plasma membrane from an intracellular storage site. *Proc Natl Acad Sci USA* 77 (5):2542–2545.

Sylow, L., T. E. Jensen, M. Kleinert, K. Hojlund, B. Kiens, J. Wojtaszewski, C. Prats, P. Schjerling, and E. A. Richter. 2013. Rac1 signaling is required for insulin-stimulated glucose uptake and is dysregulated in insulin-resistant murine and human skeletal muscle. *Diabetes* 62 (6):1865–1875.

Sylow, L., M. Kleinert, C. Pehmoller, C. Prats, T. T. Chiu, A. Klip, E. A. Richter, and T. E. Jensen. 2014. Akt and Rac1 signaling are jointly required for insulin-stimulated glucose uptake in skeletal muscle and downregulated in insulin resistance. *Cell Signal* 26 (2):323–331.

Sylow, L., I. L. Nielsen, M. Kleinert, L. L. Moller, T. Ploug, P. Schjerling, P. J. Bilan, A. Klip, T. E. Jensen, and E. A. Richter. 2016. Rac1 governs exercise-stimulated glucose uptake in skeletal muscle through regulation of GLUT4 translocation in mice. *J Physiol* 594:4997–5008.

Takata, K., H. Hirano, and M. Kasahara. 1997. Transport of glucose across the blood-tissue barriers. *Int Rev Cytol* 172:1–53.

Takenaka, N., R. Izawa, J. Wu, K. Kitagawa, Y. Nihata, T. Hosooka, T. Noguchi, W. Ogawa, A. Aiba, and T. Satoh. 2014. A critical role of the small GTPase Rac1 in Akt2-mediated GLUT4 translocation in mouse skeletal muscle. *FEBS J* 281 (5):1493–1504.

Thai, M. V., S. Guruswamy, K. T. Cao, J. E. Pessin, and A. L. Olson. 1998. Myocyte enhancer factor 2 (MEF2)-binding site is required for GLUT4 gene expression in transgenic mice. Regulation of MEF2 DNA binding activity in insulin-deficient diabetes. *J Biol Chem* 273 (23):14285–14292.

Thamotharan, M., M. Garg, S. Oak, L. M. Rogers, G. Pan, F. Sangiorgi, P. W. Lee, and S. U. Devaskar. 2007. Transgenerational inheritance of the insulin-resistant phenotype in embryo-transferred intrauterine growth-restricted adult female rat offspring. *Am J Physiol Endocrinol Metab* 292 (5):E1270–E1279.

Thamotharan, M., R. A. McKnight, S. Thamotharan, D. J. Kao, and S. U. Devaskar. 2003. Aberrant insulin-induced GLUT4 translocation predicts glucose intolerance in the offspring of a diabetic mother. *Am J Physiol Endocrinol Metab* 284 (5):E901–E914.

Thamotharan, M., B. C. Shin, D. T. Suddirikku, S. Thamotharan, M. Garg, and S. U. Devaskar. 2005. GLUT4 expression and subcellular localization in the intrauterine growth-restricted adult rat female offspring. *Am J Physiol Endocrinol Metab* 288 (5):E935–E947.

Thoidis, G., and K. V. Kandror. 2001. A Glut4-vesicle marker protein, insulin-responsive aminopeptidase, is localized in a novel vesicular compartment in PC12 cells. *Traffic* 2 (8):577–587.

Thorn, S. R., T. R. Regnault, L. D. Brown, P. J. Rozance, J. Keng, M. Roper, R. B. Wilkening, W. W. Hay, Jr., and J. E. Friedman. 2009. Intrauterine growth restriction increases fetal hepatic gluconeogenic capacity and reduces messenger ribonucleic acid translation initiation and nutrient sensing in fetal liver and skeletal muscle. *Endocrinology* 150 (7):3021–3030.

Tomi, M., Y. Zhao, S. Thamotharan, B. C. Shin, and S. U. Devaskar. 2013. Early life nutrient restriction impairs blood-brain metabolic profile and neurobehavior predisposing to
Alzheimer's disease with aging. *Brain Res* 1495:61–75.

Tontonoz, P., E. Hu, R. A. Graves, A. I. Budavari, and B. M. Spiegelman. 1994. mPPAR gamma
2: Tissue-specific regulator of an adipocyte enhancer. *Genes Dev* 8 (10):1224–1234.

Treadway, J. L., D. E. James, E. Burcel, and N. B. Ruderman. 1989. Effect of exercise on
insulin receptor binding and kinase activity in skeletal muscle. *Am J Physiol* 256
(1 Pt 1):E138–E144.

Trobec, K., S. von Haehling, S. D. Anker, and M. Lainscak. 2011. Growth hormone, insulin-
like growth factor 1, and insulin signaling–a pharmacological target in body wasting and
cachexia. *J Cachexia Sarcopenia Muscle* 2 (4):191–200.

Tsao, T. S., A. E. Stenbit, S. M. Factor, W. Chen, L. Rossetti, and M. J. Charron. 1999.
Prevention of insulin resistance and diabetes in mice heterozygous for GLUT4 ablation
by transgenic complementation of GLUT4 in skeletal muscle. *Diabetes* 48 (4):775–782.

Tsirka, A. E., E. M. Gruetzmacher, D. E. Kelley, V. H. Ritov, S. U. Devaskar, and R. H. Lane.
2001. Myocardial gene expression of glucose transporter 1 and glucose transporter 4 in
response to uteroplacental insufficiency in the rat. *J Endocrinol* 169 (2):373–380.

Tuuli, M. G., A. Cahill, D. Stamilio, G. Macones, and A. O. Odibo. 2011. Comparative efficiency of measures of early fetal growth restriction for predicting adverse perinatal outcomes. *Obstet Gynecol* 117 (6):1331–1340.

Vidal-Puig, A., M. Jimenez-Linan, B. B. Lowell, A. Hamann, E. Hu, B. Spiegelman, J. S. Flier,
and D. E. Moller. 1996. Regulation of PPAR gamma gene expression by nutrition and
obesity in rodents. *J Clin Invest* 97 (11):2553–2561.

Vidal-Puig, A. J., R. V. Considine, M. Jimenez-Linan, A. Werman, W. J. Pories, J. F. Caro, and
J. S. Flier. 1997. Peroxisome proliferator-activated receptor gene expression in human
tissues. Effects of obesity, weight loss, and regulation by insulin and glucocorticoids.
J Clin Invest 99 (10):2416–2422.

Wali, J. A., H. A. de Boo, J. G. Derraik, H. H. Phua, M. H. Oliver, F. H. Bloomfield, and
J. E. Harding. 2012. Weekly intra-amniotic IGF-1 treatment increases growth of growth-
restricted ovine fetuses and up-regulates placental amino acid transporters. *PLoS One*
7 (5):e37899.

Wallberg-Henriksson, H., and J. R. Zierath. 2001. GLUT4: A key player regulating glucose
homeostasis? Insights from transgenic and knockout mice (review). *Mol Membr Biol* 18
(3):205–211.

Wang, H., E. B. Arias, and G. D. Cartee. 2016a. Calorie restriction leads to greater Akt2 activity and glucose uptake by insulin-stimulated skeletal muscle from old rats. *Am J Physiol
Regul Integr Comp Physiol* 310 (5):R449–R458.

Wang, H., N. Sharma, E. B. Arias, and G. D. Cartee. 2016b. Insulin signaling and glucose
uptake in the soleus muscle of 30-month-old rats after calorie restriction with or without
acute exercise. *J Gerontol A Biol Sci Med Sci* 71 (3):323–332.

Wells, J. C., S. Chomtho, and M. S. Fewtrell. 2007. Programming of body composition by
early growth and nutrition. *Proc Nutr Soc* 66 (3):423–434.

Wojtaszewski, J. F., Y. Higaki, M. F. Hirshman, M. D. Michael, S. D. Dufresne, C. R. Kahn,
and L. J. Goodyear. 1999. Exercise modulates postreceptor insulin signaling and glucose transport in muscle-specific insulin receptor knockout mice. *J Clin Invest* 104
(9):1257–1264.

Wolf, G. 2003. Adult type 2 diabetes induced by intrauterine growth retardation. *Nutr Rev* 61
(5 Pt 1):176–179.

Wu, G., F. W. Bazer, J. M. Wallace, and T. E. Spencer. 2006. Board-invited review: Intrauterine
growth retardation: Implications for the animal sciences. *J Anim Sci* 84 (9):2316–2337.

Wu, X., and H. H. Freeze. 2002. GLUT14, a duplicon of GLUT3, is specifically expressed in
testis as alternative splice forms. *Genomics* 80 (6):553–557.

Xie, X., T. Lin, M. Zhang, L. Liao, G. Yuan, H. Gao, Q. Ning, and X. Luo. 2015. IUGR with infantile overnutrition programs an insulin-resistant phenotype through DNA methylation of peroxisome proliferator-activated receptor-gamma coactivator-1alpha in rats. *Pediatr Res* 77 (5):625–632.

Yates, D. T., D. S. Clarke, A. R. Macko, M. J. Anderson, L. A. Shelton, M. Nearing, R. E. Allen, R. P. Rhoads, and S. W. Limesand. 2014. Myoblasts from intrauterine growth-restricted sheep fetuses exhibit intrinsic deficiencies in proliferation that contribute to smaller semitendinosus myofibres. *J Physiol* 592 (14):3113–3125.

Zambrano, E., P. M. Martinez-Samayoa, C. J. Bautista, M. Deas, L. Guillen, G. L. Rodriguez-Gonzalez, C. Guzman, F. Larrea, and P. W. Nathanielsz. 2005. Sex differences in transgenerational alterations of growth and metabolism in progeny (F2) of female offspring (F1) of rats fed a low protein diet during pregnancy and lactation. *J Physiol* 566 (Pt 1):225–236.

Zeng, Y., P. Gu, K. Liu, and P. Huang. 2013. Maternal protein restriction in rats leads to reduced PGC-1alpha expression via altered DNA methylation in skeletal muscle. *Mol Med Rep* 7 (1):306–312.

Zhang, L. N., L. Xu, H. Y. Zhou, L. Y. Wu, Y. Y. Li, T. Pang, C. M. Xia, B. Y. Qiu, M. Gu, T. C. Dong, J. Y. Li, J. K. Shen, and J. Li. 2013a. Novel small-molecule AMP-activated protein kinase allosteric activator with beneficial effects in db/db mice. *PLoS One* 8 (8):e72092.

Zhang, L. N., H. Y. Zhou, Y. Y. Fu, Y. Y. Li, F. Wu, M. Gu, L. Y. Wu, C. M. Xia, T. C. Dong, J. Y. Li, J. K. Shen, and J. Li. 2013b. Novel small-molecule PGC-1alpha transcriptional regulator with beneficial effects on diabetic db/db mice. *Diabetes* 62 (4):1297–1307.

Zhao, F. Q., and A. F. Keating. 2007. Functional properties and genomics of glucose transporters. *Curr Genomics* 8 (2):113–128.

Zheng, S., M. Rollet, and Y. X. Pan. 2012. Protein restriction during gestation alters histone modifications at the glucose transporter 4 (GLUT4) promoter region and induces GLUT4 expression in skeletal muscle of female rat offspring. *J Nutr Biochem* 23 (9):1064–1071.

Zhou, Y., P. Gu, W. Shi, J. Li, Q. Hao, X. Cao, Q. Lu, and Y. Zeng. 2016. MicroRNA-29a induces insulin resistance by targeting PPARdelta in skeletal muscle cells. *Int J Mol Med* 37 (4):931–938.

7 Impact of Maternal Obesity and Diabetes on Fetal Pancreatic Development

Jens H. Nielsen, Caroline Jaksch,
Isabela Iessi, and Débora C.Damasceno

CONTENTS

7.1   INTRODUCTION

The global epidemics of obesity and type 2 diabetes (T2D) are serious threats to human health and health-care expenses. Although genetics is an important factor, it does not explain this dramatic increase that involves environmental factors such as nutrients, gut microbiota, and lifestyles. Twenty-five years ago, the concept of "fetal programming" or "Developmental Origins of Health and Disease" was introduced stating that the intrauterine environment during pregnancy has an impact on gene expression that may persist through adulthood and be transmitted to the next generations. It was found that both under- and overnutrition before and during pregnancy may cause metabolic diseases like obesity and T2D. Studies in humans have shown that offspring of mothers with obesity, type 1 diabetes (T1D), T2D, or gestational diabetes mellitus (GDM) are prone to develop metabolic disorders such as obesity, T2D, and GDM in adult life (Carrapato 2003; Hummel et al. 2013; Ruchat et al. 2013; Yan and Yang 2014). In certain populations, up to 15% of pregnant women develop GDM (King 1998) and offspring of GDM mothers has an up to eightfold increased risk of developing T2D or prediabetes later in life (Clausen et al. 2008). Obesity is a risk factor for development of GDM (Black et al. 2013; Fox et al. 2014), and the prevalence of obesity in women of reproductive age (20–44 years) in the United States is around 33% (Huda et al. 2010). Among pregnant women in 20 U.S. states, 20.5% were pre-pregnant obese in 2009 (Fisher et al. 2013). The clinical consequences of obesity and diabetes in pregnancy for the offspring will be dealt with in Chapters 13 and 14 of this book.

As the pancreatic β-cells are crucial in the regulation of metabolism, this chapter describes the influence of maternal obesity and diabetes on the development and function of the endocrine pancreas in the offspring. As the access to pancreatic tissue from humans is limited, most of the studies mentioned in this chapter have been performed in animals. The effects of undernutrition during pregnancy and modified nutrients in the early postnatal period on programming of the endocrine pancreas are discussed elsewhere in this book.

In healthy pregnancy, there is a marked increase in the β-cell mass in order to compensate for the increased demand for insulin in late pregnancy. In rodents, this is accomplished mainly by increased proliferation of the existing β-cells due to increased levels of the somatolactogenic hormones placental lactogen and placental growth hormone as well as an increased expression of the receptors for prolactin and growth hormone in the endocrine pancreas (Parsons et al. 1992; Rieck and Kaestner 2010; Nielsen et al. 2016). It was recently confirmed that β-cell-specific inactivation of the PRL receptor resulted in GDM in pregnant mice (Banerjee et al. 2016). In human pregnancy, there is an increase in the β-cell mass but the mechanism may rather be by neogenesis than by proliferation of existing β-cells (Butler et al. 2010). There is also evidence for neogenesis in rodent pregnancy (Sostrup et al. 2014; Hakonen et al. 2014). It is conceivable that lack of this compensatory increase in β-cell mass is involved in the pathogenesis of GDM. It has been known for a long time that the offspring of pregnant women with diabetes in particular T1D are at risk of macrosomia and malformations, which has been suggested to be due to the increased delivery of nutrients in particular glucose and lipids to the fetus (Freinkel 1980).

Women with GDM have a sevenfold increased risk of developing T2D later in life (Bellamy et al. 2009). The mechanisms involved in the development of GDM are not clarified. Most probably it is an imbalance between insulin resistance and insulin delivery. Thus, a reduction in the β-cell mass by a low-dose streptozotocin (STZ) treatment before pregnancy in the rats resulted in hyperglycemia during pregnancy, suggesting that the prepregnancy β-cell mass is a determining factor (Devlieger et al. 2008). The β-cell mass depends on genetic and environmental factors during early life that influences the programming of the endocrine pancreas (Nielsen et al. 2014). Both the lack of β-cell stimulating factors and occurrence of β-cell inhibitory factors like abnormal metabolites or toxins from food or microbiota may lead to impaired β-cell growth and function during pregnancy (Prentice et al. 2014). The regulation of the β-cell mass under normal and pathological condition is illustrated in Figure 7.1.

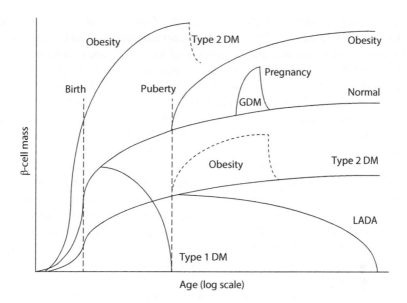

FIGURE 7.1   Schematic changes in the functional β-Cell mass in normal growth, microsomia, macrosomia, obesity, pregnancy, gestational diabetes (GDM), type 1 diabetes (T1D), type 2 diabetes (T2D), and latent autoimmune diabetes in adults (LADA).

7.2   EFFECT OF MATERNAL OBESITY ON THE ENDOCRINE PANCREAS IN THE OFFSPRING

In many countries around the world, a Western lifestyle has led to an increased consumption of a high-fat/high-sucrose food and an increase in maternal obesity. The risk of giving birth to a macrosomic neonate increases with increasing body mass index (BMI) in women even with normal glucose tolerance (Sewell et al. 2006; Ovesen et al. 2011). These children have increased risk of developing T2D later in life (Berends and Ozanne 2012; Dowling and McAuliffe 2013). The diet can influence fetal growth by altering the concentrations of circulating key metabolic hormones that regulate placental nutrient transport and therefore fetal growth (Jansson et al. 2008). Maternal obesity and excess nutrients *in utero* may affect several organs including the β-cells (O'Dowd and Stocker 2013).

Animal studies have confirmed the effects of maternal overnutrition during gestation and/or lactation on the adult offspring observed in humans. A maternal high-fat diet (HFD) during gestation in the rat predisposed the offspring to develop a metabolic syndrome-like phenotype with insulin resistance, glucose intolerance, and increased body weight in adulthood (Dowling and McAuliffe 2013; Srinivasan et al. 2006). Cerf et al. (2005) showed that 1-day-old neonatal rats exposed to maternal HFD *in utero* were hyperglycemic and had reduced β-cell volume and number. However, other studies in rats have shown that maternal overnutrition increased the β-cell mass and glucose-induced insulin secretion (GSIS) in the offspring early in life but impaired glucose tolerance in adulthood (Srinivasan et al. 2006) associated with mitochondrial dysfunction (Taylor et al. 2005). HFD in pregnant mice showed increased β-cell proliferation, insulin content, and expression of key islet genes (insulin 1 [Ins1], pancreatic and duodenal homeobox 1 [Pdx-1], glucose transporter 2 [GLUT-2], glucokinase [GK], ATP-sensitive potassium channel subunit 2 [Kir6.2]) but reduced GSIS and expression of vesicle-associated membrane protein 2 (VAMP2) involved in exocytosis (Tuohetimulati et al. 2012). Increased islet protein, DNA, and insulin content but impaired insulin secretion were also found in adult female offspring of HFD fed obese mice (Han et al. 2005). A time-dependent effect has also been demonstrated in sheep where diet-induced obesity (DIO) in ewes resulted in midgestation fetuses with hyperglycemia, hyperinsulinemia, and increased β-cell numbers, whereas fetuses at term had decreased β-cell numbers and increased β-cell apoptosis but similar birth weights suggesting a declining functional β-cell mass and/or β-cell exhaustion that may lead to T2D later in life (Zhang et al. 2011). Thus, depending on timing, short-term HFD may lead to β-cell compensation by proliferation and/or neogenesis, whereas long-term HFD may lead to β-cell exhaustion, hypoplasia, and/ or dedifferentiation (Cerf 2015). In 1-day-old rats born by HFD-fed obese dams, no change in the messenger RNA (mRNA) levels of GLUT-2, GK, and Pdx-1 was seen but a reduction of GK and Pdx-1 at the protein level was found as well as a reduced GSIS in the isolated islets (Cerf et al. 2009). After 3 weeks lactation by dams on HFD, Pdx-1 mRNA was increased, whereas GK mRNA and protein were reduced and the animals were hyperglycemic. It has also been reported that maternal HFD caused reduced GLUT-2 expression and mitochondrial dysfunction in the female offspring resulting in islet dysfunction at 12 weeks postpartum (Theys et al. 2011). If HFD is continued in the offspring up to 20 weeks, insulin content and Pdx-1 mRNA levels were lower in males but increased in females and oxidative stress was increased in islets from males but not from females indicating a marked sex difference in the metabolic programming (Yokomizo et al. 2014). This was also reflected in studies on the effect of HFD on the inflammation and cytokine expression in the placenta in late pregnant mice, which was more pronounced in the placentas accompanying male fetuses than female fetuses (Kim et al. 2014). HFD in mice 8 weeks before conception, during pregnancy, and during lactation resulted in reduced β-cell mass in the offspring at birth but a recovery by increased proliferation in the suckling period (Bringhenti et al. 2013) and a remodeling of the islets in the 6-month-old offspring with increases in both β- and α-cell masses and migration of some α-cells to the islet core but a decrease in Pdx-1, GLUT-2, insulin receptor substrate 1 (IRS-1) and phosphatidyl-inositol-3-kinase (PI3K) protein expression indicating β-cell dysfunction (Bringhenti et al. 2016). Mice on HFD before gestation and during gestation and lactation resulted in increased body weight, energy intake, and glucose intolerance with hyperinsulinemia, hyperleptinemia, decreased adiponectin levels, and increased β- and α-cell mass but reduced Pdx-1 expression in male F1 and F2 progeny implying intergenerational transmission (Graus-Nunes et al. 2015). The fetal programming of the pancreas does not only depend on maternal obesity but also on paternal obesity (Ng et al. 2010; Rando and Simmons 2015) as discussed in Chapter 18 of this book.

In our studies, we have used the rat model of Barry Levin (Levin et al. 1997) who derived two substrains of Sprague–Dawley rats that were bred for their propensity to resist (DR) or develop DIO when fed a high-energy (HE) diet consisting of 31% fat and 25% sucrose. At the time of weaning, the DR rats had a higher β-cell mass than the DIO rats. Both DR and DIO rats increased their β-cell mass up to 6 months of age but at 12 months of age, the DIO rats on HE diet had a decline in glucose tolerance (Paulsen et al. 2010). In order to investigate if there was a difference in fetal programming of endocrine pancreas between the DR and DIO rats, we studied the offspring of DR and DIO dams fed HE or chow during pregnancy. As the growth and maturation of the β-cells are most pronounced in the perinatal period, we studied the gene expression profile of the pancreas from 2-day-old pups. There was an increase in body weight of the DIO HE pups and the tendency to an increase in islet mass and size. There were no significant differences in the mRNA levels of insulin, musculoaponeurotic fibrosarcoma oncogene homolog A (MafA), musculoaponeurotic oncogene homolog B (MafB). Pdx-1, and neurogenin 3 (Ngn3) between the groups (Jaksch 2016). However, this does not exclude that there are differences at the protein level that may affect the β-cell function.

7.3   EFFECTS OF MATERNAL DIABETES ON THE ENDOCRINE PANCREAS IN THE OFFSPRING

Diabetes induced by STZ in pregnant rats has been studied extensively by Van Assche et al. (Devlieger et al. 2008; Rando and Simmons 2015; Aerts et al. 1997). Severe maternal diabetes resulted in acute hyperglycemia in the fetus leading to β-cell hyperplasia mainly due to formation of numerous small islets followed by early hyperinsulinemia and later hypoinsulinemia due to exhaustion of the β-cells leading to growth retardation and microsomia. In mildly diabetic pregnant rats, the fetal β-cell mass was also increased but hyperinsulinemia was maintained leading to macrosomia. The induction of experimental diabetes using a β-cytotoxic drug such as STZ is well characterized (Ward et al. 2001). This cytotoxin is derived from *Streptomyces achromogenes* and results in degranulation and necrosis of β-cells causing insulin deficiency. Depending on species, age, dose, and route of administration, different degrees of β-cell destruction may occur. Both *in vivo* and in isolated islets *in vitro*, adult rats are very susceptible to STZ, whereas adult mice are less susceptible and humans are resistant (Nielsen 1984). Mild diabetes in rats with blood glucose levels between 120 and 200–300 mg/dL can be obtained by a low dose of STZ or by treatment of neonatal rats with STZ (Portha et al. 1974; Gelardi et al. 1990; Merzouk et al. 2000; Sinzato et al. 2011; Damasceno et al. 2013), whereas severe diabetes with blood glucose levels above 300 mg/dL can be obtained by a single high-dose STZ in adult rats (de Souza et al. 2010; Rudge et al. 2007; Eriksson et al. 2003; Damasceno et al. 2014; Corvino et al. 2015; Volpato et al. 2015). Interestingly, multiple injections of low doses of STZ can induce autoimmune destruction of β-cells in mice that resembles T1D (Like and Rossini 1976). Studies in experimental animals may lead to a better understanding of pathophysiological mechanisms involved in the effect of diabetes during pregnancy on the development of the endocrine pancreas in the offspring.

Diabetes induced by low- and high-dose STZ in pregnant rats at the day of mating has been studied extensively by Van Assche et al. (1991) (Devlieger et al. 2008; Aerts et al. 1997). The partial destruction of β-cells in rats induced by low-dose STZ resulted in moderately increased blood glucose, which is transferred to fetus through placenta by facilitated diffusion (Aerts et al. 1997). During the fetal endocrine pancreas development, there is evidence of islet hypertrophy, hyperplasia of the fetal β-cells, and increased insulin synthesis due to the increased maternal glucose supply (Kervran et al. 1978). In order to investigate the role of diabetic intrauterine environment on circulating levels of insulin, glucagon, and somatostatin, fetuses of diabetic mothers were investigated as follows. Offspring of Wistar female rats were subjected to subcutaneous injection of STZ either at birth (mild diabetes) (Sinzato et al. 2011) or at adulthood (severe diabetes) (Corvino et al. 2015). The adult rats were mated and killed in order to study the fetal endocrine pancreas. The hyperglycemic intrauterine environment contributes to fetal hyperinsulinemia and higher anabolism, leading to a fetal and perinatal macrosomia as expected (Corvino et al. 2015). Iessi et al. (2016) demonstrated that this model of STZ-induced mild diabetes presented a size distribution between small and large islets with a lower percentage of large islets in fetuses of mildly diabetic mothers. At term, these fetuses presented a decreased number of proliferating cells and a decreased number of cells stained for somatostatin and increased number of apoptotic cells (Iessi et al. 2015). The fetuses also showed a lower circulating level of somatostatin as compared with that of the control fetuses. The fetal insulin/glucagon and insulin/somatostatin ratios were higher as compared with those of the control mothers. The pancreata were analyzed by number of stained cells and by ratio of stained area and total area of islets (Iessi et al. 2016). These results indicate that the maternal diabetic condition impaired the fetal pancreatic development by reduction of number of islets and abnormal number and organization of hormone-containing cells (insulin, glucagon, and somatostatin). It is known that somatostatin is indirectly involved in glycemic regulation by allowing fine adjustments in the control of insulin and glucagon secretion (Bousquet et al. 2004). The results of our research group, therefore, suggest that the somatostatin cells are more susceptible to changes in the intrauterine environment than the insulin and glucagon cells (Iessi et al. 2015).

Pancreatic organogenesis and differentiation of the endocrine pancreas require the tightly regulated control of a number of genes. Pdx-1 is crucial for the early development of the pancreatic lineage. Genetic ablation of Pdx-1 results in the absence of pancreatic development, but in the mature pancreas its expression is mainly restricted to differentiated β-cells (Kaneto et al. 2008). Pdx-1 is a transcription factor involved in embryonic development in mice and humans (Ohlsson et al. 1993; Jonsson et al. 1994; Offield et al. 1996) and controls a number of genes involved in the maintenance of β-cell identity and insulin synthesis and secretion (Chakrabarti et al. 2002; Le Lay et al. 2004), including Glut2 (Waeber et al. 1996; Lottmann et al. 2001), GK (Watada et al. 1996), and Pdx-1 (Gerrish et al. 2001). Previous results revealed that there was reduction of this marker in islets of fetuses from mildly diabetic mothers, contributing to decrease in the number of endocrine pancreatic cells in this group (Iessi et al. 2015). During perinatal life, the maternal hyperglycemic stimulus disappears causing hypoplasia of the pup's endocrine pancreas during the weaning period (Aerts et al. 1990). These adult pups from mothers with mild diabetes present normal distribution of islet-cell types leading to normoglycemia and insulin levels in endocrine pancreas (Aerts et al. 1997). However, under glucose challenge these animals exhibit an impaired insulin response.

When diabetes is induced in adult rats by a single high-dose STZ, the majority of β-pancreatic cells are destroyed, resulting in severe hyperglycemia. Maternal
severe diabetes leads to an acute hyperglycemia in the fetus causing β-cell hyperplasia mainly due to formation of numerous small islets followed by early hyperinsulinemia and later hypoinsulinemia due to exhaustion of the β-cells leading to growth
retardation and microsomia (Van Assche et al. 2001).

In our experimental model, the diabetic rats presented exacerbated oxidative
stress and hypoxia, and this was further exacerbated at term pregnancy in severely
diabetic rats. The reduced β-cell mass explains not only the development of severe
and chronic hyperglycemia but also other maternal changes. Islet number per unit
area and the number of cells per islet were significantly reduced in fetuses from
severely diabetic dams on days 18 and 21 of pregnancy. These alterations were related
to higher blood glucose level, oxidative stress, and hypoxia at term pregnancy. The
size distribution between small and large islets has revealed a higher fraction of large
islets in fetuses from severely diabetic mothers than those from mildly diabetic rats
(Iessi et al. 2015).

Interestingly, fetal islets from severely diabetic rats had a significantly reduced
relative number of cells stained by Pdx-1–positive cells on day 21 of pregnancy
and a reduced number of proliferating cells and an increased incidence of apoptosis on days 18 and 21 of pregnancy, supporting a reduced number of insulin-
positive β-cells in this period. These findings corroborate reduced β-cell mass and
growth-retarded fetuses of diabetic rats compared to control (Iessi et al., unpub-
lished data). The plasma glucagon concentration was diminished in fetuses from
the severe diabetic dams with a marked increase of the insulin/glucagon ratio and
a reduction of insulin/somatostatin ratio in fetuses in relation to the control group.
These ratios were reversed in the newborns when the glucose level was reduced
to below normal (Iessi et al. 2016), indicating that the interactions between the
islet hormones play important roles in metabolic programming. It has been shown
that pregnant diabetic women may experience impaired embryofetal development
due to hypoxia and oxidative stress (Ornoy et al. 2010). The relationship between
number of islets and cells per islets in fetuses with maternal hyperglycemia, oxidative stress markers, and maternal hypoxia suggests that these mechanisms are
involved in the reduction of the number of fetal islets as well as the number of
cells per islet.

Offspring of mothers with T1D only have a low risk of T1D (Buschard et al. 1989)
but it has recently been reported that maternal obesity without diabetes is associated
with a higher prevalence of T1D (Hussen et al 2015). It has also been shown that
female nonobese diabetic (NOD) mice fed HFD during pregnancy gave rise to more
severe lymphocytic infiltration in the islets and lower insulin levels in their female
offspring (Wang et al. 2014), suggesting that the inflammatory intrauterine environment under some circumstances may give rise to T1D. However, further human studies are required to confirm these findings.

When the offspring became pregnant, both those that were born from severely
diabetic mothers and those born from mildly diabetic mothers developed GDM
(Aerts et al. 1997), which may continue to the following generations (Chavey
et al. 2014).

7.4   ROLE OF INFLAMMATION

Obesity and diabetes are characterized by a low-grade inflammation in several tissues, including the pancreatic islets (Gregor and Hotamisligil 2011; Donath and Shoelson 2011). It has been reported (Desai et al. 2013) that fetuses of high calorie fed rat mothers had elevated plasma levels of interleukin 6 (IL-6), tumor necrosis factor α (TNFα), and chemokine ligand 2. Pups born by obese mouse dams or suckled by obese dams were found to develop nonalcoholic fatty pancreas disease (NAFPD) (Oben et al. 2010). NAFPD involves fat deposition and inflammation with resultant pancreatic fibrosis, with the accumulation of collagen being the major extracellular matrix component produced by the activation of pancreatic stellate cells. Gene expression profiling of pancreas in offspring of DIO and DR rats fed HE diet or chow during pregnancy showed differences in expression of genes involved in pro- and anti-inflammatory pathways between the groups. Thus, the expression of the proinflammatory phospholipase A2 group 2a (Pla2g2a) was twofold higher in DIO pups than in DR pups independent of the diet, whereas the anti-inflammatory phospholipase A2 group 2d (Pla2g2d) was increased more in DIO pups than in the DR pups on HE diet. Interleukin 1β stimulated the expression of Pla2g2a in both rat isles and INS-1E cells (Jaksch 2016) and the expression of the anti-inflammatory interleukin 1 receptor antagonist gene (IL-1ra) was upregulated in both DR and DIO pups on HE diet supporting the role in the inflammatory processes in the islets that may lead to β-cell dysfunction later in life.

Although maternal obesity is associated with inflammatory responses in several organs (Segovia et al. 2014), including the placenta where it has been found that Toll-like receptors TLR2 and TLR4, macrophage markers CD14 and CD68, TNFα, IL-6, IL-8, and nuclear factor kappa B (NF-κB) were upregulated in midgestational ewes that may be transmitted to the fetus (Zhu et al. 2010), pregnancy is also associated with anti-inflammatory reactions. Thus, the low-grade inflammation in adipose tissue, liver, and placenta induced in female mice fed an obesogenic diet for 6 weeks before conception was reversed on day 18 of gestation (Ingvorsen et al. 2014). It has also been reported that some women with T1D have increased levels of C-peptide during pregnancy and reduced circulating levels of IL-6, IL-8, and MCP-1 compared to the levels after delivery (Nalla 2012), suggesting a suppression of the autoimmune reaction in T1D. This has also been observed in T1D in pregnant rats and in women with GDM (Yessoufou et al. 2011). It is known that pregnancy is associated with a switch from Th1 response characterized by production of proinflammatory cytokines (IL-2, IL-12, interferon γ [IFNγ]) toward Th2 response characterized by production of anti-inflammatory cytokines (IL-4, IL-5, IL-10, IL-13) that may be due to the increased levels of pregnancy hormones including human chorionic gonadotrophin (hCG) (Furcron et al. 2016). However, after delivery the Th1/Th2 ratio is rebound and the adverse effects of inflammatory reactions in the offspring of obese or diabetic mothers will precipitate.

Another family of genes that was upregulated in the pancreas of pups from DIO rats on HE diet was the Reg genes Reg3α and Reg3γ (Jaksch 2016) that have been found to be increased in pancreatitis (Zenilman et al. 2000) and so they have been implicated in pancreas development (Xiong et al. 2011) and β-cell regeneration (Terazono et al. 1988; Kapur et al. 2012). Thus, they may be involved in the compensatory increase in β-cell mass in the offspring of obese mothers, although this is still controversial.

7.5 ROLE OF IMPRINTED GENES AND NONCODING RNAS

Interestingly, the long noncoding RNA gene Bsr was found to be downregulated two-fold in the DIO pups on HE diet compared to DR pups on HE or chow (Jaksch 2016). It is located in the delta-like 1 (DLK1)-type 3-iodothyronine deiodinase (DIO3) genomic region that contains the paternally expressed protein-coding genes DLK1 (also called preadipocyte factor 1 [Pref-1]), retrotransposon-like 1 (RTL1), and DIO3 and maternally expressed noncoding transcription unit containing maternally expressed 3 (MEG3), MEG8 (called brain specific repetitive long noncoding RNA [Bsr] in the rat), and antisense RTL1 and a very large microRNA (miRNA) cluster (Benetatos et al. 2013). It is expressed in human β-cells and has been reported to be strongly repressed in islets from T2D donors (Kameswaran et al. 2014). Recently, it was shown that the expression of MEG3 was decreased in islets from NOD mice and db/db mice and that knockdown of MEG3 in mice resulted in impaired glucose tolerance and decreased expression of Pdx-1 and MafA (You et al. 2016).

DLK1 was previously shown to be highly expressed in islets from 2-day-old rats (Carlsson et al. 1997) and there was a tendency to lower the expression of DLK1 in DIO pups on HE diet in the microarray analysis (Jaksch 2016). DLK1/Pref-1 is highly expressed in embryonic tissues and seems to be a maintenance factor for undifferentiated cells and be permissive for fetal growth. Thus, it acts an inhibitor of differentiation in preadipocytes to mature adipocytes. In adulthood, it is only expressed in the endocrine pancreas, the pituitary, and the adrenal cells. It is highly expressed in human β-cells (Dorrell et al. 2011). DLK1 expression is upregulated by growth hormone and prolactin in rat islets and during pregnancy (Carlsson et al. 1997; Friedrichsen et al. 2003). It is highly expressed in fetal and neonatal β-cells and it does not seem to act as a growth factor for β-cells but may be permissive for allowing cell proliferation and maturation in response to other factors (Martens et al. 2014). Recently, it was shown that overexpression of DLK1 activates Pdx-1 that leads to differentiation of human pancreatic ductal cells into β-like cells (Rhee et al. 2016). Transgenic mice overexpressing DLK1 showed an increase in insulin secretion and islet mass with a higher proportion of large islets and improved glucose tolerance (Wang et al. 2015). Thus, DLK1 may be a positive regulator of β-cells and insulin production. However, DLK1 knockout mice had normal β-cell development, suggesting that compensatory mechanisms exist (Appelbe et al. 2013).

Some of the miRNAs in the DLK1-DIO3 cluster were downregulated in the DIO–HE pups, including miR495 that previously reported to be downregulated in islets from T2D patients. This resulted in increased expression of p53-induced nuclear protein 1 (TP53INP1), which in turn increased the susceptibility to apoptosis (Kameswaran et al. 2014). Although much more research is needed in this field, these results indicate that noncoding RNAs play important roles in fetal programming of the β-cells (Kameswaran and Kaestner 2014; Singer et al. 2015). Chapters 16 an 17 in this book describe epigenetic mechanisms involved in fetal and early programming of other organs in more detail.

7.6 CONCLUSIONS

This chapter has focused on the fetal programming of the endocrine pancreas in various animal models of obesity and diabetes. Figure 7.2 summarizes some of the

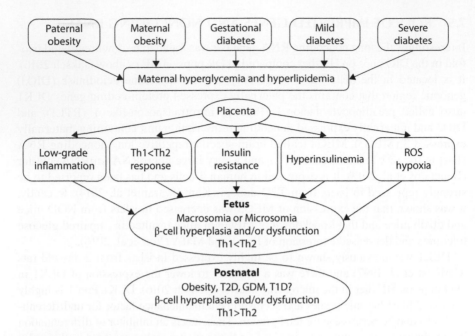

FIGURE 7.2 Schematic representation of the mechanism involved in fetal programming of the β-cells in maternal obesity and diabetes.

factors and processes that are involved. With regard to metabolism, pregnancy is associated with an opposing effect as it increases the demand for insulin as insulin resistance in the mother contributes to the delivery of nutrients to the fetus. If the capacity of the insulin production is compensated by an increase in the β-cell mass, euglycemia is maintained, but if the capacity of the β-cells is compromised by genetic and/or malnutrition, GDM may occur. Then the fetus will be exposed to high concentrations of glucose and lipids that will cause increased fetal insulin production that will lead to macrosomia or exhaustion of the fetal β-cells that will lead to microsomia. Thus, overnutrition is a common denominator for the adverse effect of maternal obesity and diabetes on the health of the offspring in several generations. It should also be stressed that pregnancy in itself has a protective role in the health of the fetus via the placenta and the modulation of the innate and adaptive immune reactions that prevent rejection of the fetus but also protects against infections and toxic agents and adverse effects of inflammatory reactions. These protective effects disappear after delivery and may even be promoted both in the mother and in the offspring. In order to prevent the adverse effects of obesity and diabetes on the offspring lifestyle intervention is required for both parents, preferably before conception. Adequate calorie intake and physical activity should be compulsory from childhood.

REFERENCES

Aerts L, Holemans K, Van Assche FA. Maternal diabetes during pregnancy: Consequences for the offspring. *Diabetes/Metabolism Reviews*. 1990;6:147–67.

Aerts L, Vercruysse L, Van Assche FA. The endocrine pancreas in virgin and pregnant offspring of diabetic pregnant rats. *Diabetes Research and Clinical Practice.* 1997;38:9–19.

Appelbe OK, Yevtodiyenko A, Muniz-Talavera H, Schmidt JV. Conditional deletions refine the embryonic requirement for Dlk1. *Mechanisms of Development.* 2013;130:143–59.

Banerjee RR, Cyphert HA, Walker EM, Chakravarthy H, Peiris H, Gu X, et al. Gestational diabetes mellitus from inactivation of prolactin receptor and MafB in islet beta-cells. *Diabetes.* 2016;65:2331–41.

Bellamy L, Casas JP, Hingorani AD, Williams D. Type 2 diabetes mellitus after gestational diabetes: A systematic review and meta-analysis. *Lancet.* 2009;373:1773–9.

Benetatos L, Hatzimichael E, Londin E, Vartholomatos G, Loher P, Rigoutsos I, et al. The microRNAs within the DLK1-DIO3 genomic region: Involvement in disease pathogenesis. *Cellular and Molecular Life Sciences: CMLS.* 2013;70:795–814.

Berends LM, Ozanne SE. Early determinants of type-2 diabetes. *Best Practice & Research Clinical Endocrinology & Metabolism.* 2012;26:569–80.

Black MH, Sacks DA, Xiang AH, Lawrence JM. The relative contribution of prepregnancy overweight and obesity, gestational weight gain, and IADPSG-defined gestational diabetes mellitus to fetal overgrowth. *Diabetes Care.* 2013;36:56–62.

Bousquet C, Guillermet J, Vernejoul F, Lahlou H, Buscail L, Susini C. Somatostatin receptors and regulation of cell proliferation. *Digestive and Liver Disease.* 2004;36 Suppl 1:S2–7.

Bringhenti I, Moraes-Teixeira JA, Cunha MR, Ornellas F, Mandarim-de-Lacerda CA, Aguila MB. Maternal obesity during the preconception and early life periods alters pancreatic development in early and adult life in male mouse offspring. *PLoS One.* 2013;8:e55711.

Bringhenti I, Ornellas F, Mandarim-de-Lacerda CA, Aguila MB. The insulin-signaling pathway of the pancreatic islet is impaired in adult mice offspring of mothers fed a high-fat diet. *Nutrition.* 2016;32:1138–43.

Buschard K, Kuhl C, Molsted-Pedersen L, Lund E, Palmer J, Bottazzo GF. Investigations in children who were in utero at onset of insulin-dependent diabetes in their mothers. *Lancet.* 1989;1:811–4.

Butler AE, Cao-Minh L, Galasso R, Rizza RA, Corradin A, Cobelli C, et al. Adaptive changes in pancreatic beta cell fractional area and beta cell turnover in human pregnancy. *Diabetologia.* 2010;53:2167–76.

Carlsson C, Tornehave D, Lindberg K, Galante P, Billestrup N, Michelsen B, et al. Growth hormone and prolactin stimulate the expression of rat preadipocyte factor-1/delta-like protein in pancreatic islets: Molecular cloning and expression pattern during development and growth of the endocrine pancreas. *Endocrinology.* 1997;138:3940–8.

Carrapato MRG. The offspring of gestational diabetes. *Journal of Perinatal Medicine.* 2003;31:5–11.

Cerf ME, Chapman CS, Muller CJ, Louw J. Gestational high-fat programming impairs insulin release and reduces Pdx-1 and glucokinase immunoreactivity in neonatal Wistar rats. *Metabolism: Clinical and Experimental.* 2009;58:1787–92.

Cerf ME, Williams K, Nkomo XI, Muller CJ, Du Toit DF, Louw J, et al. Islet cell response in the neonatal rat after exposure to a high-fat diet during pregnancy. *American Journal of Physiology. Regulatory, Integrative and Comparative Physiology.* 2005;288:R1122–8.

Cerf ME. High fat programming of beta cell compensation, exhaustion, death and dysfunction. *Pediatric Diabetes.* 2015;16:71–8.

Chakrabarti SK, James JC, Mirmira RG. Quantitative assessment of gene targeting in vitro and in vivo by the pancreatic transcription factor, Pdx1. Importance of chromatin structure in directing promoter binding. *Journal of Biological Chemistry.* 2002;277:13286–93.

Chavey A, Ah Kioon MD, Bailbe D, Movassat J, Portha B. Maternal diabetes, programming of beta-cell disorders and intergenerational risk of type 2 diabetes. *Diabetes & Metabolism.* 2014;40:323–30.

Clausen TD, Mathiesen ER, Hansen T, Pedersen O, Jensen DM, Lauenborg J, et al. High prevalence of type 2 diabetes and pre-diabetes in adult offspring of women with gestational diabetes mellitus or type 1 diabetes: The role of intrauterine hyperglycemia. *Diabetes Care.* 2008;31:340–6.

Corvino SB, Netto AO, Sinzato YK, Campos KE, Calderon IM, Rudge MV, et al. Intrauterine growth restricted rats exercised at pregnancy: Maternal–fetal repercussions. *Reproductive Sciences.* 2015;22:991–9.

Damasceno DC, Netto AO, Iessi IL, Gallego FQ, Corvino SB, Dallaqua B, et al. Streptozotocin-induced diabetes models: Pathophysiological mechanisms and fetal outcomes. *BioMed Research International.* 2014;2014:819065.

Damasceno DC, Sinzato YK, Bueno A, Netto AO, Dallaqua B, Gallego FQ, et al. Mild diabetes models and their maternal-fetal repercussions. *Journal of Diabetes Research.* 2013;2013:473575.

de Souza MSS Sinzato YK, Lima PH, Calderon IM, Rudge MV, Damasceno DC. Oxidative stress status and lipid profiles of diabetic pregnant rats exposed to cigarette smoke. *Reproductive Biomedicine Online.* 2010;20:547–52.

Desai N, Roman A, Rochelson B, Gupta M, Xue X, Chatterjee PK, et al. Maternal metformin treatment decreases fetal inflammation in a rat model of obesity and metabolic syndrome. *American Journal of Obstetrics and Gynecology.* 2013;209:136.e1–9.

Devlieger R, Casteels K, Van Assche FA. Reduced adaptation of the pancreatic B cells during pregnancy is the major causal factor for gestational diabetes: Current knowledge and metabolic effects on the offspring. *Acta Obstetricia et Gynecologica Scandinavica.* 2008;87:1266–70.

Donath MY, Shoelson SE. Type 2 diabetes as an inflammatory disease. *Nature Reviews Immunology.* 2011;11:98–107.

Dorrell C, Schug J, Lin CF, Canaday PS, Fox AJ, Smirnova O, et al. Transcriptomes of the major human pancreatic cell types. *Diabetologia.* 2011;54:2832–44.

Dowling D, McAuliffe FM. The molecular mechanisms of offspring effects from obese pregnancy. *Obesity Facts.* 2013;6:134–45.

Eriksson UJ, Cederberg J, Wentzel P. Congenital malformations in offspring of diabetic mothers—Animal and human studies. *Reviews in Endocrine & Metabolic Disorders.* 2003;4:79–93.

Fisher SC, Kim SY, Sharma AJ, Rochat R, Morrow B. Is obesity still increasing among pregnant women? Prepregnancy obesity trends in 20 states, 2003–2009. *Preventive Medicine.* 2013;56:372–8.

Fox NS, Roman AS, Saltzman DH, Klauser CK, Rebarber A. Obesity and adverse pregnancy outcomes in twin pregnancies. *Journal of Maternal-Fetal & Neonatal Medicine.* 2014;27:355–9.

Freinkel N. Banting Lecture 1980. Of pregnancy and progeny. *Diabetes.* 1980;29:1023–35.

Friedrichsen BN, Carlsson C, Moldrup A, Michelsen B, Jensen CH, Teisner B, et al. Expression, biosynthesis and release of preadipocyte factor-1/ delta-like protein/fetal antigen-1 in pancreatic beta-cells: Possible physiological implications. *Journal of Endocrinology.* 2003;176:257–66.

Furcron AE, Romero R, Mial TN, Balancio A, Panaitescu B, Hassan SS, et al. Human chorionic gonadotropin has anti-inflammatory effects at the maternal-fetal interface and prevents endotoxin-induced preterm birth, but causes dystocia and fetal compromise in mice. *Biology of Reproduction.* 2016;94:136.

Gelardi NL, Cha CJ, Oh W. Glucose metabolism in adipocytes of obese offspring of mild hyperglycemic rats. *Pediatric Research.* 1990;28:641–5.

Gerrish K, Cissell MA, Stein R. The role of hepatic nuclear factor 1 alpha and PDX-1 in transcriptional regulation of the Pdx-1 gene. *Journal of Biological Chemistry.* 2001;276:47775–84.

Graus-Nunes F, Dalla Corte Frantz E, Lannes WR, da Silva Menezes MC, Mandarim-de-Lacerda CA, Souza-Mello V. Pregestational maternal obesity impairs endocrine pancreas in male F1 and F2 progeny. *Nutrition.* 2015;31:380–7.

Gregor MF, Hotamisligil GS. Inflammatory mechanisms in obesity. *Annual Review of Immunology.* 2011;29:415–45.

Hakonen E, Ustinov J, Palgi J, Miettinen PJ, Otonkoski T. EGFR signaling promotes beta-cell proliferation and surviving expression during pregnancy. *PLoS One.* 2014;9:e93651.

Han J, Xu J, Epstein PN, Liu YQ. Long-term effect of maternal obesity on pancreatic beta cells of offspring: Reduced beta cell adaptation to high glucose and high-fat diet challenges in adult female mouse offspring. *Diabetologia.* 2005;48:1810–8.

Huda SS, Brodie LE, Sattar N. Obesity in pregnancy: Prevalence and metabolic consequences. *Seminars in Fetal & Neonatal Medicine.* 2010;15:70–6.

Hummel S, Much D, Rossbauer M, Ziegler AG, Beyerlein A. Postpartum outcomes in women with gestational diabetes and their offspring: POGO study design and first-year results. *Review of Diabetic Studies: RDS.* 2013;10:49–57.

Hussen HI, Persson M, Moradi T. Maternal overweight and obesity are associated with increased risk of type 1 diabetes in offspring of parents without diabetes regardless of ethnicity. *Diabetologia.* 2015;58:1464–73.

Iessi IL, Sinzato YK, Gallego FQ, Dallaqua B, Amorim RL, Alves CEF, Calderon IMP, Rudge MVC, Nielsen JH, Damaceno DC. In vitro analysis of oxidative sress status on pancreas development in fetuses from diabetic rats. In: Islet cell plasticity in diabetes therapy. *2nd BBDC-Joslin-UCPH Conference,* Copenhagen, Denmark, 2015. Abstract.

Iessi IL, Sinzato YK, Gallego FQ, Nielsen JH, Damasceno DC. Effect of diabetes on circulating pancreatic hormones in pregnant rats and their offspring. *Hormone and Metabolic Research* 2016;48:682–686.

Ingvorsen C, Thysen AH, Fernandez-Twinn D, Nordby P, Nielsen KF, Ozanne SE, et al. Effects of pregnancy on obesity-induced inflammation in a mouse model of fetal programming. *International Journal of Obesity* 2014;38:1282–9.

Jaksch C. The role of maternal high energy feeding on expression of inflammatory genes and the DLK1-DIO3 locus in pancreas of DR and DIO offspring: University of Copenhagen; 2016.

Jansson N, Nilsfelt A, Gellerstedt M, Wennergren M, Rossander-Hulthen L, Powell TL, et al. Maternal hormones linking maternal body mass index and dietary intake to birth weight. *American Journal of Clinical Nutrition.* 2008;87:1743–9.

Jonsson J, Carlsson L, Edlund T, Edlund H. Insulin-promoter-factor 1 is required for pancreas development in mice. *Nature.* 1994;371:606–9.

Kameswaran V, Bramswig NC, McKenna LB, Penn M, Schug J, Hand NJ, et al. Epigenetic regulation of the DLK1-MEG3 microRNA cluster in human type 2 diabetic islets. *Cell Metabolism.* 2014;19:135–45.

Kameswaran V, Kaestner KH. The missing lnc(RNA) between the pancreatic beta-cell and diabetes. *Frontiers Genetics.* 2014;5:200.

Kaneto H, Miyatsuka T, Kawamori D, Yamamoto K, Kato K, Shiraiwa T, et al. PDX-1 and MafA play a crucial role in pancreatic beta-cell differentiation and maintenance of mature beta-cell function. *Endocrine Journal.* 2008;55:235–52.

Kapur R, Hojfeldt TW, Hojfeldt TW, Ronn SG, Karlsen AE, Heller RS. Short-term effects of INGAP and Reg family peptides on the appearance of small beta-cells clusters in non-diabetic mice. *Islets.* 2012;4:40–8.

Kervran A, Guillaume M, Jost A. The endocrine pancreas of the fetus from diabetic pregnant rat. *Diabetologia.* 1978;15:387–93.

Kim DW, Young SL, Grattan DR, Jasoni CL. Obesity during pregnancy disrupts placental morphology, cell proliferation, and inflammation in a sex-specific manner across gestation in the mouse. *Biology of Reproduction.* 2014;90:130.

King H. Epidemiology of glucose intolerance and gestational diabetes in women of childbearing age. *Diabetes Care*. 1998;21(Suppl 2):B9–13.

Le Lay J, Matsuoka TA, Henderson E, Stein R. Identification of a novel PDX-1 binding site in the human insulin gene enhancer. *Journal of Biological Chemistry*. 2004;279: 22228–35.

Levin BE, Dunn-Meynell AA, Balkan B, Keesey RE. Selective breeding for diet-induced obesity and resistance in Sprague-Dawley rats. *American Journal of Physiology*. 1997;273:R725–30.

Like AA, RossinI AA. Streptozotocin-induced pancreatic insulitis: New model of diabetes mellitus. *Science*. 1976;193:415–7.

Lottmann H, Vanselow J, Hessabi B, Walther R. The Tet-On system in transgenic mice: Inhibition of the mouse Pdx-1 gene activity by antisense RNA expression in pancreatic beta-cells. *Journal of Molecular Medicine*. 2001;79:321–8.

Martens GA, Motte E, Kramer G, Stange G, Gaarn LW, Hellemans K, et al. Functional characteristics of neonatal rat beta cells with distinct markers. *Journal of Molecular Endocrinology*. 2014;52:11–28.

Merzouk H, Madani S, Chabane Sari D, Prost J, Bouchenak M, Belleville J. Time course of changes in serum glucose, insulin, lipids and tissue lipase activities in macrosomic offspring of rats with streptozotocin-induced diabetes. *Clinical Science*. 2000;98:21–30.

Nalla A. Adaptation of pancreatic beta cells to pregnancy: Role of circulating factors from pregnant women without and with autoimmune diabetes on beta cell growth and survival in vitro PhD Thesis, University of Copenhagen; 2012.

Ng SF, Lin RC, Laybutt DR, Barres R, Owens JA, Morris MJ. Chronic high-fat diet in fathers programs beta-cell dysfunction in female rat offspring. *Nature*. 2010;467:963–6.

Nielsen JH, editor. Destruction of insulin producing cells by diabetogenic agents in vitro: Differences in susceptibility and mechanisms of action. Immunology in Diabetes 84 International Symposium; 1984; Rome, Italy.

Nielsen JH, Haase TN, Jaksch C, Nalla A, Sostrup B, Nalla AA, et al. Impact of fetal and neonatal environment on beta cell function and development of diabetes. *Acta Obstetricia et Gynecologica Scandinavica*. 2014;93:1109–22.

Nielsen JH, Horn S, Kirkegaard J, Nalla A, Søstrup B. Beta cell adaptability during pregnancy. In: Hill DJ, editor. Control of pancreatic beta cell function and plasticity in health and diabetes. Current and future development in physiology, Vol. 1, Bentham Science Publishers, 2016.

O'Dowd JF, Stocker CJ. Endocrine pancreatic development: Impact of obesity and diet. *Frontiers Physiology*. 2013;4:170.

Oben JA, Patel T, Mouralidarane A, Samuelsson AM, Matthews P, Pombo J, et al. Maternal obesity programmes offspring development of non-alcoholic fatty pancreas disease. *Biochemical and Biophysical Research Communications*. 2010;394:24–8.

Offield MF, Jetton TL, Labosky PA, Ray M, Stein RW, Magnuson MA, et al. PDX-1 is required for pancreatic outgrowth and differentiation of the rostral duodenum. *Development*. 1996;122:983–95.

Ohlsson H, Karlsson K, Edlund T. IPF1, a homeodomain-containing transactivator of the insulin gene. *The EMBO Journal*. 1993;12:4251–9.

Ornoy A, Rand SB, Bischitz N. Hyperglycemia and hypoxia are interrelated in their teratogenic mechanism: Studies on cultured rat embryos. *Birth Defects Research Part B, Developmental and Reproductive Toxicology*. 2010;89:106–15.

Ovesen P, Rasmussen S, Kesmodel U. Effect of prepregnancy maternal overweight and obesity on pregnancy outcome. *Obstetric Gynecology*. 2011;118:305–12.

Parsons JA, Brelje TC, Sorenson RL. Adaptation of islets of Langerhans to pregnancy: Increased islet cell proliferation and insulin secretion correlates with the onset of placental lactogen secretion. *Endocrinology*. 1992;130:1459–66.

Paulsen SJ, Jelsing J, Madsen AN, Hansen G, Lykkegaard K, Larsen LK, et al. Characterization of beta-cell mass and insulin resistance in diet-induced obese and diet-resistant rats. *Obesity*. 2010;18:266–73.

Portha B, Levacher C, Picon L, Rosselin G. Diabetogenic effect of streptozotocin in the rat during the perinatal period. *Diabetes*. 1974;23:889–95.

Prentice KJ, Luu L, Allister EM, Liu Y, Jun LS, Sloop KW, et al. The furan fatty acid metabolite CMPF is elevated in diabetes and induces beta cell dysfunction. *Cell Metabolism*. 2014;19:653–66.

Rando OJ, Simmons RA. I'm eating for two: Parental dietary effects on offspring metabolism. *Cell*. 2015;161:93–105.

Rhee M, Lee SH, Kim JW, Ham DS, Park HS, Yang HK, et al. Preadipocyte factor 1 induces pancreatic ductal cell differentiation into insulin-producing cells. *Scientific Reports*. 2016;6:23960.

Rieck S, Kaestner KH. Expansion of beta-cell mass in response to pregnancy. *Trends Endocrinology and Metabolism*. 2010;21:151–8.

Ruchat SM, Hivert MF, Bouchard L. Epigenetic programming of obesity and diabetes by in utero exposure to gestational diabetes mellitus. *Nutrition Reviews*. 2013;71(Suppl 1):S88–94.

Rudge MV, Damasceno DC, Volpato GT, Almeida FC, Calderon IM, Lemonica IP. Effect of Ginkgo biloba on the reproductive outcome and oxidative stress biomarkers of streptozotocin-induced diabetic rats. *Brazilian Journal of Medical and Biological Research* 2007;40:1095–9.

Segovia SA, Vickers MH, Gray C. Maternal obesity, inflammation, and developmental programming. *BioMed Research International*. 2014:Article ID418975.

Sewell MF, Huston-Presley L, Super DM, Catalano P. Increased neonatal fat mass, not lean body mass, is associated with maternal obesity. *American Journal of Obstetrics and Gynecology*. 2006;195:1100–3.

Singer RA, Arnes L, Sussel L. Noncoding RNAs in beta cell biology. *Current Opinion in Endocrinology, Diabetes, and Obesity*. 2015;22:77–85.

Sinzato YK, Damasceno DC, Laufer-Amorim R, Rodrigues MM, Oshiiwa M, Taylor KN, et al. Plasma concentrations and placental immunostaining of interleukin-10 and tumor necrosis factor-alpha as predictors of alterations in the embryo-fetal organism and the placental development of diabetic rats. *Brazilian Journal of Medical and Biological Research* 2011;44:206–11.

Sostrup B, Gaarn LW, Nalla A, Billestrup N, Nielsen JH. Co-ordinated regulation of neurogenin-3 expression in the maternal and fetal pancreas during pregnancy. *Acta Obstetricia et Gynecologica Scandinavica*. 2014;93:1190–7.

Srinivasan M, Katewa SD, Palaniyappan A, Pandya JD, Patel MS. Maternal high-fat diet consumption results in fetal malprogramming predisposing to the onset of metabolic syndrome-like phenotype in adulthood. *American Journal of Physiology Endocrinology and Metabolism*. 2006;291:E792–9.

Taylor PD, McConnell J, Khan IY, Holemans K, Lawrence KM, Asare-Anane H, et al. Impaired glucose homeostasis and mitochondrial abnormalities in offspring of rats fed a fat-rich diet in pregnancy. *American Journal of Physiology. Regulatory, Integrative and Comparative Physiology*. 2005;288:R134–9.

Terazono K, Yamamoto H, Takasawa S, Shiga K, Yonemura Y, Tochino Y, et al. A novel gene activated in regenerating islets. *Journal of Biological Chemistry*. 1988; 263:2111–4.

Theys N, Ahn MT, Bouckenooghe T, Reusens B, Remacle C. Maternal malnutrition programs pancreatic islet mitochondrial dysfunction in the adult offspring. *Journal of Nutritional Biochemistry*. 2011;22:985–94.

Tuohetimulati G, Uchida T, Toyofuku Y, Abe H, Fujitani Y, Hirose T, et al. Effect of maternal high-fat diet on pancreatic beta cells of the offspring. *Diabetology International*. 2012;3:217–23.

Van Assche FA, Aerts L, Holemans K. The effects of maternal diabetes on the offspring. *Baillieres Clinical Obstetrics and Gynaecology*. 1991;5:485–92.

Van Assche FA, Holemans K, Aerts L. Long-term consequences for offspring of diabetes during pregnancy. *British Medical Bulletin*. 2001;60:173–82.

Volpato GT, Damasceno DC, Sinzato YK, Ribeiro VM, Rudge MV, Calderon IM. Oxidative stress status and placental implications in diabetic rats undergoing swimming exercise after embryonic implantation. *Reproductive Sciences*. 2015;22:602–8.

Waeber G, Thompson N, Nicod P, Bonny C. Transcriptional activation of the GLUT2 gene by the IPF-1/STF-1/IDX-1 homeobox factor. *Molecular Endocrinology*. 1996;10:1327–34.

Wang H, Xue Y, Wang B, Zhao J, Yan X, Huang Y, et al. Maternal obesity exacerbates insulitis and type 1 diabetes in non-obese diabetic mice. *Reproduction*. 2014;148:73–9.

Wang Y, Lee K, Moon YS, Ahmadian M, Kim KH, Roder K, et al. Overexpression of Pref-1 in pancreatic islet beta-cells in mice causes hyperinsulinemia with increased islet mass and insulin secretion. *Biochemical and Biophysical Research Communications*. 2015;461:630–5.

Ward DT, Yau SK, Mee AP, Mawer EB, Miller CA, Garland HO, et al. Functional, molecular, and biochemical characterization of streptozotocin-induced diabetes. *Journal of the American Society of Nephrology*. 2001;12:779–90.

Watada H, Kajimoto Y, Miyagawa J, Hanafusa T, Hamaguchi K, Matsuoka T, et al. PDX-1 induces insulin and glucokinase gene expressions in alphaTC1 clone 6 cells in the presence of betacellulin. *Diabetes*. 1996;45:1826–31.

Xiong X, Wang X, Li B, Chowdhury S, Lu Y, Srikant CB, et al. Pancreatic islet-specific overexpression of Reg3beta protein induced the expression of pro-islet genes and protected the mice against streptozotocin-induced diabetes mellitus. *American Journal of Physiology Endocrinology and Metabolism*. 2011;300:E669–80.

Yan J, Yang H. Gestational diabetes mellitus, programing and epigenetics. *Journal of Maternal-Fetal & Neonatal Medicine*. 2014;27:1266–9.

Yessoufou A, Moutairou K. Maternal diabetes in pregnancy: Early and long-term outcomes on the offspring and the concept of "metabolic memory". *Experimental Diabetes Research*. 2011;2011:218598.

Yokomizo H, Inoguchi T, Sonoda N, Sakaki Y, Maeda Y, Inoue T, et al. Maternal high-fat diet induces insulin resistance and deterioration of pancreatic beta-cell function in adult offspring with sex differences in mice. *American Journal of Physiology Endocrinology and Metabolism*. 2014;306:E1163–75.

You L, Wang N, Yin D, Wang L, Jin F, Zhu Y, et al. Downregulation of long noncoding RNA Meg3 affects insulin synthesis and secretion in mouse pancreatic beta cells. *Journal of Cellular Physiology*. 2016;231:852–862.

Zenilman ME, Tuchman D, Zheng Q, Levine J, Delany H. Comparison of reg I and reg III levels during acute pancreatitis in the rat. *Annals of Surgery*. 2000;232:646–52.

Zhang L, Long NM, Hein SM, Ma Y, Nathanielsz PW, Ford SP. Maternal obesity in ewes results in reduced fetal pancreatic beta-cell numbers in late gestation and decreased circulating insulin concentration at term. *Domestic Animal Endocrinology*. 2011;40:30–9.

Zhu MJ, Du M, Nathanielsz PW, Ford SP. Maternal obesity up-regulates inflammatory signaling pathways and enhances cytokine expression in the mid-gestation sheep placenta. *Placenta*. 2010;31:387–91.

8 Integrative Metabolism and Circadian Rhythms— Contributions of Maternal Programming

Umesh D. Wankhade, Keshari M. Thakali, and Kartik Shankar

CONTENTS

8.1 INTRODUCTION

Circadian rhythms govern a wide variety of physiological and metabolic processes in organisms ranging from cyanobacteria to humans. The 24-hour cycle of light and dark drives cyclic changes in most organisms, which anticipate and coordinate their behavioral and metabolic functions in response to the changing environment. Most organisms modulate their metabolism over a 24-hour period via an endogenous phenomenon called a circadian rhythm. This biological circadian clock in vertebrate species provides time cues for various physiological activities and synchronizes metabolic, endocrine, and behavioral functions associated with the activities (Brainard et al. 1983; Meng et al. 2011; Brainard et al. 1984). The master clock regulating circadian rhythm is located in the suprachiasmatic nucleus (SCN) of the hypothalamus (Swanson and Cowan 1975; Lydic et al. 1980). The SCN synchronizes many circadian rhythm-related processes in humans and other vertebrates (Gillette and Tischkau 1999; Hofman 2000) and these circadian rhythms control a wide array of physiological events, including metabolism, feeding, sleep, and hormonal secretions. Metabolic homeostasis at the systemic level is dependent upon an accurate and collaborative harmony of circadian rhythms in individual cells and tissues of the body. Misalignment or disruption of the circadian rhythm is associated with a number of detrimental metabolic conditions such as obesity, metabolic syndrome, and cardiovascular disease.

At the molecular level, the circadian clock is a highly conserved and coordinated transcription–translation feedback system that modulates messenger RNA (mRNA) expression, protein stability, chromatin state, and metabolite production, utilization, and turnover to keep correct physiological functions occurring in a chronological order. Recent findings show that regulation of metabolism by the circadian clock and its components is a reciprocal process. Specifically, components of the circadian clock sense alterations in the cellular metabolism and respond accordingly. Moreover, unhealthy diets, irregular timing of eating, or lifestyle factors such as sleep deprivation or night-shift work are known to alter circadian rhythms and alter metabolism. Importantly, disruption of the circadian clock gene network (as seen in *Clock* mutant mice) leads to the development of obesity secondary to hyperphagia. In addition, these mice are hyperleptinemic, hyperlipidemic, hyperglycemic, and develop hepatic steatosis (Turek et al. 2005). Thus, it is evident that disruption of circadian rhythms leads to severe metabolic consequences. However, the influence of gestational insults (such as maternal obesity and poor quality diets) on circadian rhythms in offspring remains poorly understood. Maternal obesity is associated with increased risk of offspring obesity, insulin resistance, glycemic dysregulation, hepatic steatosis, and cardiovascular disease. Moreover, maternal diet and obesity during pregnancy have been shown to influence offspring metabolism, appetite, and adiposity. In this context, altered circadian rhythms could be contributing mediators (Shankar et al. 2008; Wankhade et al. 2016). Gestational obesity and prenatal nutritional status have been shown to affect the circadian machinery of key organs in offspring such as the liver, brain, and adipose tissue (Mouralidarane et al. 2015; Borengasser et al. 2014; Sutton et al. 2010). This chapter provides a brief overview of the physiology of circadian rhythms and an up-to-date review on the literature examining how the maternal body habitus and diet during gestation affect offspring circadian rhythms, metabolism, and health.

8.2   AN OVERVIEW OF CIRCADIAN RHYTHMS

A common feature of all organisms, from bacteria, fungi, plants, birds, animals, is the temporal organization of biological processes into daily cycles. These circadian (*circa diem* is Latin for "about a day") rhythms, or internal clocks, include many biological processes—physical, mental, and/or behavioral—that follow approximately a 24-hour cycle and often occur in response to light and dark patterns in the environment (Partch et al. 2014; Bell-Pedersen et al. 2005). Circadian rhythms or clocks are regulated by an internal circadian oscillator that is comprised of positive and negative autoregulatory feedback loops that generate daily (24-hour) timing circuits. In response to environmental input, the positive elements of the feedback loops activate the transcription of "clock genes" that encode for the negative elements of the system. Thus, this interconnected network of positive and negative feedback loops maintains the stability and robustness of the oscillator and generates rhythmic transcription and biological activity.

In mammals, such as rodents and humans, a circadian pacemaker or "master" clock is located in the SCN of the hypothalamus. This master clock in the SCN is unique from peripheral molecular clocks as the SCN receives input directly via the retinohypothalamic tract to allow entrainment, or synchronization, of mammalian circadian rhythms to environmental light/dark cycles. Peripheral clocks are phase delayed to the time it takes for signals (circulating hormones and other metabolic cues) to be sent from the SCN to the periphery. Thus, the SCN coordinates clocks in peripheral tissues that have their own intrinsic circadian rhythms.

Through early microarray studies, it was discovered that peripheral clocks regulate numerous transcriptional programs and lead to a peak in gene expression once a day for clock-controlled genes. Both SCN and peripheral circadian clocks share similar molecular elements: (1) negative elements such as the period homologues 1 and 2 (*PER1* and *PER2*) and cryptochromes 1 and 2 (*CRY1* and *CRY2*) and (2) positive acting proteins such as the basic helix–loop–helix transcription factors *CLOCK* and brain and muscle ARNT-like protein 1 (*BMAL*). The *CLOCK:BMAL* heterodimeric complex acts as a positive regulator of circadian transcription by binding at consensus E-box DNA motifs and recruiting transcriptional repressors (*PER1*, *PER2*, *CRY1*, and *CRY2*) to repress *CLOCK:BMAL* activity in a cyclical fashion. Thus, circadian output is controlled primarily at the transcriptional level, but there is also evidence for posttranscriptional regulatory processes to play a role in circadian rhythms. For example, for some genes, circadian control of poly-A tail length regulates translation independently of steady-state mRNA levels. In addition, the epigenetic landscape also plays an important part in circadian transcriptional activation as histone modifications and RNA polymerase II recruitment are another level of circadian regulation of transcription.

8.3   CIRCADIAN REGULATION OF METABOLISM

Since integrative metabolism is exquisitely coordinated with feeding, food-seeking behavior, and energy expenditure associated with locomotion, it is no surprise that numerous metabolic mediators show prominent circadian rhythms (summarized in Figure 8.1). The main neural output pathways of the SCN that drive the circadian pacemaker are the subparaventricular zone (SPZ) and dorsomedial hypothalamus (DMH) (Saper et al. 2005). The SCN also has efferent targets in the arcuate nucleus of the ventromedial hypothalamus (VMH) and the ventral part of the lateral hypothalamus (LH), suggesting an interaction of circadian pathways with neural pathways involved in food intake and physical activity (Yi et al. 2006). Downstream of the SPZ and DMH are the paraventricular nucleus (PVN), the LH, the ventrolateral preoptic nucleus, and the medial preoptic area. These brain regions regulate corticosteroid release, feeding, sleep, and thermoregulation, respectively (Chou et al. 2003; Lu et al. 2001). Ablation of DMH regions, which receive inputs from both the SCN and the SPZ, results in severe impairment of circadian-regulated sleep–wakefulness, locomotor activity, corticosteroid secretion, and feeding (Chou et al. 2003). Thus, the DMH and VMH constitute a gateway between the master pacemaker neurons of the SCN and cell bodies located within brain centers in the hypothalamus (Ramsey et al. 2007). Moreover, preautonomic nervous system neurons are located in the

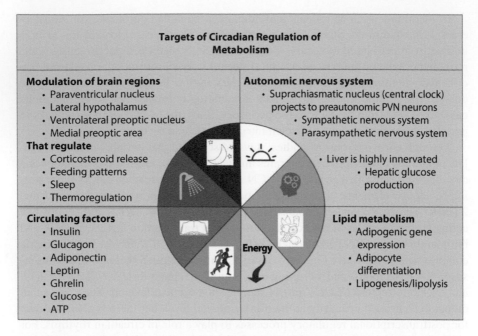

FIGURE 8.1 Physiological targets of circadian rhythm regulation of metabolism include specific brain regions downstream of the suprachiasmatic nucleus, the autonomic nervous system, the liver, adipose tissue, and various circulating factors. These systems influence biochemical pathways and behavioral functions in an integrated manner.

ventral and dorsal borders of the PVN and are selectively innervated by fibers of SCN (Buijs et al. 1999). Thus, one mechanism by which the SCN controls energy homeostasis is through the innervation of preautonomic neurons in the PVN, which are connected to the parasympathetic and sympathetic nervous systems (Buijs et al. 2006). For example, in the rat, lesions of the SCN impair diurnal variations in whole-body glucose homeostasis, which results in defective glucose utilization rates and endogenous hepatic glucose production. Importantly, the liver is highly innervated by both sympathetic and parasympathetic nerve fibers, and autonomic input is critical in regulating hepatic glucose production. Transneural viral tracing combined with selective denervation demonstrated that SCN neurons project to preautonomic PVN neurons, providing evidence that the central clock via the autonomic nervous system plays a critical role in controlling hepatic glucose production (Kalsbeek et al. 2006). Neuronal projections from the SCN to the PVN contain gamma-aminobutyric acid (GABA) as the primary neurotransmitter and neurotransmitter release inhibit PVN function (Roland and Sawchenko 1993). Thus, the SCN is capable of controlling peripheral tissues not only by the secretion of humoral signals but also by affecting both branches of the autonomic nervous system.

Gene expression and circulating plasma levels of insulin, glucagon, adiponectin, leptin, and ghrelin also exhibit circadian oscillation. Leptin, an adipocyte-derived circulating hormone that acts at specific receptors in the hypothalamus to suppress appetite and increase metabolism, is elevated in obesity (Ahima et al. 1998). Leptin exhibits remarkable circadian patterns in both gene expression and protein secretion, which spikes during sleep (Kalra et al. 2003). Ablation of SCN regions impairs circadian leptin expression in rodents, suggesting that the central circadian clock regulates leptin expression (Kalsbeek et al. 2001). Circadian rhythms also control energy homeostasis in peripheral tissues by mediating the expression and/or activity of specific metabolic enzymes and transporters involved in cholesterol, amino acid, and glucose metabolism (Ramsey et al. 2007; La Fleur et al. 1999; La Fleur 2003; Davidson et al. 2004). Glucose uptake and adenosine triphosphate (ATP) concentrations in the brain and peripheral tissues also fluctuate around the circadian cycle (Kalsbeek et al. 2006; La Fleur 2003), and several nuclear receptors involved in lipid and glucose metabolism, such as peroxisome proliferator-activated receptor gamma (*PPARα*), alpha (*PPARγ*), and delta (*PPARδ*), and estrogen receptor alpha (*ERRα*), exhibit circadian patterns of expression (Yang et al. 2006). While disturbances in circadian rhythms affect metabolism, dysregulation of metabolism due to feeding, food metabolites, or hormones whose secretion is controlled by food or its absence also impacts circadian rhythms. Glucose, amino acids, minerals, and vitamins all are known to reset circadian rhythms (Stephan and Davidson 1998; Iwanaga et al. 2005; Mohri et al. 2003; Langlais and Hall 1998). Hormones responsive to the metabolic state also tend to induce or reset circadian rhythms through the regulation of clock gene expression. Thus, coordination of circadian rhythms and metabolism occur in conjunction with each other to respond to the host environment.

As mentioned earlier, at the cellular level, both the central and peripheral clocks are controlled through positive and negative transcriptional and translational feedback loops that involve genes such as *BMAL1*, *CLOCK*, *PER1*, *PER2*, *PER3*, *CRY1*, *CRY2*, and *REV-ERB* (Gekakis et al. 1998; Prasai et al. 2008). *PER2* is an important intermediary between metabolic and circadian pathways as it has been shown to control lipid metabolism through the regulation of *PPARγ*. In addition, leptin induces upregulation of *PER2* and *CLOCK* gene expression in mouse osteoblasts that exhibit endogenous circadian rhythms (Fu et al. 2005). Importantly, it has been reported that *PER2*-deficient mice display profound reductions in triacylglycerol and nonesterified fatty acids; thus, *PER2* acts to inhibit lipid metabolism and potentiate hepatic steatosis (Grimaldi et al. 2010).

Circadian rhythms impact lipid metabolism through other important genes as well. Transcriptome studies in mice revealed the rhythmic expression of clock and adipokine genes, such as resistin, adiponectin, and visfatin in visceral fat tissue (Ando et al. 2005), and in humans, expression of these mediators is reduced with obesity (Kalsbeek et al. 2001; Saad et al. 1998; Gavrila et al. 2003). Fatty acid transport protein 1 (*Fatp1*), fatty acyl-CoA synthetase 1 (*Acs1*), and adipocyte differentiation-related protein (*Adrp*) exhibit diurnal variations in expression, suggesting that nocturnal expression of *Fatp1*, *Acs1*, and *Adrp* may promote higher rates of fatty acid uptake and storage of triglyceride in rodents (Bray and Young 2007). *Bmal1*, the gene encoding the core clock mechanism, is involved in the control of adipogenesis and lipid metabolism in mature adipocytes as loss of *Bmal1* leads to defective adipocyte differentiation and adipogenesis in embryonic fibroblasts. Moreover, loss of *Bmal1* in 3T3-L1 adipocytes leads to downregulation of several key adipogenic genes such *PPARγ2*, adipocyte fatty acid binding protein 2 (*aP2*), CCAAT enhancer binding proteins (*C/EBPα* and *C/EBPβ*), sterol regulatory element-binding protein 1a (*SREBP-1a*), phosphoenolpyruvate carboxykinase, and fatty acid synthase, whereas overexpression of *Bmal1* in adipocytes increases lipid synthesis activity. These results indicate that *Bmal1*, a master regulator of circadian rhythm, also plays a critical role in the regulation of adipose differentiation and lipogenesis in mature adipocytes (Shimba et al. 2005). Thus, circadian rhythms influence metabolism through the autonomic nervous system and also by affecting the expression of genes involved in key metabolic processes such as glucose and lipid metabolism (Figure 8.1).

8.4 MATERNAL PROGRAMMING OF OFFSPRING CIRCADIAN RHYTHMS

Since maternal diet and obesity during pregnancy can influence offspring metabolism, food intake, and adiposity, it is possible that altered circadian rhythms could be causal mediators of offspring metabolic dysfunction (summarized in Figure 8.2). The proximity of the SCN to the arcuate nucleus and the PVN, which is mainly responsible for food intake, satiety, and physical activity behavior, highlights the possibility that developmental programming of hyperphagia and physical inactivity may occur at early fetal stages of development. Rodent models have been instrumental in analyzing the mechanisms responsible for the developmental programming of obesity and its comorbidities. For example, Samuelsson et al. demonstrated that offspring of obese mouse dams are hyperphagic from 4 to 6 weeks of age, and have reduced locomotor activity and increased adiposity. Moreover, in this model,

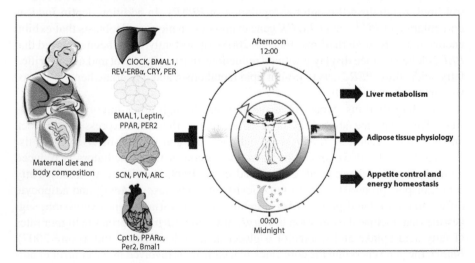

FIGURE 8.2 Maternal obesity and obesogenic diets influence the expression and regulation of several core circadian rhythm-related genes in metabolic tissues such as liver, adipose tissue, brain, and heart. These changes presumably could contribute to the modulation of metabolism and generally enhanced sensitivity of offspring to metabolic disease.

exposure to maternal obesity during fetal development in the mouse leads to adult offspring adiposity and cardiovascular and metabolic dysfunction (Samuelsson et al. 2008). In another mouse model, exposure to a maternal low protein diet during gestation followed by a postweaning obesogenic diet was associated with higher offspring blood pressure and heart rate and loss of circadian rhythmicity of blood pressure and heart rate in offspring exposed to maternal low protein diet during gestation (Bol et al. 2010). These rodent studies suggest that the *in utero* environment plays an important role in the circadian regulation of energy balance and obesity-related comorbidities such as cardiovascular disease.

Previously, our group has shown that an obesogenic *in utero* environment during fetal development interacts with postnatal obesogenic challenges to induce permanent changes in the hepatic molecular chronobiological network. Borengasser et al. demonstrated that the oscillatory amplitude of both hepatic core clock regulators and circadian metabolic regulators was altered in offspring when challenged with high-fat diet (HFD), and this response to postnatal HFD was further exacerbated in offspring exposed to maternal obesity. In particular, exposure to both maternal obesity and 2-week postweaning HFD challenge resulted in the greatest impairment of gene transcription of hepatic core clock machinery and metabolic and epigenetic targets (Borengasser et al. 2014). Changes in *PPARα* mRNA expression were specifically linked to decreased rates of mRNA synthesis and increased rates of degradation as determined by mathematical modeling. Additionally, epigenomic changes were evident as seen by differences in enrichment of histone H3 lysine 4 trimethylation (H3K4me3) and H3K27me3 histone marks on the *PPARα* promoter. In agreement with mRNA expression, the coupling of maternal obesity and postweaning HFD exposure led to the most dramatic changes in the mathematical model and histone mark enrichment. In addition to its central role as a pleiotropic regulator of lipid metabolism, *PPARα* directly interacts with core clock components in a circadian fashion. These findings clearly indicate that maternal obesity impairs the underlying circadian mechanisms regulating transcriptional induction of *PPARα*. Consequently, offspring of obese dams are unable to adequately mount a response to metabolic demands that require mobilization of lipids (viz. fasting and HFDs), specifically via an inability to induce *PPARα* and its downstream targets (Borengasser et al. 2014).

Consistent with the above-mentioned findings, Mourlidarane et al. demonstrated that exposure to maternal obesity led to the development of severe nonalcoholic fatty liver disease (NAFLD) phenotype in offspring. Further dietary challenge in postnatal life induced a biphasic rhythmic pattern of *Clock* expression, with peaks observed in both the light and dark phases (Mouralidarane et al. 2015). Rhythmic disruption of *Clock* transcription in the liver may therefore be partially responsible for the observed dysmetabolic and fatty liver phenotype in offspring born to obese dams. Such a causal association is supported by earlier reports of adiposity, impaired lipid metabolism, and insulin resistance in *Clock* mutant mice (Turek et al. 2005; Oishi et al. 2003). Rhythmic 24-hour expression of *Bmal1*, a coactivator of the circadian molecular network, was similarly disrupted following exposure to maternal obesity and a postweaning obesogenic diet. Observations of arrhythmic *Bmal1* transcription are in line with previous reports of impaired adipogenesis and hepatic carbohydrate metabolism in rodents with

Bmal1 ablation (Shimba et al. 2005; Rudic et al. 2004). Exposure to maternal obesity induces a significant increase in *Cry2* transcription in offspring, which further worsens in the context of a postweaning obesogenic diet in the dark phase. Therefore, and most importantly, offspring exposure to maternal obesity significantly induces arrhythmic expression of *Cry2* and as such may be in part responsible for the observed NAFLD phenotype. This is further supported by reports of cryptochrome-mediated regulation of hepatic gluconeogenesis and cyclic adenosine monophosphate (cAMP) signaling, reaffirming the association between core clock genes and their control of metabolic pathways (Zhang et al. 2010). It is evident that these canonical clock genes affect metabolic physiology and that circadian-related genes regulate hepatic inflammatory and fibrogenic pathways implicated in NAFLD pathogenesis. It is tempting to speculate that the resulting asynchrony not only affects metabolic homeostasis but also impacts hepatic proinflammatory and profibrogenic pathways involved in NAFLD as possible clock output pathways.

In addition to the liver, other organ systems, such as the heart and pancreas, are also targets for maternal obesity-associated disruption of circadian rhythms. For example, Wang et al. observed that at postnatal day 17, offspring exposed to maternal obesity exhibited antiphase oscillations in cardiac gene expression of *Cpt1β*, *PPARα*, and *Per2*, and greater oscillation amplitude of hepatic *Bmal1*, tumor necrosis factor alpha (*Tnfα*), and interleukin 6 (*IL-6*) (Wang et al. 2015). Moreover, Carter et al. observed that when offspring exposed to maternal obesity were fed a postweaning obesogenic diet, the offspring developed fatty pancreas and increased pancreatic inflammation that was associated with phase shifts in pancreatic *Clock*, *REV-ERBα*, and *Per2* expression and a decreased oscillatory amplitude of *Bmal1* and *Per2* expression (Carter et al. 2014). Thus, the maternal environment during fetal development affects offspring circadian rhythms in multiple organ systems involved in energy balance and metabolism (Figure 8.2).

8.5   MECHANISMS LINKING MATERNAL PROGRAMMING TO OFFSPRING CIRCADIAN RHYTHMS

While it is evident that maternal nutritional status during pregnancy has lasting consequences on offspring circadian rhythms and metabolism, the mechanisms linking *in utero* environment and offspring circadian rhythms are considerably less well characterized. The placenta is an integral organ linking fetal growth and development to maternal habitus as it plays a key role in nutrient transport, hormone production, and immunologic barrier function (Jansson and Powell 2013; Diaz et al. 2014). Moreover, as a nutrient sensing organ, the placenta integrates both maternal and fetal information to appropriately match fetal growth with maternal nutrient supply. Thus, the placenta plays an important role in sensing changes in the maternal environment (e.g., hypoxia, stress, obesity, gestational diabetes) and inducing changes in fetal growth and development accordingly. The key molecular components of the clock gene machinery have been identified in rodent and human placenta but, in the rodent placenta, there appears to be significantly less rhythmicity or coordination with day/light cycles when compared to other central and peripheral clocks (Waddell et al. 2012). In both humans and nonhuman primates, placental steroidogenesis occurs in a rhythmic fashion, and in rodents, placental glucocorticoid production, glucocorticoid receptor expression, and proinflammatory cytokine production occur rhythmically, suggesting that circadian rhythms are an important part of normal placental function. Importantly, disruption of circadian rhythms is linked with compromised placental function, suggesting that the placenta may play a significant role in the development of the fetal circadian system (Waddell et al. 2012).

Another possible mechanism linking the *in utero* environment and offspring circadian rhythms is via epigenetic modification of offspring DNA or regulators of chromatin structure such as histone modifications during critical periods of development. Several groups have reported that chromatin remodeling of the DNA landscape follows circadian patterns, and enzymes such as histone acetyltransferases (HATs), histone methyltransferases (HMTs), and histone deacetylases (HDACs) are key mediators of chromatin remodeling. In the mouse liver, there are rhythmic changes in H3K4me3 and histone H3 lysine 9 acetylation (H3K9ac), histone modifications that are associated with active promoters, and recruitment of RNA polymerase II also exhibits circadian modulation (Koike et al. 2012). However, elongation marks such as H3K36me3 and H3K79me2 demonstrate low-amplitude circadian modulation (Koike et al. 2012). Additionally, in the mouse liver, genomic recruitment of *HDAC3* follows a circadian pattern that is synchronized to the expression pattern of the circadian nuclear receptor *REV-ERBα*, which recruits nuclear corepressor (*NCoR*) and *HDAC3* to deacetylate and repress transcription (Feng et al. 2011; Feng and Lazar 2012). Moreover, these circadian-related changes in chromatin landscape are associated with metabolic consequences as deletion of either HDAC3 or *REV-ERBα* induces hepatosteatosis (Feng et al. 2011). The *Bmal1/Clock* heterodimer interacts with sirtuin 1 (*SIRT1*), a nicotinamide adenine dinucleotide (NAD)-dependent HDAC, while *Bmal1* also binds to the transcriptional coactivators with HAT activity p300 and CREB-binding protein (CBP) and *Clock* binds to p300 and p300/CBP-associated protein (pCAF) (Feng and Lazar 2012). Importantly, *Clock* itself is a HAT that controls rhythmic acetylation of the *Per1* promoter (Feng and Lazar 2012). In a nonhuman primate model, maternal HFD during gestation was associated with altered fetal liver *Npas2* (a paralog of *Clock*) expression and hyperacetylation of H3K14ac in the *Npas2* promoter (Suter et al. 2011), suggesting that epigenetic modification of fetal circadian genes is determined by the maternal environment during fetal development.

Change in DNA methylation is another possible epigenetic mechanism involved in fetal programming of metabolism. Relative to other genes, regulatory regions of circadian genes are enriched in CpG motifs (Ripperger and Merrow 2011). Also, during development there is a clearly defined role of CpG methylation of circadian genes. For example, for specific CpGs within regulatory regions of *Per1*, methylation status was dependent on development stage (Ripperger and Merrow 2011). Adiposity has an effect on methylation status of specific CpGs in core canonical clock genes as hypermethylation of the *Bmal1* and *Per2* promoters was observed in white blood cells of overweight/obese women compared to lean women (Milagro et al. 2012). Since DNA methylation is established early in development, it is possible to speculate that maternal obesity-associated alterations in the methylation status of fetal circadian genes could have long-lasting effects on offspring metabolism.

8.6 CONCLUSIONS AND PERSPECTIVES

Since the fetal peripheral clocks develop earlier than the master fetal SCN clock and maternal SCN ablation induces asynchrony of circadian rhythms in offspring, it is clear that the gestational maternal environment is crucial for the development of fetal clocks and preparing the fetus for the postnatal environment. The field of maternal programming of offspring circadian rhythms and metabolism is still nascent and many unanswered questions remain. For example, how the maternal *in utero* environment programs offspring hypothalamic circuitry to regulation of energy intake and expenditure and circadian rhythms needs to be further explored. In addition, while maternal melatonin and corticosteroids have been postulated to regulate fetal circadian rhythms, the maternal signals that drive fetal peripheral oscillators are still unknown. In conclusion, we have summarized the existing literature on how circadian rhythms are involved in the regulation of metabolism and how perturbations to the maternal environment during gestation could affect the development of offspring circadian rhythms with long-term metabolic consequences.

ACKNOWLEDGMENTS

The authors acknowledge funding from the USDA–Agriculture Research Service Project 6251-51000-010-05S and National Institutes of Health NIDDK Grant R01-DK-084225 (to K. Shankar).

REFERENCES

Ahima, R. S., Prabakaran, D., and Flier, J. S. (1998) Postnatal leptin surge and regulation of circadian rhythm of leptin by feeding. Implications for energy homeostasis and neuro-endocrine function. *J Clin Invest* 101, 1020–1027.
Ando, H., Yanagihara, H., Hayashi, Y., Obi, Y., Tsuruoka, S., Takamura, T., Kaneko, S., and Fujimura, A. (2005) Rhythmic messenger ribonucleic acid expression of clock genes and adipocytokines in mouse visceral adipose tissue. *Endocrinology* 146, 5631–5636.
Bell-Pedersen, D., Cassone, V. M., Earnest, D. J., Golden, S. S., Hardin, P. E., Thomas, T. L., and Zoran, M. J. (2005) Circadian rhythms from multiple oscillators: Lessons from diverse organisms. *Nat Rev Genet* 6, 544–556.
Bol, V., Desjardins, F., Reusens, B., Balligand, J. L., and Remacle, C. (2010) Does early mis-matched nutrition predispose to hypertension and atherosclerosis, in male mice? *PLoS One* 5, e12656.
Borengasser, S. J., Kang, P., Faske, J., Gomez-Acevedo, H., Blackburn, M. L., Badger, T. M., and Shankar, K. (2014) High fat diet and in utero exposure to maternal obesity disrupts circadian rhythm and leads to metabolic programming of liver in rat offspring. *PLoS One* 9, e84209.
Brainard, G. C., Richardson, B. A., King, T. S., and Reiter, R. J. (1984) The influence of different light spectra on the suppression of pineal melatonin content in the Syrian hamster. *Brain Res* 294, 333–339.

Brainard, G. C., Richardson, B. A., King, T. S., Matthews, S. A., and Reiter, R. J. (1983) The suppression of pineal melatonin content and N-acetyltransferase activity by different light irradiances in the Syrian hamster: A dose-response relationship. *Endocrinology* 113, 293–296.

Bray, M. S., and Young, M. E. (2007) Circadian rhythms in the development of obesity: Potential role for the circadian clock within the adipocyte. *Obes Rev* 8, 169–181.

Buijs, R. M., Scheer, F. A., Kreier, F., Yi, C., Bos, N., Goncharuk, V. D., and Kalsbeek, A. (2006) Organization of circadian functions: Interaction with the body. *Prog Brain Res* 153, 341–360.

Buijs, R. M., Wortel, J., Van Heerikhuize, J. J., Feenstra, M. G., Ter Horst, G. J., Romijn, H. J., and Kalsbeek, A. (1999) Anatomical and functional demonstration of a multisynaptic suprachiasmatic nucleus adrenal (cortex) pathway. *Eur J Neurosci* 11, 1535–1544.

Carter, R., Mouralidarane, A., Soeda, J., Ray, S., Pombo, J., Saraswati, R., Novelli, M., Fusai, G., Rappa, F., Saracino, C., Pazienza, V., Poston, L., Taylor, P. D., Vinciguerra, M., and Oben, J. A. (2014) Non-alcoholic fatty pancreas disease pathogenesis: A role for developmental programming and altered circadian rhythms. *PLoS One* 9, e89505.

Chou, T. C., Scammell, T. E., Gooley, J. J., Gaus, S. E., Saper, C. B., and Lu, J. (2003) Critical role of dorsomedial hypothalamic nucleus in a wide range of behavioral circadian rhythms. *J Neurosci* 23, 10691–10702.

Davidson, A. J., Castanon-Cervantes, O., and Stephan, F. K. (2004) Daily oscillations in liver function: Diurnal vs circadian rhythmicity. *Liver Int* 24, 179–186.

Diaz, P., Powell, T. L., and Jansson, T. (2014) The role of placental nutrient sensing in maternal-fetal resource allocation. *Biol Reprod* 91, 82.

Feng, D., and Lazar, M. A. (2012) Clocks, metabolism, and the epigenome. *Mol Cell* 47, 158–167.

Feng, D., Liu, T., Sun, Z., Bugge, A., Mullican, S. E., Alenghat, T., Liu, X. S., and Lazar, M. A. (2011) A circadian rhythm orchestrated by histone deacetylase 3 controls hepatic lipid metabolism. *Science* 331, 1315–1319.

Fu L., Patel M. S., Bradley A., Wagner E. F., and Karsenty G. (2005) The molecular clock mediates leptin-regulated bone formation. *Cell* 122, 803–815.

Gavrila, A., Peng, C. K., Chan, J. L., Mietus, J. E., Goldberger, A. L., and Mantzoros, C. S. (2003) Diurnal and ultradian dynamics of serum adiponectin in healthy men: Comparison with leptin, circulating soluble leptin receptor, and cortisol patterns. *J Clin Endocrinol Metab* 88, 2838–2843.

Gekakis, N., Staknis, D., Nguyen, H. B., Davis, F. C., Wilsbacher, L. D., King, D. P., Takahashi, J. S., and Weitz, C. J. (1998) Role of the CLOCK protein in the mammalian circadian mechanism. *Science* 280, 1564–1569.

Gillette, M. U., and Tischkau, S. A. (1999) Suprachiasmatic nucleus: The brain's circadian clock. *Recent Prog Horm Res* 54, 33–58; discussion 58–39.

Grimaldi, B., Bellet, M. M., Katada, S., Astarita, G., Hirayama, J., Amin, R. H., Granneman, J. G., Piomelli, D., Leff, T., and Sassone-Corsi, P. (2010) PER2 controls lipid metabolism by direct regulation of PPARgamma. *Cell Metab* 12, 509–520.

Hofman, M. A. (2000) The human circadian clock and aging. *Chronobiol Int* 17, 245–259.

Iwanaga, H., Yano, M., Miki, H., Okada, K., Azama, T., Takiguchi, S., Fujiwara, Y., Yasuda, T., Nakayama, M., Kobayashi, M., Oishi, K., Ishida, N., Nagai, K., and Monden, M. (2005) Per2 gene expressions in the suprachiasmatic nucleus and liver differentially respond to nutrition factors in rats. *JPEN J Parenter Enteral Nutr* 29, 157–161.

Jansson, T., and Powell, T. L. (2013) Role of placental nutrient sensing in developmental programming. *Clin Obstet Gynecol* 56, 591–601.

Kalra, S. P., Bagnasco, M., Otukonyong, E. E., Dube, M. G., and Kalra, P. S. (2003) Rhythmic, reciprocal ghrelin and leptin signaling: New insight in the development of obesity. *Regul Pept* 111, 1–11.

Kalsbeek, A., Fliers, E., Romijn, J. A., La Fleur, S. E., Wortel, J., Bakker, O., Endert, E., and Buijs, R. M. (2001) The suprachiasmatic nucleus generates the diurnal changes in plasma leptin levels. *Endocrinology* 142, 2677–2685.

Kalsbeek, A., Ruiter, M., La Fleur, S. E., Cailotto, C., Kreier, F., and Buijs, R. M. (2006) The hypothalamic clock and its control of glucose homeostasis. *Prog Brain Res* 153, 283–307.

Koike, N., Yoo, S. H., Huang, H. C., Kumar, V., Lee, C., Kim, T. K., and Takahashi, J. S. (2012) Transcriptional architecture and chromatin landscape of the core circadian clock in mammals. *Science* 338, 349–354.

La Fleur, S. E. (2003) Daily rhythms in glucose metabolism: Suprachiasmatic nucleus output to peripheral tissue. *J Neuroendocrinol* 15, 315–322.

La Fleur, S. E., Kalsbeek, A., Wortel, J., and Buijs, R. M. (1999) A suprachiasmatic nucleus generated rhythm in basal glucose concentrations. *J Neuroendocrinol* 11, 643–652.

Langlais, P. J., and Hall, T. (1998) Thiamine deficiency-induced disruptions in the diurnal rhythm and regulation of body temperature in the rat. *Metab Brain Dis* 13, 225–239.

Lu, J., Zhang, Y. H., Chou, T. C., Gaus, S. E., Elmquist, J. K., Shiromani, P., and Saper, C. B. (2001) Contrasting effects of ibotenate lesions of the paraventricular nucleus and sub-paraventricular zone on sleep-wake cycle and temperature regulation. *J Neurosci* 21, 4864–4874.

Lydic, R., Schoene, W. C., Czeisler, C. A., and Moore-Ede, M. C. (1980) Suprachiasmatic region of the human hypothalamus: Homolog to the primate circadian pacemaker? *Sleep* 2, 355–361.

Meng, Y., He, Z., Yin, J., Zhang, Y., and Zhang, T. (2011) Quantitative calculation of human melatonin suppression induced by inappropriate light at night. *Med Biol Eng Comput* 49, 1083–1088.

Milagro, F. I., Gomez-Abellan, P., Campion, J., Martinez, J. A., Ordovas, J. M., and Garaulet, M. (2012) CLOCK, PER2 and BMAL1 DNA methylation: Association with obesity and metabolic syndrome characteristics and monounsaturated fat intake. *Chronobiol Int* 29, 1180–1194.

Mohri, T., Emoto, N., Nonaka, H., Fukuya, H., Yagita, K., Okamura, H., and Yokoyama, M. (2003) Alterations of circadian expressions of clock genes in Dahl salt-sensitive rats fed a high-salt diet. *Hypertension* 42, 189–194.

Mouralidarane, A., Soeda, J., Sugden, D., Bocianowska, A., Carter, R., Ray, S., Saraswati, R., Cordero, P., Novelli, M., Fusai, G., Vinciguerra, M., Poston, L., Taylor, P. D., and Oben, J. A. (2015) Maternal obesity programs offspring non-alcoholic fatty liver disease through disruption of 24-h rhythms in mice. *Int J Obes* 39, 1339–1348.

Oishi, K., Miyazaki, K., Kadota, K., Kikuno, R., Nagase, T., Atsumi, G., Ohkura, N., Azama, T., Mesaki, M., Yukimasa, S., Kobayashi, H., Iitaka, C., Umehara, T., Horikoshi, M., Kudo, T., Shimizu, Y., Yano, M., Monden, M., Machida, K., Matsuda, J., Horie, S., Todo, T., and Ishida, N. (2003) Genome-wide expression analysis of mouse liver reveals CLOCK-regulated circadian output genes. *J Biol Chem* 278, 41519–41527.

Partch, C. L., Green, C. B., and Takahashi, J. S. (2014) Molecular architecture of the mammalian circadian clock. *Trends Cell Biol* 24, 90–99.

Prasai, M. J., George, J. T., and Scott, E. M. (2008) Molecular clocks, type 2 diabetes and cardiovascular disease. *Diab Vasc Dis Res* 5, 89–95.

Ramsey, K. M., Marcheva, B., Kohsaka, A., and Bass, J. (2007) The clockwork of metabolism. *Annu Rev Nutr* 27, 219–240.

Ripperger, J. A., and Merrow, M. (2011) Perfect timing: Epigenetic regulation of the circadian clock. *FEBS Lett* 585, 1406–1411.

Roland, B. L., and Sawchenko, P. E. (1993) Local origins of some GABAergic projections to the paraventricular and supraoptic nuclei of the hypothalamus in the rat. *J Comp Neurol* 332, 123–143.

Rudic, R. D., McNamara, P., Curtis, A. M., Boston, R. C., Panda, S., Hogenesch, J. B., and Fitzgerald, G. A. (2004) BMAL1 and CLOCK, two essential components of the circadian clock, are involved in glucose homeostasis. *PLoS Biol* 2, e377.

Saad, M. F., Riad-Gabriel, M. G., Khan, A., Sharma, A., Michael, R., Jinagouda, S. D., Boyadjian, R., and Steil, G. M. (1998) Diurnal and ultradian rhythmicity of plasma leptin: Effects of gender and adiposity. *J Clin Endocrinol Metab* 83, 453–459.

Samuelsson, A. M., Matthews, P. A., Argenton, M., Christie, M. R., McConnell, J. M., Jansen, E. H., Piersma, A. H., Ozanne, S. E., Twinn, D. F., Remacle, C., Rowlerson, A., Poston, L., and Taylor, P. D. (2008) Diet-induced obesity in female mice leads to offspring hyperphagia, adiposity, hypertension, and insulin resistance: A novel murine model of developmental programming. *Hypertension* 51, 383–392.

Saper, C. B., Lu, J., Chou, T. C., and Gooley, J. (2005) The hypothalamic integrator for circadian rhythms. *Trends Neurosci* 28, 152–157.

Shankar, K., Harrell, A., Liu, X., Gilchrist, J. M., Ronis, M. J., and Badger, T. M. (2008) Maternal obesity at conception programs obesity in the offspring. *Am J Physiol Regul Integr Comp Physiol* 294, R528–R538.

Shimba, S., Ishii, N., Ohta, Y., Ohno, T., Watabe, Y., Hayashi, M., Wada, T., Aoyagi, T., and Tezuka, M. (2005) Brain and muscle Arnt-like protein-1 (BMAL1), a component of the molecular clock, regulates adipogenesis. *Proc Natl Acad Sci USA* 102, 12071–12076.

Stephan, F. K., and Davidson, A. J. (1998) Glucose, but not fat, phase shifts the feeding-entrained circadian clock. *Physiol Behav* 65, 277–288.

Suter, M., Bocock, P., Showalter, L., Hu, M., Shope, C., McKnight, R., Grove, K., Lane, R., and Aagaard-Tillery, K. (2011) Epigenomics: Maternal high-fat diet exposure in utero disrupts peripheral circadian gene expression in nonhuman primates. *FASEB J* 25, 714–726.

Sutton, G. M., Centanni, A. V., and Butler, A. A. (2010) Protein malnutrition during pregnancy in C57BL/6J mice results in offspring with altered circadian physiology before obesity. *Endocrinology* 151, 1570–1580.

Swanson, L. W., and Cowan, W. M. (1975) The efferent connections of the suprachiasmatic nucleus of the hypothalamus. *J Comp Neurol* 160, 1–12.

Turek, F. W., Joshu, C., Kohsaka, A., Lin, E., Ivanova, G., McDearmon, E., Laposky, A., Losee-Olson, S., Easton, A., Jensen, D. R., Eckel, R. H., Takahashi, J. S., and Bass, J. (2005) Obesity and metabolic syndrome in circadian Clock mutant mice. *Science* 308, 1043–1045.

Waddell, B. J., Wharfe, M. D., Crew, R. C., and Mark, P. J. (2012) A rhythmic placenta? Circadian variation, clock genes and placental function. *Placenta* 33, 533–539.

Wang, D., Chen, S., Liu, M., and Liu, C. (2015) Maternal obesity disrupts circadian rhythms of clock and metabolic genes in the offspring heart and liver. *Chronobiol Int* 32, 615–626.

Wankhade, U. D., Thakali, K. M., and Shankar, K. (2016) Persistent influence of maternal obesity on offspring health: Mechanisms from animal models and clinical studies. *Mol Cell Endocrinol* 435, 7–19.

Yang, X., Downes, M., Yu, R. T., Bookout, A. L., He, W., Straume, M., Mangelsdorf, D. J., and Evans, R. M. (2006) Nuclear receptor expression links the circadian clock to metabolism. *Cell* 126, 801–810.

Yi, C. X., van der Vliet, J., Dai, J., Yin, G., Ru, L., and Buijs, R. M. (2006) Ventromedial arcuate nucleus communicates peripheral metabolic information to the suprachiasmatic nucleus. *Endocrinology* 147, 283–294.

Zhang, E. E., Liu, Y., Dentin, R., Pongsawakul, P. Y., Liu, A. C., Hirota, T., Nusinow, D. A., Sun, X., Landais, S., Kodama, Y., Brenner, D. A., Montminy, M., and Kay, S. A. (2010) Cryptochrome mediates circadian regulation of cAMP signaling and hepatic gluconeogenesis. *Nat Med* 16, 1152–1156.

Section III

Early Postnatal Programming

9 Perinatal Nutrition and Programming of the Hypothalamic Regulation of Feeding Behavior and Energy Homeostasis

Francisco Bolaños-Jimenez, Rosalio Mercado-Camargo, and Héctor Urquiza-Marín

CONTENTS

9.1 INTRODUCTION

The interest for the study of the influence of malnutrition on the development and function of the central nervous system (CNS) dates back to the mid-1960s when a large proportion of children all over the world were undernourished. These early investigations were essentially focused on the study of the consequences on learning and other cognitive functions of early nutrient deficiency and the analysis of the hippocampus as anatomical substrate. Economic development followed by the implementation of appropriate public health policy allowed a gradual reduction of the incidence of childhood malnutrition in most countries such that the studies about the impact of *in utero* or neonatal undernutrition on brain function became marginal by the 1980s. The thrifty phenotype hypothesis proposed by Hales and Barker in 1992 linking perinatal malnutrition to metabolic disease risk (Hales and Barker 1992) has led to a resurgence of interest for this topic and placed the hypothalamus in the focus of the investigations aimed at determining the effects of maternal nutrient deficiency on the offspring's CNS development and function. This interest is justified by the central role played by the hypothalamus in the regulation of feeding behavior and metabolic homeostasis. The "thrifty phenotype" hypothesis eventually evolved into the Developmental Origins of Health and Disease (DOHaD) hypothesis, also called metabolic or nutritional programming, to include the fact that over- and high-calorie nutrition during early life also predisposes to the development of the metabolic syndrome in adulthood (Barker 2004). This, and the fact that obesity is currently a health problem of pandemic proportion worldwide, has also stimulated the analysis of the impact of maternal obesity and overnutrition on the structural and functional properties of the hypothalamus of the offspring. The purpose of this chapter is to provide an overview of the hypothalamic regulation of energy homeostasis and of our actual knowledge about the impact of early malnutrition (under- or overnutrition) on the morphological and functional characteristics of the hypothalamic neuronal circuits regulating food intake and energy homeostasis. This overview will be essentially limited to the description and discussion of data generated in rodents as is in these species where the mechanisms underlying the metabolic programming of the hypothalamus are best understood.

9.2   HYPOTHALAMIC REGULATION OF FOOD INTAKE AND ENERGY HOMEOSTASIS

Historically, the involvement of the hypothalamus in the regulation of energy homeostasis, that is the physiological status where the amount of energy obtained though the ingestion of nutrients and their metabolism equals the amount of energy expended by the body, was uncovered during the 40s and 50s when it was observed that the lesion of the ventromedial nucleus of the hypothalamus (VMH) induced hyperphagia, while, in contrast, lesioning the lateral hypothalamus (LH) resulted in reduced food intake (Hetherington and Ranson 1940; Anand 1951). These observations led to the suggestion that feeding results from the stimulation of the LH, the feeding center, whose activity decreases as eating reaches satiety due to an increase in VMH activity, the satiety center. It soon became clear, however, that energy homeostasis is modulated by complex regulatory mechanisms driven by both nutritional (homeostatic) and cognitive (nonhomeostatic) signals. The former category comprises cellular signals triggered in response to the absence or presence of nutrients (hunger, satiety) that inform the brain of the energy needs of the body and involve a bidirectional communication network between the CNS and the peripheral organs (liver, intestine, pancreas, adipose tissue, etc.) in which the absorption, digestion, and metabolism of nutrients take place. The second category includes signals elicited by cognitive processes, such as emotional processing, decision making, and learning, engaged by the sensory systems in response to environmental factors. All these cognitive processes play an important role in the regulation of feeding behavior. For example, ingestion of food provides subjective pleasure, especially sweet or high-fat food, such that eating can be a source of comfort in depressive or stressful states (Dallman et al. 2003). Similarly, learned behavioral responses modulate the motivation to eat through the association of pleasant or aversive effects events to the ingestion of food (Petrovich et al. 2002). Thus, cognitive processing of visual or olfactory sensory stimuli may evoke the desire for food even in the absence of an energy deficit. This desire is regulated in large part by the mesolimbic system and in particular by the dopaminergic projections from the ventral tegmental area (VTA) to the nucleus accumbens, as well as by the neural networks of the prefrontal cortex and the amygdala. All these structures are associated with the expression of motivation and reward (Berthoud 2004; Kelley et al. 2005). Therefore, various brain regions in addition to the hypothalamus are involved in the regulation of feeding and energy metabolism via the release of neuronal signals reflecting the mood, emotions, a state of anxiety or psychological stress, memory of previous experiences, or educational, family, or social conditioning. Nevertheless, all homeostatic or nonhomeostatic signals converge at one moment or another to the hypothalamus that acts as the master regulator of whole-body energy balance and food intake (Figure 9.1). Also, the concept that feeding is a process held in balance by the opposite action of stimulatory and inhibitory networks is still valid today.

Actually, there exist two main neuronal populations within the arcuate nucleus (ARC) of the hypothalamus, which are able to detect nutritional and hormonal signals and direct food intake and energy metabolism (Morton et al. 2006; Coll et al. 2007). One group of neurons coexpresses neuropeptide Y (NPY) and agouti-related protein (AgRP), whereas the other group coexpresses proopiomelanocortin (POMC) and the cocaine and amphetamine-regulated transcript (CART). These two groups of neurons send extensive projections to other nuclei of the hypothalamus including the VMH, the LH, the paraventricular nucleus (PVN), and the dorsomedial hypothalamus (DMH). POMC can be cleaved to numerous peptides known collectively as melanocortins. These include adrenocorticotrophic hormone (ACTH), β-endorphin, and α-melanocyte stimulating hormone (α-MSH). This latter peptide inhibits food intake and increases energy expenditure through the stimulation of melanocortin 3 (MC3R) and melanocortin 4 (MC4R) receptors that are highly expressed in the PVN. The effects of α-MSH on food intake and energy expenditure are blocked by AgRP, which acts as an endogenous antagonist of MC4R receptors and, therefore, stimulates feeding and reduces energy expenditure. NPY induces identical effects via its binding to specific NPY receptors. Indeed, NPY neurons establish synaptic contacts with POMC neurons and reduce their activity via the release of the inhibitory neurotransmitter gamma aminobutyric acid (GABA) (Cowley et al. 2001).

Therefore, stimulation of NPY and AgRP neurons promotes food intake and reduces energy expenditure, while activation of POMC and CART neurons leads to a decrease in food intake together with reduced energy expenditure (Figure 9.2a).

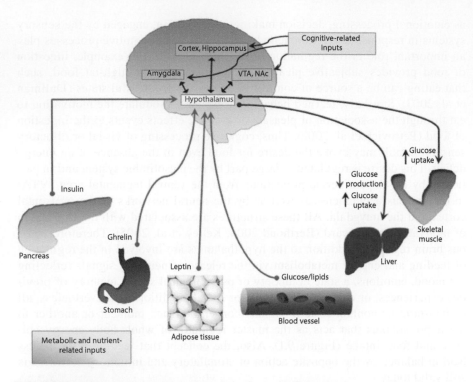

FIGURE 9.1   Schematic representation of the flow of information between the central nervous system and the main peripheral organs involved in the regulation of energy homeostasis. A large number of hormonal and nutritional signals generated at the peripheral level converge to the hypothalamus informing the brain about the energy needs of the body. The integration and processing of this information in a coordinated manner by the various hypothalamic nuclei result in the generation of cellular signals that in turn regulate food intake and the use of energetic substrates by the skeletal muscle, liver, or adipose tissue. The hypothalamus also incorporates the information associated with the hedonic value and the perception of food generated in other brain regions involved in the modulation of reward and motivated behaviors.

More than 40 hormone and neurotransmitter molecules have been shown to interact with NPY/AgRP and POMC/CART neurons as well as with other neuronal populations located in other hypothalamic nuclei to regulate food intake and energy expenditure (Atkinson 2008). A detailed description of all these factors is off-topic for this review and so we will only summarize the characteristics and mechanisms for action of the peptides and neurotransmitters whose expression and/or function has been shown to be affected by perinatal malnutrition.

9.3   INSULIN

Insulin is a hormone secreted by pancreatic β-cells in response to an increase in the circulating levels of glucose. It rapidly lowers blood glucose by promoting glucose uptake and reducing endogenous glucose production by the liver. Insulin also crosses

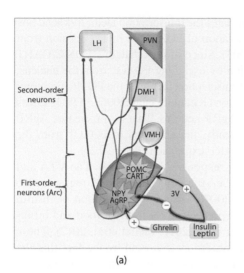
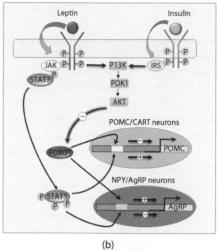

(a)   (b)

FIGURE 9.2 Schematic illustration of the cellular and molecular mechanisms involved in the hypothalamic regulation of food intake and energy homeostasis. (a) The arcuate nucleus is composed of two main neuronal populations. One of these neuronal groups coexpresses the agouti-related protein (AgRP) and neuropeptide Y (NPY) peptides that stimulate food intake (orexigenic effect). The other neuronal population coexpresses proopiomelanocortin (POMC) and cocaine and amphetamine-regulated transcript (CART) peptides that, in contrast, reduce food intake (anorexigenic effect). These first-order neurons establish extensive synaptic contacts with so-called second-order neurons located in other hypothalamic areas including the ventromedial (VMH), the paraventricular (PVH), and dorsomedial hypothalamus (DMH) nuclei, as well as the lateral hypothalamic area (LHA). Both AgRP/NPY and POMC/CART neurons express on their surface specific receptors for many orexigenic and anorexigenic cellular signals, including the receptors for leptin, insulin, and ghrelin. It is through their combined action on these two types of neurons that these hormones and other cellular factors inhibit or promote food intake and energy expenditure. (b) Via the stimulation of their respective receptors, insulin and leptin activate the PIK3 signaling pathway that eventually leads to the translocation of the phosphorylated form of the protein kinase B (Akt) to the cell nucleus where it inactivates and excludes from the nucleus the transcription factor forkhead box protein 1 (FOXO1) by phosphorylation. In POMC/CART neurons, FOXO1 inhibits the expression of POMC, whereas in AgRP/NPY neurons it stimulates AgRP gene expression. Thus, the activation of PIK3 by insulin and leptin reduces food intake and increased energy expenditure through the simultaneous stimulation and repression of, respectively, POMC and AgRP. In addition to the activation of PIK3, leptin stimulates the activator of transcription signal transducer and activator of transcription 3 (STAT3) that once in the nucleus activates the expression of POMC and inhibits that of AgRP.

the blood–brain barrier (BBB) and reaches several brain structures including the hypothalamus where it inhibits food intake through the stimulation of specific insulin receptors expressed by POMC/CART and AgRP/NPY neurons. The suppressive effects of insulin on feeding involve a signaling cascade that starts with the recruitment of insulin receptor substrate (IRS) proteins after the binding of insulin to its membrane receptor (Plum et al. 2006). This leads to the activation of phosphoinositide 3-kinase (PI3K). The phosphorylated form of PIK3 then activates phosphoinositide-dependent kinase-1 (PDK1). In turn, the activated form of PDK1 phosphorylates the serine threonine kinase

Akt that enters into the nucleus and phosphorylates the transcription factor forkhead box protein 1 (FOXO1). This results in the inactivation of FOXO and in its exclusion from the nucleus (Guo et al. 1999; Gan et al. 2005). Since in hypothalamic POMC/CART neurons FOXO1 reduces POMC transcription by excluding FOXO1 from the nucleus, insulin relieves the inhibitory effect of this transcription factor on the POMC promoter and, therefore, enhances POMC gene expression (Kitamura et al. 2006). FOXO1 exerts opposite effects on gene expression in NPY/AgRP neurons. That is, it increases AgRP expression (Kitamura et al. 2006). Consequently, the exclusion of FOXO1 from the nucleus by insulin also results in decreased AgRP expression (Figure 9.2b).

The hypothalamus is not the only insulin-responsive brain region. The VTA and the central bed nucleus of the amygdala (CeA), among other brain regions, also contain insulin receptors (Figlewicz et al. 2003). Direct administration of insulin into the VTA decreases food intake reduces preference for high-fat food and inhibits reward-based feeding behaviors (Könner et al. 2011; Mebel et al. 2012). These effects are mediated by the dopaminergic system as indicated by the fact that the specific inactivation of insulin receptor gene expression in catecholaminergic neurons (which include dopamine neurons) results in increased food intake and fat mass accretion (Könner et al. 2011). The administration of insulin in the CeA also reduces food intake and this effect is abolished by high-fat feeding (Boghossian et al. 2009).

9.4 LEPTIN

Leptin is a hormone predominantly produced by white adipose tissue and released into the circulation in proportion to the amount of total body fat mass. As insulin, it inhibits food intake and enhances energy expenditure by stimulating the phosphoinositide 3-kinase (PI3K)/AKT signaling pathway within POMC/CART and NPY/AgRP hypothalamic neurons though by a different signaling mechanism involving, as a first step, the binding of leptin to a selective leptin receptor (Figure 9.2b). There are six different types of leptin receptors in rodents, from Ob-Ra to Ob-Rf, which are encoded by one single leptin receptor gene. However, only the Ob-Rb has the structural requirements allowing the transduction of leptin binding into the activation of intracellular signals (Baumann et al. 1996) and, therefore, is the only one involved in the regulatory effects of leptin on food intake and energy homeostasis. The binding of leptin to the Ob-Rb receptor induces a conformational change that favors its interaction with the Janus-activated kinase (JAK) protein, which, in turn phosphorylates the Ob-Rb receptor in different tyrosine residues (Tyr) that serve as binding sites for specific Src homology 2 (SH2) binding proteins. Thus, the binding of the Src protein SH2B1 to the leptin receptor increases JAK activity leading to the recruitment of IRS proteins and subsequent PI3K activation (Duan et al. 2004; Ren et al. 2005). On the other hand, phosphorylation of Tyr_{1138} results in the binding of the signal transducer and activator of transcription 3 (STAT3) to the Ob-Rb receptor followed by its activation (Banks et al. 2000). Once activated, STAT3 translocates to the nucleus where it stimulates POMC gene expression while inhibiting that of AgRP (Kitamura et al. 2006). As insulin, leptin also modulates food reward-related behaviors through its interaction with Ob-Rb receptors expressed by dopaminergic neurons in the VTA and the nucleus accumbens (Hommel et al. 2006). At the cellular level, the binding of leptin to these receptors results in reduced firing of mesolombic dopaminergic neurons, reduced dopamine release, and decreased dopamine concentration, while, in behavioral terms, the intraventricular administration of leptin reduces the self-administration of sucrose (Figlewicz et al. 2006).

9.5 GHRELIN

Ghrelin is a peptide synthesized by the endocrine X/A-like cells of the fundus mucosa of the stomach but is also expressed in other parts of the gastrointestinal tract as well as in the heart, pancreas, and hypothalamus. Its circulating levels increase before meals (Cummings et al. 2001; Sugino et al. 2002) as well as following food deprivation and after weight loss (Tanaka et al. 2003; Soriano-Guillén et al. 2004). These latter observations together with the fact that ghrelin stimulates feeding (Wren et al. 2000) indicate that ghrelin acts as a starvation signal. However, in addition to stimulating appetite and food intake, ghrelin possesses many other physiological functions including the secretion of growth hormone, the modulation of intestinal motility, and the regulation of gastric acid and pancreatic secretions (Muccioli et al. 2002).

The effects of ghrelin are mediated by a unique receptor called the growth hormone secretagogue receptor (GHSR1a), which belongs to the G-protein coupled receptors (GPCRs) superfamily and is localized in many cerebral structures including the hippocampus, hypothalamus, midbrain, cortex, VTA, and amygdala. The stimulation of GHSR1a receptor by ghrelin leads to the activation of phospholipase C, the production of inositols triphosphate, and an increased concentration of intracellular calcium (Sun et al. 2004). Of note, the acylation of ghrelin by the enzyme ghrelin O-acyl transferase (GOAT) is essential for its binding to the GHSR1a receptor.

The orexigenic effects of ghrelin are directly related to its capacity to stimulate the activity of NPY/AgRP hypothalamic neurons. Indeed, the central administration of ghrelin increases the expression of NPY and AgRP within the ARC (Kamegai et al. 2001) and the stimulating effects of ghrelin on feeding are completely abolished in NPY/AgRP double knockout animals (Chen et al. 2004). In addition, it has been shown that the selective disruption of GABA release from AgRP neurons through the inactivation of vesicular GABA transporter gene expression cancels the anorexic effects of ghrelin (Tong et al. 2008). These data have led to a proposal that ghrelin stimulates food intake via two interrelated mechanisms, which are both mediated by NPY/AgRP neurons. Thus, the stimulation of these neurons by ghrelin leads to the production and release of the anorexic peptides NPY and AgRP and of GABA. This latter neurotransmitter would reinforce the positive effects on feeding of NPY and AgRP through its inhibitory action on POMC neurons. It should be noted, however, that the GHSR1a receptor is also expressed in other hypothalamic nuclei and in several structures of the limbic system (hippocampus, amygdala, VTA, substantia nigra) and that the direct administration of ghrelin in these nuclei also triggers food intake (Naleid et al. 2005; Alvarez-Crespo et al. 2012).

9.6 SEROTONIN

Serotonin, or 5-hydroxytryptamine (5-HT), is a monoamine synthesized from the essential amino acid L-tryptophan that regulates a multitude of brain functions including the control of body temperature, hormone secretion, sexual behavior, learning, and memory and food intake. Thus, an increase of brain serotonin activity results in reduced food consumption and decreased weight gain (Voigt and Fink 2015). These effects have been observed after the central or peripheral administration of serotonin agonists or of pharmacological compounds that increase the synaptic availability of 5-HT through the inhibition of its reuptake by serotoninergic neurons or by facilitating its release. Behavioral studies have shown that the anorexic effects of the 5-HT are the result of its specific action in the hypothalamus and are associated with alterations in the process of satiety. In particular, it has been shown that the hypothalamic administration of serotonergic agonists results in a significant decrease in the amount of food consumed at a meal and the length of the meal (Shor-Posner et al. 1986; Leibowitz and Alexander 1988). In contrast, these pharmacological manipulations do not alter meal frequency or the latency to eat after the presentation of food. These results, together with the observations indicating that the circulating levels of tryptophan, the precursor of serotonin synthesis, are increased in animals fed a high-carbohydrate diet, have led to suggestions that 5-HT is at the heart of a negative feedback circuit modulating the intake of food (Leibowitz and Alexander 1988). Thus, an excessive stimulation of the hypothalamus by serotonin would produce anorexia, while a deficient serotoninergic transmission would lead to overeating and obesity.

The anorectic effects of serotonin are attributed to its ability to modulate the activity of POMC/CART and NPY/AgRP neurons as determined by the combined use of anatomical, electrophysiological, and behavioral techniques. Namely, serotonin increases the firing rate of POMC neurons in the ARC and this effect is abolished by the pharmacological blocking or gene inactivation of melanocortin receptors (Heisler et al. 2003). At the cellular level, this effect would be the result of the interaction of serotonin with 5-HT1B and 5-HT2C receptors (Heisler et al. 2006). 5-HT activates the release of α-MSH through the stimulation of 5-HT2C receptors expressed by POMC/CART neurons. Simultaneously, by stimulating 5-HT1B receptors expressed in NPY/AgRP neurons, serotonin blocks the release of NPY and AgRP and abolishes the inhibitory effect of GABA on POMC neurons (Heisler et al. 2006). Interestingly, serotonin improves glucose tolerance and hyperinsulinemia via the stimulation of the melanocortonin system independently of its effects on food intake (Zhou et al. 2007).

In addition to its action on the ARC, 5-HT participates in the regulation of energy balance by interacting with serotonin receptors localized in other brain regions than the hypothalamus. In particular, it has been shown that stimulation of 5-HT4 receptors in the nucleus accumbens blocks the motivational stimulus of food both in fed and fasted mice and, in parallel, increases the mRNA levels encoding the anorexic peptide CART (Jean et al. 2007).

9.7 IMPACT OF EARLY MALNUTRITION ON FOOD INTAKE AND HYPOTHALAMIC GENE EXPRESSION

After the proposal of the thrifty phenotype hypothesis by Hales and Barker, several groups reported that maternal undernutrition results in increased food intake. Thus, Vickers et al. were among the first to show that the offspring born to dams provided

30% of the amount of food consumed by control dams ate more food per body weight than the offspring of dams fed ad libitum (Vickers et al. 2000). These observations were confirmed and extended by other authors who also demonstrated that calorie or protein restriction during early life induces a preference for the consumption of high-fat food in addition to enhanced food intake (Cambraia et al. 2001; Bellinger et al. 2004; Desai et al. 2005).

Meal pattern analysis further showed that the increased food intake presented by the offspring of protein-restricted rats is due to the delayed appearance of satiety, an increase in meal size, and a reduced latency to eat (Orozco-Sólis et al. 2009). At the molecular level, these changes are associated with an increased expression of NPY and AgRP along with reduced expression of POMC in the hypothalamus (Ikenasio-Thorpe et al. 2007; Coupé et al. 2009, 2012; Orozco-Sólis et al. 2009), indicating that the higher food intake of early undernourished rats relative to control animals is the result of both an enhanced function of the positive signals that initiate and maintain eating and a decreased action of negative feedback signals critical to meal termination (satiety). In support of this contention, the anorexic actions of insulin, leptin, and serotonin have been shown to be reduced in adult animals born to food-restricted dams (Sardinha et al. 2006; Desai et al. 2007; Lopes de Souza et al. 2008). In addition, ghrelin induces a higher firing frequency of ARC and VMH neurons in hypothalamic slices from early malnourished rats as compared with controls (Yousheng Jia et al. 2008). The reduced anorexic effects of leptin can be explained by impaired Ob-Rb gene expression and signaling as indicated by the decreased levels of Ob-Rb mRNA levels and reduced Akt and STAT3 phosphorylation after leptin administration in perinatally malnourished rats (Desai et al. 2007; Coupé et al. 2012). On the other hand, the reduced anorexic effects of 5-HT in malnourished animals are associated to a decreased sensitivity, but to a reduced expression, of 5-HT1B receptors (Lopes de Souza et al. 2008).

The preference for the consumption of high-fat food exhibited by the offspring of malnourished dams suggested that the cognitive circuits regulating food intake are also affected by maternal malnutrition. This was confirmed by Vucetic et al. (2010) who showed that maternal protein restriction in the mice enhances the expression levels of several genes involved in the synthesis, reuptake, degradation, and signaling of dopamine in several brain regions associated with food reward including the VTA, nucleus accumbens, and prefrontal cortex (Vucetic et al. 2010). Strikingly, however, these molecular changes were correlated with a decreased preference for sucrose. An increased expression of tyrosine hydroxylase, the key enzyme in dopamine synthesis, has also been reported in the nucleus accumbens of adult offspring from calorie-restricted rats (Alves et al. 2015).

Though hyperphagia seems to be a trend of early nutrient restriction, some studies have reported no differences in food intake between the offspring of control and malnourished mothers (Petry et al. 1997; Bieswal et al. 2006). Moreover, it has been shown that after 2–3 months of age early malnourished rats consume daily the same amount of food as control animals (Desai et al. 2007; Coupé et al. 2009; Orozco-Sólis et al. 2009). However, these animals develop with aging clear metabolic and body composition disturbances indicative of obesity including elevated levels of triglycerides and fatty acids in serum along with increased visceral fat (Petry et al.

1997; Bieswal et al. 2006; Orozco-Sólis et al. 2009). This indicates that perinatal malnutrition programs obesity through a mechanism independent of its effects on feeding behavior. The hyperphagia exhibited by perinatal nutrient-restricted animals might in fact correspond to a homeostatic mechanism operating to accelerate the restoration of body weight during the phase of nutritional rehabilitation in which increased food intake is a necessary condition for the supply of the high quantity of energy required for tissue growth and differentiation. As animals get older, the needs in energy for growth diminish leading to the normalization of food intake.

The development of obesity and associated metabolic perturbations induced by maternal undernutrition might implicate the cross talk, via the autonomic nervous system, between the hypothalamus and peripheral organs controlling carbohydrates and lipids metabolism (Lam et al. 2009; Sandoval et al. 2009). This bidirectional network involves the same neuronal populations and signaling pathways regulating food intake. As an example, insulin inhibits hepatic glucose production via the stimulation of ATP-dependent potassium channels located in hypothalamic AgRP neurons (Könner et al. 2007), and the selective ablation of these neurons shifts energy metabolism toward the use of lipids in liver and skeletal muscle without altering food intake (Joly-Amado et al. 2012). Also, the accumulation of nutrients and their metabolites in the hypothalamus activates nutrient-sensing mechanisms that regulate glucose homeostasis in the periphery. Thus, an acute increase in glucose or lipids and lipid-derived metabolites, such as long-chain fatty acyl CoA in brain, reduces hepatic glucose production (Lam et al. 2005) and favors skeletal muscle glucose uptake (Cha et al. 2006). The relevance of these regulatory mechanisms for the development of metabolic disorders is illustrated by the fact that a high-fat diet impairs the ability of the hypothalamic administration of oleic acid, a long-chain fatty acid, to reduce hepatic glucose production (Morgan et al. 2004).

Interestingly, nutrient sensing in the hypothalamus is impaired by early malnutrition. Thus, perinatal protein restriction alters the hypothalamic expression of the nutrient sensor sirtuin 1 (SIRT1) (Desai et al. 2014) as well as that of several nuclear receptors and coregulators of transcription involved in the detection and use of lipid nutrients as fuel, which, in addition, link temporal and nutritional cues to metabolism through their tight interaction with the circadian clock (Orozco-Solís et al. 2010). In addition, adult rats born to food-restricted dams show enhanced phosphorylation levels of hypothalamic AMP-activated protein kinase (AMPK) in the fed state together with decreased activation of Akt (Fukami et al. 2012). Moreover, whereas fasting induced a significant activation of AMPK in the hypothalamus of control rats, no change in AMPK phosphorylation levels in response to fasting was detected in malnourished rats (Fukami et al. 2012). Similarly, the adult offspring of dams fed a low protein diet during gestation and lactation exhibit enhanced activation in the hypothalamus of the protein kinase mammalian target of rapamycin (mTOR) in the fed state as well as impaired mTOR responses to fasting and refeeding (Guzmán-Quevedo et al. 2013). The protein kinase AMPK is a nutrient sensor, which is activated by energy depletion and once activated regulates a wide range of cellular processes that synergistically inhibit protein and lipid biosynthesis and stimulate β-oxidation, glucose uptake, and glycolysis (Lopez et al. 2016). In contrast, mTOR is a downstream component of the PI3K/Akt signaling pathway that acts as nutrient sensor of high nutrient supply in different tissues where it regulates positively protein synthesis and lipogenesis (Haissaguerre et al. 2014). mTOR is also involved in the control of feeding behavior by integrating hormonal and nutrient signals in the hypothalamus (Cota et al. 2006) and, therefore, regulates energy homeostasis at the whole-body level. Combined, these data strongly suggest that altered nutrient sensing in response to an inadequate fetal and neonatal energetic environment is one of the basic mechanisms of the developmental programming of metabolic disorders induced by malnutrition during early life.

Similar to the offspring of calorie or protein-restricted dams, rodents born to obese or overfed mothers are hyperphagic and exhibit altered expression patterns in the hypothalamus of key genes regulating food intake. However, there are conflicting results as to whether the expression of anorexigenic genes is upregulated or downregulated and in some studies the gene expression changes are difficult to reconcile with the observed feeding phenotype. Thus, while the group of Morris has reported reduced levels of mRNAs encoding for NPY and AgRP along with decreased expression of POMC in pups and adult offspring born to dams fed a high-fat diet (Morris and Chen 2008; Chen et al. 2009), other authors observed increased gene expression levels of NPY and AgRP using a very similar experimental paradigm (Gupta et al. 2009; Desai et al. 2016). Postnatally overfed rats from small litters also exhibit an increased of immune-positive NPY hypothalamic neurons (Plagemann et al. 1999). The hyperphagic effects induced by maternal obesity or neonatal overfeeding have been attributed to a reduced sensitivity to leptin and insulin (Rodrigues et al. 2011), altered neuronal responses to anorexigenic (CART, α-MSH) and orexigenic (NPY, melanin-concentrating hormone) peptides (Davidowa et al. 2003), and central ghrelin resistance (Collden et al. 2015). However, it was recently shown that maternal obesity also impairs the expression in the hypothalamus of the offspring of several nutrient sensors including mTOR and SIRT1 (Desai et al. 2016) further sustaining the hypothesis that altered nutrient sensing contributes to metabolic programming of hyperphagia.

In addition to modifying the homeostatic control of food intake, maternal obesity interferes with the cognitive regulation of feeding as indicated by the increased preference for fat and sugar intake in the offspring of obese dams (Bayol et al. 2007; Teegarden et al. 2009; Vucetic et al. 2010). These feeding preferences are associated with an upregulation of the dopamine reuptake transporter as well as of the μ-opioid receptor and preproenkephalin in the nucleus accumbens and prefrontal cortex (Vucetic et al. 2010).

9.8 IMPACT OF EARLY MALNUTRITION ON HYPOTHALAMIC STRUCTURE

Embryonic and neonatal development is characterized by the existence of several successive phases of proliferation and cell differentiation whereby, from a relatively small number of multipotent cells, the various organs and tissues of an organism are formed. The quantity and quality of the maternal diet during pregnancy and lactation can affect these processes inducing alterations in the number and type of cells in different tissues and organs with physiological consequences in the long term. Here we provide an overview of the ontogeny of the hypothalamus and provide some examples of the deleterious effects of maternal malnutrition on this process.

Birth-dating studies in rodents using 5-bromo-2'-deoxyuridine (BrdU) or [³H] thymidine labeling have shown that the majority of hypothalamic neurons are generated between the 11th and 16th day of embryonic development (E11–E16) from the rostral diencephalic neuroepithelium lining the third ventricle. Postmitotic neurons then migrate perpendicularly from the third ventricle during the radial migration phase to reach their final location within the hypothalamus during a second tangential intrahypothalamic migration phase. The first neurons to leave the cell-division cycle (E12–E13) form the LH structures, while the later generated neurons (E16–E17) form the median structures (Ifft 1972; Shimada and Nakamura 1973). Cell proliferation in the hypothalamus extends until birth and the temporal differentiation of the new cells into neurons differs from one hypothalamic nucleus to another. For example, neurogenesis within the ARC and VMH expands from E12 to E16, whereas PVH neurogenesis is restricted to E12 (Bouret et al. 2004a; Bouret and Simerly 2004). Axon elongation and synaptogenesis of the new generated cells take place during the first weeks of postnatal life with separate temporary phases. Namely, the dorsomedial nuclei are innervated on postnatal day 6 (P6), whereas the innervation of the PVN (P8–P10), followed by the innervation the lateral area (P12), takes place in a second phase.

The development of the hypothalamus is regulated by several cellular factors some of which are also involved in the modulation of energy homeostasis. This is the case of leptin (Bouret and Simerly 2004) and ghrelin (Steculorum et al. 2015). Indeed, experiments conducted in mice revealed the existence of a transient increase in the circulating levels of leptin during the second week of life (the leptin surge), which coincides with the period of synaptogenesis in the hypothalamus and neurite outgrowth from the ARC to the other hypothalamic nuclei (Ahima et al. 1998). These neuronal projections are disrupted in leptin-deficient mice (Lep^{ob}/Lep^{ob}), and the administration of leptin early after birth, but not in adulthood, restores ARC projections to normal levels (Bouret et al. 2004b).

In pups born to nutrient- or protein-restricted dams, the leptin surge is advanced (Yura et al. 2005; Coupé et al. 2010) and reduced in magnitude (Delahaye et al. 2008; Coupé et al. 2010), and these alterations are associated with a decreased number of AgRP and α-MSH fibers in the PVN together with an increased density of NPY and CART nerve terminals. Rats underfed during lactation due to rearing in large litters also exhibit an increased number of NPY in the ARC (Plagemann et al. 1999a). The aforementioned morphological abnormalities could be the result of the impaired neurotrophic effects of insulin and leptin as indicated by fact that the proliferation and neuronal differentiation of hypothalamic neurosphere progenitor cells in response to these two hormones *in vitro* are decreased in malnourished pups as compared with controls (Desai et al. 2011). Interestingly, the simulation of the shift in the leptin surge in control pups via the systemic injection of leptin reproduces the metabolic phenotype of animals born to undernourished mothers (Yura et al. 2005). Similarly, leptin administration from birth to 10 days of age results in hyperphagia, increased body weight, and hyperleptinemia at adulthood (Toste et al. 2006). These observations indicate that leptin is a key programming factor of the metabolic disorders induced by malnutrition during early life. However, it remains to be determined how the manipulation in two opposite directions of the leptin system results in the same metabolic phenotype. Actually, blocking leptin function during the first 2 weeks of neonatal life by the systemic administration of a leptin antagonist leads to leptin resistance at adulthood and to enhanced body fat as compared with control animals (Attig et al. 2008).

The development of the hypothalamic circuits regulating food intake is also affected by maternal overfeeding. Thus, increased proliferation, migration, and neuronal differentiation of the hypothalamic neuronal precursor cells has been observed in the embryos of dams fed a high-fat diet (Chang et al. 2008). Neonatally overfed rats also exhibit a higher number of galanin neurons in the PVN coupled to a reduced density of cholecystokinin-8S-neurons (Plagemann et al. 1998, 1999b,c). Moreover, mice born to dams fed a high-fat diet during lactation present a significant reduction in the number of α-MSH and AgRP fibers in several hypothalamic nuclei regulating energy homeostasis including the PVN, the median, and the LH (Vogt et al. 2014). Notably, the specific inactivation of the insulin receptor in POMC neurons prevents the deleterious effects of maternal high-fat feeding on the density of α-MSH fibers in the PVN but this genetic manipulation is without effect on the reduced number of AgRP fibers (Vogt et al. 2014).

9.9   EPIGENETIC MECHANISMS AND TRANSGENERATIONAL PROGRAMMING

At the molecular level, a number of studies indicate that the alteration of the epigenetic mechanisms regulating gene expression might be the link between under- (or over-) nutrition in early life and the development of a pathological phenotype in adulthood (Gabory et al. 2011; Pinney and Simmons 2011; Desai et al. 2015). The term epigenetics refers to biologic processes that regulate mitotically or meiotically heritable changes in gene expression without altering the DNA sequence. These include DNA modification by methylation of cytosine residues in CpG dinucleotides, the posttranslational modifications of the N-terminal tails of histone proteins, and the regulation by microRNAs (miRNAs) of enzymatic effectors involved in epigenetic modulation.

Interestingly, some of the physiological and epigenetic alterations resulting from under- or overnutrition in early life can be transmitted to the offspring of the second generation (F2), though they have never suffered from nutrient deficiency or nutritional excess (Zambrano et al. 2005; Reyes-Castro et al. 2015; see Aiken and Ozanne 2014 for review). This transgenerational programming process could be explained by a defective development of the reproductive tract in the female animals of the first generation (F1), which would lead to the establishment of an abnormal intrauterine environment at the time of pregnancy and, consequently, to altered embryonic development of F2 animals. However, the fact that metabolic alterations in the offspring are determined not only by the nutritional status of the mother but also by the nutritional status of the father (Ng and Morris 2010) strongly suggests the existence of a transgenerational transmission via germ cells. In agreement with this idea, altered gene expression and epigenetic profiles have been documented in the sperm of adult male offspring born to malnourished dams (Carone et al. 2010; Radford et al. 2014). Metabolic programming is therefore a transgenerational phenomenon by which parental undernutrition or parental obesity increases the risk of developing metabolic disorders not only in the first (F1) but also in the second (F2) generation in the absence of adverse nutritional conditions, thus initiating a vicious cycle to perpetuate noncommunicable diseases. Interestingly, the increased hypothalamic expression of NPY induced in the first generation by feeding the dam a low protein diet is transferred to the second generation via the maternal lineage (Peixoto-Silva et al. 2011). Maternal undernutrition during gestation or the lactation period also induces transgenerational programming of the hypothalamic–pituitary–adrenal axis (Bertram et al. 2008), as well as of the hypothalamic neuronal circuits regulating reproduction function (Kaczmarek et al. 2016).

Several studies have documented epigenetic modifications in the hypothalamus as a result of maternal or neonatal malnutrition. Nevertheless, our knowledge about how an imbalanced nutritional environment during early life impacts on the epigenetic profile of the hypothalamus and how these epigenetic modifications relate to the alterations in hypothalamic gene expression and function exhibited by perinatally malnourished animals remains limited.

Actually, there are less than 10 studies in which the epigenetic alterations in the hypothalamus of the offspring as a result of maternal over- or undernutrition have been examined and most of these studies have focused on the analysis of POMC. Thus, feeding a reduced protein diet to pregnant rats or inducing neonatal overfeeding of pups born to dams fed a standard diet results in reduced expression of POMC and hypermethylation of its promoter region (Plagemann et al. 2009; Coupé et al. 2010). Similarly, maternal food restriction in sheep (Stevens et al. 2010) or maternal supplementation with conjugated linolenic acids during the first 2 weeks of lactation in mice (Zhang et al. 2014) increases the methylation level of the POMC promoter in the hypothalamus. In contrast, feeding a high-folate diet during pregnancy results in reduced POMC DNA methylation (Cho et al. 2013). Neonatal overfeeding also induces hypermethylation in the promoter of the hypothalamic insulin receptor (Plagemann et al. 2010) or hypomethylation of the NPY promoter region (Mahmood et al. 2013).

9.10   CONCLUDING REMARKS

Given its central role in the regulation of feeding behavior and energy homeostasis, the hypothalamus has been the subject of multiple studies aimed at determining the cellular and molecular basis of the nutritional programming of metabolic disorders. Globally, these studies show that nutrient restriction or overfeeding during *in utero* development or neonatal life results in gene expression changes that drive the homeostatic control of energy homeostasis toward enhanced food intake and reduced energy expenditure. However, although the rodent offspring born to malnourished dams exhibit hyperphagia, the question remains as to whether this alteration contributes in the long term to the development of obesity and associated metabolic disorders. In this respect, it is important to underline that the same hypothalamic neuronal circuits and signaling pathways regulating food intake modulate energy homeostasis via nutrient-sensing mechanisms that, when activated, send efferent signals via the autonomic nervous system to the liver, skeletal muscle, and other peripheral organs to regulate glucose and lipid metabolism (Lam et al. 2009; Sandoval et al. 2009). These central sensing mechanisms are disrupted in obesity and/or diabetes (Morgan et al. 2004) and several reports indicate that the offspring of undernourished (Orozco-Solís et al. 2010; Fukami et al. 2012) or obese dams (Desai et al. 2016) exhibit modified gene expression and function of nutrient-sensing systems both under basal conditions and in response to a nutritional challenge. Thus, instead of, or in addition to, altered food intake, impaired hypothalamic nutrient sensing might underpin the development of metabolic disorders induced by malnutrition during early life. However, the metabolic consequences at the peripheral level, that is, decrease in blood glucose and insulin levels and suppression of hepatic glucose production, of impaired hypothalamic nutrient sensing in early malnourished animals remain to be explored.

One inherent limitation of all hypothalamic epigenetic and gene expression changes associated with metabolic programming reported to date is their lack of cellular resolution. This is of important concern for the establishment of a mechanistic link between a given molecular alteration and a behavioral or metabolic phenotype. Actually, the vast majority of genes within the hypothalamus display nucleus-specific patterns of regulation and the same gene within the same nucleus might be submitted to different regulatory processes depending on the type of cell it is expressed. For instance, although leptin enhances PI3K activity in POMC neurons, it inhibits PI3K in AgRP-expressing neurons (Xu et al. 2005). Similarly, the specific deletion of AMPK from POMC neurons leads to an increased expression ratio of orexigenic versus anorexigenic genes (Claret et al. 2007). In contrast, no changes in gene expression are observed after the targeted loss-of-function mutation of AMPK in AgRP neurons (Claret et al. 2007). These data were obtained using a combination of pharmacological, molecular genetics, and electrophysiological techniques that allow cell-specific genetic deletion and single-cell recordings of activity. The use of these experimental approaches should allow for establishment of the cellular and physiological output of the hypothalamic epigenetic and gene expression changes induced by malnutrition during early life.

ACKNOWLEDGMENTS

This work was supported by a grant from the ECOS Nord/ANUIES/CONACyT/SEP Program, Action Number M12-S01.

REFERENCES

Ahima, R. S., D. Prabakaran, et al. (1998). Postnatal leptin surge and regulation of circadian rhythm of leptin by feeding. Implications for energy homeostasis and neuroendocrine function. *Journal of Clinical Investigation* 101(5): 1020–1027.
Aiken, C. E. and S. E. Ozanne (2014). Transgenerational developmental programming. *Human Reproduction Update* 20(1): 63–75.
Alvarez-Crespo, M., K. P. Skibicka, et al. (2012). The amygdala as a neurobiological target for ghrelin in rats: Neuroanatomical, electrophysiological and behavioral evidence. *PLoS ONE* 7(10): e46321.

Alves, M. B., R. Dalle Molle, et al. (2015). Increased palatable food intake and response to food cues in intrauterine growth-restricted rats are related to tyrosine hydroxylase content in the orbitofrontal cortex and nucleus accumbens. *Behavioural Brain Research* 287: 73–81.

Anand, B. K., Brobeck, J.R. (1951). Localization of a "feeding center" in the hypothalamus of the rat. *Proceedings of the Society for Experimental Biology and Medicine. Society for Experimental Biology and Medicine* 77: 323–324.

Atkinson, T. J. (2008). Central and peripheral neuroendocrine peptides and signalling in appetite regulation: Considerations for obesity pharmacotherapy. *Obesity Reviews* 9(2): 108–120.

Attig, L., G. Solomon, et al. (2008). Early postnatal leptin blockage leads to a long-term leptin resistance and susceptibility to diet-induced obesity in rats. *International Journal of Obesity* 32(7): 1153–1160.

Banks, A. S., S. M. Davis, et al. (2000). Activation of downstream signals by the long form of the leptin receptor. *Journal of Biological Chemistry* 275(19): 14563–14572.

Barker, D. J. P. (2004). Developmental origins of adult health and disease. *Journal of Epidemiology and Community Health* 58(2): 114–115.

Baumann, H., K. K. Morella, et al. (1996). The full-length leptin receptor has signaling capabilities of interleukin 6-type cytokine receptors. *Proceedings of the National Academy of Sciences of the United States of America* 93(16): 8374–8378.

Bayol, S. A., S. J. Farrington, et al. (2007). A maternal 'junk food' diet in pregnancy and lactation promotes an exacerbated taste for 'junk food' and a greater propensity for obesity in rat offspring. *British Journal of Nutrition* 98(04): 843–851.

Bellinger, L., C. Lilley, et al. (2004). Prenatal exposure to a maternal low-protein diet programmes a preference for high-fat foods in the young adult rat. *British Journal of Nutrition* 92(03): 513–520.

Berthoud, H.-R. (2004). Neural control of appetite: Cross-talk between homeostatic and non-homeostatic systems. *Appetite* 43(3): 315–317.

Bertram, C., O. Khan, et al. (2008). Transgenerational effects of prenatal nutrient restriction on cardiovascular and hypothalamic-pituitary-adrenal function. *Journal of Physiology* 586(8): 2217–2229.

Bieswal, F., M.-T. Ahn, et al. (2006). The importance of catch-up growth after early malnutrition for the programming of obesity in male rat. *Obesity* 14(8): 1330–1343.

Boghossian, S., K. Lemmon, et al. (2009). High-fat diets induce a rapid loss of the insulin anorectic response in the amygdala. *American Journal of Physiology—Regulatory, Integrative and Comparative Physiology* 297(5): R1302–R1311.

Bouret, S. G., S. J. Draper, et al. (2004a). Formation of projection pathways from the arcuate nucleus of the hypothalamus to hypothalamic regions implicated in the neural control of feeding behavior in mice. *Journal of Neuroscience* 24(11):2797–2805.

Bouret, S. G., S. J. Draper, et al. (2004b). Trophic action of leptin on hypothalamic neurons that regulate feeding. *Science* 304(5667): 108–110.

Bouret, S. G. and R. B. Simerly (2004). Minireview: Leptin and development of hypothalamic feeding circuits. *Endocrinology* 145(6): 2621–2626.

Cambraia, R. P. B., H. Vannucchi, et al. (2001). Effects of malnutrition during early lactation on development and feeding behavior under the self-selection paradigm. *Nutrition* 17(6): 455–461.

Carone, B. R., L. Fauquier, et al. (2010). Paternally induced transgenerational environmental reprogramming of metabolic gene expression in mammals. *Cell* 143(7): 1084–1096.

Cha, S.-H., J. T. Rodgers, et al. (2006). Hypothalamic malonyl-CoA triggers mitochondrial biogenesis and oxidative gene expression in skeletal muscle: Role of PGC-1α. *Proceedings of the National Academy of Sciences* 103(42): 15410–15415.

Chang, G.-Q., V. Gaysinskaya, et al. (2008). Maternal high-fat diet and fetal programming: Increased proliferation of hypothalamic peptide-producing neurons that increase risk for overeating and obesity. *Journal of Neuroscience* 28(46): 12107–12119.

Chen, H., D. Simar, et al. (2009). Hypothalamic neuroendocrine circuitry is programmed by maternal obesity: Interaction with postnatal nutritional environment. *PLOS ONE* 4(7): e6259.

Chen, H. Y., M. E. Trumbauer, et al. (2004). Orexigenic action of peripheral ghrelin is mediated by neuropeptide Y and agouti-related protein. *Endocrinology* 145(6): 2607–2612.

Cho, C. E., D. Sánchez-Hernández, et al. (2013). High folate gestational and post-weaning diets alter hypothalamic feeding pathways by DNA methylation in Wistar rat offspring. *Epigenetics* 8(7): 710–719.

Claret, M., M. A. Smith, et al. (2007). AMPK is essential for energy homeostasis regulation and glucose sensing by POMC and AgRP neurons. *Journal of Clinical Investigation* 117(8): 2325–2336.

Coll, A. P., I. S. Farooqi, et al. (2007). The hormonal control of food intake. *Cell* 129(2): 251–262.

Collden, G., E. Balland, et al. (2015). Neonatal overnutrition causes early alterations in the central response to peripheral ghrelin. *Molecular Metabolism* 4(1): 15–24.

Cota, D., K. Proulx, et al. (2006). Hypothalamic mTOR signaling regulates food intake. *Science* 312(5775): 927–930.

Coupé, B., V. Amarger, et al. (2010). Nutritional programming affects hypothalamic organization and early response to leptin. *Endocrinology* 151(2): 702–713.

Coupé, B., I. Grit, et al. (2009). The timing of catch-up growth affects metabolism and appetite regulation in male rats born with intrauterine growth restriction. *American Journal of Physiology—Regulatory, Integrative and Comparative Physiology* 297(3): R813–R824.

Coupé, B., I. Grit, et al. (2012). Postnatal growth after intrauterine growth restriction alters central leptin signal and energy homeostasis. *PLOS ONE* 7(1): e30616.

Cowley, M. A., J. L. Smart, et al. (2001). Leptin activates anorexigenic POMC neurons through a neural network in the arcuate nucleus. *Nature* 411(6836): 480–484.

Cummings, D. E., J. Q. Purnell, et al. (2001). A preprandial rise in plasma ghrelin levels suggests a role in meal initiation in humans. *Diabetes* 50(8): 1714–1719.

Dallman, M. F., N. Pecoraro, et al. (2003). Chronic stress and obesity: A new view of "comfort food". *Proceedings of the National Academy of Sciences* 100(20): 11696–11701.

Davidowa, H., Y. Li, et al. (2003). Altered responses to orexigenic (AGRP, MCH) and anorexigenic (α-MSH, CART) neuropeptides of paraventricular hypothalamic neurons in early postnatally overfed rats. *European Journal of Neuroscience* 18(3): 613–621.

Delahaye, F., C. Breton, et al. (2008). Maternal perinatal undernutrition drastically reduces postnatal leptin surge and affects the development of arcuate nucleus proopiomelanocortin neurons in neonatal male rat pups. *Endocrinology* 149(2): 470–475.

Desai, M., D. Gayle, et al. (2005). Programmed obesity in intrauterine growth-restricted newborns: Modulation by newborn nutrition. *American Journal of Physiology—Regulatory, Integrative and Comparative Physiology* 288(1): R91–R96.

Desai, M., D. Gayle, et al. (2007). Programmed hyperphagia due to reduced anorexigenic mechanisms in intrauterine growth-restricted offspring. *Reproductive Sciences* 14(4): 329–337.

Desai, M., G. Han, et al. (2016). Programmed hyperphagia in offspring of obese dams: Altered expression of hypothalamic nutrient sensors, neurogenic factors and epigenetic modulators. *Appetite* 99: 193–199.

Desai, M., J. K. Jellyman, et al. (2015). Epigenomics, gestational programming and risk of metabolic syndrome. *International Journal of Obesity* 39(4): 633–641.

Desai, M., T. Li, et al. (2011). Hypothalamic neurosphere progenitor cells in low birth-weight rat newborns: Neurotrophic effects of leptin and insulin. *Brain Research* 1378: 29–42.

Desai, M., T. Li, et al. (2014). Programmed hyperphagia secondary to increased hypothalamic SIRT1. *Brain Research* 1589: 26–36.

Duan, C., M. Li, et al. (2004). SH2-B Promotes insulin receptor substrate 1 (IRS1)- and IRS2-mediated activation of the phosphatidylinositol 3-kinase pathway in response to leptin. *Journal of Biological Chemistry* 279(42): 43684–43691.

Figlewicz, D. P., J. L. Bennett, et al. (2006). Intraventricular insulin and leptin decrease sucrose self-administration in rats. *Physiology & Behavior* 89(4): 611–616.

Figlewicz, D. P., S. B. Evans, et al. (2003). Expression of receptors for insulin and leptin in the ventral tegmental area/substantia nigra (VTA/SN) of the rat. *Brain Research* 964(1): 107–115.

Fukami, T., X. Sun, et al. (2012). Mechanism of programmed obesity in intrauterine fetal growth restricted offspring: Paradoxically enhanced appetite stimulation in fed and fasting states. *Reproductive Sciences* 19(4): 423–430.

Gabory, A., L. Attig, et al. (2011). Developmental programming and epigenetics. *American Journal of Clinical Nutrition* 94(6 Suppl): 1943S-1952S.

Gan, L., W. Zheng, et al. (2005). Nuclear/cytoplasmic shuttling of the transcription factor FoxO1 is regulated by neurotrophic factors. *Journal of Neurochemistry* 93(5): 1209–1219.

Guo, S., G. Rena, et al. (1999). Phosphorylation of serine 256 by protein kinase B disrupts transactivation by FKHR and mediates effects of insulin on insulin-like growth factor-binding protein-1 promoter activity through a conserved insulin response sequence. *Journal of Biological Chemistry* 274(24): 17184–17192.

Gupta, A., M. Srinivasan, et al. (2009). Hypothalamic alterations in fetuses of high fat diet-fed obese female rats. *Journal of Endocrinology* 200(3): 293–300.

Guzmán-Quevedo, O., R. Da Silva Aragão, et al. (2013). Impaired hypothalamic mTOR activation in the adult rat offspring born to mothers fed a low-protein diet. *PLOS ONE* 8(9): e74990.

Haissaguerre, M., N. Saucisse, et al. (2014). Influence of mTOR in energy and metabolic homeostasis. *Molecular and Cellular Endocrinology* 397(1–2): 67–77.

Hales, C. N., Barker, D.J. (1992). Type 2 (non-insulin-dependent) diabetes mellitus: The thrifty phenotype hypothesis. *Diabetologia.* 35: 595–601.

Heisler, L. K., M. A. Cowley, et al. (2003). Central serotonin and melanocortin pathways regulating energy homeostasis. *Annals of the New York Academy of Sciences* 994(1): 169–174.

Heisler, L. K., E. E. Jobst, et al. (2006). Serotonin reciprocally regulates melanocortin neurons to modulate food intake. *Neuron* 51(2): 239–249.

Hetherington, A. W., Ranson, S.W. (1940). Hypothalamic lesions and adiposity in the rat. *The Anatomical Record* 78: 149.

Hommel, J. D., R. Trinko, et al. (2006). Leptin receptor signaling in midbrain dopamine neurons regulates feeding. *Neuron* 51(6): 801–810.

Ifft, J. D. (1972). An autoradiographic study of the time of final division of neurons in rat hypothalamic nuclei. *Journal of Comparative Neurology* 144(2): 193–204.

Ikenasio-Thorpe, B. A., B. H. Breier, et al. (2007). Prenatal influences on susceptibility to diet-induced obesity are mediated by altered neuroendocrine gene expression. *Journal of Endocrinology* 193(1): 31–37.

Jean, A., G. Conductier, et al. (2007). Anorexia induced by activation of serotonin 5-HT4 receptors is mediated by increases in CART in the nucleus accumbens. *Proceedings of the National Academy of Sciences* 104(41): 16335–16340.

Joly-Amado, A., R. G. P. Denis, et al. (2012). Hypothalamic AgRP-neurons control peripheral substrate utilization and nutrient partitioning. *The EMBO Journal* 31(22): 4276–4288.

Kaczmarek, M. M., T. Mendoza, et al. (2016). Lactation undernutrition leads to multigenerational molecular programming of hypothalamic gene networks controlling reproduction. *BMC Genomics* 17(1): 1–18.

Kamegai, J., H. Tamura, et al. (2001). Chronic central infusion of ghrelin increases hypothalamic neuropeptide Y and agouti-related protein mRNA levels and body weight in rats. *Diabetes* 50(11): 2438–2443.

Kelley, A. E., B. A. Baldo, et al. (2005). Corticostriatal-hypothalamic circuitry and food motivation: Integration of energy, action and reward. *Physiology & Behavior* 86(5): 773–795.

Kitamura, T., Y. Feng, et al. (2006). Forkhead protein FoxO1 mediates Agrp-dependent effects of leptin on food intake. *Nature Medicine* 12(5): 534–540.

Könner, A. C., S. Hess, et al. (2011). Role for insulin signaling in catecholaminergic neurons in control of energy homeostasis. *Cell Metabolism* 13(6): 720–728.

Könner, A. C., R. Janoschek, et al. (2007). Insulin action in AgRP-expressing neurons is required for suppression of hepatic glucose production. *Cell Metabolism* 5(6): 438–449.

Lam, C. K. L., M. Chari, et al. (2009). CNS regulation of glucose homeostasis. *Physiology* 24(3): 159–170.

Lam, T. K. T., A. Pocai, et al. (2005). Hypothalamic sensing of circulating fatty acids is required for glucose homeostasis. *Nature Medicine* 11(3): 320–327.

Leibowitz, S. F. and J. T. Alexander (1988). Hypothalamic serotonin in control of eating behavior, meal size, and body weight. *Biological Psychiatry* 44(9): 851–864.

Lopes de Souza, S., R. Orozco-Solís, et al. (2008). Perinatal protein restriction reduces the inhibitory action of serotonin on food intake. *European Journal of Neuroscience* 27(6): 1400–1408.

Lopez, M., R. Nogueiras, et al. (2016). Hypothalamic AMPK: A canonical regulator of whole-body energy balance. *Nature Reviews Endocrinology* 12(7):421-432.

Mahmood, S., D. J. Smiraglia, et al. (2013). Epigenetic changes in hypothalamic appetite regulatory genes may underlie the developmental programming for obesity in rat neonates subjected to a high-carbohydrate dietary modification. *Journal of Developmental Origins of Health and Disease* 4(06): 479–490.

Mebel, D. M., J. C. Y. Wong, et al. (2012). Insulin in the ventral tegmental area reduces hedonic feeding and suppresses dopamine concentration via increased reuptake. *European Journal of Neuroscience* 36(3): 2336–2346.

Morgan, K., S. Obici, et al. (2004). Hypothalamic responses to long-chain fatty acids are nutritionally regulated. *Journal of Biological Chemistry* 279(30): 31139–31148.

Morris, M. J. and H. Chen (2008). Established maternal obesity in the rat reprograms hypothalamic appetite regulators and leptin signaling at birth. *International Journal of Obesity* 33(1): 115–122.

Morton, G. J., D. E. Cummings, et al. (2006). Central nervous system control of food intake and body weight. *Nature* 443(7109): 289–295.

Muccioli, G., M. Tschöp, et al. (2002). Neuroendocrine and peripheral activities of ghrelin: Implications in metabolism and obesity. *European Journal of Pharmacology* 440(2–3): 235–254.

Naleid, A. M., M. K. Grace, et al. (2005). Ghrelin induces feeding in the mesolimbic reward pathway between the ventral tegmental area and the nucleus accumbens. *Peptides* 26(11): 2274–2279.

Orozco-Sólis, R., S. Lopes de Souza, et al. (2009). Perinatal undernutrition-induced obesity is independent of the developmental programming of feeding. *Physiology & Behavior* 96(3): 481–492.

Orozco-Solís, R., R. J. B. Matos, et al. (2010). Nutritional programming in the rat is linked to long-lasting changes in nutrient sensing and energy homeostasis in the hypothalamus. *PLOS ONE* 5(10): e13537.

Peixoto-Silva, N., E. D. C. Frantz, et al. (2011). Maternal protein restriction in mice causes adverse metabolic and hypothalamic effects in the F1 and F2 generations. *British Journal of Nutrition* 106(09): 1364–1373.

Petrovich, G. D., B. Setlow, et al. (2002). Amygdalo-hypothalamic circuit allows learned cues to override satiety and promote eating. *Journal of Neuroscience* 22(19): 8748–8753.

Petry, C. J., S. E. Ozanne, et al. (1997). Early protein restriction and obesity independently induce hypertension in 1-year-old rats. *Clinical Science* 93(2): 147–152.

Pinney, S. E. and R. A. Simmons (2011). Metabolic programming, epigenetics, and gestational diabetes mellitus. *Current Diabetes Reports* 12(1): 67–74.

Plagemann, A., T. Harder, et al. (1999a). Observations on the orexigenic hypothalamic neuro-peptide Y-system in neonatally overfed weanling rats. *Journal of Neuroendocrinology* 11(7): 541–546.

Plagemann, A., T. Harder, et al. (1999b). Increased number of galanin-neurons in the para-ventricular hypothalamic nucleus of neonatally overfed weanling rats. *Brain Research* 818(1): 160–163.

Plagemann, A., T. Harder, et al. (1999c). Perinatal elevation of hypothalamic insulin, acquired malformation of hypothalamic galaninergic neurons, and syndrome X-like alterations in adulthood of neonatally overfed rats. *Brain Research* 836(1–2): 146–155.

Plagemann, A., T. Harder, et al. (2009). Hypothalamic proopiomelanocortin promoter meth-ylation becomes altered by early overfeeding: An epigenetic model of obesity and the metabolic syndrome. *Journal of Physiology* 587(20): 4963–4976.

Plagemann, A., A. Rake, et al. (1998). Reduction of cholecystokinin-8S-neurons in the para-ventricular hypothalamic nucleus of neonatally overfed weanling rats. *Neuroscience Letters* 258(1): 13–16.

Plagemann, A., K. Roepke, et al. (2010). Epigenetic malprogramming of the insulin receptor promoter due to developmental overfeeding. *Journal of Perinatal Medicine* 38: 393.

Plum, L., B. F. Belgardt, et al. (2006). Central insulin action in energy and glucose homeosta-sis. *Journal of Clinical Investigation* 116(7): 1761–1766.

Radford, E. J., M. Ito, et al. (2014). In utero undernourishment perturbs the adult sperm methy-lome and intergenerational metabolism. *Science* 345(6198): 1255903.

Ren, D., M. Li, et al. (2005). Identification of SH2-B as a key regulator of leptin sensitivity, energy balance, and body weight in mice. *Cell Metabolism* 2(2): 95–104.

Reyes-Castro, L. A., G. L. Rodríguez-González, et al. (2015). Paternal line multigenerational passage of altered risk assessment behavior in female but not male rat offspring of moth-ers fed a low protein diet. *Physiology & Behavior* 140: 89–95.

Rodrigues, A. L., E. G. de Moura, et al. (2011). Postnatal early overfeeding induces hypo-thalamic higher SOCS3 expression and lower STAT3 activity in adult rats. *Journal of Nutritional Biochemistry* 22(2): 109–117.

Sandoval, D. A., S. Obici, et al. (2009). Targeting the CNS to treat type 2 diabetes. *Nature Reviews Drug Discovery* 8(5): 386–398.

Sardinha, F. L. C., M. M. Telles, et al. (2006). Gender difference in the effect of intrauter-ine malnutrition on the central anorexigenic action of insulin in adult rats. *Nutrition* 22(11–12): 1152–1161.

Shimada, M. and T. Nakamura (1973). Time of neuron origin in mouse hypothalamic nuclei. *Experimental Neurology* 41(1): 163–173.

Shor-Posner, G., J. A. Grinker, et al. (1986). Hypothalamic serotonin in the control of meal patterns and macronutrient selection. *Brain Research Bulletin* 17(5): 663–671.

Soriano-Guillén, L., V. Barrios, et al. (2004). Ghrelin levels in obesity and anorexia nervosa: Effect of weight reduction or recuperation. *Journal of Pediatrics* 144(1): 36–42.

Steculorum, S. M., G. Collden, et al. (2015). Neonatal ghrelin programs development of hypo-thalamic feeding circuits. *Journal of Clinical Investigation* 125(2): 846–858.

Stevens, A., G. Begum, et al. (2010). Epigenetic changes in the hypothalamic proopiomelano-cortin and glucocorticoid receptor genes in the ovine fetus after periconceptional under-nutrition. *Endocrinology* 151(8): 3652–3664.

Sugino, T., Y. Hasegawa, et al. (2002). A transient ghrelin surge occurs just before feeding in a scheduled meal-fed sheep. *Biochemical and Biophysical Research Communications* 295(2): 255–260.

Sun, Y., P. Wang, et al. (2004). Ghrelin stimulation of growth hormone release and appe-tite is mediated through the growth hormone secretagogue receptor. *Proceedings of the National Academy of Sciences of the United States of America* 101(13): 4679–4684.

Tanaka, M., T. Naruo, et al. (2003). Fasting plasma ghrelin levels in subtypes of anorexia nervosa. *Psychoneuroendocrinology* 28(7): 829–835.

Teegarden, S. L., A. N. Scott, et al. (2009). Early life exposure to a high fat diet promotes long-term changes in dietary preferences and central reward signaling. *Neuroscience* 162(4): 924–932.

Tong, Q., C.-P. Ye, et al. (2008). Synaptic release of GABA by AgRP neurons is required for normal regulation of energy balance. *Nature Neuroscience* 11(9): 998–1000.

Toste, F. P., E. G. de Moura, et al. (2006). Neonatal leptin treatment programmes leptin hypothalamic resistance and intermediary metabolic parameters in adult rat. *British Journal of Nutrition* 95(04): 830–837.

Vickers, M. H., B. H. Breier, et al. (2000). Fetal origins of hyperphagia, obesity, and hypertension and postnatal amplification by hypercaloric nutrition. *American Journal of Physiology—Endocrinology and Metabolism* 279(1): E83–E87.

Vogt, M. C., L. Paeger, et al. (2014). Neonatal insulin action impairs hypothalamic neurocircuit formation in response to maternal high-fat feeding. *Cell* 156(3): 495–509.

Voigt, J.-P. and H. Fink (2015). Serotonin controlling feeding and satiety. *Behavioural Brain Research* 277: 14–31.

Vucetic, Z., J. Kimmel, et al. (2010). Maternal high-fat diet alters methylation and gene expression of dopamine and opioid-related genes. *Endocrinology* 151(10): 4756–4764.

Wren, A. M., C. J. Small, et al. (2000). The novel hypothalamic peptide ghrelin stimulates food intake and growth hormone secretion. *Endocrinology* 141(11): 4325–4328.

Xu, A. W., C. B. Kaelin, et al. (2005). PI3K integrates the action of insulin and leptin on hypothalamic neurons. *Journal of Clinical Investigation* 115(4): 951–958.

Yousheng Jia, T., Nguyen, et al. (2008). Programmed alterations in hypothalamic neuronal orexigenic responses to ghrelin following gestational nutrient restriction. *Reproductive Sciences* 15(7): 702–709.

Yura, S., H. Itoh, et al. (2005). Role of premature leptin surge in obesity resulting from intrauterine undernutrition. *Cell Metabolism* 1(6): 371–378.

Zambrano, E., P. M. Martínez-Samayoa, et al. (2005). Sex differences in transgenerational alterations of growth and metabolism in progeny (F2) of female offspring (F1) of rats fed a low protein diet during pregnancy and lactation. *Journal of Physiology* 566(1): 225–236.

Zhang, X., R. Yang, et al. (2014). Hypermethylation of Sp1 binding site suppresses hypothalamic POMC in neonates and may contribute to metabolic disorders in adults: Impact of maternal dietary CLAs. *Diabetes* 63(5): 1475–1487.

Zhou, L., G. M. Sutton, et al. (2007). Serotonin 2C receptor agonists improve type 2 diabetes via melanocortin-4 receptor signaling pathways. *Cell Metabolism* 6(5): 398–405.

10 Nutritional Modifications in the Immediate Postnatal Period Can Cause Metabolic Programming in Adulthood

Mulchand S. Patel, Saleh Mahmood,
Todd C. Rideout, and Suzanne G. Laychock

CONTENTS

10.1 INTRODUCTION

The prevalence of adult obesity is steadily increasing in the United States and other westernized countries, and obesity and its associated complications represent one of the most daunting health challenges of the 21st century (Kopelman 2000). Childhood obesity is also increasing at an alarming rate in the United States (8% of 2–5-year olds and 17% of 6–11 year olds) (Ogden et al. 2015). Although poor dietary habits with increased calorie intake and sedentary lifestyles accompanied by reduced energy expenditure are the major contributors to the obesity epidemic, the recent emergence of this enormous rise in obesity over the past few decades suggests that there are other contributing factors in the etiology of the obesity epidemic.

The contribution of developmental programming due to nutritional experience (undernutrition and overnutrition) during the early phases of life (fetal and infancy) to long-term predisposition for obesity and associated health complications in adulthood is now supported by compelling evidence from epidemiological observations, as well as some human studies and extensive animal investigations (Alfaradhi and Ozanne 2011; Williams et al. 2014; Dearden and Ozanne 2015; Marchi et al. 2015; Wahlqvist et al. 2015; Luque et al. 2015). Barker's hypothesis of the "Fetal Origins of Adult Diseases" recognized that maternal nutritional status (largely undernutrition) during gestation is a strong determinant of the metabolic phenotype of adult offspring (Hales et al. 1991; Barker 1995). Presently, maternal obesity represents another extreme in the nutritional experience of the developing fetus for metabolic programming. Relevant information on fetal programming from human and animal studies can be found in recent reviews, and this topic is covered extensively elsewhere in this book (Alfaradhi and Ozanne 2011; Williams et al. 2014; Marchi et al. 2015; Woo Baidal et al. 2016). Since the development of many organs and biological systems in mammalian newborns continues in the immediate postnatal period (during infancy), these systems could be subject to plasticity due to any nutritional interventions imposed during infancy only. Animal studies have well documented that insult or stimuli (such as maternal undernutrition or protein restriction, pup's undernourishment or overnourishment, feeding of modified milk or milk formulas, etc.) during the immediate postnatal period (the suckling period) alone can function as independent cues for the metabolic programming of adult-onset metabolic disorders (McCance 1962; Moura et al. 2002; Fahrenkrog et al. 2004; Plagemann 2006; Neu et al. 2007; Patel et al. 2009). For example, overnourishment of rat pups by reducing the litter size results in increased weight gain and development of hyperinsulinemia during the suckling period, which is sustained in the postweaning period causing adult-onset obesity and associated metabolic complications (Plagemann 2006). In contrast, early postnatal undernutrition due to large litter sizes leads to reductions in weight gain and in plasma leptin levels (Kappeler et al. 2009). Consumption of a modified milk formula enriched in carbohydrate-derived energy during the suckling period also mal-programs the pancreatic β-cells and the hypothalamic neurons in the rat (Patel and Srinivasan 2011). In another dietary modification, reduction in food consumption by 30% in lactating mice from days 1 to 21 following parturition resulted in lower body weight gains as well as lower levels of plasma triglycerides, cholesterol, and leptin in the progeny at weaning compared to the progeny of mothers fed *ad libitum* (AL). The undernourished juvenile progeny also demonstrated changes in locomotor activity and anxiety behavior with improvement in catch-up growth and behavior in adulthood (Kumon et al. 2010).

The focus of our research has been on metabolic programming of rat pups during the suckling period by two different protocols: (1) increasing carbohydrate-derived calories in milk formula without increasing daily total calorie intake (the "pup-in-cup" rat model; HC rats) and (2) overnourishment by providing increased level of mother's milk by reducing litter size to 3 pups/dam (small litter model; SL rats). Both these nutritional modifications during the suckling period have been shown to result in metabolic programming at the level of pancreatic β-cells and hypothalamic neurons. These two dietary modifications result in increased levels of serum insulin due to malprogramming of the pancreatic β-cells during the suckling period. This early hyperinsulinemic state has been shown to mal-program brain function, particularly the hypothalamic neurons and the autonomic nervous system (Figure 10.1) (Plagemann 2005, 2006; Patel et al. 2009). After weaning,

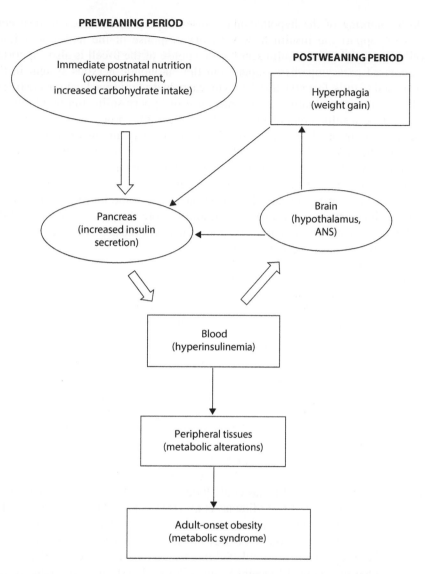

FIGURE 10.1 Possible major mechanisms involved in developmental programming due to increased consumption of carbohydrates or overnourishment by rat pups during the suckling period. Early events in the preweaning period included (shown with heavy open arrows): programming of pancreatic β-cells with increased insulin secretion in response to early dietary modifications; development of hyperinsulinemia; and programming of the hypothalamus and the autonomic nervous systems. Later events in the postweaning period include development of hyperphagia due to programmed hypothalamic nuclei, hypersecretory response of β-cells due to increased parasympathetic input, maintenance of hyperinsulinemia and resulting in increased body fat mass and obesity.

malprogramming of the hypothalamus causes hyperphagia, which in turn continues to support the insulin hypersecretory response of the mal-programmed β-cells. The heightened insulin secretory response of the β-cell is also supported by increased parasympathetic input from the autonomic nervous system in the rat exposed to milk formula enriched with carbohydrate-derived calories (Mitrani et al. 2007a,b), perpetuating the maintenance of hyperinsulinemia in adulthood. In turn, hyperinsulinemia enhances anabolic metabolic processes in various tissues, resulting in the development of adult-onset obesity and its associated metabolic complications (Figure 10.1). Of great importance to the long-term health and well-being of future generations is the examination of dietary manipulations during the postweaning period to reduce or reverse the ill effects of early metabolic malprogramming. In this chapter, we summarize the findings of metabolic programming in these two rodent models and explore the possible reversal of the metabolic effects by nutritional interventions that vary the degree of calorie reduction in the postweaning period.

10.2 MODIFIED INFANT FEEDING PRACTICES AND POSSIBLE METABOLIC PROGRAMMING

There has been a significant change in infant feeding practice in westernized societies over the past five or six decades, largely due to women joining the workforce as a postwar phenomenon. Breast milk is species specific and hence human milk is an ideal food for human babies as it supports optimal growth as well as provides bioactive compounds and immune protection during the suckling period. It should be noted that specific differences exist in macronutrient content (especially protein content) and bioactive factors between human breast milk and milk-based formulas. Furthermore, although the composition of formula remains relatively constant, the composition of breast milk varies widely between mothers as well as by time of day and duration of lactation (Mitoulas et al. 2002). This could have significant impact on infant growth (Dewey 1998; Mitoulas et al. 2002; Smith 2007; Gale et al. 2012). Furthermore, overnourishment may be caused by unrestricted availability of formula at each feeding compared to breastfeeding, which depends on the mother's milk supply. It has been reported that formula-fed infants are on average 400–600 g heavier than breast-fed infants by 12 months of age (Dewey 1998). In a systematic review (15 studies) and meta-analysis of 11 studies (Gale et al. 2012), body composition of breast-fed and formula-fed infants were analyzed. Compared to breast-fed infants, fat mass in formula-fed infants was reduced at 3–4 and 6 months but was increased at 12 months. Interestingly, fat-free mass was increased in formula-fed infants compared to breast-fed infants at 3–4, 8–9, and 12 months. The latter finding could be due to increased protein content of commercial milk formulas compared to human milk (Heinig et al. 1993). The authors suggested that these changes in body composition in formula-fed infants could be indicative of nutritional programming (Gale et al. 2012).

Introduction of infant milk formulas and complementary infant foods could result in altered nutrient composition as well as total calorie intake during infancy and early childhood. Infant formulas are devoid of bioactive compounds and could result in overnutrition due to unrestricted supply of milk formula as well as by its nutrient content (i.e., increased protein). Compared to cow's milk-based infant formulas, human milk contains lower protein content (Luque et al. 2015). This may, in part, explain a slower growth rate of breast-fed infants. A high-protein intake may enhance secretion of insulin, insulin-like growth factor 1, and incretin hormones such as glucagon-like peptide 1 due to increased levels of amino acids (such as insulin-releasing leucine and arginine) (Axelsson et al. 1989; Koletzko et al. 2009; Socha et al. 2011; Pesta and Samuel 2014). This, in turn, may stimulate growth and adipogenic activity and predispose to later onset of obesity and associated health risks.

The American Diabetes Association recommends exclusive breastfeeding of infants for the first 6 months. However, formula feeding and even early introduction of complementary infant foods and sugar-loaded drinks/juices are widely practiced in the United States and other westernized societies. Breast milk and infant formulas have higher levels of calories derived from fats compared to carbohydrates. In contrast, complementary infant foods (juices, fruits, cereals) are highly enriched with carbohydrate-derived calories (from simple sugars) with fewer calories from fats and proteins. Hence, it is possible that early introduction of complementary infant foods prior to 6 months of age can distort the composition of daily macronutrient-derived calories in favor of carbohydrates. Additionally, early introduction of carbohydrate-rich complementary infant foods could further contribute to increased daily total calorie intake and also alter the calorie ratio of carbohydrate to fats, possibly contributing to metabolic programming during early childhood. A previous study estimates that as many as 40% of infants may be provided solid foods before 4 months of age (Clayton et al. 2013). Although the findings on the association between age at first introduction of solid foods and later development of obesity have been inconsistent (Daniels et al. 2015; Patro-Golab et al. 2016), a review of several studies recently found that introduction of complementary solid foods to formula-fed infants prior to 4 months of age was associated with obesity in childhood (Barrera et al. 2016).

10.3 INCREASED CARBOHYDRATE-DERIVED CALORIES DURING THE SUCKLING PERIOD CAUSE METABOLIC PROGRAMMING IN THE RAT PUP

To investigate possible effects of increased intake of carbohydrate-derived calories on metabolic programming in the rat pup, we employed an artificial rearing technique to feed a modified milk formula high in carbohydrate-derived calories during the suckling period. The artificial rearing procedure combined with intragastric feeding is a challenging experimental approach to feed modified milk formulas to rat neonates (Srinivasan et al. 2003; Patel et al. 2009). To investigate the effects of increased carbohydrate intake in rat pups, a milk formula high in carbohydrate-derived calories (HC formula; percent calorie distribution: 56% carbohydrate, 20%

fats, and 24% protein) was fed to rat pups from postnatal days 4 to 24. For artificial rearing, rat neonates fitted with intragastric cannulas were individually housed in Styrofoam cups floating in a 37°C water bath. Hence, this rat model is referred to as "Pup-in-a-Cup" model. The details for automated milk delivery and daily cleaning were reported previously (Hiremagalur et al. 1993; Patel et al. 1994). For comparison, we also included a group of artificially reared rats on a high-fat (HF) formula (percent calorie distribution: 8% carbohydrate, 68% fats, and 24% protein), which was similar in macronutrient composition to that of rat milk, and a group of mother-reared (mother-fed [MF]) rat pups as an additional control. Outcomes of several parameters for HF rats reared artificially were not different when compared with that of naturally reared MF rats, indicating that the observed metabolic programming effects in HC rats were due to the HC dietary modification and not due to the artificial rearing technique *per se* employed in this rat model.

Adaptive changes at the cellular level were measured in pancreatic β-cells, hypothalamic neurons, and the autonomic nervous system in pups and adult HC rats. In response to HC formula, hyperinsulinemia was observed in HC pups within a day after initiation of the diet (postnatal day 4) and persisted for the duration of the HC formula feeding period (until postnatal day 24), indicating that development of hyperinsulinemia is in direct response to HC formula (Haney and Patel 1985). Hence, alterations were investigated at the cellular and molecular levels in HC rats to account for developmental programming leading to chronic hyperinsulinemia during the suckling period and maintenance of hyperinsulinemia in the postweaning period and development of adult-onset obesity due to hyperphagia. Islet number per unit area and percent of small islets were significantly increased in HC pups (Petrik et al. 2001). Furthermore, a reduction in the area occupied by glucagon-positive α-cells with an increased area occupied by β-cells was observed, resulting in an increased β/α-cell ratio in HC islets at 2 weeks of age (Petrik et al. 2001). Glucose-stimulated insulin secretion by isolated HC islets at varying concentrations of glucose was markedly different compared to islets from age-matched control pups. In contrast to control islets, HC islets secreted significantly higher levels of insulin at sub-basal, basal, and high-glucose concentrations, indicating a leftward shift in their responsiveness to glucose. This response was supported by an increased content of glucose transporter 2 protein as well as increased activities of cytoplasmic hexokinase and glucokinase (Aalinkeel et al. 1999). The low Km (<1 mM) of hexokinase and the increased hexokinase activity observed support increased insulin secretion by HC islets at sub-basal and basal glucose concentrations (Schuit et al. 2001). Moderate levels of insulin secretion by HC islets in the absence of Ca^{2+} or in the presence of Ca^{2+} channel blockers suggested the presence of glucose- and calcium-independent insulin secretory mechanisms in HC islets (Aalinkeel et al. 1999). Similarly, employing specific agonists and antagonists of the parasympathetic and sympathetic nervous systems exposed alterations in glucose-stimulated insulin secretion in HC rats with increased cholinergic potentiation of secretion via the parasympathetic nervous system and a reduction in adrenergic receptor-induced inhibition of secretion via sympathetic input (Mitrani et al. 2007a,b).

Adaptive changes at the molecular level in pancreatic β-cells and hypothalamic neurons were also observed. Increased levels of *Pdx-1* messenger RNA (mRNA) and its protein as well as its increased DNA-binding activity supported the increased level of insulin biosynthesis by islets from HC pups (Srinivasan et al. 2001). Furthermore, increased mRNA expression of insulin receptor substrate-1 (IRS-1), IRS-2, glucose transporter 2, and acetyl CoA carboxylase was observed in HC islets (Song et al. 2001). The protein products of these mRNAs are involved in intracellular signaling and coupling for insulin secretion.

The effects of high-carbohydrate feeding to neonates were also reflected in changes in specific areas of the brain. Hypothalami from HC rats showed increased mRNA expression of orexigenic neuropeptide Y (*Npy*), agouti-related protein, and reduced mRNA expression of proopiomelanocortin, cocaine- and amphetamine-regulated transcripts, corticotrophin-releasing factor, and melano-cortin-4-receptor, supporting a hyperphagic response of HC rats after weaning (Srinivasan et al. 2008). Alterations in methylation pattern of specific CpG dinu-cleotides in the proximal promoter region of the *Npy* gene, as well as increased acetylation of lysine 9 in histone 3 (H3K9) for the *Npy* gene from adult HC rat hypothalami, were consistent with increased *Npy* gene expression (Mahmood et al. 2013).

10.4 IS IT POSSIBLE TO REVERSE METABOLIC PROGRAMMING IN HC RATS IN ADULTHOOD?

To evaluate this possibility, HC and MF rats were reared during the preweaning period as described above. On postnatal day 24, these rats were weaned on a lab chow with the following dietary treatments: (1) MF rats on lab chow AL, (2) HC rat on lab chow AL, (3) HC rats pair-fed (PF) lab chow based on daily food consumption by age-matched MF (HC/PF), (4) HC rats PF chow until postnatal day 90 and then switched over to AL feeding (HC/PF/AL) (Srinivasan et al. 2013). As expected, HC rats fed AL consumed more food, gained body weight at a higher rate (Figure 10.2), and had higher levels of serum insulin and leptin compared to MF controlled rats (Figure 10.3a,b). Pair feeding normalized the weight gains (Figure 10.2) and serum and leptin levels of HC/PF rats similar to that of MF rats (Figure 10.3a,b), suggesting possible normalization on the gross metabolic pheno-type in HC/PF rats. However, HC/PF/AL rats restored body weight gains and food intake (Figure 10.2) as well as serum insulin and leptin levels (Figure 10.3a,b). It should be noted that the higher insulin secretory responses of isolated islets from both HC/PF and HC/PF/AL to glucose, acetylcholine, and oxymetazoline remained unaltered and were similar to that of islets from HC rats (Figure 10.3c–f) (Srinivasan et al. 2013). Similarly, the mRNA expression profiles of *Npy* and proo-piomelanocortin in the hypothalamus were not significantly different for HC/PF and HC/PF/AL rats compared to that of HC rats (Figure 10.3g,h). The results clearly showed that although calorie reduction by pair feeding (about 14% compared to that of HC rats) normalized weight gains and serum hormonal profiles

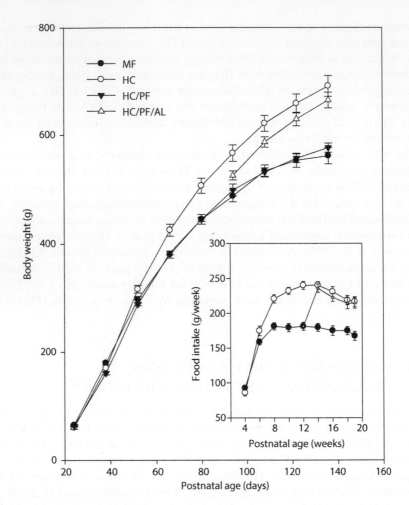

FIGURE 10.2 Effect of pair feeding (PF) with or without *ad libitum* (AL) regimen on body weights and food intake (insert) of mother-fed (MF) control and high-carbohydrate (HC) milk formula-fed rats in the postweaning period. MF: mother-fed control rats on a chow diet AL; HC: artificially reared rats on HC milk formula and then fed a chow diet AL. HC/PF: HC rats PF to MF rats from postnatal days 24 to 140; and HC/PF/AL: HC/PF rats PF from days 24 to 90 and then switched over to AL feeding until day 140. The results are means ± standard error (SE) (*n* = 8 rats/group). (From Srinivasan, M. et al., *Am J Physiol Endocrinol Metab*, 304, E486–E494, 2013.)

for insulin and leptin, the mal-programmed hypersecretory capacity of islets and the hypothalamic energy homeostasis mechanism in the HC/PF rats could not be erased by the pair feeding for a period of nearly 4 months (Srinivasan et al. 2013). It is possible that a more severe caloric restriction (CR) would be necessary to erase malprogramming effects of early postnatal dietary exposure to increased carbohydrate intake.

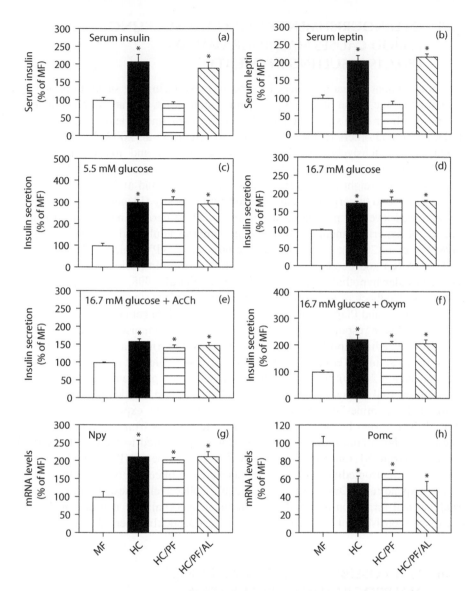

FIGURE 10.3 Serum insulin (a), serum leptin (b), insulin secretion by isolated islets for 60 minutes at 5.5 mM glucose (c), at 16.7 mM glucose (d), at 16.7 mM glucose + 100 μM acetylcholine (AcCh) (e), and at 16.7 mM glucose + 10 μM oxymetazoline (Oxym) (f), and mRNA levels of neuropeptide Y (*Npy*) (g) and proopiomelanocortin (*Pomc*) (h) in the hypothalami from MF, HC, HC/PF, HC/PF/AL rats, as described in Figure 10.2. The results are means ± 6–8 animals/group. (From Srinivasan, M. et al., *Am J Physiol Endocrinol Metab,* 304, E486–E494, 2013.)

10.5 OVERNOURISHMENT DURING THE SUCKLING PERIOD CAUSES MALPROGRAMMING EFFECTS RESULTING IN OBESITY

Overnourishment is readily induced in rodent pups during the suckling period by reducing the size of the litter to 3 pups/dam (Small Litter, SL rat model) compared to a normal litter (NL) size of 10 pups/dam. Plagemann and colleagues (Plagemann 2005, 2006) and others (Lopez et al. 2005; Rodrigues et al. 2009, 2011; Liu et al. 2013a) have extensively investigated malprogramming and mal-functioning of hypothalamic neurons in SL rats. Some of their findings are summarized below: (1) increased body weight gains during the suckling period and also in the postweaning period due to hyperphagia causing adult-onset obesity (Plagemann et al. 1998); (2) increased levels of plasma insulin in the suckling period and continued maintenance of hyperinsulinemia and hyperleptinemia in adulthood (Plagemann et al. 1998; Liu et al. 2013a); (3) increase in the number of NPY neurons in the arcuate nucleus (ARC) and decreased number of cholecystokinin-positive neurons in the paraventricular hypothalamic nucleus (Plagemann et al. 1998, 1999); (4) reduction in negative feedback of leptin and insulin as a result of resistance in the ARC in SL rats (Davidowa and Plagemann 2000a,b; Davidowa and Plagemann 2001, 2007); (5) differential leptin response in hypothalamic nucleus as demonstrated by leptin activated ventromedial hypothalamic (VMH) neurons in normal rats versus inhibitory leptin response in VMH neurons of juvenile SL rats (Heidel et al. 1999; Davidowa and Plagemann 2000b); (6) inhibition of neurons in the paraventricular nuclei and the ventromedial nucleus by NPY, agouti-related protein, corticotrophin-releasing factor, and dopamine-favoring feeding and reduced energy expenditure (Davidowa et al. 2002a; Li et al. 2002); (7) medial arcuate neurons from SL rats were activated by melanin-concentrating hormone (MCH) compared to the effect observed on neurons from NL rats, inducing feeding through release of NPY (Davidowa et al. 2002b), and ventromedial neurons of SL rats were inhibited, contributing to reduced energy expenditure (Davidowa et al. 2002b). Collectively, these findings clearly establish mal-formation and mal-functioning of hypothalamic neurons in SL rats due to overnourishment by mother's milk during the suckling period.

10.6 IS IT POSSIBLE TO REVERSE METABOLIC MALPROGRAMMING IN SL RATS IN THE POSTWEANING PERIOD?

As discussed above, overnourishment in SL rat pups due to a reduction in the litter size resulted in increased levels of serum insulin and leptin and also increased body weight gains by the end of the suckling period (postnatal day 21) (Plagemann et al. 1998; Lopez et al. 2005; Liu et al. 2013a). These modifications persisted in the postweaning period, resulting in hyperphagia and adult-onset obesity. The Plagemann group has extensively documented the mal-formation and mal-functioning of the hypothalamic neurons in the SL rats, supporting the development of insulin and leptin resistance in the hypothalamus and subsequent development of hyperphagia (as discussed above). We wondered if CR from the time of weaning could have a positive impact on the reversal of the malprogramming effects in the SL rats. Since the degree of CR required for a positive outcome cannot be predetermined, we investigated its effects at two different levels: (1) mild CR (by pair-feeding to equalize daily caloric intake to that of age-matched NL rats and amounting to ~14% reduction in daily caloric intake compared to age-matched AL-fed SL rats) and (2) moderate CR (initially at the level of about 10% from days 24 to 44 to slow down their weight gains and then increased to ~24% to that of AL-fed SL rats) (Liu et al. 2013b). As expected, weekly food intake and body weight gains (Figure 10.4a,b) as well as the levels of serum insulin and leptin (Figure 10.5a,b) were higher in SL rats compared to age-matched NL rats in the postweaning period. A postweaning pair-feeding regimen

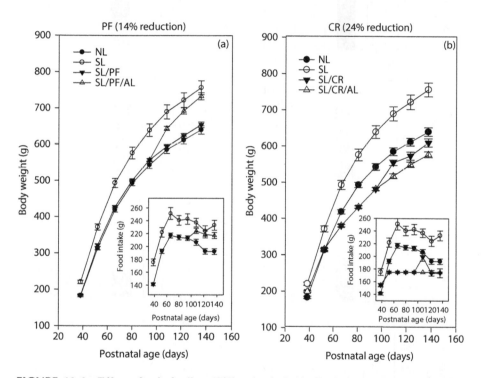

FIGURE 10.4 Effect of pair feeding (14% reduction) (a) or calorie restriction (CR; 24% reduction) (b) with or without AL regimen on body weights and food intakes (inserts) of MF rats in normal litter (NL) size (12 male pups/dam) or in small litter (SL) size (3 male pups/dam) in the postweaning period. (a and b) NL: rat pups reared in a NL size and then fed chow AL from postnatal days 21 to 140; (a and b) SL: rat pups reared in a SL size and then fed chow AL from days 21 to 140; (a) SL/PF: SL rats PF (14% reduction) to the NL rats from days 21 to 140; SL/PF/AL: SL rats PF to NL rats to days 21 to 94 and then switched over to AL feeding until day 140; (b) SL/CR: SL rats consumed 10% less food compared to SL rats from days 21 to 45 and then increased CR to the level of 24% to that of the SL rats from days 46 to 140; SL/CR/AL: SL/CR rats were switched over to AL feedings from days 94 to 140. The results are means ± SE (*n* = 10–12 rats/group). (From Liu, H.W. et al., *Am J Physiol Endocrinol Metab*, 305, E785–E794, 2013b.)

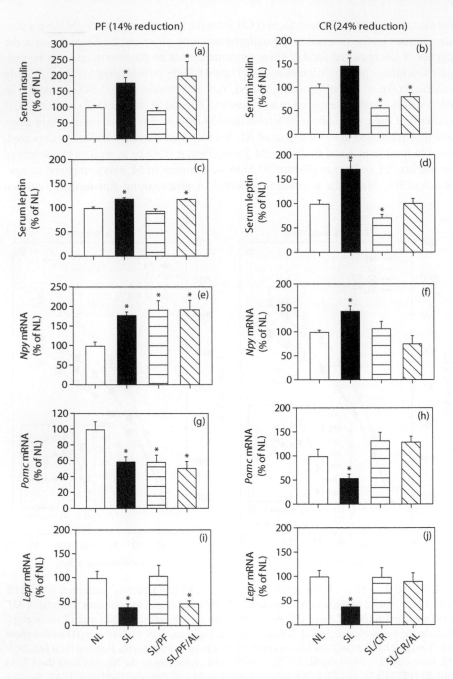

FIGURE 10.5 Serum insulin (a, b), serum leptin (c, d), messenger RNA (mRNA) levels of Npy (e, f), proopiomelanocortin (Pomc) (g, h), and leptin receptor (Lepr) (i, j) in NL, SL, SL/ PF, SL/PF/AL, SL/CR, and SL/CR/AL rats, as described in the legend to Figure 10.4. The results are means ± SE (*n* = 5–6 rats/group). (From Liu, H.W. et al., *Am J Physiol Endocrinol Metab,* 305, E785–E794, 2013b.)

normalized the body weight gains (Figure 10.4a) as well as the levels of serum insulin and leptin in SL/PF rats compared to NL rats (Figure 10.5a,c). However, after switching to AL feeding from days 94 to 140, SL/PF/AL rats demonstrated significant increases in food intake and body weight gains (Figure 10.4a) as well as increases in the levels of serum insulin and leptin (Figure 10.5a,c), which compared nearly equal with that of SL rats (Liu et al. 2013b).

A significant increase in *Npy* mRNA expression and a significant decrease in *Pomc* mRNA expression were observed in hypothalami from SL rats compared to that of NL rats (Figure 10.5e,g), supporting hyperphagia observed in SL rats. Interestingly, pair feeding failed to restore the levels of *Npy* mRNA and *Pomc* mRNA in SL/PF rats (Figure 10.5e,g), although pair-feeding was effective in normalizing the serum insulin and leptin levels in these rats (Figure 10.5a,c) (Liu et al. 2013b). Similarly, the mRNA levels of *Npy* and *Pomc* remained unchanged in SL/PF/AL rats and they were similar to that of SL rats (Figure 10.5e,g). Interestingly, the levels of *Lepr* mRNA were negatively associated with the serum leptin levels of the four groups of rats (Figure 10.5i), whereas *Insr* mRNA expression remained similar among these groups (Liu et al. 2013b). These findings clearly showed that mild CR (by pair feeding to equalize calorie intake to that of NL rats) resulted in suppression of the mal-programmed effects on gross metabolic parameters such as body weight gains and serum hormonal profiles only while it was implemented. Mild CR (at ~14%), however, had no effect on the mal-programmed effects on the hypothalamus, indicating that this level of CR was not sufficient for a permanent reversal of the mal-program for the obese phenotype in SL rats (Liu et al. 2013b).

For implementation of moderate CR (about 24% reduction), SL/CR rats initially received 10% CR in daily food intake starting from the postnatal days 25 to 45 to slow down their body growth rate, and then increased to 24% reduction in daily intake from days 46 to 140. SL/CR rats gained less body weight from days 24 to 45, reaching body weights similar to age-matched NL rats (Figure 10.4b). On a 24% dietary reduction regimen, SL/CR rats grew at an even slower rate compared to NL rats until the end of the experiment (Figure 10.4b). The levels of serum hormones in SL/CR rats were nearly similar to that of NL rats (Figure 10.5b,d). Consistent with the deprogramming effect, moderate CR restored *Npy*, *Pomc*, and *Lepr* mRNA expression in the hypothalamus of SL/CR rats to that of NL rats (Figure 10.5f,h), showing that this level of CR was sufficient to erase malprogramming effects of overnourishment in SL rats in the immediate postnatal period. When SL/CR/AL rats were switched over to AL feeding from days 95 to 140, their calorie intake increased immediately reaching the level of age-matched NL rats but not to the level of food intake by SL rats (Figure 10.4b) (Liu et al. 2013b). SL/CR/AL rats immediately started gaining more body weight, reaching that of NL rats by day 140. Their body weight, however, remained significantly lower than that of SL rats (Figure 10.4b), indicating deprogramming of hyperphagic response in SL/CR/AL rats. This observation was also supported by normalization of the levels of serum insulin and leptin in SL/CR/AL rats (Figure 10.5b,d). Furthermore, expression of *Npy*, *Pomc*, and *Lepr* mRNAs in the hypothalamus remained at the normal level to that of NL rats, indicating that SL/CR/AL rats were deprogrammed at the hypothalamic neurons (Figure 10.5f,h).

Epigenetic mechanism(s) could contribute to metabolic programming (Plagemann et al. 2009; Pinney and Simmons 2010). Hence, DNA methylation analysis of specific dinucleotides in the proximal promoter regions of the *Npy* and *Pomc* genes in the hypothalami from the four groups of rats was performed. Methylation level of the *Npy* proximal promoter region (from +103 to –242 bp harboring 24 CpG dinucleotides) at CpG positions 20 and 22–23 was significantly decreased in SL rats compared to the corresponding positions in NL and SL/CR rats, whereas methylation level at CpG position 15 was increased in SL rats compared to NL rats (Liu et al. 2013b). Interestingly, methylation of CpG dinucleotides in the proximal promoter region (from +43 to –298 bp and harboring 23 CpG dinucleotides) of the *Pomc* gene remained unaltered among the four groups of rats. In contrast, no changes were observed in either mRNA expression or the CpG dinucleotide methylation pattern in the *Npy* promoter region in the hypothalamus from 21-day-old SL rats (Plagemann et al. 2009). The changes in the methylation status of the *Npy* proximal promoter region in SL/CR and SL/CR/AL rats observed in our study (Liu et al. 2013b) could modify the binding ability of specific transcription factors and hence contribute to normalization of *Npy* gene expression.

Collectively, the results from two levels of CRs demonstrate that a mild level (~14%) of CR (by pair-feeding technique resulting in normalization of caloric intake to that of age-matched NL rats) resulted in normalization of gross metabolic phenotype, including growth trajectory and serum hormonal profiles as long as CR was implemented. There was, however, no reversal of the malprograming effects at the cellular levels (at the hypothalamus and the autonomic nervous system) because the ill effects of malprogramming reappeared when CR was removed (Liu et al. 2013b). In contrast, a moderate level of CR (~24%) resulted in not only normalization of the gross metabolic phenotype of obese-prone SL rats, but also erased the mal-program at the cellular and molecular levels, indicating that it is possible to erase the mal-programmatic effects in SL rats using this level of CR for a sufficient length of time (Liu et al. 2013b). At a translational level, it may be very difficult, if not impossible, to institute this level of CR in children and adolescence during growing years. Hence, other approaches for deprogramming need to be explored to erase malprogramming effects of overnutrition during infancy.

10.7   CONCLUSION AND HUMAN RELEVANCE

The findings from numerous animal models involving different types of nutritional modifications during the suckling period may have relevance to human infant feeding practices resulting in overnutrition and other dietary modifications. Infant feeding has remarkably changed from exclusive breastfeeding for at least first 6 months to breastfeeding or milk-based formula feeding with introduction of complementary infant foods (such as fruits, juices, cereals, etc.) prior to the age of 6 months. Formula feeding has a potential to introduce increased calorie intake due to unrestricted supply at each feeding and parental influence on feeding experience. Furthermore, cow milk-based formulas have a higher level of protein compared to human milk, which could cause an increase in growth rate of infants. Additionally, early introduction of complementary infant foods can result in an increased level of carbohydrate-derived calories and could also contribute to overnourishment. So, individually, each of these three modifications may contribute to a smaller extent to possible malprogramming effects in infants. But, it is quite possible that some combination of all three modifications in infant feeding could lead to a higher degree of malprogramming, resulting in the development of childhood obesity and also contributing to the development of adult-onset obesity. Breastfeeding needs to be encouraged and supported by all sectors of the society. As an alternative, development of better milk-based formulas and maternal education for later introduction of complementary infant foods are warranted for curtailment of childhood obesity in westernized societies.

ACKNOWLEDGMENTS

Work performed in the authors' laboratories and summarized in this chapter was supported in part by the National Institutes of Health Grants HD-11089, DK-51601, DK-25705, and DK-61518.

REFERENCES

Aalinkeel, R., Srinivasan, M., Kalhan, S.C., Laychock, S.G., Patel, M.S., 1999. A dietary intervention (high carbohydrate) during the neonatal period causes islet dysfunction in rats. *Am J Physiol* 277, E1061–E1069.

Alfaradhi, M.Z., Ozanne, S.E., 2011. Developmental programming in response to maternal overnutrition. *Front Genet* 2, 27. Doi: 10.3389/fgene.2011.00027.

Axelsson, I.E., Ivarsson, S.A., Raiha, N.C., 1989. Protein intake in early infancy: Effects on plasma amino acid concentrations, insulin metabolism, and growth. *Pediatr Res* 26, 614–617.

Barker, D.J., 1995. The fetal and infant origins of disease. *Eur J Clin Invest* 25, 457–463.

Barrera, C.M., Perrine, C.G., Li, R., Scanlon, K.S., 2016. Age at Introduction to solid foods and child obesity at 6 years. *Child Obes* 12, 188–192.

Clayton, H.B., Li, R., Perrine, C.G., Scanlon, K.S., 2013. Prevalence and reasons for introducing infants early to solid foods: Variations by milk feeding type. *Pediatrics* 131, e1108–e1114.

Daniels, L., Mallan, K.M., Fildes, A., Wilson, J., 2015. The timing of solid introduction in an 'obesogenic' environment: A narrative review of the evidence and methodological issues. *Aust N Z J Public Health* 39, 366–373.

Davidowa, H., Li, Y., Plagemann, A., 2002a. Differential response to NPY of PVH and dopamine-responsive VMH neurons in overweight rats. *Neuroreport* 13, 1523–1527.

Davidowa, H., Li, Y., Plagemann, A., 2002b. Hypothalamic ventromedial and arcuate neurons of normal and postnatally overnourished rats differ in their responses to melanin-concentrating hormone. *Regul Pept* 108, 103–111.

Davidowa, H., Plagemann, A., 2000a. Decreased inhibition by leptin of hypothalamic arcuate neurons in neonatally overfed young rats. *Neuroreport* 11, 2795–2798.

Davidowa, H., Plagemann, A., 2000b. Different responses of ventromedial hypothalamic neurons to leptin in normal and early postnatally overfed rats. *Neurosci Lett* 293, 21–24.

Davidowa, H., Plagemann, A., 2001. Inhibition by insulin of hypothalamic VMN neurons in rats overweight due to postnatal overfeeding. *Neuroreport* 12, 3201–3204.

Davidowa, H., Plagemann, A., 2007. Insulin resistance of hypothalamic arcuate neurons in neonatally overfed rats. *Neuroreport* 18, 521–524.

Dearden, L., Ozanne, S.E., 2015. Early life origins of metabolic disease: Developmental programming of hypothalamic pathways controlling energy homeostasis. *Front Neuroendocrinol* 39, 3–16.

Dewey, K.G., 1998. Growth characteristics of breast-fed compared to formula-fed infants. *Biol Neonate* 74, 94–105.

Fahrenkrog, S., Harder, T., Stolaczyk, E., Melchior, K., Franke, K., Dudenhausen, J.W., Plagemann, A., 2004. Cross-fostering to diabetic rat dams affects early development of mediobasal hypothalamic nuclei regulating food intake, body weight, and metabolism. *J Nutr* 134, 648–654.

Gale, C., Logan, K.M., Santhakumaran, S., Parkinson, J.R., Hyde, M.J., Modi, N., 2012. Effect of breastfeeding compared with formula feeding on infant body composition: A systematic review and meta-analysis. *Am J Clin Nutr* 95, 656–669.

Hales, C.N., Barker, D.J., Clark, P.M., Cox, L.J., Fall, C., Osmond, C., Winter, P.D., 1991. Fetal and infant growth and impaired glucose tolerance at age 64. *BMJ* 303, 1019–1022.

Haney, P.M., Patel, M.S., 1985. Regulation of succinyl-CoA:3-oxoacid CoA-transferase in developing rat brain: Responsiveness associated with prenatal but not postnatal hyperketonemia. *Arch Biochem Biophys* 240, 426–434.

Heidel, E., Plagemann, A., Davidowa, H., 1999. Increased response to NPY of hypothalamic VMN neurons in postnatally overfed juvenile rats. *Neuroreport* 10, 1827–1831.

Heinig, M.J., Nommsen, L.A., Peerson, J.M., Lonnerdal, B., Dewey, K.G., 1993. Energy and protein intakes of breast-fed and formula-fed infants during the first year of life and their association with growth velocity: The DARLING Study. *Am J Clin Nutr* 58, 152–161.

Hiremagalur, B.K., Vadlamudi, S., Johanning, G.L., Patel, M.S., 1993. Long-term effects of feeding high carbohydrate diet in pre-weaning period by gastrostomy: A new rat model for obesity. *Int J Obes Relat Metab Disord* 17, 495–502.

Kappeler, L., De Magalhaes Filho, C., Leneuve, P., Xu, J., Brunel, N., Chatziantoniou, C., Le Bouc, Y., Holzenberger, M., 2009. Early postnatal nutrition determines somatotropic function in mice. *Endocrinology* 150, 314–323.

Koletzko, B., von Kries, R., Closa, R., Escribano, J., Scaglioni, S., Giovannini, M., Beyer, J., Demmelmair, H., Anton, B., Gruszfeld, D., Dobrzanska, A., Sengier, A., Langhendries, J.P., Rolland Cachera, M.F., Grote, V., 2009. Can infant feeding choices modulate later obesity risk? *Am J Clin Nutr* 89, 1502S–1508S.

Kopelman, P.G., 2000. Obesity as a medical problem. *Nature* 404, 635–643.

Kumon, M., Yamamoto, K., Takahashi, A., Wada, K., Wada, E., 2010. Maternal dietary restriction during lactation influences postnatal growth and behavior in the offspring of mice. *Neurochem Int* 57, 43–50.

Li, Y., Plagemann, A., Davidowa, H., 2002. Increased inhibition by agouti-related peptide of ventromedial hypothalamic neurons in rats overweight due to early postnatal overfeeding. *Neurosci Lett* 330, 33–36.

Liu, H.W., Mahmood, S., Srinivasan, M., Smiraglia, D.J., Patel, M.S., 2013a. Developmental programming in skeletal muscle in response to overnourishment in the immediate postnatal life in rats. *J Nutr Biochem* 24, 1859–1869.

Liu, H.W., Srinivasan, M., Mahmood, S., Smiraglia, D.J., Patel, M.S., 2013b. Adult-onset obesity induced by early life overnutrition could be reversed by moderate caloric restriction. *Am J Physiol Endocrinol Metab* 305, E785–E794.

Lopez, M., Seoane, L.M., Tovar, S., Garcia, M.C., Nogueiras, R., Dieguez, C., Senaris, R.M., 2005. A possible role of neuropeptide Y, agouti-related protein and leptin receptor isoforms in hypothalamic programming by perinatal feeding in the rat. *Diabetologia* 48, 140–148.

Luque, V., Closa-Monasterolo, R., Escribano, J., Ferre, N., 2015. Early programming by protein intake: The effect of protein on adiposity development and the growth and functionality of vital organs. *Nutr Metab Insights* 8, 49–56.

Mahmood, S., Smiraglia, D.J., Srinivasan, M., Patel, M.S., 2013. Epigenetic changes in hypothalamic appetite regulatory genes may underlie the developmental programming for obesity in rat neonates subjected to a high-carbohydrate dietary modification. *J Dev Orig Health Dis* 4, 479–490.

Marchi, J., Berg, M., Dencker, A., Olander, E.K., Begley, C., 2015. Risks associated with obesity in pregnancy, for the mother and baby: A systematic review of reviews. *Obes Rev* 16, 621–638.

McCance, R.A., 1962. Food, growth, and time. *Lancet* 2, 671–676.

Mitoulas, L.R., Kent, J.C., Cox, D.B., Owens, R.A., Sherriff, J.L., Hartmann, P.E., 2002. Variation in fat, lactose and protein in human milk over 24 h and throughout the first year of lactation. *Br J Nutr* 88, 29–37.

Mitrani, P., Srinivasan, M., Dodds, C., Patel, M.S., 2007a. Autonomic involvement in the permanent metabolic programming of hyperinsulinemia in the high-carbohydrate rat model. *Am J Physiol Endocrinol Metab* 292, E1364–E1377.

Mitrani, P., Srinivasan, M., Dodds, C., Patel, M.S., 2007b. Role of the autonomic nervous system in the development of hyperinsulinemia by high-carbohydrate formula feeding to neonatal rats. *Am J Physiol Endocrinol Metab* 292, E1069–E1078.

Moura, A.S., Franco de Sa, C.C., Cruz, H.G., Costa, C.L., 2002. Malnutrition during lactation as a metabolic imprinting factor inducing the feeding pattern of offspring rats when adults. The role of insulin and leptin. *Braz J Med Biol Res* 35, 617–622.

Neu, J., Hauser, N., Douglas-Escobar, M., 2007. Postnatal nutrition and adult health programming. *Semin Fetal Neonatal Med* 12, 78–86.

Ogden, C.L., Carroll, M. D., Fryar, C. D., and Flegal, K. M., 2015. Prevalence of obesity among adults and youth: United States, 2011-2014. *National Center for Health Statistics Data Brief* 219, 1–7.

Patel, M.S., Srinivasan, M., 2011. Metabolic programming in the immediate postnatal life. *Ann Nutr Metab* 58(Suppl 2), 18–28.

Patel, M.S., Srinivasan, M., Laychock, S.G., 2009. Metabolic programming: Role of nutrition in the immediate postnatal life. *J Inherit Metab Dis* 32, 218–228.

Patel, M.S., Vadlamudi, S., Johanning, G.L., 1994. Artificial rearing of rat pups: Implications for nutrition research. *Annu Rev Nutr* 14, 21–40.

Patro-Golab, B., Zalewski, B.M., Kouwenhoven, S.M., Karas, J., Koletzko, B., Bernard van Goudoever, J., Szajewska, H., 2016. Protein concentration in milk formula, growth, and later risk of obesity: A systematic review. *J Nutr* 146, 551–564.

Pesta, D.H., Samuel, V.T., 2014. A high-protein diet for reducing body fat: Mechanisms and possible caveats. *Nutr Metab (Lond)* 11, 53.

Petrik, J., Srinivasan, M., Aalinkeel, R., Coukell, S., Arany, E., Patel, M.S., Hill, D.J., 2001. A long-term high-carbohydrate diet causes an altered ontogeny of pancreatic islets of Langerhans in the neonatal rat. *Pediatr Res* 49, 84–92.

Pinney, S.E., Simmons, R.A., 2010. Epigenetic mechanisms in the development of type 2 diabetes. *Trends Endocrinol Metab* 21, 223–229.

Plagemann, A., 2005. Perinatal programming and functional teratogenesis: Impact on body weight regulation and obesity. *Physiol Behav* 86, 661–668.

Plagemann, A., 2006. Perinatal nutrition and hormone-dependent programming of food intake. *Horm Res* 65(Suppl 3), 83–89.

Plagemann, A., Harder, T., Brunn, M., Harder, A., Roepke, K., Wittrock-Staar, M., Ziska, T., Schellong, K., Rodekamp, E., Melchior, K., Dudenhausen, J.W., 2009. Hypothalamic proopiomelanocortin promoter methylation becomes altered by early overfeeding: An epigenetic model of obesity and the metabolic syndrome. *J Physiol* 587, 4963–4976.

Plagemann, A., Harder, T., Rake, A., Waas, T., Melchior, K., Ziska, T., Rohde, W., Dorner, G., 1999. Observations on the orexigenic hypothalamic neuropeptide Y-system in neonatally overfed weanling rats. *J Neuroendocrinol* 11, 541–546.

Plagemann, A., Rake, A., Harder, T., Melchior, K., Rohde, W., Dorner, G., 1998. Reduction of cholecystokinin-8S-neurons in the paraventricular hypothalamic nucleus of neonatally overfed weanling rats. *Neurosci Lett* 258, 13–16.

Rodrigues, A.L., de Moura, E.G., Passos, M.C., Dutra, S.C., Lisboa, P.C., 2009. Postnatal early overnutrition changes the leptin signalling pathway in the hypothalamic-pituitary-thyroid axis of young and adult rats. *J Physiol* 587, 2647–2661.

Rodrigues, A.L., de Moura, E.G., Passos, M.C., Trevenzoli, I.H., da Conceicao, E.P., Bonono, I.T., Neto, J.F., Lisboa, P.C., 2011. Postnatal early overfeeding induces hypothalamic higher SOCS3 expression and lower STAT3 activity in adult rats. *J Nutr Biochem* 22, 109–117.

Schuit, F.C., Huypens, P., Heimberg, H., Pipeleers, D.G., 2001. Glucose sensing in pancreatic beta-cells: A model for the study of other glucose-regulated cells in gut, pancreas, and hypothalamus. *Diabetes* 50, 1–11.

Smith, J., 2007. The contribution of infant food marketing to the obesogenic environment in Australia. *Breastfeed Rev* 15, 23–35.

Socha, P., Grote, V., Gruszfeld, D., Janas, R., Demmelmair, H., Closa-Monasterolo, R., Subias, J.E., Scaglioni, S., Verduci, E., Dain, E., Langhendries, J.P., Perrin, E., Koletzko, B., 2011. Milk protein intake, the metabolic-endocrine response, and growth in infancy: Data from a randomized clinical trial. *Am J Clin Nutr* 94, 1776S-1784S.

Song, F., Srinivasan, M., Aalinkeel, R., Patel, M.S., 2001. Use of a cDNA array for the identification of genes induced in islets of suckling rats by a high-carbohydrate nutritional intervention. *Diabetes* 50, 2053–2060.

Srinivasan, M., Laychock, S.G., Hill, D.J., Patel, M.S., 2003. Neonatal nutrition: Metabolic programming of pancreatic islets and obesity. *Exp Biol Med* 228, 15–23.

Srinivasan, M., Mahmood, S., Patel, M.S., 2013. Metabolic programming effects initiated in the suckling period predisposing for adult-onset obesity cannot be reversed by calorie restriction. *Am J Physiol Endocrinol Metab* 304, E486–E494.

Srinivasan, M., Mitrani, P., Sadhanandan, G., Dodds, C., Shbeir-ElDika, S., Thamotharan, S., Ghanim, H., Dandona, P., Devaskar, S.U., Patel, M.S., 2008. A high-carbohydrate diet in the immediate postnatal life of rats induces adaptations predisposing to adult-onset obesity. *J Endocrinol* 197, 565–574.

Srinivasan, M., Song, F., Aalinkeel, R., Patel, M.S., 2001. Molecular adaptations in islets from neonatal rats reared artificially on a high carbohydrate milk formula. *J Nutr Biochem* 12, 575–584.

Wahlqvist, M.L., Krawetz, S.A., Rizzo, N.S., Dominguez-Bello, M.G., Szymanski, L.M., Barkin, S., Yatkine, A., Waterland, R.A., Mennella, J.A., Desai, M., Ross, M.G., Krebs, N.F., Young, B.E., Wardle, J., Wrann, C.D., Kral, J.G., 2015. Early-life influences on obesity: From preconception to adolescence. *Ann N Y Acad Sci* 1347, 1–28.

Williams, L., Seki, Y., Vuguin, P.M., Charron, M.J., 2014. Animal models of in utero exposure to a high fat diet: A review. *Biochim Biophys Acta* 1842, 507–519.

Woo Baidal, J.A., Locks, L.M., Cheng, E.R., Blake-Lamb, T.L., Perkins, M.E., Taveras, E.M., 2016. Risk factors for childhood obesity in the first 1,000 days: A systematic review. *Am J Prev Med* 50, 761–779.

Section IV

---

*Human Studies on
Early Programming*

11 Vitamins and Programming of Noncommunicable Diseases

Chittaranjan Yajnik and Tejas Limaye

CONTENTS

11.1 INTRODUCTION

The conventional model of noncommunicable diseases (NCDs) envisages a genetic (and therefore nonmodifiable) susceptibility and precipitation by unfavorable life-style (unhealthy diet, physical inactivity, stress, and other). Therefore, prevention is usually equated with lifestyle change in adult life. Recent research has demonstrated an association between altered growth and development in early life and later susceptibility to NCDs.

The Developmental Origins of Health and Disease (DOHaD) hypothesis originated in the work of Prof. David Barker. DOHaD proposes that environmental factors that influence growth and development affect risk of NCD across the life course (Barker 2007). Maternal factors influencing intrauterine environment are of particular importance but postnatal factors affecting growth and development during infancy, childhood, and adolescence also contribute. A range of environmental factors are involved (Figure 11.1).

Environmental influences during critical stages of development permanently alter the structure and function of the cells, tissues, organs, and systems, which is called "programming" (Lucas 1991) (Figure 11.2). The idea originated in the demonstration of a link between small birth size and risk of chronic diseases in adulthood (Hales et al. 1991).

199

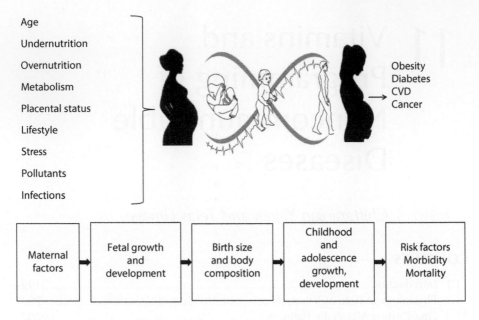

FIGURE 11.1   Concept of Developmental Origins of Health and Disease (DOHaD).

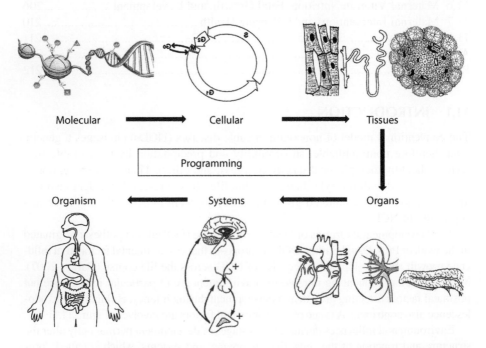

FIGURE 11.2   Programming involves "epigenetic changes," including DNA (methylation), altered chromatin structure, and RNA (microRNA or miRNA), which reflect in cellular structure and function in different tissues, organs, and systems.

Natural experiments of exposure to famine *in utero* are associated with a greater risk of chronic disease in later life (Roseboom et al. 2001). Fetal overnutrition in obese and diabetic pregnancies has a similar effect (Freinkel 1980; Dabelea and Pettitt 2001).

Maternal nutrition plays a critical role in fetal growth and development. The fetus depends on the mother for its nutritional needs, and, therefore, any disturbance in the maternal nutritional status or its supply to the fetus adversely impacts fetal growth. When nutrition is limited, it is preferentially used for the growth of the fetal brain by increased blood flow to the cephalic (preductal) system at the cost of caudal (post-ductal) and subdiaphragmatic organs like lungs, heart, liver, pancreas, and kidneys (Yajnik 2004). It makes the individual susceptible to a range of diseases, including sarcopenic adiposity, reduced β-cell mass, insulin resistance, and renal dysfunction. When challenged with adverse lifestyle these manifest as various NCDs.

Given the orchestrated nature of growth and development, there are periods (windows) when certain organs and systems are susceptible to environmental influences. Periconceptional, intrauterine, and postnatal periods may be the most influential in programming. The periconceptional period encompasses the natural "wiping out" of the inherited epigenome and the "reestablishment" of a new one (Morgan 2005). This period also covers vital processes, such as gametogenesis, fertilization, implantation, morphogenesis, embryogenesis, organogenesis, and placentation, all of which have a profound influence on the growth, development, differentiation, and phenotype of an individual (Steegers-Theunissen et al. 2013). A further window appears to be the adolescence when sexual development occurs. If the environment is not ideal (e.g., nutritional imbalance, altered metabolism, stress, infections, exposure to environmental pollutants), this might lead to undesirable programming and increase the risk for later disease (Figure 11.3).

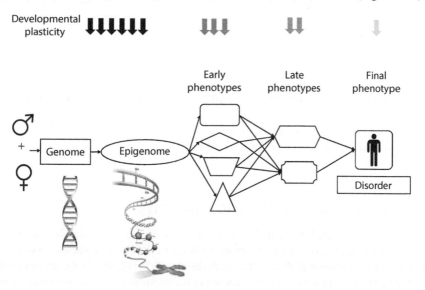

FIGURE 11.3 Evolution of a phenotype over the life course involves an interaction between the inherited genetic information and environment. The interaction involves modification in gene expression (programming). The developmental plasticity (capacity for unrestricted development) is maximum in early life and decreases with time. The phenotype changes accordingly.

There is increasing recognition of an important role for micronutrients in these phenomena (Rao et al. 2001; Fall 2012). Micronutrients (vitamins and minerals) are essential for human health and development. It has been estimated that at least half of the children worldwide suffer from one or more micronutrient deficiency and globally more than two billion people are affected (Global Report 2009). Although micronutrient deficiencies during pregnancy have been associated with adverse pregnancy outcomes (Allen 2005), their effects on the long-term health of the offspring are only beginning to be understood. This chapter reviews some of the effects of maternal vitamin nutrition on the health of the offspring.

11.2 PHYSIOLOGICAL ROLE OF VITAMINS

Vitamins play an important role in the cellular function and metabolism and therefore affect practically all the processes in cells, tissues, organs, and systems. They act as antioxidants, coenzymes for many enzymes, and contribute to cell regulation, growth, and differentiation (Rolig 1986).

Vitamin A (retinol) is essential for normal vision, growth, reproduction, immunity, and epithelial tissue maintenance. Its influence is particularly critical during periods when cells proliferate rapidly and differentiate, such as during pregnancy and early childhood.

B-complex vitamins affect the functions of various enzymes and influence a wide range of metabolic processes. This affects growth and development. Vitamins, which affect methyl group transfer, are particularly important (folate and vitamin B_{12}, B_6, B_2) in modifying functions of various molecules (DNA, proteins, and lipids). This affects numerous biological processes like DNA biosynthesis, regulation of gene expression, chromatin structure, genomic repair, and stability.

Vitamin C (ascorbic acid) acts as a cofactor in a number of enzymatic reactions. Vitamin C is required for the synthesis of collagen, carnitine, catecholamine, and the neurotransmitter norepinephrine. It also acts as an antioxidant (protects against oxidative stress).

Vitamin D (cholecalciferol) regulates functions of various genes and influences cellular calcium metabolism. It plays a role in the function of the islet cells of pancreas, muscles, and immune system.

11.3 ONE-CARBON METABOLIC PATHWAYS

One-carbon (1-C) metabolism includes reactions, including the addition, transfer, or removal of 1-C units in cellular metabolic pathways (Kalhan and Marczewski 2012). The central methylation pathway, the methylation cycle (Figure 11.4), occurs in the cytoplasm of every cell where the S-adenosyl methionine (SAM) is generated from adenosine triphosphate (ATP) and methionine and is involved in a multitude of methylation reactions. In this process, SAM is converted to S-adenosyl homocysteine (SAH) and then to homocysteine. Methionine is regenerated when a methyl group from 5-CH3-tetrahydofolate is transferred to homocysteine by methionine synthase,

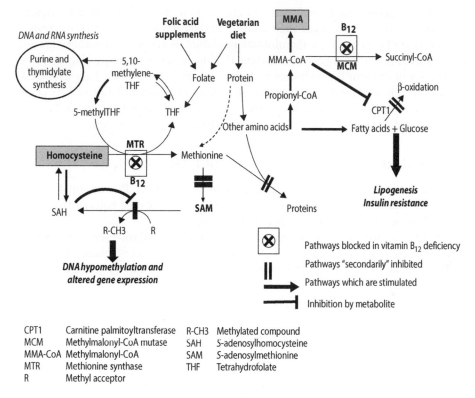

FIGURE 11.4 A simplified view of metabolic pathways influenced by folate and vitamin B_{12}. Deficiency or imbalance affects various metabolic pathways including nucleic acids, gene expression, protein synthesis, and vital cellular functions. Homocysteine is raised in deficiency of both vitamins, while methylmalonic acid (MMA) is a specific marker for vitamin B_{12} deficiency.

which requires vitamin B_{12} as a cofactor. When concentrations of vitamin B_{12} are insufficient, folate becomes trapped as 5-methyl tetrahydrofolate, the regeneration of methionine is inhibited, and the concentrations of homocysteine are increased.

Raised concentrations of homocysteine within the cell are toxic and actively regulated by (1) remethylation, which requires vitamins B_{12} and B_2, (2) transsulfuration, which requires vitamin B_6, and (3) the transfer of one of the methyl groups of betaine to homocysteine to form methionine.

The remethylation of homocysteine to methionine is linked with the folate cycle, which generates methyl tetrahydrofolate, which is a cosubstrate for the methylation of homocysteine to methionine. The folate cycle is essential for purine and pyrimidine nucleotide synthesis, which is essential for the formation and stability of DNA, RNA, and nucleoside triphosphates such as ATP.

Methylation of DNA nucleotides is an important epigenetic mechanism for the control of gene expression. This control of gene expression is particularly important during critical periods of growth and development and may help explain why nutritional imbalances are associated with fetal phenotypes, which increase the risk for subsequent diseases (Rush et al. 2013; Yajnik and Deshmukh 2012).

In the mitochondria, β-oxidation of fatty acids requires that they are sequentially broken down into small even number carbon units, which enter the tricarboxylic acid (TCA) cycle for the ultimate oxidation of acetyl (two-carbon) groups derived from lipids. This generates carbon dioxide, water, and energy (Figure 11.4). Deficiency of vitamin B_{12} interferes with the transfer of long-chain fatty acyl-CoA into the mitochondria and inhibits β-oxidation, leading to accumulation of fatty acids in the cytosol and increased inclusion into glycerolipids. Thus, vitamin B_{12} influences folate-dependent reactions as well as mitochondrial energy generation.

11.4   SOURCES OF VITAMINS (FAO 2001; FIGURE 11.5)

Vitamin A is present in animal tissues, especially fish and liver. Provitamin A (carotenoids) is obtained from green leafy vegetables and red–orange colored fruits and vegetables and converted to vitamin A in the human body.

Folates are present in many natural foods, including dark-green vegetables, whole grains, and some nonvegetarian foods. It is also synthesized by intestinal bacteria. Vitamin B_{12} (cyanocobalamin) is synthesized exclusively by

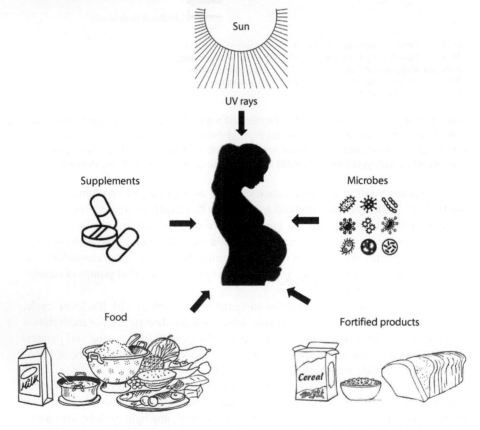

FIGURE 11.5   Vitamins are obtained from different foods (practically all vitamins), sunlight (vitamin D), microbes (folate, vitamin B_{12}), supplements, and fortified products (all vitamins).

microorganisms and is obtained in the diet through consumption of animal source foods. Vitamin B_{12}-containing plant-derived food sources include green and purple lavers (Nori) and blue–green algae/cyanobacteria (spirulina), but they may not suitable for humans due to the presence of biologically inactive pseudovitamin B_{12} (Watanabe 2007). Therefore, milk remains the only acceptable animal source of B_{12} for vegetarians.

Vitamin C is present in fresh fruits and vegetables.

Vitamins except vitamin D are not produced in the body and must be derived from the diet (Sight and Life 2011). Vitamin D is a prohormone produced in the skin under the effect of ultraviolet rays in the sunlight. Synthesis of vitamin D varies markedly by season in temperate climes. It is metabolized in the liver and kidneys to its active form. It is also present in low concentration in some natural foods and in many artificially fortified food products.

Supplements and fortified foods are also important sources of several vitamins in the modern diets (de Lourdes Samaniego-Vaesken et al. 2012). Some examples of commonly fortified foods are breakfast cereals, bread, milk, fruit juices, cooking oils, etc. Care needs to be exercised to avoid "overdose" of vitamins.

11.5   CAUSES OF VITAMIN DEFICIENCY IN PREGNANCY AND LACTATION

Vitamin deficiencies are widely prevalent in these critical stages of life especially in developing countries (Muller 2005). Inadequate (suboptimal) intake is the major reason. Requirements for almost all vitamins increase during pregnancy and lactation (Table 11.1) and therefore vegans and vegetarians (who eat little or no meat) are particularly affected. Social, cultural, and religious factors and income influence dietary practices (Dietary Reference Intakes 2010).

Fetal vitamin nutrition is mainly dependent on maternal concentrations and stores. Placental transfer of vitamins and nutrients is an important aspect of fetal nutrition. Specific transporters are present for macronutrients and many vitamins may be regulated to match fetal requirements. Maternal vitamin

---

TABLE 11.1

Recommended Dietary Allowances (RDAs) for Nonpregnant, Pregnant, and Lactating Women (Recommended by the Institute of Medicine)

Vitamins	Nonpregnant Women	Pregnant Women	Lactating Women
Vitamin A (µg/day)	700	770	1300
Folate (µg/day)	400	600	500
Vitamin B_{12} (µg/day)	2.4	2.6	2.8
Vitamin C (mg/day)	75	85	120
Vitamin D (µg/day)	15	15	15

Different countries might have their own RDAs.

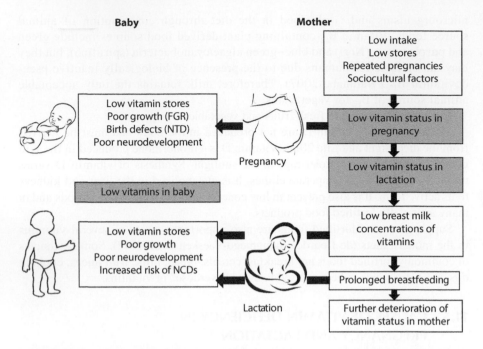

FIGURE 11.6   Direct intergenerational transfer of vitamins from mother to baby. Transfer is mediated by the placenta during pregnancy and through milk in the postnatal period. Various factors affect these processes.

deficiency thus reflects in fetal vitamin deficiency and inadequate stores in infants. Exclusive breastfeeding for prolonged periods and late introduction of complementary foods further deteriorate the deficiency in both mother and infants (National Guidelines on Infant and Young Child Feeding—Ministry of Human Resource Development, Food and Nutrition Board, Government of India 2004) (Figure 11.6).

11.6   MATERNAL VITAMIN NUTRITION, FETAL GROWTH, AND DEVELOPMENT

Inadequate maternal nutrition increases the risk of pregnancy-related complications and lifelong consequences for the health of the offspring. The role of preconceptional nutrition cannot be overemphasized because it determines the adequacy of maternal stores for the pregnancy. In turn, maternal stores and intake during pregnancy and lactation contribute to neonatal stores (Finkelstein et al. 2015; Murphy et al. 2007).

1. **Vitamin A:** Both vitamin A deficiency and excess have been associated with congenital malformations in human and animal studies (Clagett-Dame et al. 2002). Development of lungs (Antipatis et al. 2000), heart (Pan and

Baker 2007), kidneys (Lelièvre-Pégorier et al. 1998), and pancreatic islets (Matthews et al. 2004) may be affected by vitamin A.

2. **Folate, vitamin B_{12}:** Folate and vitamin B_{12} are the most prominently studied vitamins in pregnancy. Success of folic acid supplementation to prevent neural tube defects (NTDs) is a major public health achievement (MRC Vitamin Study Research Group 1991). As already mentioned, recent interest in epigenetics has further enhanced the interest in these vitamins, which contribute to regulation of the 1-C metabolism. The two vitamins are intricately linked in the (1-C) metabolism and deficiency of one leads to a functional deficiency of the other. In some situations, an imbalance has been implicated in adverse outcomes.

   a. **NTDs and congenital anomalies:** Folic acid deficiency is associated with NTDs and other congenital anomalies. In a predominantly vegetarian population (e.g., Indians), vitamin B_{12} plays a similar role (Godbole et al. 2011). Substantial trial evidence has influenced clinical practice of periconceptional supplementation with folic acid to prevent NTDs. The recommended dose is 400 μg for prevention of the first NTD and 4 mg to prevent recurrence. This difference is often forgotten. It may be important to avoid higher dose in B_{12} deficient populations. The majority of pregnancies are not planned, and therefore, timely supplementation may not be achieved. This led to the policy of food fortification to improve vitamin status of the population. The United States and many other countries have introduced a mandatory flour fortification with folic acid (Oakley and Tulchinsky 2010); in other countries voluntary fortification of selected food items is practiced.

   b. **Growth and prematurity:** Some studies show that both maternal folate and vitamin B_{12} concentrations are associated with fetal growth (Deshmukh et al. 2013; Finkelstein et al. 2015). A study in urban South India reported that low maternal vitamin B_{12} status is associated with intrauterine growth retardation (IUGR) (Muthayya et al. 2006), especially if folate intake is high (Dwarkanath et al. 2013).

   The Pune Maternal Nutrition Study (PMNS) is a longitudinal study of maternal nutrition and fetal growth and their relationship to future risk of NCDs. These rural mothers were chronically undernourished (low body mass index [BMI]) and predominantly vegetarian. Two-thirds of the mothers had low vitamin B_{12} status, while folate deficiency was rare. Maternal macronutrient intake was only marginally related to birth size but intake of micronutrient rich foods (green leafy vegetables, milk, and fruits) was strongly linked (Rao et al. 2001). Circulating folate concentrations were directly related to birth size, while B_{12} was not related. Higher homocysteine concentrations in the mother predicted smaller birth size, and mothers with methylene tetrahydrofolate reductase (MTHFR) 677TT genotype (Yajnik et al. 2014) produced smaller babies. A Mendelian randomization analysis suggested that this association may be causal and that (1-C) metabolism disturbance may be an important contributor to fetal growth restriction (Yajnik et al. 2014).

Meta-analyses have suggested that maternal low vitamin B_{12} status is associated with small birth size and a preterm delivery (Sukumar et al. 2016; Rogne 2017) both of which have a potential to increase the risk of NCDs.

c. **Body composition:** PMNS also showed that maternal folate status in pregnancy is related to higher adiposity in the child at 6 years of age (Yajnik et al. 2008). The Parthenon study in Mysore made similar observations in a longitudinal follow-up of the children at 5, 9, and 13 years (Krishnaveni et al. 2005; Krishnaveni et al. 2010). Similar findings were also made in a Spanish study. Low maternal vitamin B_{12} status is also related to the offspring adiposity (Yajnik et al. 2015).

d. **Cardiometabolic:** Folate and vitamin B_{12} deficiency and associated hyperhomocysteinemia are linked with increased cardiovascular risk in adults though the causality is in doubt because interventions to improve these factors have not resulted in a reduction in cardiovascular events. This may be due to the fact that the cardiovascular risk is already programmed by these factors in early life and that the secondary and tertiary interventions are not able to reverse it. There is an inverse association between vitamin B_{12} concentrations and a number of cardiovascular risk markers in the cord blood (Adaikalakoteswari et al. 2015). In the PMNS and Parthenon study, higher maternal folate concentrations predicted higher insulin resistance in the child (Yajnik et al. 2008; Krishnaveni et al. 2013); in the PMNS, the most insulin-resistant children were born to mothers with low-B_{12} and high-folate concentrations (Yajnik et al. 2008). Association of low maternal B_{12} with insulin resistance in the child was also seen in rural Nepal (Stewart et al. 2011). These findings suggest a possible role for maternal nutrition of these two vitamins in influencing the risk of diabetes in the offspring. The classic studies of Barker and his colleagues showed an association between low birth weight and future risk of coronary artery disease and stroke.

e. **Neurocognitive:** Traditionally, vitamin B_{12} and folate are associated with hematological and neurological systems. There is considerable evidence to associate maternal vitamin B_{12} and folate nutrition with brain development and neurocognitive function of the child. In addition to the closure of the neural tube, many other aspects of brain development are affected. A number of studies have associated these vitamins with neurocognitive performance of the child. Different aspects of brain function are influenced. Poor folate status in the mother is associated with autistic spectrum disorders, smaller brain volume, and attention deficit hyperactivity disorder (Surén et al. 2013; Steenweg-de Graaff et al. 2014; Julvez et al. 2009; Schlotz et al. 2009). Similarly, many studies have associated poor maternal vitamin B_{12} status with a number of neurological and cognitive problems in the child including infantile tremor syndrome, and poor mental and motor development (Dror and Allen 2008; Veena et al. 2010; Bhate et al. 2008;

Del Rio Garcia et al. 2009). Children born to mothers with specific conditions affecting folate and B_{12} nutrition (vegans, pernicious anemia, methylene tetrahydrofolate reductase (MTHFR) 677TT genotype) are at increased risk of neurocognitive problems. It will be of interest to follow up with the offspring for risk of various brain disorders (vascular, degenerative) in later life. It is of note that individuals exposed to Dutch winter hunger *in utero* are at an increased risk of schizophrenia.

f. **Mechanisms:** In the present state of knowledge, the exact role of (1-C) metabolism, and the vitamins which regulate it, may be difficult to pinpoint. Methylation is vital for various cellular metabolic functions and a range of processes may be affected: myelination of nerve cells, synthesis of neurotransmitters, protection from oxidative damage, etc. The role in nucleic acid metabolism has already been stressed. Currently, there is a lot of excitement in the role of epigenetic mechanisms (DNA methylation) in growth, development, and differentiation.

Studies in adults who faced intrauterine famine during Dutch winter hunger showed a different pattern of methylation of insulin-like growth factor 2 (IGF-2) gene compared to those not exposed (Heijmans et al. 2008). Babies of mothers supplemented with folic acid and other micronutrients showed a different DNA methylation pattern in the cord blood compared to those whose mothers were not supplemented. Studies in Gambia have shown that blood levels of several key nutrients and (1-C) metabolites vary by season as do the DNA methylation of metastable epialleles in their offspring (Dominguez-Salas et al. 2014; Waterland et al. 2010).

Exciting findings have been made in animal models, the classic one being change in obesity and coat color in the agouti mice offspring after a "methyl donor cocktail" (folate + vitamin B_{12} + choline + betaine) treatment of the mothers (Waterland and Jirtle 2004).

3. **Vitamin C:** Low maternal vitamin C intake during pregnancy may compromise maternal weight gain, placental function, and intrauterine development (Schjoldager et al. 2014).

4. **Vitamin D:** Vitamin D has been variably associated with fetal growth parameters and prematurity (Gernand et al. 2013; Rodriguez et al. 2014; Miliku et al. 2016). Vitamin D deficiency during pregnancy can lead to fetal hypovitaminosis D, neonatal rickets and tetany, neonatal hypocalcaemia, infantile rickets, defective tooth enamel formation, dental cavities, acute lower respiratory tract infections, asthma, and schizophrenia (Sachan et al. 2005; Hewison and Adams 2010, Karras et al. 2016). Maternal ultraviolet rays exposure during pregnancy has been positively associated with bone mass in childhood, and seasonal differences in neonatal bone mineral content have been reported. Maternal vitamin D insufficiency may influence fetal femoral development as early as 19 weeks gestation (Mahon et al. 2009) and reflects in IUGR and growth failure in later years (Kaushal and Navneet 2013; Khalessi et al. 2015; Chen et al. 2015). Role of fetal vitamin D nutrition in susceptibility to type 1 diabetes is still not clear (Sørensen et al. 2011; Miettinen et al. 2012; Marjamäki et al. 2010).

11.7   MATERNAL INTERVENTIONS AND OFFSPRING HEALTH

A number of interventions have been implemented in mothers to improve the offspring health. The most celebrated example is the success of periconceptional folic acid supplementation and reduction in the rate of NTDs. There is a growing recognition of the importance of periconceptional period in fetal programming and therefore the need to start before conception. An important consideration is to do a follow-up of the children for long periods to demonstrate the effects. Unfortunately, this is still rare. For example, most of the reviews stop at pregnancy and perinatal outcomes (De-Regil et al. 2012; McCauley et al. 2015; Rumbold et al. 2015; De-Regil et al. 2010; Lassi et al. 2013).

The majority of the trials started in pregnancy, many times in the third trimester, have measured outcomes only during pregnancy or at birth. Only a few trials have shown an effect, but the long-term implications are not clear (Table 11.2). There is an urgent need to devise new trials taking these shortcomings into consideration.

TABLE 11.2
Summary of Some of the Human Interventions and Their Results (Excluding the NTD Trials)

Author, Country	N, Subjects	Intervention	Outcomes, Findings
Vitamin A			
West et al. (2003), rural Nepal	44,646 pregnant women	7000 µg retinol equivalents for 3½ years	Low pregnancy-related mortality
Christian et al. (2003b), rural Nepal	4926 pregnant women	1000 µg retinol equivalents plus FA 400; FA + iron (60 mg); FA + iron + zinc (30 mg); MMN	No reduction in fetal loss/infant mortality
Kirkwood et al. (2010), Ghana	39,601 pregnant women	25,000 IU retinol equivalents once a week	No reduction in pregnancy related and all-cause mortality
West et al. (2011), rural Bangladesh	59,666 pregnant women	7000 µg retinol equivalents weekly first trimester to 12 weeks postpartum	No reduction in all-cause maternal, fetal, or infant mortality
Christian et al. (2012), rural Bangladesh	18,250 pregnant women	7000 µg retinol equivalents once a week until 3 months postpartum	No effect on birth outcomes
Stewart et al. (2010), rural Nepal	44,646 pregnant women	7000 µg retinol equivalents once a week until 3 months postpartum	No impact on cardiovascular risk factors at preadolescent age
Checkley et al. (2010), rural Nepal	2459 pregnant women	7000 µg retinol equivalents once a week until 3 months postpartum	Improved lung function in the offspring (9–13 years)
Folate, Vitamin B$_{12}$/MMN			
Christian et al. (2003a), rural Nepal	4926 pregnant women	FA 400; FA + iron (60 mg); FA + iron + zinc (30 mg); MMN plus 1000 µg retinol equivalents	Reduction in the risk of low birth weight

(Continued)

TABLE 11.2 (*Continued*)
Summary of Some of the Human Interventions and Their Results (Excluding the NTD Trials)

Author, Country	N, Subjects	Intervention	Outcomes, Findings
SUMMIT Study Group et al. (2008), Indonesia	31,290 pregnant women	IFA or MMN daily, from enrollment to 90 days postpartum	Reduction in early infant mortality in MMN group, especially in undernourished and anemic women
Stewart et al. (2009), rural Nepal	4926 pregnant women	FA 400; FA + iron (60 mg); FA + iron + zinc (30 mg); MMN plus 1000 μg retinol equivalents	Reduced risk of kidney dysfunction and metabolic syndrome in children
Duggan et al. (2014), India	366 pregnant women	50 μg Vitamin B_{12} daily through 6-week postpartum	Improvement in vitamin B_{12} status of mothers and infants, lower plasma MMA and Hcy concentrations in infants
Srinivasan et al. (2016), India	366 pregnant women	50 μg Vitamin B_{12} through 6-week postpartum	No effects on cognitive development at 9 months; elevated maternal tHcy associated with poor cognitive performance
Vitamin C			
McEvoy et al. (2014), Pacific Northwest	179 pregnant smokers	500 mg vitamin C daily	Improvement in newborn pulmonary function tests and decreased wheezing
Vitamin D			
Marya et al. (1988), India	200 pregnant women	600,000 IU vitamin D in 7th and 8th month of gestation	Fetal growth indices improved
Hashemipour et al. (2014), Iran	130 vitamin D deficient pregnant women	50,000 IU vitamin D per week for 8 weeks	Fetal growth indices and maternal weight gain improved
Cooper et al. (2016), UK	1134 pregnant women	1000 IU vitamin D daily until delivery	Overall no effect on whole-body bone mineral content. Subgroup analysis showed interaction with season

FA, folic acid; IFA, iron folic acid; MMN, multiple micronutrients; tHcy, total homocysteine.

11.8 SUMMARY

There is a paradigm shift in our thinking about susceptibility to NCDs. In addition to the nonmodifiable genetic susceptibility, we now know of a modifiable "epigenetic" susceptibility. A substantial component of this is established in early life (periconceptional period, pregnancy, and postnatal period). Maternal nutrition and other factors are important and vitamins appear to play a crucial role. Vitamins, which act on the genome (vitamin A, folate, vitamin B_{12}, vitamin D), are particularly important and seem to act by permanently altering the epigenome of the offspring. Such a programmed state is unable to cope with later life challenges of an unfavorable lifestyle and results in a disease. There is an exciting possibility of preventing NCDs by improving environment in early life and intergenerationally by improving the health of young girls (primordial prevention).

ACKNOWLEDGMENTS

We acknowledge participants in our research studies, colleagues, and collaborators and funding agencies (Wellcome Trust—UK, Medical Research Council—UK, Department of Biotechnology—New Delhi, Indian Council of Medical Research—New Delhi, European Union—Brussels, Nestle Foundation—Switzerland). Dr. CSY was a visiting scholar at STIαS (Stellenbosch University, South Africa) during the writing of this chapter. Dr. Sadhana Joshi commented on the manuscript.

REFERENCES

Adaikalakoteswari, A, Vatish, M, Lawson, A et al. Low maternal vitamin B_{12} status is associated with lower cord blood HDL cholesterol in white Caucasians living in the UK. *Nutrients* 7, no. 4 (2015): 2401–2414.

Allen, L. Multiple micronutrients in pregnancy and lactation: An overview. *American Journal of Clinical Nutrition* 81 (2005): S1206–S1212.

Antipatis, C, Grant, G, Ashworth, CJ. Moderate maternal vitamin A deficiency affects perinatal organ growth and development in rats. *British Journal of Nutrition* 84, no. 1 (2000): 125–132.

Barker, DJP. The origins of the developmental origins theory. *Journal of Internal Medicine* 261, no. 5 (2007): 412–417.

Bhate, V, Deshpande, S, Bhat, DS. Vitamin B_{12} status of pregnant Indian women and cognitive function in their 9-year-old children. *Food and Nutrition Bulletin* 29, no. 4 (2008): 249–254.

Checkley, W, West, KP Jr, Wise, RA et al. Maternal vitamin A supplementation and lung function in offspring. *New England Journal of Medicine* 362, no. 19 (2010): 1784–1794.

Chen, YH, Fu, L, Hao, JH et al. Maternal vitamin D deficiency during pregnancy elevates the risks of small for gestational age and low birth weight infants in Chinese population. *Journal of Clinical Endocrinology & Metabolism* 100, no. 5 (2015): 1912–1919.

Christian, P, Khatry, SK, Katz, J et al. Effects of alternative maternal micronutrient supplements on low birth weight in rural Nepal: Double blind randomised community trial. *BMJ* 326, no. 7389 (2003a): 571.

Christian, P, Klemm, R, Shamim, AA et al. Effects of vitamin A and β-carotene supplementation on birth size and length of gestation in rural Bangladesh: A cluster-randomized trial. *American Journal of Clinical Nutrition* 97, no. 1 (2012): 188–194.

Christian, P, West, KP, Khatry, SK et al. Effects of maternal micronutrient supplementation on fetal loss and infant mortality: A cluster-randomized trial in Nepal. *American Journal of Clinical Nutrition* 78, no. 6 (2003b): 1194–1202.

Clagett-Dame, M, DeLuca, HF. The role of vitamin A in mammalian reproduction and embryonic development. *Annual Review of Nutrition* 22, no. 1 (2002): 347–381.

Cooper, C, Harvey, NC, Bishop, NJ et al. Maternal gestational vitamin D supplementation and offspring bone health (MAVIDOS): A multicentre, double-blind, randomised placebo-controlled trial. *Lancet Diabetes & Endocrinology* 4, no. 5 (2016): 393–402.

Dabelea, D, Pettitt, D. Intrauterine diabetic environment confers risks for type 2 diabetes mellitus and obesity in the offspring, in addition to genetic susceptibility. *Journal of Pediatric Endocrinology and Metabolism* 14, no. 1 (2001): 1085–1091.

de Lourdes Samaniego-Vaesken, M, Alonso-Aperte, E, Varela-Moreiras, G. Vitamin food fortification today. *Food & Nutrition Research* 56, (2012), doi:10.3402/fnr.v56i0.5459.

Del Rio Garcia, C, Torres-Sanchez, L, Chen, J. Maternal MTHFR 677C>T genotype and dietary intake of folate and vitamin B_{12}: Their impact on child neurodevelopment. *Nutritional Neuroscience* 12, no. 1 (2009): 13–20.

De-Regil, LM, Fernández-Gaxiola, AC, Dowswell, T, Peña-Rosas, JP. Effects and safety of periconceptional folate supplementation for preventing birth defects. *Cochrane Database of Systematic Reviews* (2010);(10): CD007950.

De-Regil, LM, Palacios, C, Ansary, A, Kulier, R, Peña-Rosas, JP. Vitamin D supplementation for women during pregnancy. *Cochrane Database of Systematic Reviews* (2012): CD008873.

Deshmukh, U, Katre, P, Yajnik, CS. Influence of maternal vitamin B $_{12}$ and folate on growth and insulin resistance in the offspring. *Nestle Nutrition Institute Workshop Series* 74, (2013): 145–156.

Dietary Reference Intakes (Dris): Recommended Dietary Allowances and Adequate Intakes, Vitamins. Food and Nutrition Board, Institute of Medicine, National Academies. 2010. Available at https://www.ncbi.nlm.nih.gov/books/NBK278991/table/diet-treatment-obes.table15die/.

Dominguez-Salas, P, Moore, SE, Baker, MS. Maternal nutrition at conception modulates DNA methylation of human metastable epialleles. Nature Communications 5, (2014): 3746.

Dror, DK, Allen, LH. Effect of vitamin B_{12} deficiency on neurodevelopment in infants: Current knowledge and possible mechanisms. *Nutrition Reviews* 66, no. 5 (2008): 250–255.

Duggan, C, Srinivasan, K, Thomas, T et al. Vitamin B-$_{12}$ supplementation during pregnancy and early lactation increases maternal, breast milk, and infant measures of vitamin B-12 status. *Journal of Nutrition* 144, no. 5 (2014): 758–764.

Dwarkanath, P, Barzilay, JR, Thomas, T et al. High folate and low vitamin B-12 intakes during pregnancy are associated with small-for-gestational age infants in South Indian women: A prospective observational cohort study. *American Journal of Clinical Nutrition* 98, no. 6 (2013): 1450–1458.

Fall, CHD. Fetal programming and the risk of noncommunicable disease. *Indian Journal of Pediatrics* 80, no. 1 (2012): 13–20.

FAO/WHO Expert Consultation on human vitamin and mineral requirements. http://www.fao.org, 2001. http://www.fao.org/3/a-y2809e.pdf.

Finkelstein, JL, Layden, AJ, Stover, PJ. Vitamin B-12 and perinatal health. *Advances in Nutrition: An International Review Journal* 6, no. 5 (2015): 552–563.

Freinkel, N. Banting lecture 1980: Of pregnancy and progeny. *Diabetes* 29, no. 12 (1980): 1023–1035.

Gernand, AD, Simhan, HN, Klebanoff, MA, Bodnar, LM. Maternal serum 25-hydroxyvitamin D and measures of newborn and placental weight in a U.S. multicenter cohort study. *Journal of Clinical Endocrinology & Metabolism* 98, no. 1 (2013): 398–404.

Global Report. *Investing in the Future: A United Call to Action on Vitamin and Mineral Deficiencies*, 2009.

Godbole, K, Gayathri, P, Ghule, S et al. Maternal one-carbon metabolism, MTHFR and TCN2 genotypes and neural tube defects in India. *Birth Defects Research Part A: Clinical and Molecular Teratology* 91, no. 9 (2011): 848–856.

Hales, CN, Barker, DJ, Clark, PM et al. Fetal and infant growth and impaired glucose tolerance at age 64. *BMJ* 303, no. 6809 (1991): 1019–1022.

Hashemipour, S, Ziaee, A, Javadi, A et al. Effect of treatment of vitamin D deficiency and insufficiency during pregnancy on fetal growth indices and maternal weight gain: A randomized clinical trial. *European Journal of Obstetrics & Gynecology and Reproductive Biology* 172 (2014): 15–19.

Heijmans, BT, Tobi, EW, Stein, AD et al. Persistent epigenetic differences associated with prenatal exposure to famine in humans. *Proceedings of the National Academy of Sciences* 105, no. 44 (2008): 17046–17049.

Hewison, M, Adams, JS. Vitamin D insufficiency and skeletal development in utero. *Journal of Bone and Mineral Research* 25, no. 1 (2010): 11–13.

Julvez, J, Fortuny, J, Mendez, M et al. Maternal use of folic acid supplements during pregnancy and four-year-old neurodevelopment in a population-based birth cohort. *Paediatric and Perinatal Epidemiology* 23, no. 3 (2009): 199–206.

Kalhan, SC, Marczewski, SE. Methionine, homocysteine, one carbon metabolism and fetal growth. *Reviews in Endocrine and Metabolic Disorders* 13, no. 2 (2012): 109–119.

Karras, SN, Fakhoury, H, Muscogiuri, G et al. Maternal vitamin D levels during pregnancy and neonatal health: Evidence to date and clinical implications. *Therapeutic Advances in Musculoskeletal Disease* 8, no. 4 (2016): 124–135.

Kaushal, M, Navneet, M. Vitamin D in pregnancy: A metabolic outlook. *Indian Journal of Endocrinology and Metabolism* 17, no. 1 (2013): 76.

Khalessi, N, Kalani, M, Araghi, M, Farahani, Z. The relationship between maternal vitamin D deficiency and low birth weight neonates. *Journal of Family and Reproductive Health* 9, no. 3 (2015):113–117.

Kirkwood, BR, Hurt, L, Amenga-Etego, S et al. Effect of vitamin A supplementation in women of reproductive age on maternal survival in Ghana (ObaapaVitA): A cluster-randomised, placebo-controlled trial. *Lancet* 375, no. 9726 (2010): 1640–1649.

Krishnaveni, G, Hill, J, Veena, S et al. Truncal adiposity is present at birth and in early childhood in South Indian children. *Indian Pediatrics* 42, no. 6 (2005): 527–538.

Krishnaveni, GV, Veena, SR, Karat, SC, Yajnik, CS, Fall, CHD. Association between maternal folate concentrations during pregnancy and insulin resistance in Indian children. *Diabetologia* 57, no. 1 (2013): 110–121.

Krishnaveni, GV, Veena, SR, Wills, AK. Adiposity, insulin resistance and cardiovascular risk factors in 9–10-year-old Indian children: Relationships with birth size and postnatal growth. *Journal of Developmental Origins of Health and Disease* 1, no. 06 (2010): 403–411.

Lassi, ZS, Salam, RA, Haider, BA et al. Folic acid supplementation during pregnancy for maternal health and pregnancy outcomes. Cochrane Database of Systematic Reviews 3, (2013): CD006896.

Lelièvre-Pégorier, M, Vilar, J, Ferrier, M-L et al. Mild vitamin A deficiency leads to inborn nephron deficit in the rat. *Kidney International* 54, no. 5 (1998): 1455–1462.

Lucas, A. Programming by early nutrition in man. *Ciba Foundation Symposium* 156 (1991): 38–50; discussion: 50–55.

Mahon, P, Harvey, N, Crozier, S et al. Low maternal vitamin D status and fetal bone development: Cohort study. *Journal of Bone and Mineral Research: The Official Journal of the American Society for Bone and Mineral Research* 25, no. 1 (2009): 14–19.

Marjamäki, L, Niinistö, S, Kenward, MG et al. Maternal intake of vitamin D during pregnancy and risk of advanced beta cell autoimmunity and type 1 diabetes in offspring. *Diabetologia* 53, no. 8 (2010): 1599–1607.

Marya, RK, Rathee, S, Dua, V, Sangwan, K. Effect of vitamin D supplementation during pregnancy on foetal growth. *Indian Journal of Medical Research* 88 (1988): 488–492.

Matthews, K, Rhoten, W, Driscoll, H, Chertow, B. Vitamin A deficiency impairs fetal islet development and causes subsequent glucose intolerance in adult rats. *Journal of Nutrition* 134 (2004): 1958–1963.

McCauley, ME, van den Broek, N, Dou, L, Othman, M. Vitamin A supplementation during pregnancy for maternal and newborn outcomes. *Cochrane Database of Systematic Reviews* 10, (2015): CD008666.

McEvoy, CT, Schilling, D, Clay, N et al. Vitamin C supplementation for pregnant smoking women and pulmonary function in their newborn infants. *JAMA* 311, no. 20 (2014): 2074.

Micronutrient Initiative/World Bank/UNICEF. Investing in the Future: A United Call to Action on Vitamin and Mineral Deficiencies: Investing in the Future: Global Health Report. Micronutrient Initiative; Toronto, ON, Canada: 2009. ISBN:978-1-894217-31-6. Available online: http://www.micronutrient.org/english/View.asp?x=614.

Miettinen, ME, Reinert, L, Kinnunen, L et al. Serum 25-hydroxyvitamin D level during early pregnancy and type 1 diabetes risk in the offspring. *Diabetologia* 55, no. 5 (2012): 1291–1294.

Miliku, K, Vinkhuyzen, A, Blanken, LM et al. Maternal vitamin D concentrations during pregnancy, fetal growth patterns, and risks of adverse birth outcomes. *American Journal of Clinical Nutrition* 103, no. 6 (2016): 1514–1522.

Morgan, HD. Epigenetic reprogramming in mammals. *Human Molecular Genetics* 14, no. 1 (2005): R47–R58.

MRC Vitamin Study Research Group. Prevention of neural tube defects: Results of the Medical Research Council Vitamin Study: MRC Vitamin Study Research Group. Lancet 338, no. 8760 (1991): 131–137.

Muller, O. Malnutrition and health in developing countries. *Canadian Medical Association Journal* 173, no. 3 (2005): 279–286.

Murphy, M, Molloy, A, Ueland, P et al. Longitudinal study of the effect of pregnancy on maternal and fetal cobalamin status in healthy women and their offspring. *Journal of Nutrition.*137 (2007): 1863–1867.

Muthayya, S, Kurpad, A, Duggan, C et al. Low maternal vitamin B_{12} status is associated with intrauterine growth retardation in urban South Indians. *European Journal of Clinical Nutrition* 60, no. 6 (2006): 791–801.

National Guidelines on Infant and Young Child Feeding—Ministry of Human Resource Development, Food and Nutrition Board, Government of India, 2004. http://wcd.nic.in/sites/default/files/nationalguidelines.pdf.

Oakley, G, Tulchinsky, T. Folic acid and vitamin B_{12} fortification of flour: A global basic food security requirement. *Public Health Reviews* 32, no. 1 (2010): 284–295.

Pan, J, Baker, KM. Retinoic acid and the heart. *Vitamin and Hormones* 75 (2007), 257–283.

Rao, S, Kanade, A, Yajnik, C. Intake of micronutrient-rich foods in rural Indian mothers is associated with the size of their babies at birth; the Pune Maternal Nutrition Study. *Journal of Nutrition* 131 (2001): 1217–1224.

Rodriguez, A, García-Esteban, R, Basterretxea, M et al. Associations of maternal circulating 25-hydroxyvitamin D3 concentration with pregnancy and birth outcomes. *BJOG: An International Journal of Obstetrics & Gynaecology* 122, no. 12 (2014): 1695–1704.

Rogne, T. Maternal vitamin B_{12} in pregnancy and risk of preterm birth and low birth weight: A systematic review and individual participant data meta-analysis: In eating for two in pregnancy: Health outcomes in pregnant women and their children, 1st ed., 2016. *American Journal of Epidemiology* 2017 Jan 20. doi: 10.1093/aje/kww212. [Epub ahead of print].

Rolig, E. Vitamins: Physiology and deficiency states. *Journal for Nurse Practitioners* 11, no. 7 (1986): 38, 43–44, 46–48.

Roseboom, TJ, van der Meulen, JHP, Ravelli, ACJ et al. Effects of prenatal exposure to the Dutch famine on adult disease in later life: An overview. *Twin Research* 4, no. 5 (2001): 293–298.

Rumbold, A, Ota, E, Nagata, C et al. Vitamin C supplementation in pregnancy. *Cochrane Database of Systematic Reviews,* no. 9 (2015): CD004072.

Rush, E, Katre, P, Yajnik, C. Vitamin B_{12}: One carbon metabolism, fetal growth and programming for chronic disease. *European Journal of Clinical Nutrition* 68, no. 1 (2013): 2–7.

Sachan, A, Gupta, R, Das, V et al. High prevalence of vitamin D deficiency among pregnant women and their newborns in northern India. *American Journal of Clinical Nutrition* 81, no. 5 (2005): 1060–1064.

Schjoldager, JG, Paidi, MD, Lindblad, MM et al. Maternal vitamin C deficiency during pregnancy results in transient fetal and placental growth retardation in guinea pigs. *European Journal of Nutrition* 54, no. 4 (2014): 667–676.

Schlotz, W, Jones, A, Phillips, DI et al. Lower maternal folate status in early pregnancy is associated with childhood hyperactivity and peer problems in offspring. *Journal of Child Psychology and Psychiatry* 51, no. 5 (2009): 594–602.

Sight and Life: Micronutrients; macro impact, the story of vitamins and a hungry world. *Sightandlife.Org*, 2011. http://www.sightandlife.org.

Sørensen, IM, Joner, G, Jenum, PA et al. Maternal serum levels of 25-hydroxy-vitamin D during pregnancy and risk of type 1 diabetes in the offspring. *Diabetes* 61, no. 1 (2011): 175–178.

Srinivasan, K, Thomas, T, Kapanee, AR et al. Effects of maternal vitamin B_{12} supplementation on early infant neurocognitive outcomes: A randomized controlled clinical trial. *Maternal & Child Nutrition* (2016), doi: 10.1111/mcn.12325. [Epub ahead of print].

Steegers-Theunissen, RPM, Twigt, J, Pestinger, V, Sinclair, KD. The periconceptional period, reproduction and long-term health of offspring: The importance of one-carbon metabolism. *Human Reproduction Update* 19, no. 6 (2013): 640–655.

Steenweg-de Graaff, J, Ghassabian, A, Jaddoe, VWV, Tiemeier, H, Roza, SJ. Folate concentrations during pregnancy and autistic traits in the offspring. The Generation R Study. *European Journal of Public Health* 25, no. 3 (2014): 431–433.

Stewart, CP, Christian, P, Katz, J et al. Maternal supplementation with vitamin A or B-carotene and cardiovascular risk factors among pre-adolescent children in rural Nepal. *Journal of Developmental Origins of Health and Disease* 1, no. 4 (2010): 262–270.

Stewart, CP, Christian, P, LeClerq, SC et al. Antenatal supplementation with folic acid + iron + zinc improves linear growth and reduces peripheral adiposity in school-age children in rural Nepal. *American Journal of Clinical Nutrition* 90, no. 1 (2009): 132–140.

Stewart, CP, Christian, P, Schulze, KJ et al. Low maternal vitamin B-12 status is associated with offspring insulin resistance regardless of antenatal micronutrient supplementation in rural Nepal. *Journal of Nutrition* 141, no. 10 (2011): 1912–1917.

Sukumar, N, Rafnsson, SB, Kandala, N-B et al. Prevalence of vitamin B-12 insufficiency during pregnancy and its effect on offspring birth weight: A systematic review and meta-analysis. *American Journal of Clinical Nutrition* 103, no. 5 (2016): 1232–1251.

(SUMMIT) Study Group, Shankar, AH, Jahari, AB et al. Effect of maternal multiple micronutrient supplementation on fetal loss and infant death in Indonesia: A double-blind cluster-randomised trial. *Lancet* 371, no. 9608 (2008): 215–227.

Surén, P, Roth, C, Bresnahan, M et al. Association between maternal use of folic acid supplements and risk of autism spectrum disorders in children. *JAMA* 309, no. 6 (2013): 570.

Veena, SR, Krishnaveni, GV, Srinivasan, K. Higher maternal plasma folate but not vitamin B-12 concentrations during pregnancy are associated with better cognitive function scores in 9- to 10-year-old children in South India. *Journal of Nutrition* 140, no. 5 (2010): 1014–1022.

Watanabe, F. Vitamin B_{12} sources and bioavailability. *Experimental Biology and Medicine* 232, no. 10 (2007): 1266–1274.

Waterland, RA, Jirtle, RL. Early nutrition, epigenetic changes at transposons and imprinted genes, and enhanced susceptibility to adult chronic diseases. *Nutrition* 20, no. 1 (2004): 63–68.

Waterland, RA, Kellermayer, R, Laritsky, E et al. Season of conception in rural Gambia affects DNA methylation at putative human metastable epialleles. *PLOS Genetics* 6, no. 12 (2010): e1001252.

West, KP Jr, Katz, J, Khatry, SK et al. Double blind, cluster randomised trial of low dose supplementation with vitamin A or beta carotene on mortality related to pregnancy in Nepal. *BMJ* 318, no. 7183 (2003): 570–575.

West, KP, Christian, P, Labrique, AB et al. Effects of vitamin A or beta carotene supplementation on pregnancy-related mortality and infant mortality in rural Bangladesh. *JAMA* 305, no. 19 (2011).

Yajnik, C, Chandak, G, Joglekar, C et al. Maternal homocysteine in pregnancy and offspring birthweight: Epidemiological associations and Mendelian randomization analysis. *International Journal of Epidemiology* 43, no. 5 (2014): 1487–1497.

Yajnik, C, Deshpande, S, Jackson, A et al. Vitamin B12 and folate concentrations during pregnancy and insulin resistance in the offspring: The Pune Maternal Nutrition Study. *Diabetologia* 51, no. 1 (2008): 29–38.

Yajnik, C. Early life origins of insulin resistance and type 2 diabetes in India and other Asian countries. *Journal of Nutrition* 134, no. 1 (2004): 205–210.

Yajnik, CS, Deshmukh, US. Fetal programming: Maternal nutrition and role of one-carbon metabolism. *Reviews in Endocrine and Metabolic Disorders* 13, no. 2 (2012): 121–127.

Yajnik, CS, Kelkar, R, Joshi, S et al. Lifecourse associations of body fat patterns with diabetes and cardiovascular risk factors. ADA poster. 2015.

12 Developmental Programming of Insulin Resistance

Charlotte Brøns and Louise Groth Grunnet

CONTENTS

12.1 INTRODUCTION

According to the World Health Organization (WHO), diabetes is on a global scale affecting approximately 300 million people, and the prevalence of diabetes is increasing worldwide, constituting a major threat to human health as the predictable global increase is as high as 35% (Shaw et al. 2010; Wild et al. 2004). Type 2 diabetes (T2D) accounts for more than 90% of all diabetes cases (Zimmet et al. 2001). The pathophysiology of T2D involves multiple metabolic alterations and is characterized by peripheral (muscle) insulin resistance, hepatic insulin resistance, and impaired insulin secretion from the pancreatic β-cells (DeFronzo 2004). However, the order of their occurrence and the relative impact of these defects on glucose metabolism in T2D are controversial and may depend on the dominant underlying etiology. However, T2D is a multifactorial disease occurring as a result of a complicated interplay between genetic and both prenatal and postnatal environmental factors that influence several different aspects of glucose homeostasis (Defronzo 1992; Kahn 1986, 2003; Beck-Nielsen and Groop 1994). Familial aggregation of T2D has been widely demonstrated (Groop 1996; Bennett 1999; Lillioja et al. 1987), and a higher concordance rate for T2D has been found in monozygotic as compared to dizygotic twin pairs (Poulsen et al. 1999). Genome-wide association (GWA) studies have recently identified a number of novel T2D susceptibility genes; however, only up to 10% of the risk of T2D can be explained by these genes (Zeggini et al. 2008; Lango et al. 2008; Ahlqvist et al. 2011). The high prevalence of T2D and obesity in developing countries, where populations have experienced migration from rural areas to urban city life, suggests that environmental factors related to a westernized lifestyle are involved (Zimmet et al. 2001; Zimmet 1999). Interaction between genetic and nongenetic factors responsible for the development of T2D may be complex and involve epigenetic factors (Ling et al. 2007). The increased risk of insulin resistance and T2D that is associated with low birth weight (LBW) has been suggested to result from altered gene regulation patterns due to epigenetic modifications of fetal developmental genes as well as additional postnatal environmental stress factors (Woo and Patti 2008).

Epidemiologic data have shown a strong association between intrauterine growth retardation resulting in a LBW and increased risk of insulin resistance and T2D later in life (Hales et al. 1991; Valdez et al. 1994; Hales and Barker 2001). Recently, a large cross-sectional population-based study on 1458 women and 1088 men aged between 35 and 75 years showed that middle-aged adults with LBW present a higher prevalence of diabetes and obesity (Jornayvaz et al. 2016). There is convincing evidence to support the hypothesis of developmental origin of adult disease (Hales and Barker 1992, 2001; Barker et al. 1993), suggesting that a nutritional insult and/or other maternal insults, at a critical period of fetal growth, can alter the structure and/or function of an organ and consequently affect metabolic processes permanently. It has been suggested that the long-term consequences may be especially harmful if there is a divergence between nutrient supply in the early-life environment and the postnatal environment. This may be a particular problem in societies undergoing rapid economic and/or social changes.

12.2 TWIN STUDIES AS A MODEL FOR FETAL PROGRAMMING

In addition to individuals subjected to intrauterine growth retardation and thus born with LBW, twins have also often been used as a model to study the impact of fetal programming. About 2% of all births in Denmark are twin births. Two-thirds of the twin gestations are dizygotic twins and developed from the fertilization of two egg cells and therefore are genetically no more similar than siblings born after separate pregnancies. Each embryo has its own amnion, chorion, and placenta. The remaining one-third are monozygotic twins who develop from a single fertilized egg cell and are therefore genetically identical. Two-thirds of all monozygotic twins are monochorionic and diamniotic and about a third are dichorionic diamniotic, as the dizygotic twins (Hall 2003). Thus, being a monozygotic twin is especially associated with possible limited nutritional supply and limited space, and the hypothesis is, therefore, that monozygotic twins have had a more adverse intrauterine environment than dizygotic twins and that twins are more predisposed to develop metabolic diseases due to an unfavorable intrauterine programming as compared with singletons.

Since monozygotic twins have identical genotypes, twin studies have widely been used to estimate the heritability of a given trait. Heritability gives the proportion of the total variation of a trait attributable to genetic variation, and it is estimated by comparing the similarity of a given phenotype between monozygotic and dizygotic twin pairs (Neale 1992). Furthermore, twin studies can give a unique insight into whether associations between two traits are of genetic or nongenetic origin. Thus, any within-pair differences among monozygotic twins between birth weight and phenotypic traits are theoretically due to environmental factors and take into account the genetic influence and common environmental and maternal factors such as gestational age, parental height, weight, social class, and placental dysfunction.

There are some limitations that must be considered when working with, and interpreting data from, twin studies. One issue to consider when working with twins is whether results from twin studies can be generalized to the background population. Fetal growth among twins may differ from fetal growth of singletons and may not be regulated by the same mechanisms as in singletons. Twins are on average 0.8–0.9 kg lighter than singletons at birth; they are delivered 2–3 weeks earlier and do often show catch-up growth (Leon 2001). Studies have shown that fetal growth of twins resembles that of singletons until the last trimester, after which a decline in growth rate is seen among the twins (Ong et al. 2002; Harrison et al. 1993). Furthermore, it is unknown whether the putative effect of intrauterine growth restriction on the development of adult diseases is comparable in twins and singletons (Phillips 1993). However, no evidence of increased mortality in twins as compared with the general population has been observed (Vagero and Leon 1994; Christensen et al. 1995), and the quantitative impact of birth weight on blood pressure does not seem to differ between twins and singletons (McNeill et al. 2004).

12.3 LOW BIRTH WEIGHT AS A MODEL

Fetal growth and development is influenced by a genetically determined growth potential and by multiple nongenetic maternal, fetal, placental, and external environmental factors. Fetal malnutrition may be caused by several factors of different nature and amplitude (Figure 12.1) (Vaag et al. 2012). However, since adverse postnatal health is associated with compromised fetal growth, it is necessary to understand and identify factors involved in determining fetal size, and improved understanding of fetal growth may, therefore, have a significant impact on public health in general.

The relationship between maternal and fetal circulation is crucial for the efficient exchange of oxygen and nutrients dependent on uteroplacental blood flow and placental transport capacity. Consequently, reduced placental development and/or function limiting placental nutritional supply are associated with fetal growth restriction. Maternal nutrition is clearly considered a key determinant of fetal growth and development, but more often fetal growth and development is affected by nutrient imbalance, that is, malnutrition rather than true dietary deficiency—at least in the Western world. Furthermore, maternal nutrition prior to and around the time of conception and not only during pregnancy also influences fetal development. In addition, alcohol consumption, smoking, and use of drugs during pregnancy are also well-known contributors to poor birth outcomes and long-term developmental problems of varying amplitude.

Fetal programming in response to the previously mentioned insults may occur through multiple different mechanisms and at different time points during development. It may be brought about by an imbalance between nutrient demand and supply

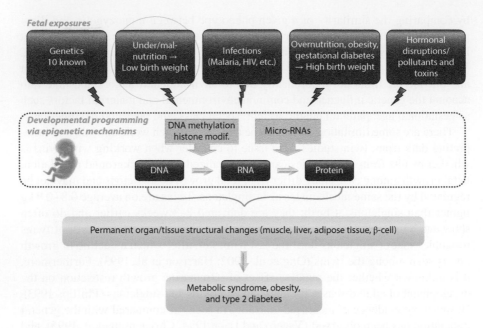

FIGURE 12.1   Fetal growth and development are influenced by a genetically determined growth potential and by multiple nongenetic maternal, fetal, placental, and external environmental factors.

causing metabolic and endocrine adaptations that benefit the fetus in the short term by reducing fetal growth, ensuring energy for brain development. However, this may cause permanent organ or tissue structural changes affecting organs and tissues such as the liver and pancreas as well as muscle and adipose tissues, which are of lower priority for nutrient partitioning during development and thus even more vulnerable (Figure 12.2) (Sutton et al. 2016). At a cellular level, programming can affect aspects of cell cycle dynamics and apoptosis, which may be reflected in numbers of cells, and at the subcellular level, telomere shortening and altered function of different enzyme systems have been demonstrated (Yajnik and Deshmukh 2008).

When studying adult human subjects, information about the reason for the LBW of the child is often unknown, and the LBW is thus merely a surrogate measure and an indicator and proxy of an unfavorable intrauterine milieu. Studies of intrauterine growth restriction in human individuals are for obvious reasons limited to observational and prospective studies. Cohorts exposed to famine during World War II and during the Chinese famine have, therefore, been studied extensively, and individuals who were *in utero* during periods of famine have provided a unique opportunity to study the effects of human maternal undernutrition during different periods of pregnancy (Li et al. 2010; Ravelli et al. 1998, 1999). In adulthood, both men and women who were exposed to famine *in utero* had significantly higher plasma glucose levels after a standard glucose tolerance test than those who were not exposed to famine *in utero*. Furthermore, there was a link between decreased glucose tolerance and decreased fetal growth for individuals exposed in late gestation as opposed to

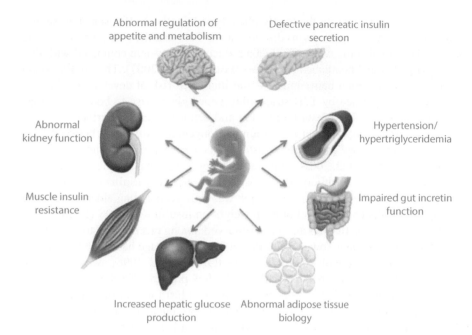

Abnormal regulation of appetite and metabolism

Defective pancreatic insulin secretion

Abnormal kidney function

Hypertension/ hypertriglyceridemia

Muscle insulin resistance

Impaired gut incretin function

Increased hepatic glucose production

Abnormal adipose tissue biology

FIGURE 12.2 The developmental origin of type 2 diabetes (T2D) explains the known multiple metabolic organ dysfunctions in T2D. (Reproduced from Vaag AA et al., *Diabetologia*, 55, 2085–2088, 2012. With permission.)

those exposed in early gestation and those not exposed to famine *in utero* (Ravelli et al. 1998).

The thrifty phenotype hypothesis formulated by Hales and Barker proposes that poor nutritional condition in early life programs a phenotype in later life, which to some extent may be beneficial to survival under poor nutritional conditions but detrimental when nutrition is abundant (Hales and Barker 2001). The long-term consequences may, therefore, be particularly harmful if there is a disagreement between nutrient supply in the early prenatal life and the postnatal environment.

12.4 INSULIN RESISTANCE IN PERIPHERAL (MUSCLE) TISSUE

Despite the substantial evidence linking early growth restriction with the subsequent development of insulin resistance and T2D, the molecular mechanisms underlying this association are not completely understood. Skeletal muscle mass accounts for the majority of insulin-stimulated whole-body glucose uptake, thereby making this tissue essential for the development of insulin resistance (Defronzo et al. 1981). Indeed, several abnormalities have been identified in insulin-resistant skeletal muscle, including impairment of insulin signaling (Schmitz-Peiffer 2000) and defective activation of glycogen synthase (Beck-Nielsen et al. 2003; Højlund et al. 2003) as well as a decreased ability of insulin to regulate fuel metabolism (Kelley and Mandarino 2000).

As proof of principle for the thrifty phenotype hypothesis, Poulsen et al. showed in a sample of monozygotic twins discordant for T2D that the twins who had developed T2D were also the twins who had a reduced birth weight compared with their genetically identical nondiabetic co-twins (Poulsen et al. 2007). This finding specifies that the association between LBW and increased risk of developing T2D may not solely be explained by T2D susceptibly genes giving rise to both a restrained fetal growth and reduced insulin secretion and action. By taking further advantage of the twin approach, Grunnet et al. found a nongenetic association between LBW and glucose intolerance and insulin resistance in elderly twins independent of degree of obesity (Grunnet et al. 2007). This was also confirmed in a sample of nondiabetic twins where insulin sensitivity was measured by the hyperinsulinemic euglycemic clamp technique. However, the association was only seen among elderly twins suggesting an age-dependent effect of birth weight on insulin sensitivity (Poulsen et al. 2002), a phenomenon that has also been observed among rats exposed to intrauterine growth restriction due to low protein, that at 3 months of age had improved glucose tolerance as compared with control offspring (Ozanne et al. 1996), whereas the glucose tolerance was worse by 15 months in the low protein offspring (Ozanne et al. 2003). Consistent with that, no association between birth weight standard deviation score and insulin action was seen among young twins, but an inverse association was found between fetal growth velocity during the third trimester and insulin action (Pilgaard et al. 2011), emphasizing the age-dependent impact. Frost et al. examined the impact of birth weight on insulin secretion and action in a selected group of monozygotic twins with the most extreme intrapair difference in birth weight. Within a twin pair, they did not find any difference in insulin action between the twins with the highest versus the lowest birth weight (Frost et al. 2012), which may be due to the U-shaped curve between birth weight and increased risk of developing metabolic disease, including T2D (Harder et al. 2007).

Brøns et al. have shown that healthy, young individuals born with LBW have a 30% lower insulin-stimulated rate of glycolytic flux, while the insulin-stimulated peripheral whole-body glucose disposal as well as substrate oxidation rates remained normal (Brøns et al. 2008). The glycolytic flux, as measured by the use of 3-H^3-glucose infusion during the clamp, is the amount of glucose that is either oxidized in the citric acid cycle (tricarboxylic acid [TCA]) or released as lactate representing the nonoxidative glycolytic flux. In support of our data, it was previously suggested that insulin resistance in subjects with LBW primarily involved an impairment of glycolysis (Taylor et al. 1995), and Jensen et al. did earlier find reduced glycolytic flux in LBW subjects during a hyperinsulinemic euglycemic clamp examination as well (Jensen et al. 2002). This finding of a reduced glycolytic flux is indicative of a primary defect associated with LBW foregoing and potentially leading to insulin resistance and T2D. Impairment of insulin-stimulated glycolysis has previously been shown to precede insulin resistance in animal studies (Kim et al. 1996; Kim and Youn 1997). Furthermore, there are data to suggest that LBW is associated with normal or even improved insulin action at a young age, and that insulin resistance occurs later in life, as demonstrated in twins where increasing age may be an important factor unmasking the effect of a deprived fetal environment on glucose metabolism (Poulsen and Vaag 2006).

12.5 HEPATIC INSULIN RESISTANCE

Nonalcoholic fatty liver disease (NAFLD) is caused by ectopic lipid accumulation in the liver and is characterized by steatosis due to hepatic triglyceride accumulation possibly serving as a protective mechanism against lipotoxicity (Cusi 2012). NAFLD affects up to 30% of the general population and is thus the most common liver disease, and it is defined as steatosis in 5–10% of the hepatocytes (Ahmed 2015). NAFLD occurs as a result of dysregulated lipid homeostasis. Insulin resistance resulting in increased *de novo* hepatic fatty acid lipogenesis and excessive fatty acid influx into the liver due to increased adipose tissue lipolysis is the major driving force for hepatic steatosis, and NAFLD is considered to be the hepatic component of the metabolic syndrome (Levene and Goldin 2012).

When using an approach comparing twins with singletons, Poulsen et al. found that elderly twins had higher basal and insulin-stimulated hepatic glucose production—an indication of hepatic insulin resistance—as compared to singletons (Poulsen and Vaag 2006). Association between LBW and NAFLD has also been shown in both human and animal studies (Desai et al. 2005; Nobili et al. 2008; Alisi et al. 2011), and in spite of undernourishment, LBW rat fetuses have excess lipid accumulation in the embryonic liver, suggesting gestational programming of NAFLD (Yamada et al. 2011). However, it is unclear whether this fatty liver development is "programmed" or secondary to the accompanying obesity. Maternal protein restriction in rats produces hepatic alterations in the offspring, including liver dysfunction, structural changes, and increased lobule size, all similar to changes observed in T2D patients (Ozanne et al. 1996).

There are studies suggesting that hepatic insulin resistance may precede skeletal muscle insulin resistance, and it is, therefore, debated whether early ectopic lipid accumulation in the liver and concurrent hepatic insulin resistance are major contributing factors for the development of T2D. In elderly twins, total muscle triglyceride content was not associated with peripheral insulin sensitivity but only with hepatic insulin resistance, suggesting that muscle triglyceride content reflects the general ectopic accumulation of triglycerides, including fat in the liver (Grunnet et al. 2012). This theory is further supported by a study showing that liver fat content measured by ^1H magnetic resonance spectroscopy was negatively correlated with insulin sensitivity in overweight men (van Herpen et al. 2011). Mice exhibiting a genetic inactivation of adipose triglyceride lipase disproved the hypothesis that triglyceride accumulation *per se* causes lipotoxicity and insulin resistance because these mice have both increased insulin sensitivity and glucose tolerance despite increased triglyceride levels in muscle and liver (Haemmerle et al. 2006). Dufour et al. showed that healthy young lean individuals born with LBW, and therefore, at increased risk of developing T2D compared to the background population, exhibited both hepatic and muscle insulin resistance independent of ectopic lipid accumulation in these organs (Dufour and Petersen 2011). In addition, when young men are overfed with a high-fat diet for only 5 days, they become insulin resistant in the liver, whereas peripheral tissue as mainly reflected by the muscles does not become insulin resistant (Brøns et al. 2012), thus providing new evidence to imply that increased hepatic lipid infiltration possibly occurs early in the pathogenesis of insulin resistance. Altogether, the role of ectopic fat in the development of insulin resistance and T2D points toward a central role of the liver as opposed to the muscle, particularly in the early pathogenesis of T2D.

12.6 INSULIN RESISTANCE IN THE SUBCUTANEOUS ADIPOSE TISSUE

It is widely acknowledged that the white adipose tissue exhibits multiple important metabolic and endocrine functions and plays a key role in regulation of the energy metabolism. Obesity is associated with changes of adipose tissue functions, which lead to an increased release of fatty acids, hormones, and proinflammatory molecules contributing to increased risk of insulin resistance and T2D.

The "adipose tissue expandability" hypothesis proposes that it is a limited capacity or a dysregulation of the adipose tissue expansion, rather than obesity *per se*, which explains the link between a positive energy balance and T2D (Lafontan 2014). All individuals possess a maximum capacity for adipose expansion determined by both genetic and environmental factors. Once this expansion limit is reached, adipose tissue ceases to store energy efficiently and lipids accumulate ectopically in nonadipocyte cells in other tissues. This phenomenon where accumulating lipids are causing lipotoxic insults, including insulin resistance, apoptosis, and inflammation, is referred to as lipotoxicity (Moreno-Indias and Tinahones 2015).

In addition to limited expandability, patients with insulin resistance and T2D generally display defects in adipocyte fatty acid metabolism and exhibit an increased rate of lipolysis, releasing free fatty acids (FFAs) into the circulation resulting in elevated plasma concentrations (Boden and Shulman 2002; Boden 2003). Altogether, the importance of normal adipose tissue development and that disturbances of adipose tissue function can result in features of T2D are well documented, supporting the adipose tissue expandability hypothesis. The importance of the adipose tissue, and especially the dynamics of adipose tissue turnover, has furthermore been illustrated by Arner et al. who showed that the lipid removal rate was positively associated with the capacity of adipocytes to break down triglycerides and inversely associated with insulin resistance in human subjects independently of the degree of obesity (Arner and Spalding 2010; Arner et al. 2011).

De Zegher et al. found that fetal growth restriction was associated with increased circulating levels of preadipocyte factor 1 (Pref-1), which inhibit adipocyte differentiation (de Zegher et al. 2012). These data suggest that Pref-1 may be a mediator of reduced adipocyte differentiation in growth-restrained fetuses and thus of a reduction in lifelong lipid-storage capacity and thereby of adult vulnerability to metabolic disease, once lipid storage becomes an issue. Following this line of thinking, Sebastiani et al. showed that 6-year-old small for gestational age (SGA) children with normal height and weight have more hepatic fat than appropriate for gestational age (AGA) children of comparable size (Sebastiani et al. 2015). Supporting the hypothesis of limited adipose tissue expandability as one reason for lipotoxicity, the authors here propose that a postnatal reduction of subcutaneous adipogenesis, followed by hyperexpansion and subsequent overfilling of subcutaneous adipocytes due to postnatal catch-up growth, may be among the mechanisms predisposing SGA children to excessive lipid storage in other organs, including in the liver (Sebastiani et al. 2015).

In adult, lean, and healthy LBW men, it has previously been shown that they exhibit increased whole-body lipolysis as well as increased lipolysis of the subcutaneous adipose tissue, possibly representing a primary metabolic defect contributing to the development of insulin resistance and perhaps later T2D (Alibegovic et al. 2010; Højbjerre et al. 2011). In addition, an inverse association between birth weight and visceral adipose tissue was found in young twins examined by magnetic resonance spectroscopy (Pilgaard et al. 2011), supporting fetal programming as a player of an adverse adipose tissue distribution later in life. In contrast, another study found no difference in intramyocellular lipid or hepatic triglyceride content between LBW and normal birth weight (NBW) subjects despite the LBW individuals being insulin resistant (Dufour and Petersen 2011). Similarly, no difference in either intramyocellular or hepatic lipid content was observed in a study of young Indian men born with LBW (<2450 g) (Livingstone et al. 2016).

Adipocytes from 3-month-old low protein rat offspring have an elevated basal and insulin-stimulated glucose uptake, and like findings in muscle, liver adipocytes at this age express more insulin receptors than the control animals (Ozanne et al. 1997). With regard to adipose tissue expandability, in a study of human subjects and rats exposed to suboptimal nutrition during fetal life, it has been shown that an increase in the *in vivo* expression of the microRNA (miRNA) miR-483-3p, programmed by early life nutrition, limits the storage of lipids in adipose tissue via translational repression of the growth differentiation factor-3 (GDF3) (Ferland-McCollough et al. 2012). Dysregulation of miR-483-3p expression could possibly affect whole-body physiology by constraining adipose tissue expandability and therefore lipid

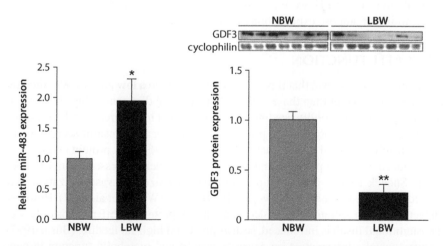

FIGURE 12.3 Programming of adipose tissue miR-483-3p and growth/differentiation factor-3 (GDF-3) expression by maternal diet in T2D. The consequence of upregulating miR-483-3p is a dysregulated expression of one of its targets GDF3 leading to an inhibition of adipocyte differentiation and maturation. This suggests that this could limit the capacity of adipose tissue to store lipids, leading to ectopic triglyceride deposition, insulin resistance, and T2D. (Reproduced from Ferland-McCollough D et al., *Cell Death Differ*, 19, 1003–1012, 2012. With permission.)

storage, promoting ectopic triglyceride storage and lipotoxicity in other tissues and thus increasing susceptibility to metabolic disease (Figure 12.3).

Schultz et al. recently found immaturity of preadipocyte stem cells from LBW subjects, reflected by impaired leptin protein synthesis and mRNA expression in these cells, which in turn was shown to be associated with a significantly increased degree of DNA methylation of the leptin promoter in the preadipocytes from LBW subjects (Schultz et al. 2013). This provides evidence of a prime role for immature adipose tissue stem cell function in the developmental programming of T2D possibly mediated by early defects in the adipose tissue and a reduced expandability resulting in ectopic lipid storage, lipotoxicity, and insulin resistance.

During pregnancy, the adipose tissue must expand rapidly in order to meet the needs for the growing fetus but also to support the future needs of the offspring through lactation. Rojas-Rodriguez et al. showed that women with gestational diabetes had greater adipocyte size and decreased capillary density in the omental fat as compared with women with a normal glucose tolerance test during pregnancy, indicating an impaired adipose tissue expandability in gestational diabetes (Rojas-Rodriguez et al. 2015). In addition, it was recently shown that the progenitor density (and thus the source of new adipocytes) was lower and accompanied by limited expansion of adipocyte number when challenged with a high-fat diet in 3-month-old rat offspring of maternal obese dams as compared with offspring of control dams. This was associated with lower DNA methylation of the zinc finger protein 423 (involved in adipogenesis) in the epididymal fat in the offspring of obese dams (Liang et al. 2016), suggesting a focus on epigenetic changes in adipocyte progenitors when looking for possible mechanisms in fetal programming of an obesogenic maternal environment. However, today, very limited knowledge exists on the fetal programming of adipose expandability in humans.

12.7 β-CELL FUNCTION

Studies in rats have shown that if pregnant dams were fed a low protein (8%) diet, the offspring were smaller than those of dams fed a control diet containing 20% protein (Hattersley and Tooke 1999). Feeding a low protein diet to the pregnant dam restricts fetal development, as protein is a primary stimulus for fetal insulin secretion, and because insulin is a fetal growth factor (Desai et al. 1996). Low protein rat offspring has a reduced weight of pancreas and muscle—even when expressed relative to body weight (Snoeck 1990)—and β-cell proliferation, islet size, and vascularization were reduced in pancreas of newborn low protein offspring (Wilson et al. 1997). However, a defect in insulin secretion from islets of adult low protein rat offspring is only seen when additional insult is introduced, such as postnatal high-fat feeding (Burns 1997).

Unfortunately, information on pancreas weight and metabolic function in newborns is not available in human studies. However, it is well known that abnormalities in insulin secretion are an important determinant of T2D and other states of glucose intolerance, and most cases of early T2D and obesity are associated with either normal or significantly increased plasma insulin concentrations (Pacini 2006; Leahy 2005). The development of obesity as well as the progression to overt T2D usually involves an intake of an energy-dense diet, and insulin secretion increases under such conditions to accommodate for the storage of excess glucose and fatty acids. β-cell failure is characterized by the inability of the β-cell to secrete sufficient insulin in response to glucose, which ultimately results in hyperglycemia. The glucose transporter GLUT-2 and the glucose phosphorylating enzyme glucokinase are both essential for glucose sensing of the pancreatic β-cell, the initial event in the pathway for glucose-stimulated insulin secretion (Reimer and Ahren 2002). A study by Jensen et al. investigated insulin secretion during both an oral and intravenous glucose tolerance test and found no differences in absolute insulin secretion between LBW and NBW subjects. However, when the corresponding insulin sensitivity was accounted for, the LBW subjects had approximately 30% reduced insulin secretion compared with the NBW subjects (Jensen et al. 2002). In healthy individuals with normal glucose tolerance, a reduction in insulin sensitivity is normally accompanied by a compensatory upregulation of insulin secretion. Simplified, this relationship between insulin sensitivity and insulin secretion is thought to be approximately hyperbolic so that the product of the two variables is constant for individuals with the same degree of glucose tolerance (Kahn et al. 1993). This is commonly known as the disposition index and therefore highlights the importance of taking insulin sensitivity into account when examining the β-cell function. In normal glucose-tolerant Pima Indians, a reduced insulin secretory capacity in LBW subjects was found, again only significant when adjusted for the degree of insulin sensitivity (Stefan et al. 2004).

In a study by Brøns et al. both LBW and NBW subjects had a significantly elevated incremental insulin response when challenged by a high-fat overfeeding diet. However, only the LBW subjects exhibited peripheral insulin resistance when overfed, suggesting that the increased insulin secretion was a compensation for the decreased whole-body insulin sensitivity (Brøns et al. 2009). Additional, a study by Storgaard et al. showed that after being exposed to a prolonged FFA infusion both the LBW and NBW subjects had an appropriate increase in insulin secretion that matched the decline in insulin sensitivity (Jensen et al. 2005). When LBW subjects are exposed to an inactivity challenge, significantly higher levels of fasting plasma insulin and C-peptide were seen in LBW subjects on the first day of bed rest exposure. However, both before and after the intervention, insulin secretion, expressed in relation to the degree of peripheral insulin action, was similar in the LBW and NBW subjects (Alibegovic et al. 2010). Thus, combined, it seems that LBW subjects have higher baseline insulin secretion as a compensatory mechanism for reduced insulin sensitivity, whereas the LBW subjects are not more susceptible to diabetogenic exposures such as energy dense diet or inactivity with regard to insulin secretion.

12.8 POSSIBLE UNDERLYING MECHANISMS

The association between fetal programming and later development of metabolic disturbances and T2D has been suggested to be explained by epigenetic mechanisms. Epigenetics refer to the study of changes in gene function caused by mechanisms other than changes in the actual, underlying DNA sequence. Epigenetic mechanisms include DNA methylations and histone modifications and these epigenetic mechanisms can be affected by miRNAs (Ling and Groop 2009). DNA methylation and histone modifications affect the DNA at the transcriptional level. miRNAs are members of a large class of noncoding RNAs of approximately 22 nucleotides in length, which regulates the translation of miRNAs into protein. The majority of evidence linking specific environmental exposures *in utero* with epigenetic changes in progeny come from animal models, or observational human studies. One important human study is the Dutch hunger winter study investigating the impact of famine during World War II in the Netherlands. The study showed that individuals who were prenatally exposed to famine had, six decades later, less DNA methylation of the imprinted insulin-like growth factor 2 (*IGF2*) gene compared with their unexposed, same sex siblings supporting that early life environmental conditions can cause epigenetic changes in humans that persist throughout life (Heijmans et al. 2008). It has been demonstrated that the fetal environment affects epigenetic prints in adult differentiated tissues, including skeletal muscle and subcutaneous fat (Brøns et al. 2010; Gillberg et al. 2014), thereby reinforcing the fetal life as a critical time for establishment and maintenance of epigenetic marks. For instance, it is shown that young LBW men exhibit increased methylation in the promoter region of the transcription factor peroxisome proliferator-activated receptor gamma coactivator 1-alpha (PGC1α) in skeletal muscle (Brøns et al. 2010). Furthermore, Jacobsen et al. investigated global DNA methylation in muscle and fat biopsies obtained from NBW controls and LBWs following 5 days of overfeeding. Overfeeding induced widespread DNA methylation changes in NBW controls affecting genes involved in inflammation, reproduction, and cancer (Jacobsen et al. 2012). However, similar short-term changes in DNA methylations were not seen in LBW subjects, suggesting that inflexibility of short-term changes of DNA methylations in response to high-fat diet may represent an epigenetic trait potentially contributing to the increased risk of developing T2D later in life among subjects born with LBW (Figure 12.1) (Jacobsen et al. 2014).

However, when global DNA methylation was examined in monozygotic twins discordant for T2D no difference in methylation patterns was found between the diabetic and nondiabetic twins in either fat or muscle tissue (Ribel-Madsen et al. 2012); thus global DNA methylation had a modest contribution to the nongenetic component of insulin resistance in these twins. Even though no global DNA methylation differences were found, a number of differences were found in known T2D-related candidate genes between the diabetic and nondiabetic twin. Another study examined twins discordant for birth weight and found that intrauterine growth differences were associated with DNA methylation changes in the IGFR1 (Tsai et al. 2015) that plays a role in childhood growth and anabolic processes.

Bork-Jensen et al. identified 20 differentially regulated miRNAs in skeletal muscle biopsies from monozygotic twins with T2D compared with their genetically identical co-twins (Bork-Jensen et al. 2015). The two most significant miRNAs associated with T2D both belong to the miR-15 family with insulin-signaling proteins being their prime predicted targets. Importantly, we found that the miRNA expression levels were associated with LBW. In another study, differential expression of mir-483 in fat biopsies from LBW subjects as well as in rats that have been protein undernourished in fetal life (Ferland-McCollough et al. 2012) was found. The increased mir-483 in LBW human subjects was associated with impaired maturation of subcutaneous fat due to reduced expression of GDF3, which promotes adipocyte differentiation (Ferland-McCollough et al. 2012).

There is also evidence to suggest that muscle and fat stem cells are involved in mediating the association between fetal programming and later risk of disease. As muscle and fat stem cells are "remnants" of the embryonic environment they could turn out to be the key entry point to investigate the effects of the intrauterine environment on adult metabolic tissues. Muscle and fat stem cells are formed during fetal life and reside quiescent in adult tissues (Charge and Rudnicki 2004; Laharrague and Casteilla 2010). Muscle and fat stem cell determination and differentiation are controlled by epigenetic mechanisms, involving DNA methylations and histone acetylations as well as small noncoding miRNAs (Ge 2012; Sousa-Victor et al. 2011). The epigenome is established early in development, during a time period where environmental insults such as different types of *in utero* stress are able to influence the developmental trajectories. Altered epigenetic regulations are, therefore, mechanisms, which could underlie programmed changes in adipose and muscle tissue in the offspring. Schultz et al. recently provided evidence of a prime role for immature adipose tissue stem cell functions, including impaired leptin release associated with increased leptin gene promoter DNA methylation among LBW subjects (Schultz et al. 2013).

12.9 CONCLUDING REMARKS

There are currently around 300 million people worldwide suffering from T2D. A mismatch between impaired development in fetal life and overfeeding combined with low physical activity throughout life, as seen in westernized societies and also in developing countries, is likely to represent the most unfortunate combination and scenario responsible for the development of T2D and its complications. Future studies should provide a transdisciplinary study approach to understand the magnitude of such a mismatch as well as the underlying physiological and molecular mechanisms involved. Understanding the mechanisms of developmental programming may lead to novel and more sustainable strategies to prevent T2D in an intergenerational manner so we can improve our knowledge about how to break the vicious cycle responsible for the current propagation of T2D all over the world.

REFERENCES

Ahlqvist E, Ahluwalia TS, Groop L. Genetics of type 2 diabetes. *Clin Chem* 2011;57(2): 241–254.

Ahmed M. Non-alcoholic fatty liver disease in 2015. *World J Hepatol* 2015;7(11):1450–1459.

Alibegovic AC, Højbjerre L, Sonne MP et al. Increased rate of whole body lipolysis before and after 9 days of bed rest in healthy young men born with low birth weight. *Am J Physiol Endocrinol Metab* 2010;298(3):E555–E564.

Alisi A, Panera N, Agostoni C, Nobili V. Intrauterine growth retardation and nonalcoholic Fatty liver disease in children. *Int J Endocrinol* 2011;2011:269853.

Arner P, Bernard S, Salehpour M et al. Dynamics of human adipose lipid turnover in health and metabolic disease. *Nature* 2011;478(7367):110–113.

Arner P, Spalding KL. Fat cell turnover in humans. *Biochem Biophys Res Commun* 2010;396(1):101–104.

Barker DJ, Hales CN, Fall CH, Osmond C, Phipps K, Clark PM. Type 2 (non-insulin-dependent) diabetes mellitus, hypertension and hyperlipidaemia (syndrome X): Relation to reduced fetal growth. *Diabetologia* 1993;36(1):62–67.

Beck-Nielsen H, Groop LC. Metabolic and genetic characterization of prediabetic states. Sequence of events leading to non-insulin-dependent diabetes mellitus. *J Clin Invest* 1994;94(5):1714–1721.

Beck-Nielsen H, Vaag A, Poulsen P, Gaster M. Metabolic and genetic influence on glucose metabolism in type 2 diabetic subjects—Experiences from relatives and twin studies. *Best Pract Res Clin Endocrinol Metab* 2003;17(3):445–467.

Bennett PH. Type 2 diabetes among the Pima Indians of Arizona: An epidemic attributable to environmental change? *Nutr Rev* 1999;57(5 Pt 2):S51–S54.

Boden G, Shulman GI. Free fatty acids in obesity and type 2 diabetes: Defining their role in the development of insulin resistance and beta-cell dysfunction. *Eur J Clin Invest* 2002;32(s3):14–23.

Boden G. Effects of free fatty acids (FFA) on glucose metabolism: Significance for insulin resistance and type 2 diabetes. *Exp Clin Endocrinol Diabetes* 2003;111:121–124.

Bork-Jensen J, Scheele C, Christophersen DV et al. Glucose tolerance is associated with differential expression of microRNAs in skeletal muscle: Results from studies of twins with and without type 2 diabetes. *Diabetologia* 2015;58(2):363–373.

Brøns C, Jacobsen S, Hiscock N et al. Effects of high-fat overfeeding on mitochondrial function, glucose and fat metabolism, and adipokine levels in low-birth-weight subjects. *Am J Physiol Endocrinol Metab* 2012;302(1):E43–E51.

Brøns C, Jacobsen S, Nilsson E et al. Deoxyribonucleic acid methylation and gene expression of PPARGC1A in human muscle Is influenced by high-fat overfeeding in a birth-weight-dependent manner. *J Clin Endocrinol Metab* 2010;95(6):3048–3056.

Brøns C, Jensen CB, Storgaard H et al. Impact of short-term high-fat feeding on glucose and insulin metabolism in young healthy men. *J Physiol* 2009;587(10):2387–2397.

Brøns C, Jensen CB, Storgaard H et al. Mitochondrial function in skeletal muscle is normal and unrelated to insulin action in young men born with low birth weight. *J Clin Endocrinol Metab* 2008;93(10):3885–3892.

Burns SP. Gluconeogenesis, glucose handling, and structural changes in livers of the adult offspring of rats partially deprived of protein during pregnancy and lactation. *J Clin Invest* 1997;100(7):1768–1774.

Charge SB, Rudnicki MA. Cellular and molecular regulation of muscle regeneration. *Physiol Rev* 2004;84(1):209–238.

Christensen K, Vaupel JW, Holm NV, Yashin AI. Mortality among twins after age 6: Fetal origins hypothesis versus twin method. *BMJ* 1995;310(6977):432–436.

Cusi K. Role of obesity and lipotoxicity in the development of nonalcoholic steatohepatitis: Pathophysiology and clinical implications. *Gastroenterology* 2012;142(4):711–725.

de Zegher F, Diaz M, Sebastiani G et al. Abundance of circulating preadipocyte factor 1 in early life. *Diabetes Care* 2012;35(4):848–849.

Defronzo RA, Jacot E, Jequier E, Maeder E, Wahren J, Felber JP. The effect of insulin on the disposal of intravenous glucose. Results from indirect calorimetry and hepatic and femoral venous catheterization. *Diabetes* 1981;30(12):1000–1007.

Defronzo RA. Pathogenesis of type 2 (non-insulin dependent) diabetes mellitus: A balanced overview. *Diabetologia* 1992;35(4):389–397.

DeFronzo RA. Pathogenesis of type 2 diabetes mellitus. *Med Clin North Am* 2004;88(4):787–835.

Desai M, Crowther NJ, Lucas A, Hales CN. Organ-selective growth in the offspring of protein-restricted mothers. *Br J Nutr* 1996;76(4):591–603.

Desai M, Gayle D, Babu J, Ross MG. Programmed obesity in intrauterine growth-restricted newborns: Modulation by newborn nutrition. *Am J Physiol Regul Integr Comp Physiol* 2005;288(1):R91–R96.

Dufour S, Petersen KF. Disassociation of liver and muscle insulin resistance from ectopic lipid accumulation in low-birth-weight individuals. *J Clin Endocrinol Metab* 2011;96(12):3873–3880.

Ferland-McCollough D, Fernandez-Twinn DS, Cannell IG et al. Programming of adipose tissue miR-483-3p and GDF-3 expression by maternal diet in type 2 diabetes. *Cell Death Differ* 2012;19(6):1003–1012.

Frost M, Petersen I, Brixen K et al. Adult glucose metabolism in extremely birthweight-discordant monozygotic twins. *Diabetologia* 2012;55(12):3204–3212.

Ge K. Epigenetic regulation of adipogenesis by histone methylation. *Biochim Biophys Acta* 2012;1819(7):727–732.

Gillberg L, Jacobsen SC, Ronn T, Brøns C, Vaag A. PPARGC1A DNA methylation in subcutaneous adipose tissue in low birth weight subjects—Impact of 5 days of high-fat overfeeding. *Metabolism* 2014;63(2):263–271.

Groop L. Metabolic consequences of a family history of NIDDM (the Botnia study): Evidence for sex-specific parental effects. *Diabetes* 1996;45:1585–1593.

Grunnet L, Vielwerth S, Vaag A, Poulsen P. Birth weight is nongenetically associated with glucose intolerance in elderly twins, independent of adult obesity. *J Intern Med* 2007;262(1):96–103.

Grunnet LG, Laurila E, Hansson O et al. The triglyceride content in skeletal muscle is associated with hepatic but not peripheral insulin resistance in elderly twins. *J Clin Endocrinol Metab* 2012;97:4571–4577.

Haemmerle G, Lass A, Zimmermann R et al. Defective lipolysis and altered energy metabolism in mice lacking adipose triglyceride lipase. *Science* 2006;312(5774):734–737.

Hales CN, Barker DJ, Clark PM et al. Fetal and infant growth and impaired glucose tolerance at age 64. *BMJ* 1991;303(6809):1019–1022.

Hales CN, Barker DJP. The thrifty phenotype hypothesis: Type 2 diabetes. *Br Med Bull* 2001;60(1):5–20.

Hales CN, Barker DJP. Type 2 (non-insulin-dependent) diabetes mellitus: The thrifty phenotype hypothesis. *Diabetologia* 1992;35(7):595–601.

Hall JG. Twinning. *Lancet* 2003;362(9385):735–743.

Harder T, Rodekamp E, Schellong K, Dudenhausen JW, Plagemann A. Birth weight and subsequent risk of type 2 diabetes: A meta-analysis. *Am J Epidemiol* 2007;165(8):849–857.

Harrison SD, Cyr DR, Patten RM, Mack LA. Twin growth problems: Causes and sonographic analysis. *Semin Ultrasound CT MR* 1993;14(1):56–67.

Hattersley AT, Tooke JE. The fetal insulin hypothesis: An alternative explanation of the association of low birthweight with diabetes and vascular disease. *Lancet* 1999;353(9166):1789–1792.

Heijmans BT, Tobi EW, Stein AD et al. Persistent epigenetic differences associated with prenatal exposure to famine in humans. *Proc Natl Acad Sci* 2008;105(44):17046–17049.

Højbjerre L, Alibegovic AC, Sonne MP et al. Increased lipolysis but diminished gene expression of lipases in subcutaneous adipose tissue of healthy young males with intrauterine growth retardation. *J Appl Physiol* 2011;111(6):1863–1870.

Højlund K, Wrzesinski K, Larsen PM et al. Proteome analysis reveals phosphorylation of ATP synthase beta—Subunit in human skeletal muscle and proteins with potential roles in type 2 diabetes. *J Biol Chem* 2003;278(12):10436–10442.

Jacobsen SC, Brøns C, Bork-Jensen J et al. Effects of short-term high-fat overfeeding on genome-wide DNA methylation in the skeletal muscle of healthy young men. *Diabetologia* 2012;55(12):3341–3349.

Jacobsen SC, Gillberg L, Bork-Jensen J et al. Young men with low birthweight exhibit decreased plasticity of genome-wide muscle DNA methylation by high-fat overfeeding. *Diabetologia* 2014;57(6):1154–1158.

Jensen CB, Storgaard H, Dela F, Holst JJ, Madsbad S, Vaag AA. Early differential defects of insulin secretion and action in 19-year-old Caucasian men who had low birth weight. *Diabetes* 2002;51(4):1271–1280.

Jensen CB, Storgaard H, Holst JJ, Dela F, Madsbad S, Vaag A. Young, low-birth-weight men are not more susceptible to the diabetogenic effects of a prolonged free fatty acid exposure than matched controls. *Metabolism* 2005;54(10):1398–1406.

Jornayvaz FR, Vollenweider P, Bochud M, Mooser V, Waeber G, Marques-Vidal P. Low birth weight leads to obesity, diabetes and increased leptin levels in adults: The CoLaus study. *Cardiovasc Diabetol* 2016;15(1):73.

Kahn CR. Insulin resistance: A common feature of diabetes mellitus. *N Engl J Med* 1986;315(4):252–254.

Kahn SE, Prigeon RL, McCulloch DK et al. Quantification of the relationship between insulin sensitivity and beta-cell function in human subjects. Evidence for a hyperbolic function. *Diabetes* 1993;42(11):1663–1672.

Kahn SE. The relative contributions of insulin resistance and beta-cell dysfunction to the pathophysiology of Type 2 diabetes. *Diabetologia* 2003;46(1):3–19.

Kelley DE, Mandarino LJ. Fuel selection in human skeletal muscle in insulin resistance: A reexamination. *Diabetes* 2000;49(5):677–683.

Kim JK, Wi JK, Youn JH. Metabolic impairment precedes insulin resistance in skeletal muscle during high-fat feeding in rats. *Diabetes* 1996;45(5):651–658.

Kim JK, Youn JH. Prolonged suppression of glucose metabolism causes insulin resistance in rat skeletal muscle. *Am J Physiol* 1997;272(2 Pt 1):E288–E296.

Lafontan M. Adipose tissue and adipocyte dysregulation. *Diabetes Metab* 2014;40(1):16–28.

Laharrague P, Casteilla L. The emergence of adipocytes. *Endocr Dev* 2010;19:21–30.

Lango H, The UT, Palmer CN et al. Assessing the combined impact of 18 common genetic variants of modest effect sizes on type 2 diabetes risk. *Diabetes* 2008;db08–0504.

Leahy JL. Pathogenesis of type 2 diabetes mellitus. *Arch Med Res* 2005;36(3):197–209.

Leon DA. The foetal origins of adult disease: Interpreting the evidence from twin studies. *Twin Res* 2001;4(5):321–326.

Levene AP, Goldin RD. The epidemiology, pathogenesis and histopathology of fatty liver disease. *Histopathology* 2012;61(2):141–152.

Li Y, He Y, Qi L et al. Exposure to the Chinese famine in early life and the risk of hyperglycemia and type 2 diabetes in adulthood. *Diabetes* 2010;59(10):2400–2406.

Liang X, Yang Q, Fu X et al. Maternal obesity epigenetically alters visceral fat progenitor cell properties in male offspring mice. *J Physiol* 2016;594(15):4453–4466.

Lillioja S, Mott DM, Zawadzki JK et al. In vivo insulin action is familial characteristic in nondiabetic Pima Indians. *Diabetes* 1987;36(11):1329–1335.

Ling C, Groop L. Epigenetics: A molecular link between environmental factors and type 2 diabetes. *Diabetes* 2009;58(12):2718–2725.

Ling C, Poulsen P, Simonsson S et al. Genetic and epigenetic factors are associated with expression of respiratory chain component NDUFB6 in human skeletal muscle. *J Clin Invest* 2007;117(11):3427–3435.

Livingstone RS, Grunnet LG, Thomas N et al. Are hepatic and soleus lipid content, assessed by magnetic resonance spectroscopy, associated with low birth weight or insulin resistance in a rural Indian population of healthy young men? *Diabet Med* 2016;33(3):365–370.

McNeill G, Tuya C, Smith WC. The role of genetic and environmental factors in the association between birthweight and blood pressure: Evidence from meta-analysis of twin studies. *Int J Epidemiol* 2004;33(5):995–1001.

Moreno-Indias I, Tinahones FJ. Impaired adipose tissue expandability and lipogenic capacities as ones of the main causes of metabolic disorders. *J Diabetes Res* 2015;2015:970375.

Neale M. In *Methodology for Genetic Studies of Twins and Familes*. Nato ASI series. Boston, London: Kluwer Academic Publishers, Dordrecht; 1992:35–53.

Nobili V, Alisi A, Panera N, Agostoni C. Low birth weight and catch-up-growth associated with metabolic syndrome: A ten year systematic review. *Pediatr Endocrinol Rev* 2008;6(2):241–247.

Ong S, Lim MN, Fitzmaurice A, Campbell D, Smith AP, Smith N. The creation of twin centile curves for size. *BJOG* 2002;109(7):753–758.

Ozanne SE, Nave BT, Wang CL, Shepherd PR, Prins J, Smith GD. Poor fetal nutrition causes long-term changes in expression of insulin signaling components in adipocytes. *Am J Physiol Endocrinol Metab* 1997;273(1):E46–E51.

Ozanne SE, Olsen GS, Hansen LL et al. Early growth restriction leads to down regulation of protein kinase C zeta and insulin resistance in skeletal muscle. *J Endocrinol* 2003;177(2):235–241.

Ozanne SE, Wang CL, Coleman N, Smith GD. Altered muscle insulin sensitivity in the male offspring of protein-malnourished rats. *Am J Physiol Endocrinol Metab* 1996;271(6):E11 28–E1134.

Pacini G. The hyperbolic equilibrium between insulin sensitivity and secretion. *Nutr Metab Cardiovasc Dis* 2006;16(Suppl 1):S22–S27.

Phillips DI. Twin studies in medical research: Can they tell us whether diseases are genetically determined? *Lancet* 1993;341(8851):1008–1009.

Pilgaard K, Hammershaimb MT, Grunnet L et al. Differential nongenetic impact of birth weight versus third-trimester growth velocity on glucose metabolism and magnetic resonance imaging abdominal obesity in young healthy twins. *J Clin Endocrinol Metab* 2011;96(9):2835–2843.

Poulsen P, Levin K, Beck-Nielsen H, Vaag A. Age-dependent impact of zygosity and birth weight on insulin secretion and insulin action in twins. *Diabetologia* 2002;45(12):1649–1657.

Poulsen P, Ohm Kyvik K, Vaag A, Beck-Nielsen H. Heritability of Type II (non-insulin-dependent) diabetes mellitus and abnormal glucose tolerance—A population-based twin study. *Diabetologia* 1999;42(2):139–145.

Poulsen P, Vaag A. The intrauterine environment as reflected by birth size and twin and zygosity status influences insulin action and intracellular glucose metabolism in an age—Or time-dependent manner. *Diabetes* 2006;55(6):1819–1825.

Poulsen P, Wojtaszewski JFP, Richter EA, Beck-Nielsen H, Vaag A. Low birth weight and zygosity status is associated with defective muscle glycogen and glycogen synthase regulation in elderly twins. *Diabetes* 2007;56(11):2710–2714.

Ravelli AC, van der Meulen JH, Osmond C, Barker DJ, Bleker OP. Obesity at the age of 50 y in men and women exposed to famine prenatally. *Am J Clin Nutr* 1999;70(5):811–816.

Ravelli ACJ, van der Meulen JHP, Michels RPJ et al. Glucose tolerance in adults after prenatal exposure to famine. *Lancet* 1998;351(9097):173–177.

Reimer MK, Ahren B. Altered {beta}-cell distribution of pdx-1 and GLUT-2 after a short-term challenge with a high-fat diet in C57BL/6J mice. *Diabetes* 2002;51(90001):S138–S143.

Ribel-Madsen R, Fraga MF, Jacobsen S et al. Genome-wide analysis of DNA methylation differences in muscle and fat from monozygotic twins discordant for type 2 diabetes. *PLOS ONE* 2012;7(12):e51302.

Rojas-Rodriguez R, Lifshitz LM, Bellve KD et al. Human adipose tissue expansion in pregnancy is impaired in gestational diabetes mellitus. *Diabetologia* 2015;58(9):2106–2114.

Schmitz-Peiffer C. Signalling aspects of insulin resistance in skeletal muscle: Mechanisms induced by lipid oversupply. *Cell Signal* 2000;12(9–10):583–594.

Schultz NS, Broholm C, Gillberg L et al. Impaired leptin gene expression and release in cultured preadipocytes isolated from individuals born with low birth weight. *Diabetes* 2013;63(1):111–121.

Sebastiani G, Diaz M, Bassols J et al. The sequence of prenatal growth restraint and post-natal catch-up growth leads to a thicker intima-media and more pre-peritoneal and hepatic fat by age 3–6 years. *Pediatr Obes* 2015;11(4):251–257.

Shaw JE, Sicree RA, Zimmet PZ. Global estimates of the prevalence of diabetes for 2010 and 2030. *Diabetes Res Clin Pract* 2010;87(1):4–14.

Snoeck A. Effect of a low protein diet during pregnancy on the fetal rat endocrine pancreas. *Biol Neonate* 1990;57(2):107–118.

Sousa-Victor P, Munoz-Canoves P, Perdiguero E. Regulation of skeletal muscle stem cells through epigenetic mechanisms. *Toxicol Mech Methods* 2011;21(4):334–342.

Stefan N, Weyer C, Levy-Marchal C et al. Endogenous glucose production, insulin sensitivity, and insulin secretion in normal glucose-tolerant Pima Indians with low birth weight. *Metabolism* 2004;53(7):904–911.

Sutton EF, Gilmore LA, Dunger DB et al. Developmental programming: State-of-the-science and future directions-Summary from a Pennington Biomedical symposium. *Obesity* 2016;24(5):1018–1026.

Taylor DJ, Thompson CH, Kemp GJ et al. A relationship between impaired fetal growth and reduced muscle glycolysis revealed by 31P magnetic resonance spectroscopy. *Diabetologia* 1995;38(10):1205–1212.

Tsai PC, Van DJ, Tan Q et al. DNA methylation changes in the IGF1R gene in birth weight discordant adult monozygotic twins. *Twin Res Hum Genet* 2015;18(6):635–646.

Vaag AA, Grunnet LG, Arora GP, Brøns C. The thrifty phenotype hypothesis revisited. *Diabetologia* 2012;55(8):2085–2088.

Vagero D, Leon D. Ischaemic heart disease and low birth weight: A test of the fetal-origins hypothesis from the Swedish Twin Registry. *Lancet* 1994;343(8892):260–263.

Valdez R, Athens MA, Thompson GH, Bradshaw BS, Stern MP. Birthweight and adult health outcomes in a biethnic population in the USA. *Diabetologia* 1994;37(6):624–631.

van Herpen NA, Schrauwen-Hinderling VB, Schaart G, Mensink RP, Schrauwen P. Three weeks on a high-fat diet increases intrahepatic lipid accumulation and decreases metabolic flexibility in healthy overweight men. *J Clin Endocrinol Metab* 2011;96(4):E691–E695.

Wild S, Roglic G, Green A, Sicree R, King H. Global prevalence of diabetes: Estimates for the year 2000 and projections for 2030. *Diabetes Care* 2004;27(5):1047–1053.

Wilson MR. The effect of maternal protein deficiency during pregnancy and lactation on glucose tolerance and pancreatic islet function in adult rat offspring. *J Endocrinol* 1997;154(1):177–185.

Woo M, Patti ME. Diabetes risk begins in utero. *Cell Metab* 2008;8(1):5–7.

Yajnik C, Deshmukh U. Maternal nutrition, intrauterine programming and consequential risks in the offspring. *Rev Endocr Metab Disord* 2008;9(3):203–211.

Yamada M, Wolfe D, Han G, French SW, Ross MG, Desai M. Early onset of fatty liver in growth-restricted rat fetuses and newborns. *Congenit Anom* 2011;51(4):167–173.

Zeggini E, Scott LJ, Saxena R et al. Meta-analysis of genome-wide association data and large-scale replication identifies additional susceptibility loci for type 2 diabetes. *Nat Genet* 2008;40(5):638–645.

Zimmet P, Alberti KGMM, Shaw J. Global and societal implications of the diabetes epidemic. *Nature* 2001;414(6865):782–787.

Zimmet PZ. Diabetes epidemiology as a tool to trigger diabetes research and care. *Diabetologia* 1999;42(5):499–518.

13 Influence of Maternal Obesity during Pregnancy on Childhood Health Outcomes

Romy Gaillard, Susana Santos, Liesbeth Duijts, Janine F. Felix, and Vincent W.V. Jaddoe

CONTENTS

13.1 INTRODUCTION

Obesity is a major public health problem in both Western and non-Western countries (WHO 1999). In recent decades, the prevalence of obesity has nearly doubled worldwide. In 2014, the World Health Organization estimated that 11% of men and 15% of women of the world's adult population were obese (WHO 1999). The strong increase in obesity prevalence has also affected women of reproductive age. A study among 66,221 births in 9 U.S. states showed that from 1993 to 2003, the rate of maternal obesity at the start of pregnancy increased from 13% in 1993/1994 to 22% around 2002/2003 (Kim et al. 2007). Similarly, a study from 1990 to 2004 among 36,821 women in the United Kingdom showed a significant increase in the proportion of maternal obesity at the start of pregnancy from approximately 10% to 16% (Heslehurst et al. 2007). To date, the obesity prevalence rate in pregnant women is estimated to be as high as 30% in Western countries (Huda et al. 2010; Flegal et al. 2012; Bahadoer et al. 2015; Devlieger et al. 2016). In addition, in these countries, even higher percentages of women gain an excessive amount of weight during pregnancy based on the U.S. Institute of Medicine (IOM) guidelines (Fraser et al. 2010;

TABLE 13.1
Institute of Medicine Criteria for Gestational Weight Gain[a]

Prepregnancy Body Mass Index	Recommended Amount of Total Gestational Weight Gain in kg
Underweight (BMI < 18.5 kg/m^2)	12.5–18
Normal weight (BMI ≥ 18.5–24.9 kg/m^2)	11.5–16
Overweight (BMI ≥ 25.0–29.9 kg/m^2)	7–11.5
Obesity (BMI ≥ 30.0 kg/m^2)	5–9

Source: Adapted from Rasmussen, K. M., A. L. Yaktine, editors, *Weight Gain during Pregnancy: Reexamining the Guidelines*, National Academies Press, Washington, DC, 2009.

[a] Recommended gestational weight gain guidelines according to women's prepregnancy BMI.

Restall et al. 2014; Bahadoer et al. 2015). In the IOM guidelines, optimal ranges of maternal weight gain during pregnancy are defined according to a mother's prepregnancy body mass index (BMI; Rasmussen et al. 2009) (Table 13.1). These guidelines have been established based on evidence from observational studies that relate gestational weight gain to various maternal and offspring outcomes (Rasmussen et al. 2009). As described previously, an accumulating body of evidence suggests that maternal obesity and excessive weight gain during pregnancy also have a long-term adverse influence on common health outcomes in the offspring (Gaillard et al. 2014a, 2016; Gaillard 2015).

In this chapter, we discuss the findings from recent observational studies and meta-analyses focused on the associations of maternal obesity and excessive weight gain during pregnancy with adiposity, cardiometabolic, respiratory, and cognitive-related health outcomes throughout childhood. We also discuss the causality and potential mechanisms underlying the observed associations. This chapter is based on our previously written reviews (Gaillard et al. 2014a, 2016; Gaillard 2015).

13.2   FETAL OUTCOMES

Maternal prepregnancy obesity and excessive gestational weight gain are important risk factors for multiple fetal pregnancy complications (Poston et al. 2011; (Gaillard et al. 2014a, 2016; Gaillard 2015). (Figure 13.1). Two large meta-analyses among 9 and 38 observational studies, respectively, showed that a higher maternal prepregnancy or early pregnancy BMI is associated with an increased risk of fetal death, stillbirth, and neonatal death (Chu et al. 2007; Aune et al. 2014). These associations remained present when analyses were restricted to studies that adjusted for potential confounders or excluded women who developed gestational hypertensive disorders or gestational diabetes (Chu et al. 2007; Aune et al. 2014). Maternal obesity is an important risk factor for the development of several congenital anomalies, including neural tube defects, cardiovascular anomalies, cleft palate, hydrocephaly, and limb reduction anomalies, which was shown in a meta-analysis among 18 observational studies (Stothard et al. 2009). A meta-analysis among 13 studies showed

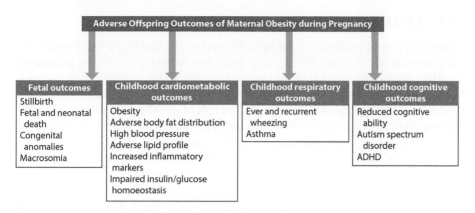

Adverse Offspring Outcomes of Maternal Obesity during Pregnancy

Fetal outcomes	Childhood cardiometabolic outcomes	Childhood respiratory outcomes	Childhood cognitive outcomes
Stillbirth Fetal and neonatal death Congenital anomalies Macrosomia	Obesity Adverse body fat distribution High blood pressure Adverse lipid profile Increased inflammatory markers Impaired insulin/glucose homoeostasis	Ever and recurrent wheezing Asthma	Reduced cognitive ability Autism spectrum disorder ADHD

FIGURE 13.1 Maternal obesity during pregnancy and adverse childhood outcomes.

that compared with a normal maternal prepregnancy weight, maternal prepregnancy obesity was associated with a twofold higher risk of delivering a large size for gestational age infant (Gaudet et al. 2014). A meta-analysis among 11 observational studies including a total of 2,586,265 participants showed that maternal obesity was associated with an increased odds ratio of 1.40 (95% confidence interval [CI]: 1.27–1.54) of a Apgar score <7 at 5 minutes (Zhu et al. 2015). In this meta-analysis, no association with cord blood pH was present.

Next to maternal prepregnancy BMI, excessive gestational weight gain may independently affect the risk of fetal pregnancy complications (Poston et al. 2011; Gaillard et al. 2013). However, compared with the associations of maternal prepregnancy BMI, the associations for excessive maternal gestational weight gain with several adverse fetal outcomes seem to be weaker and less consistent (Poston et al. 2011; Gaillard et al. 2013). Excessive gestational weight gain is most consistently associated with an increased risk of delivering a large size for gestational age infant. A meta-analysis among 15 cohort and case–control studies showed that excessive gestational weight gain based on the IOM criteria was associated with a 2.35 (95% CI: 1.95, 2.85) higher risk of macrosomia (Tian et al. 2016). Studies that assessed the associations of gestational weight gain in specific periods of pregnancy showed that especially higher second and third trimester maternal weight gain were associated with an increased risk of delivering a large size for gestational age infant (Gaillard et al. 2013; Karachaliou et al. 2015). Thus far, increased gestational weight gain seems not to be associated with fetal death or stillbirth but may be associated with adverse neonatal outcomes, such as preterm birth, low 5-minute Apgar score, and neonatal hypoglycemia, although results are inconsistent (Rydhstrom et al. 1994; Stephansson et al. 2001; Stotland et al. 2006; McDonald et al. 2011; Gaillard et al. 2013).

Thus, both maternal prepregnancy obesity and excessive gestational weight gain lead to increased risks of fetal complications. Overall, the associations for maternal prepregnancy obesity with adverse pregnancy outcomes seem to be more consistent and stronger than for excessive gestational weight gain (Poston et al. 2011; Gaillard et al. 2013).

13.3   CHILDHOOD CARDIOMETABOLIC OUTCOMES

A large number of previous studies have focused on the childhood cardiometabolic consequences of maternal obesity and excessive weight gain during pregnancy (Gaillard 2015) (Figure 13.1). Most studies focused on the associations with childhood adiposity outcomes. Maternal prepregnancy obesity and excessive gestational weight gain are associated with an increased risk of obesity throughout childhood (Schack-Nielsen et al. 2010). Two meta-analyses among 4 and 12 observational studies, respectively, showed that maternal prepregnancy obesity and excessive gestational weight gain according to the IOM criteria were associated with a three-fold higher risk of childhood obesity compared with normal weight women and a recommended amount of gestational weight gain, respectively (Yu et al. 2013; Tie et al. 2014). In addition, several studies showed that a higher maternal prepregnancy BMI and total gestational weight gain are independently associated with a higher childhood waist circumference, total body fat mass, and abdominal fat mass levels, although the associations for total gestational weight gain are less consistent (Crozier et al. 2010; Fraser et al. 2010; Gaillard et al. 2014b, 2015; Kaar et al. 2014; Oostvogels et al. 2014; Perng et al. 2014). Critical periods of maternal weight during pregnancy for the development of childhood adiposity have been identified. A study performed among 5154 UK mother–offspring pairs showed that especially gestational weight gain in the first 14 weeks of pregnancy was positively associated with offspring adiposity measures at 9 years of age (Fraser et al. 2010). Among 5908 mothers and their children participating within the Generation R Study, a population-based prospective cohort study from early pregnancy onwards in Rotterdam, the Netherlands, we observed that independent from maternal prepregnancy weight and weight gain in later pregnancy, early pregnancy weight gain was associated with a higher childhood BMI, total fat mass, android/gynoid fat mass ratio, and abdominal subcutaneous fat mass level at the age of 6 years (Gaillard et al. 2015). A study among 977 mother–child pairs from Greece showed that maternal first trimester weight gain was associated with an increased risk of childhood obesity (Karachaliou et al. 2015).

Both maternal prepregnancy obesity and excessive gestational weight gain seem to be associated with a suboptimal cardiometabolic profile in childhood. A Dutch study among 1459 mother–child pairs showed that a higher maternal prepregnancy BMI was associated with higher childhood systolic blood pressure and overall metabolic score, as a measure of a metabolic syndrome like phenotype, at the age of 5–6 years (Oostvogels et al. 2014). In the same cohort, no associations of maternal prepregnancy BMI with childhood sympathetic drive, parasympathetic drive, or heart rate measured by electrocardiography and impedance cardiography at rest were present (Gademan et al. 2013). Within the Generation R Study, we observed that a higher maternal prepregnancy BMI was associated with a higher childhood systolic blood pressure, left ventricular mass, aortic root diameter, and insulin levels, and lower high-density lipoprotein (HDL) cholesterol levels at the age of 6 years (Gaillard et al. 2014b; Toemen et al. 2016). Compared with children from normal weight mothers, children from obese mothers had an increased risk of clustering of cardiometabolic risk factors (odds ratio [OR] 3.00 [95%CI: 2.09, 4.34]), a measure of a metabolic syndrome-like phenotype in childhood (Gaillard et al. 2014b). Similarly, higher maternal early pregnancy weight gain, but not weight gain later in pregnancy, was associated with an increased risk of childhood clustering of cardiometabolic risk factors (Gaillard et al. 2015). A study among 5154 UK mother–offspring pairs showed that higher maternal prepregnancy weight and gestational weight gain in mid-pregnancy were associated with higher childhood levels of triglycerides, HDL cholesterol, apolipoprotein A1, and interleukin 6 (IL-6) at the age of 9 years (Fraser et al. 2010). A study among 1090 mother–child pairs participating in a prebirth cohort in the United States showed that a higher maternal prepregnancy BMI was associated with higher midchildhood leptin, high-sensitivity C-reactive protein, and IL-6 levels, and lower adiponectin levels, whereas a higher total gestational weight gain was only associated with higher mid-childhood leptin levels (Perng et al. 2014). Across different studies, these associations are not explained by birth weight. However, these associations seem to be largely mediated by childhood BMI (Gaillard 2015).

Thus, in line with the risks of pregnancy complications, maternal prepregnancy obesity and excessive gestational weight gain also lead to increased risks of adiposity and adverse cardiometabolic-related outcomes in children. These associations seem not to be restricted to obesity or excessive gestational weight gain but present across the full range of BMI and gestational weight gain. Maternal weight gain in early pregnancy, when maternal fat accumulation forms a relatively large component of gestational weight gain, may be an especially critical period for an adverse childhood cardiometabolic risk profile.

13.4 CHILDHOOD RESPIRATORY OUTCOMES

Maternal obesity during pregnancy may affect respiratory outcomes throughout childhood (Gaillard et al. 2014a) (Figure 13.1). A meta-analysis among 85,509 mothers and their children from 14 European birth cohort studies showed that maternal overweight and obesity during pregnancy were associated with the risk of ever wheezing and with recurrent wheezing until age 2 years (Zugna et al. 2015). In this meta-analysis, multiple socioeconomic and lifestyle factors and birth characteristics were taken into account. A more recent meta-analysis among 14 studies with more than 108,000 mother–child pairs also reported associations of maternal prepregnancy overweight and obesity with childhood asthma, with a 31% increased risk of asthma or ever wheezing in children aged 14 months to 16 years (Forno et al. 2014). Each 1 kg/m^2 increase in maternal BMI was associated with a 3% increase in childhood asthma risk. Similarly, increased gestational weight gain was associated with an increased risk of childhood asthma. Children whose mothers were in the higher gestational weight gain categories had a 1.16 (95% CI: 1.00–1.34) higher risk of ever asthma or wheeze but not of current asthma or wheeze. These associations tended to be stronger when the prevalence of maternal asthma was lower (Leermakers et al. 2013). The observed associations could not be explained by birth weight or by the child's BMI at the time of assessment of the outcome. Few studies examined the influence of maternal obesity during pregnancy on childhood lung function directly (Scholtens et al. 2010; Pike et al. 2013). A study among 940 mother–offspring pairs showed that maternal prepregnancy obesity was not associated with spirometry parameters or levels of fractional exhaled nitric oxide, a measure of eosinophilic airway inflammation, at the age of 6 years (Pike et al. 2013). Also, no associations of maternal prepregnancy overweight with bronchial hyperresponsiveness at the age of 8 years were found among 3963 mother–offspring pairs (Scholtens et al. 2010). Asthma is partly considered an atopic disorder. For other atopic disorders, maternal prepregnancy obesity is not or inconsistently associated with allergic rhinitis, hay fever, atopic dermatitis, or inhalant and food allergen sensitization up to age 16 years (Kumar et al. 2010; Scholtens et al. 2010; Harpsoe et al. 2013; Pike et al. 2013; Ekstrom et al. 2015).

Thus, in line with associations with childhood cardiometabolic outcomes, maternal obesity during pregnancy may also lead to increased risks of childhood wheezing and asthma.

13.5 CHILDHOOD COGNITIVE OUTCOMES

Fewer studies have examined the relationship of maternal BMI during pregnancy with cognitive outcomes in the offspring (Neggers et al. 2003; Heikura et al. 2008; Brion et al. 2011; Hinkle et al. 2012; Basatemur et al. 2013; Casas et al. 2013; Eriksen et al. 2013; Mann et al. 2013; Tanda et al. 2013; Bliddal et al. 2014; Pugh et al. 2015) (Figure 13.1). Although results are inconsistent, most studies have reported that maternal prepregnancy obesity is associated with a lower cognitive function in children (Neggers et al. 2003; Hinkle et al. 2012; Basatemur et al. 2013; Casas et al. 2013; Eriksen et al. 2013; Mann et al. 2013; Tanda et al. 2013; Bliddal et al. 2014; Pugh et al. 2015). In more recent European cohort studies, no consistent associations were observed between maternal prepregnancy overweight and obesity and maternal reported childhood cognitive ability (Brion et al. 2011). However, maternal overweight and obesity were associated with a lower intelligence quotient (IQ) assessed by a psychologist at 8 years (Brion et al. 2011). A meta-analysis among five observational studies showed that maternal obesity during pregnancy was associated with a 1.47 (95% CI 1.24–1.74) higher odds of childhood autism spectrum disorder (Li et al. 2016). A study among 12,556 school-aged children and their mothers from three prospective Scandinavian cohorts showed that maternal prepregnancy obesity was associated with an increased risk of childhood attention deficit hyperactivity disorder (ADHD) symptoms rated by teachers (Rodriguez et al. 2008).

Next to maternal prepregnancy BMI, gestational weight gain may be associated with childhood cognitive-related health outcomes (Keim and Pruitt 2012; Gage et al. 2013; Mann et al. 2013, Pugh et al. 2015; Hinkle et al. 2016). Three previous studies have reported no associations between total weight gain during pregnancy and cognitive outcomes during childhood (Keim and Pruitt 2012; Mann et al. 2013; Pugh et al. 2015). However, a study of term deliveries from Avon Longitudinal Study of Parents and Children (ALSPAC), a population-based prospective cohort study from Bristol, UK, reported small positive associations between weight gain in each trimester of pregnancy and child IQ scores at 8 years of age, with no clear differences in strength of the effect estimates for different periods of maternal weight gain (Gage et al. 2013). Among normal weight Scandinavian mothers and their children, maternal trimester-specific gestational weight gain was not associated with child IQ scores at 5 years of age. However, when the sample was limited to term deliveries, third trimester weight gain was positively associated with child IQ scores (Hinkle et al. 2016). In a large Swedish study, both low and high maternal gestational weight gain were associated with an increased risk of autism spectrum disorder in children (Gardner et al. 2015).

Thus, maternal obesity during pregnancy may affect offspring cognitive development but the associations seem to be less consistent and weaker compared with the associations with childhood cardiometabolic and respiratory outcomes.

13.6   CAUSALITY OR CONFOUNDING

Despite the large number of observational studies reporting these strong associations with a variety of childhood health outcomes, it remains unclear whether these associations of maternal prepregnancy obesity or excessive gestational weight gain with childhood outcomes are explained by direct intrauterine mechanisms (Gaillard et al. 2014a, 2016; Gaillard 2015). The observed associations may also be explained by environmental, lifestyle-related, or genetic characteristics. Despite extensive adjustment for potential confounding factors in observational studies, residual confounding may still be an important issue (Gaillard et al. 2014a, 2016; Gaillard 2015).

Several approaches can be used in epidemiological research to better control for confounding. Multiple studies have compared the strength of associations of maternal and paternal BMI with childhood outcomes as an aid to further disentangle underlying mechanisms (Gaillard 2015). Stronger associations for maternal BMI suggest direct intrauterine mechanisms, whereas similar or stronger associations for paternal BMI suggest a role for shared family-based, lifestyle-related characteristics or genetic factors (Gaillard 2015). Stronger associations for maternal prepregnancy BMI with birth weight have been reported than for paternal prepregnancy BMI (Durmus et al. 2013). Thus far, studies comparing associations of maternal and paternal BMI with childhood BMI have shown conflicting results (Patro et al. 2013). However, studies examining these associations with more detailed childhood fat mass measures and other cardiometabolic risk factors have shown that maternal prepregnancy BMI tends to be more strongly associated with childhood total fat mass, android/gynoid fat mass ratio, and clustering of cardiometabolic risk factors than paternal BMI (Lawlor et al. 2008; Gaillard et al. 2014b). No such studies have yet been performed with childhood respiratory outcomes. With regard to childhood cognitive outcomes, maternal and paternal comparison studies did not show strong evidence for an intrauterine effect. A study among 1783 Danish parent–offspring pairs observed similar effect estimates for the associations of maternal and paternal BMI with childhood IQ at the age of 5 years (Bliddal et al. 2014). A study among 2379 infants, aged 11–22 months, and their parents from two Southern European birth cohorts did not find an association between paternal BMI and childhood cognition, which suggests that the effects of maternal BMI on offspring cognition may be due to intrauterine mechanisms (Casas et al. 2013). However, the effect estimates of the maternal and paternal associations had overlapping confidence intervals and thus seem not to be statistically different. Thus, overall these findings suggest that maternal prepregnancy

BMI may, at least partly, influence the cardiometabolic health of offspring through direct intrauterine mechanisms (Gaillard et al. 2014a, 2016; Gaillard 2015). However, this remains to be further explored for other childhood health outcomes.

A second approach to establish causality is a sibling comparison study, which enables better control for environmental characteristics as well as maternal genotype that are shared among siblings (Gaillard 2015). Sibling studies among offspring from mothers who had high levels of prepregnancy weight loss due to biliopancreatic diversion bariatric surgery observed a lower risk of macrosomia, lower prevalence of obesity, improved insulin sensitivity, and lipid levels among children born to mothers after surgery than those born to mothers before surgery (Kral et al. 2006). These findings suggest that some of the effect of maternal obesity on offspring outcomes may be through direct intrauterine mechanisms. However, it remains unclear whether this effect is also present for less extreme maternal prepregnancy BMI levels and a variety of childhood health outcomes. A sibling comparison study among 513,501 mothers and their 1,164,750 children showed that children born to mothers who gained a large amount of weight during pregnancy had a higher birth weight than children born to mothers who gained less weight during pregnancy (Ludwig and Currie 2010). A sibling comparison study among 42,133 mothers who had more than one singleton pregnancy and their 91,045 offspring showed that every additional kilogram of maternal gestational weight gain increased childhood BMI of the offspring by 0.0220 kg/m^2 (95% CI 0.01–0.03) (Ludwig et al. 2013). This association was only partly mediated by offspring birth weight. A study using a sibling comparison design among 280,866 singleton-born Swedish men showed that a higher maternal BMI in early pregnancy was only in the whole cohort and between non-siblings associated with higher offspring BMI at the age of 18 years, but not within siblings, which suggests that the association may be explained by confounding factors (Lawlor et al. 2011b). However, among the same study population it was shown that among overweight and obese mothers, higher total gestational weight gain was associated with higher offspring BMI at the age of 18 years among siblings, which suggests a possible intrauterine effect for gestational weight gain (Lawlor et al. 2011a). A study among 4908 brother pairs from Sweden showed no associations of maternal gestational weight gain and offspring blood pressure or risk of hypertension at 18 years among siblings (Scheers Andersson et al. 2015). Thus far, no sibling comparison studies have focused on childhood respiratory outcomes and only two sibling comparison studies focused on childhood cognitive outcomes. These studies suggested that the association of maternal BMI with autism spectrum disorder and ADHD may be attributed to unmeasured familial confounding, but excessive gestational weight gain was associated with the risk of autism spectrum disorder within a matched sibling analysis (Chen et al. 2014; Gardner et al. 2015). Thus, findings from sibling comparison studies among less extreme obese populations suggest that especially gestational weight gain may affect offspring health outcomes through direct intrauterine mechanisms. However, the results are not consistent and remain to be further assessed in large population based studies. An important limitation of sibling comparison studies is that next to the major exposures of interest, maternal prepregnancy BMI and gestational weight gain, other lifestyle-related characteristics may also differ between pregnancies (Gaillard 2015, Gaillard et al. 2016).

A third approach to obtain further insight in causality is a Mendelian randomization approach (Gaillard et al. 2014a, 2016; Gaillard 2015). This approach uses genetic variants, which are robustly associated with the exposure of interest and not affected by confounding, as an instrumental variable for a specific exposure (Gaillard 2015). A study among 30,487 mothers and their newborns from 18 cohort studies showed that a 1 SD (≈ 4 points) genetically higher maternal BMI was associated with a 55-g higher offspring birth weight (95% CI, 17–93 g), which suggests that genetically elevated maternal BMI may be causally related with offspring birth weight (Tyrrell et al. 2016). A study among 4091 mother–offspring pairs showed no association of maternal (FTO gene) with childhood fat mass at the age of 9 years, which suggest that maternal obesity may not be causally related to childhood adiposity outcomes (Lawlor et al. 2008). However, this study may be limited by a relatively small sample size. The findings from these studies mark the importance for further Mendelian randomization studies with a larger sample size and using multiple maternal genetic variants as instruments focused on a variety of childhood health outcomes.

Finally, randomized controlled trials are considered as the golden standard to assess causality (Gaillard et al. 2014a, 2016; Gaillard 2015). Previous randomized controlled trials have focused on influencing determinants of maternal obesity and excessive weight gain during pregnancy, such as dietary factors and physical activity levels, since directly randomized studies are difficult to perform with maternal prepregnancy obesity and excessive gestational weight gain as major exposures of interest (Gaillard 2015). A recent randomized controlled trial providing a 6-month lifestyle intervention program for obese infertile women prior to fertility treatment showed a small reduction in maternal prepregnancy weight but no effect on rates of healthy singleton life born children (Mutsaerts et al. 2016). A meta-analysis among 44 randomized controlled trials focused on dietary and physical activity interventions during pregnancy suggested that especially dietary interventions during pregnancy, and not physical activity interventions, may lead to a small reduction in the amount of gestational weight gain and to a slightly lower risk of adverse pregnancy outcomes (Thangaratinam et al. 2012). However, whether they also have a beneficial effect on childhood outcomes remains unclear. A small randomized controlled trial among 254 mothers and their children, which provided both dietary advice and exercise to obese women during pregnancy, observed no effect on BMI or metabolic risk factors in infant offspring (Tanvig et al. 2015). Long-term follow-up of participants in these trials will provide further insight into the causality of these observed associations as well as the effectiveness of maternal lifestyle interventions during pregnancy for improving long-term health of offspring.

Altogether, results from studies specifically designed to explore the causality for the associations of maternal obesity with offspring outcomes are not conclusive yet.

13.7 POTENTIAL MECHANISMS

The mechanisms underlying the associations of maternal prepregnancy obesity or excessive gestational weight gain with offspring health outcomes remain unclear. Maternal prepregnancy obesity and excessive gestational weight are complex traits

(Gaillard 2015). Maternal prepregnancy obesity not only reflects maternal fat accumulation, but also other maternal characteristics, such as maternal nutritional status, insulin and glucose metabolism, and low-grade systemic inflammation (Gaillard 2015). Similarly, maternal weight gain during pregnancy reflects maternal fat accumulation, but also maternal and amniotic fluid expansion and growth of the fetus, placenta, and uterus (Gaillard 2015). Both maternal prepregnancy obesity and excessive gestational weight gain as well as the correlated maternal exposures may lead to programming effects in the offspring through several pathways (Gaillard et al. 2014a, 2016; Gaillard 2015).

There is accumulating evidence which suggests that epigenetic modifications play a key role as the underlying pathway in these observed associations. Epigenetic modifications are mitotically heritable changes to the DNA that do not affect the DNA sequence, but may influence its function (Groom et al. 2011). DNA methylation is the most studied epigenetic mechanism and refers to the binding of a methyl group to specific positions in the DNA, the cytosine–phosphate–guanine (CpG) sites, where a cytosine is located next to a guanine. Fetal exposures, such as maternal smoking and folic acid levels, have been shown to be associated with changes in DNA methylation (Joubert et al. 2016a,b). Thus far, animal studies provide support for epigenetic modifications due to maternal obesity or a high-fat diet, but this has not been explored in large human studies (Alfaradhi et al. 2011; Gaillard 2015; Gaillard et al. 2016).

Previous studies have found that maternal BMI is associated with methylation of specific, predefined CpG sites (Gemma et al. 2009; Soubry et al. 2015). Recently, techniques have become available to analyze methylation at hundreds of thousands of CpG sites, spread across the genome, simultaneously, enabling "epigenome-wide" analyses of larger sample sizes (Moran et al. 2016). A number of epigenome-wide association studies have focused specifically on associations of maternal prepregnancy BMI or gestational weight gain with DNA methylation in offspring cord blood (Guenard et al. 2013; Liu et al. 2014; Morales et al. 2014; Bohlin et al. 2015; Sharp et al. 2015). An early study in 308 mother–infant pairs showed an association of maternal BMI with methylation at a single CpG sites, but did not attempt replication (Liu et al. 2014). Comparing siblings born before and after gastrointestinal bypass surgery, Guénard et al reported differential DNA methylation of 5698 genes, many of which were related to glucose metabolism, inflammation, and cardiovascular disease (Guenard et al. 2013). A study in 88 mother–offspring pairs did not find significantly associated CpG site for maternal prepregnancy BMI, but did show increased methylation of four sites associated with first trimester gestational weight gain, although none replicated (Morales et al. 2014; Bohlin et al. 2015). A second, larger analysis of 1018 participants from the same study found 28 differentially methylated CpG sites in newborns of obese mothers and 1621 differentially methylated CpG sites in newborns of underweight mothers compared with normal weight mothers (Sharp et al. 2015). No associations were found for gestational weight gain. Some of the identified CpG sites were also nominally associated with measures of childhood and adolescent adiposity. In this study, maternal obesity showed stronger associations with cord blood DNA methylation than did paternal obesity, which is in line with a potential direct intrauterine mechanism. A longitudinal analysis of the associated CpG sites, using data from ages 7 and 17 years, showed that the differences in DNA methylation in cord blood of offspring of obese or underweight mothers mostly resolved over time (Sharp et al. 2015). Although sample sizes are still relatively small, the epigenome-wide association studies on maternal BMI and gestational weight gain published to date highlight the potential of epigenome-wide approaches to discover differentially methylated sites and underline the need for larger, population-based studies. Altogether, epigenetic modifications together with other mechanisms may thus be involved in adiposity, cardiometabolic, respiratory, and cognitive developmental adaptations in response to maternal obesity during pregnancy (Gaillard 2015).

It has been suggested that the influence of maternal obesity during pregnancy on birth weight may act as an underlying pathway for the associations of maternal obesity during pregnancy with cardiometabolic health outcomes in childhood (Gaillard 2015). However, many observational studies have shown that additional adjustment for birth weight does not explain the observed associations (Gaillard 2015). The lack of effect of adjustment for birth weight may partly be explained by birth weight not accurately reflecting neonatal fat mass, but might also suggest that other mechanisms are involved in these associations. Animal studies have suggested that maternal obesity during pregnancy may affect offspring adipocyte morphology and metabolism and lead to altered appetite control (Drake et al. 2010). The associations of maternal prepregnancy BMI and gestational weight gain with adverse childhood cardiometabolic outcomes appear to be largely mediated through offspring adiposity (Gaillard 2015). However, direct cardiovascular and metabolic programming effects of maternal obesity during pregnancy may also be present. Thus far, mainly animal studies have shown that maternal obesity, a maternal high-fat diet, and increased maternal glucose transport during pregnancy are associated with offspring high blood pressure, endothelial dysfunction, increased aortic stiffness, cardiac hypertrophy, impaired glucose and insulin homoeostasis, and nonalcoholic fatty liver disease (Drake et al. 2010).

Both inflammatory and immunological mechanisms influenced by maternal obesity during pregnancy may contribute to the increased risk of adverse respiratory related health outcomes in offspring. Levels of proinflammatory cytokines are increased in the amniotic fluid, surrounding and breathed in by the developing fetus of obese mothers, which may affect fetal lung development and allergic responses (Bugatto et al. 2010). Also, increased leptin and adipokines levels during fetal development may directly affect the developing lung. Leptin and adiponectin receptors are expressed in the lung, and leptin regulates the maturation of fetal lung cells (Bruno et al. 2009; Miller et al. 2009). In mice, it has been shown that administration of leptin enhanced ozone-induced airway inflammation and responsiveness, whereas adiponectin administration attenuates allergen-induced airway hyperreactivity and inflammation (Shore et al. 2003, 2006).

Maternal obesity during pregnancy may affect fetal brain development through various influences. Adipose tissue of obese women may contain higher levels of neurotoxins that may negatively affect fetal brain development (Rodriguez et al. 2008). Maternal obesity impairs brain-derived neurotrophic factor production, which plays an important role in neuronal proliferation and differentiation, and in hippocampus-dependent cognitive functions such as spatial learning and memory (Bilbo et al. 2010; Tozuka et al. 2010). Also, increased oxidative stress and inflammation and decreased neurogenesis have been observed in the fetal brain of obese mothers and can result in cognitive disruption.

Thus, multiple mechanisms may be involved in the intrauterine pathways leading from maternal obesity and excessive weight gain during pregnancy to long-term adverse childhood health outcomes (Gaillard 2015). Currently, epigenetic mechanisms are considered one of the major underlying pathways of interest. These underlying mechanisms have mainly been studied in animal models and remain to be further explored in large human studies.

13.8 CONCLUSIONS

Maternal prepregnancy obesity and excessive weight gain during pregnancy are common and important risk factors for adverse fetal pregnancy outcomes and childhood adiposity, cardiometabolic, respiratory, and cognitive-related health outcomes. Parent–offspring studies, sibling comparison studies, Mendelian randomization studies, and randomized controlled trials can be used to explore the causality of these associations. Further mechanistic studies in human populations are needed to obtain insight in the underlying mechanisms. Finally, the potential for prevention of common diseases in future generations by reducing maternal obesity and excessive weight gain during pregnancy needs to be explored.

ACKNOWLEDGMENTS

The authors received funding from the European Union's Seventh Framework Programme (FP7/2007-2013), Project Early Nutrition under Grant Agreement No. 289346. Vincent Jaddoe received an additional grant from the Netherlands Organization for Health Research and Development (NWO, ZonMw-VIDI 016.136.361) and a European Research Council Consolidator Grant (ERC-2014-CoG-648916). Liesbeth Duijts received funding from the Lung Foundation Netherlands (No. 3.2.12.089; 2012). Janine Felix has received funding from the European Union's Horizon 2020 Research and Innovation Program under Grant Agreement No. 633595 (DynaHEALTH).

REFERENCES

Alfaradhi, M. Z., S. E. Ozanne (2011). Developmental programming in response to maternal overnutrition. *Front Genet* 2: 27.
Aune, D., O. D. Saugstad, T. Henriksen, S. Tonstad (2014). Maternal body mass index and the risk of fetal death, stillbirth, and infant death: A systematic review and meta-analysis. *JAMA* 311(15): 1536–1546.
Bahadoer, S., R. Gaillard, J. F. Felix et al. (2015). Ethnic disparities in maternal obesity and weight gain during pregnancy. The Generation R Study. *Eur J Obstet Gynecol Reprod Biol* 193: 51–60.
Basatemur, E., J. Gardiner, C. Williams et al. (2013). Maternal prepregnancy BMI and child cognition: A longitudinal cohort study. *Pediatrics* 131(1): 56–63.
Bilbo, S. D., V. Tsang (2010). Enduring consequences of maternal obesity for brain inflammation and behavior of offspring. *FASEB J* 24(6): 2104–2115.
Bliddal, M., J. Olsen, H. Stovring et al. (2014). Maternal pre-pregnancy BMI and intelligence quotient (IQ) in 5-year-old children: A cohort based study. *PLoS One* 9(4): e94498.

Bohlin, J., B. K. Andreassen, B. R. Joubert et al. (2015). Effect of maternal gestational weight gain on offspring DNA methylation: A follow-up to the ALSPAC cohort study. *BMC Res Notes* 8: 321.

Brion, M. J., M. Zeegers, V. Jaddoe et al. (2011). Intrauterine effects of maternal prepregnancy overweight on child cognition and behavior in 2 cohorts. *Pediatrics* 127(1): e202–211.

Bruno, A., E. Pace, P. Chanez et al. (2009). Leptin and leptin receptor expression in asthma. *J Allergy Clin Immunol* 124(2): 230–237, 237 e231–234.

Bugatto, F., A. Fernandez-Deudero, A. Bailen et al. (2010). Second-trimester amniotic fluid proinflammatory cytokine levels in normal and overweight women. *Obstet Gynecol* 115(1): 127–133.

Casas, M., L. Chatzi, A. E. Carsin et al. (2013). Maternal pre-pregnancy overweight and obesity, and child neuropsychological development: Two Southern European birth cohort studies. *Int J Epidemiol* 42(2): 506–517.

Chen, Q., A. Sjolander, N. Langstrom et al. (2014). Maternal pre-pregnancy body mass index and offspring attention deficit hyperactivity disorder: A population-based cohort study using a sibling-comparison design. *Int J Epidemiol* 43(1): 83–90.

Chu, S. Y., S. Y. Kim, J. Lau et al. (2007). Maternal obesity and risk of stillbirth: A metaanalysis. *Am J Obstet Gynecol* 197(3): 223–228.

Crozier, S. R., H. M. Inskip, K. M. Godfrey et al. (2010). Weight gain in pregnancy and childhood body composition: Findings from the Southampton Women's Survey. *Am J Clin Nutr* 91(6): 1745–1751.

Devlieger, R., K. Benhalima, P. Damm et al. (2016). Maternal obesity in Europe: Where do we stand and how to move forward?: A scientific paper commissioned by the European Board and College of Obstetrics and Gynaecology (EBCOG). *Eur J Obstet Gynecol Reprod Biol* 201: 203–208.

Drake, A. J., M. Reynolds (2010). Impact of maternal obesity on offspring obesity and cardiometabolic disease risk. *Reproduction* 140(3): 387–398.

Durmus, B., L. R. Arends, L. Ay et al. (2013). Parental anthropometrics, early growth and the risk of overweight in pre-school children: The Generation R Study. *Pediatr Obes* 8(5): 339–350.

Ekstrom, S., J. Magnusson, I. Kull et al. (2015). Maternal body mass index in early pregnancy and offspring asthma, rhinitis and eczema up to 16 years of age. *Clin Exp Allergy* 45(1): 283–291.

Eriksen, H. L., U. S. Kesmodel, M. Underbjerg et al. (2013). Predictors of intelligence at the age of 5: Family, pregnancy and birth characteristics, postnatal influences, and postnatal growth. *PLoS One* 8(11): e79200.

Flegal, K. M., M. D. Carroll, B. K. Kit, C. L. Ogden (2012). Prevalence of obesity and trends in the distribution of body mass index among US adults, 1999–2010. *JAMA* 307(5): 491–497.

Forno, E., O. M. Young, R. Kumar, H. Simhan, J. C. Celedon (2014). Maternal obesity in pregnancy, gestational weight gain, and risk of childhood asthma. *Pediatrics* 134(2): e535–e546.

Fraser, A., K. Tilling, C. Macdonald-Wallis et al. (2010). Association of maternal weight gain in pregnancy with offspring obesity and metabolic and vascular traits in childhood. *Circulation* 121(23): 2557–2564.

Gademan, M. G., M. van Eijsden, T. J. Roseboom et al (2013). Maternal prepregnancy body mass index and their children's blood pressure and resting cardiac autonomic balance at age 5 to 6 years. *Hypertension* 62(3): 641–647.

Gage, S. H., D. A. Lawlor, K. Tilling, A. Fraser (2013). Associations of maternal weight gain in pregnancy with offspring cognition in childhood and adolescence: Findings from the Avon Longitudinal Study of Parents and Children. *Am J Epidemiol* 177(5): 402–410.

Gaillard, R. (2015). Maternal obesity during pregnancy and cardiovascular development and disease in the offspring. *Eur J Epidemiol* 30(11): 1141–1152.

Gaillard, R., B. Durmus, A. Hofman et al. (2013). Risk factors and outcomes of maternal obesity and excessive weight gain during pregnancy. *Obesity* 21(5): 1046–1055.

Gaillard, R., J. F. Felix, L. Duijts, V. W. Jaddoe (2014a). Childhood consequences of maternal obesity and excessive weight gain during pregnancy. *Acta Obstet Gynecol Scand* 93(11): 1085–1089.

Gaillard R., S. Santos, L. Duijts, J.F. Felix (2016). Childhood health consequences of maternal obesity during pregnancy: A narrative review. *Ann Nutr Metab* 69:171–180.

Gaillard, R., E. A. Steegers, L. Duijts et al. (2014b). Childhood cardiometabolic outcomes of maternal obesity during pregnancy: The Generation R Study. *Hypertension* 63(4): 683–691.

Gaillard, R., E. A. Steegers, O. H. Franco, A. Hofman, V. W. Jaddoe (2015). Maternal weight gain in different periods of pregnancy and childhood cardio-metabolic outcomes. The Generation R Study. *Int J Obes* 39(4): 677–685.

Gardner, R. M., B. K. Lee, C. Magnusson et al. (2015). Maternal body mass index during early pregnancy, gestational weight gain, and risk of autism spectrum disorders: Results from a Swedish total population and discordant sibling study. *Int J Epidemiol* 44(3): 870–883.

Gaudet, L., Z. M. Ferraro, S. W. Wen, M. Walker (2014). Maternal obesity and occurrence of fetal macrosomia: A systematic review and meta-analysis. *Biomed Res Int* 2014: 640291.

Gemma, C., S. Sookoian, J. Alvarinas et al. (2009). Maternal pregestational BMI is associated with methylation of the PPARGC1A promoter in newborns. *Obesity* 17(5): 1032–1039.

Groom, A., H. R. Elliott, N. D. Embleton, C. L. Relton (2011). Epigenetics and child health: Basic principles. *Arch Dis Child* 96(9): 863–869.

Guenard, F., Y. Deshaies, K. Cianflone et al. (2013). Differential methylation in glucoregulatory genes of offspring born before vs. after maternal gastrointestinal bypass surgery. *Proc Natl Acad Sci USA* 110(28): 11439–11444.

Harpsoe, M. C., S. Basit, P. Bager et al. (2013). Maternal obesity, gestational weight gain, and risk of asthma and atopic disease in offspring: A study within the Danish National Birth Cohort. *J Allergy Clin Immunol* 131(4): 1033–1040.

Heikura, U., A. Taanila, A. L. Hartikainen et al. (2008). Variations in prenatal sociodemographic factors associated with intellectual disability: A study of the 20-year interval between two birth cohorts in northern Finland. *Am J Epidemiol* 167(2): 169–177.

Heslehurst, N., L. J. Ells, H. Simpson et al. (2007). Trends in maternal obesity incidence rates, demographic predictors, and health inequalities in 36,821 women over a 15-year period. *BJOG* 114(2): 187–194.

Hinkle, S. N., P. S. Albert, L. A. Sjaarda, J. Grewal, K. L. Grantz (2016). Trajectories of maternal gestational weight gain and child cognition assessed at 5 years of age in a prospective cohort study. *J Epidemiol Community Health* 70(7): 696–703.

Hinkle, S. N., L. A. Schieve, A. D. Stein et al. (2012). Associations between maternal prepregnancy body mass index and child neurodevelopment at 2 years of age. *Int J Obes* 36(10): 1312–1319.

Huda, S. S., L. E. Brodie, N. Sattar (2010). Obesity in pregnancy: Prevalence and metabolic consequences. *Semin Fetal Neonatal Med* 15(2): 70–76.

Joubert, B. R., H. T. den Dekker, J. F. Felix et al. (2016a). Maternal plasma folate impacts differential DNA methylation in an epigenome-wide meta-analysis of newborns. *Nat Commun* 7: 10577.

Joubert, B. R., J. F. Felix, P. Yousefi et al. (2016b). DNA methylation in newborns and maternal smoking in pregnancy: Genome-wide consortium meta-analysis. *Am J Hum Genet* 98(4): 680–696.

Kaar, J. L., T. Crume, J. T. Brinton et al. (2014). Maternal obesity, gestational weight gain, and offspring adiposity: The exploring perinatal outcomes among children study. *J Pediatr* 165(3): 509–515.

Karachaliou, M., V. Georgiou, T. Roumeliotaki et al. (2015). Association of trimester-specific gestational weight gain with fetal growth, offspring obesity, and cardiometabolic traits in early childhood. *Am J Obstet Gynecol* 212(4): 502 e501–514.

Keim, S. A., N. T. Pruitt (2012). Gestational weight gain and child cognitive development. *Int J Epidemiol* 41(2): 414–422.

Kim, S. Y., P. M. Dietz, L. England, B. Morrow, W. M. Callaghan (2007). Trends in pre-pregnancy obesity in nine states, 1993–2003. *Obesity* 15(4): 986–993.

Kral, J. G., S. Biron, S. Simard et al. (2006). Large maternal weight loss from obesity sur-gery prevents transmission of obesity to children who were followed for 2 to 18 years. *Pediatrics* 118(6): e1644–1649.

Kumar, R., R. E. Story, J. A. Pongracic et al. (2010). Maternal pre-pregnancy obesity and recur-rent wheezing in early childhood. *Pediatr Allergy Immunol Pulmonol* 23(3): 183–190.

Lawlor, D. A., P. Lichtenstein, A. Fraser, N. Langstrom (2011a). Does maternal weight gain in pregnancy have long-term effects on offspring adiposity? A sibling study in a prospective cohort of 146,894 men from 136,050 families. *Am J Clin Nutr* 94(1): 142–148.

Lawlor, D. A., P. Lichtenstein, N. Langstrom (2011b). Association of maternal diabetes mel-litus in pregnancy with offspring adiposity into early adulthood: Sibling study in a pro-spective cohort of 280,866 men from 248,293 families. *Circulation* 123(3): 258–265.

Lawlor, D. A., N. J. Timpson, R. M. Harbord et al. (2008). Exploring the developmental over-nutrition hypothesis using parental-offspring associations and FTO as an instrumental variable. *PLOS Med* 5(3): e33.

Leermakers, E. T., A. M. Sonnenschein-van der Voort, R. Gaillard et al. (2013). Maternal weight, gestational weight gain and preschool wheezing: The Generation R Study. *Eur Respir J* 42(5): 1234–1243.

Li, Y. M., J. J. Ou, L. Liu et al. (2016). Association between maternal obesity and autism spectrum disorder in offspring: A meta-analysis. *J Autism Dev Disord* 46(1): 95–102.

Liu, X., Q. Chen, H. J. Tsai et al. (2014). Maternal preconception body mass index and offspring cord blood DNA methylation: Exploration of early life origins of disease. *Environ Mol Mutagen* 55(3): 223–230.

Ludwig, D. S., J. Currie (2010). The association between pregnancy weight gain and birth-weight: A within-family comparison. *Lancet* 376(9745): 984–990.

Ludwig, D. S., H. L. Rouse, J. Currie (2013). Pregnancy weight gain and childhood body weight: A within-family comparison. *PLOS Med* 10(10): e1001521.

Mann, J. R., S. W. McDermott, J. Hardin, C. Pan, Z. Zhang (2013). Pre-pregnancy body mass index, weight change during pregnancy, and risk of intellectual disability in children. *BJOG* 120(3): 309–319.

McDonald, S. D., Z. Han, S. Mulla et al. (2011). High gestational weight gain and the risk of preterm birth and low birth weight: A systematic review and meta-analysis. *J Obstet Gynaecol Can* 33(12): 1223–1233.

Miller, M., J. Y. Cho, A. Pham, J. Ramsdell, D. H. Broide (2009). Adiponectin and functional adiponectin receptor 1 are expressed by airway epithelial cells in chronic obstructive pulmonary disease. *J Immunol* 182(1): 684–691.

Morales, E., A. Groom, D. A. Lawlor, C. L. Relton (2014). DNA methylation signatures in cord blood associated with maternal gestational weight gain: Results from the ALSPAC cohort. *BMC Res Notes* 7: 278.

Moran, S., C. Arribas, M. Esteller (2016). Validation of a DNA methylation microarray for 850,000 CpG sites of the human genome enriched in enhancer sequences. *Epigenomics* 8(3): 389–399.

Mutsaerts, M. A., A. M. van Oers, H. Groen et al. (2016). Randomized trial of a lifestyle program in obese infertile women. *N Engl J Med* 374(20): 1942–1953.

Neggers, Y. H., R. L. Goldenberg, S. L. Ramey, S. P. Cliver (2003). Maternal prepregnancy body mass index and psychomotor development in children. *Acta Obstet Gynecol Scand* 82(3): 235–240.

Oostvogels, A. J., K. Stronks, T. J. Roseboom et al. (2014). Maternal prepregnancy BMI, offspring's early postnatal growth, and metabolic profile at age 5-6 years: The ABCD Study. *J Clin Endocrinol Metab* 99(10): 3845–3854.

Patro, B., A. Liber, B. Zalewski et al. (2013). Maternal and paternal body mass index and off-spring obesity: A systematic review. *Ann Nutr Metab* 63(1–2): 32–41.

Perng, W., M. W. Gillman, C. S. Mantzoros, E. Oken (2014). A prospective study of maternal prenatal weight and offspring cardiometabolic health in midchildhood. *Ann Epidemiol* 24(11): 793–800 e791.

Pike, K. C., H. M. Inskip, S. M. Robinson et al. (2013). The relationship between maternal adiposity and infant weight gain, and childhood wheeze and atopy. *Thorax* 68(4): 372–379.

Poston, L., L. F. Harthoorn, E. M. Van Der Beek (2011). Obesity in pregnancy: Implications for the mother and lifelong health of the child. A consensus statement. *Pediatr Res* 69(2): 175–180.

Pugh, S. J., G. A. Richardson, J. A. Hutcheon et al. (2015). Maternal obesity and excessive gestational weight gain are associated with components of child cognition. *J Nutr* 145(11): 2562–2569.

Rasmussen, K. M., A. L. Yaktine, editors (2009). Institute of Medicine (U.S.) and National Research Council (US) Committee to Reexamine IOM Pregnancy Weight Guidelines. *Weight Gain During Pregnancy: Reexamining the Guidelines.* Washington, DC: National Academies Press (U.S.).

Restall, A., R. S. Taylor, J. M. Thompson et al. (2014). Risk factors for excessive gestational weight gain in a healthy, nulliparous cohort. *J Obes* 2014: 148391.

Rodriguez, A., J. Miettunen, T. B. Henriksen et al. (2008). Maternal adiposity prior to pregnancy is associated with ADHD symptoms in offspring: Evidence from three prospective pregnancy cohorts. *Int J Obes* 32(3): 550–557.

Rydhstrom, H., T. Tyden, A. Herbst, U. Ljungblad, B. Walles (1994). No relation between maternal weight gain and stillbirth. *Acta Obstet Gynecol Scand* 73(10): 779–781.

Schack-Nielsen, L., K. F. Michaelsen, M. Gamborg, E. L. Mortensen, T. I. Sorensen (2010). Gestational weight gain in relation to offspring body mass index and obesity from infancy through adulthood. *Int J Obes* 34(1): 67–74.

Scheers Andersson, E., P. Tynelius, E. A. Nohr, T. I. Sorensen, F. Rasmussen (2015). No association of maternal gestational weight gain with offspring blood pressure and hypertension at age 18 years in male sibling-pairs: A prospective register-based cohort study. *PLoS One* 10(3): e0121202.

Scholtens, S., A. H. Wijga, B. Brunekreef et al. (2010). Maternal overweight before pregnancy and asthma in offspring followed for 8 years. *Int J Obes* 34(4): 606–613.

Sharp, G. C., D. A. Lawlor, R. C. Richmond et al. (2015). Maternal pre-pregnancy BMI and gestational weight gain, offspring DNA methylation and later offspring adiposity: Findings from the Avon Longitudinal Study of Parents and Children. *Int J Epidemiol* 44(4): 1288–1304.

Shore, S. A., Y. M. Rivera-Sanchez, I. N. Schwartzman, R. A. Johnston (2003). Responses to ozone are increased in obese mice. *J Appl Physiol* 95(3): 938–945.

Shore, S. A., R. D. Terry, L. Flynt, A. Xu, C. Hug (2006). Adiponectin attenuates allergen-induced airway inflammation and hyperresponsiveness in mice. *J Allergy Clin Immunol* 118(2): 389–395.

Soubry, A., S. K. Murphy, F. Wang et al. (2015). Newborns of obese parents have altered DNA methylation patterns at imprinted genes. *Int J Obes* 39(4): 650–657.

Stephansson, O., P. W. Dickman, A. Johansson, S. Cnattingius (2001). Maternal weight, pregnancy weight gain, and the risk of antepartum stillbirth. *Am J Obstet Gynecol* 184(3): 463–469.

Stothard, K. J., P. W. Tennant, R. Bell, J. Rankin (2009). Maternal overweight and obesity and the risk of congenital anomalies: A systematic review and meta-analysis. *JAMA* 301(6): 636–650.

Stotland, N. E., Y. W. Cheng, L. M. Hopkins, A. B. Caughey (2006). Gestational weight gain and adverse neonatal outcome among term infants. *Obstet Gynecol* 108(3 Pt 1): 635–643.

Tanda, R., P. J. Salsberry, P. B. Reagan, M. Z. Fang (2013). The impact of prepregnancy obesity on children's cognitive test scores. *Matern Child Health J* 17(2): 222–229.

Tanvig, M., C. A. Vinter, J. S. Jorgensen et al. (2015). Effects of lifestyle intervention in pregnancy and anthropometrics at birth on offspring metabolic profile at 2.8 years: Results from the Lifestyle in Pregnancy and Offspring (LiPO) study. *J Clin Endocrinol Metab* 100(1): 175–183.

Thangaratinam, S., E. Rogozinska, K. Jolly et al. (2012). Effects of interventions in pregnancy on maternal weight and obstetric outcomes: Meta-analysis of randomised evidence. *BMJ* 344: e2088.

Tian, C., C. Hu, X. He et al. (2016). Excessive weight gain during pregnancy and risk of macrosomia: A meta-analysis. *Arch Gynecol Obstet* 293(1): 29–35.

Tie, H. T., Y. Y. Xia, Y. S. Zeng et al. (2014). Risk of childhood overweight or obesity associated with excessive weight gain during pregnancy: A meta-analysis. *Arch Gynecol Obstet* 289(2): 247–257.

Toemen, L., O. Gishti, L. van Osch-Gevers et al. (2016). Maternal obesity, gestational weight gain and childhood cardiac outcomes: Role of childhood body mass index. *Int J Obes* 40(7): 1070–1078.

Tozuka, Y., M. Kumon, E. Wada et al. (2010). Maternal obesity impairs hippocampal BDNF production and spatial learning performance in young mouse offspring. *Neurochem Int* 57(3): 235–247.

Tyrrell, J., R. C. Richmond, T. M. Palmer et al. (2016). Genetic evidence for causal relationships between maternal obesity-related traits and birth weight. *JAMA* 315(11): 1129–1140.

World Health Organization. Obesity and overweight fact sheet. http://www.who.int/mediacentre/factsheets/fs311/en/. Accessed 06-06-2016

Yu, Z., S. Han, J. Zhu et al. (2013). Pre-pregnancy body mass index in relation to infant birth weight and offspring overweight/obesity: A systematic review and meta-analysis. *PLoS One* 8(4): e61627.

Zhu, T., J. Tang, F. Zhao, Y. Qu, D. Mu (2015). Association between maternal obesity and offspring Apgar score or cord pH: A systematic review and meta-analysis. *Sci Rep* 5: 18386.

Zugna, D., C. Galassi, I. Annesi-Maesano et al. (2015). Maternal complications in pregnancy and wheezing in early childhood: A pooled analysis of 14 birth cohorts. *Int J Epidemiol* 44(1): 199–208.

14 Long-Term Impact of Diabetes in Pregnancy on Human Offspring Metabolism

Louise Kelstrup, Tine Dalgaard Clausen,
Azadeh Houshmand-Oeregaard,
Elisabeth R. Mathiesen, and Peter Damm

CONTENTS

14.1 INTRODUCTION

Elevated blood glucose or *hyperglycemia* is the main clinical characteristic of all types of diabetes mellitus (DM). If a pregnant woman has diabetes, her fetus is exposed to intrauterine hyperglycemia as glucose is an essential nutrient and transfers freely across the placental barrier. This earliest environmental exposure to maternal hyperglycemia *in utero* affects the individual adversely in both short- and long-time life span (Dabelea and Crume 2011; Metzger et al. 2008; Metzger 2007). From the early 1950s, the first literature on short-term clinical adverse outcomes in newborn children of mothers with type 1 diabetes mellitus (T1DM) emerged. In the same decade, increased focus on pathophysiological mechanisms began and later the question arose on how exposure to intrauterine hyperglycemia affects the individual in the long-term perspective. Various clinical parameters related to obesity, glucose metabolism, cardiovascular profile, and cognitive function have been investigated so far and the field expanded over the years to include gestational diabetes mellitus (GDM) as well as T1DM.

The aim of this chapter is to give an overview of the present knowledge on long-term metabolic consequences for offspring from pregnancies complicated by either T1DM or GDM with a focus on literature from this century.

Our own data will be presented originating from the Copenhagen cohort, a cohort of adult subjects exposed to intrauterine hyperglycemia (Clausen et al. 2008, 2009; Kelstrup et al. 2012, 2013, 2015, 2016a,b). The Copenhagen cohort consists of offspring (O) exposed to maternal GDM (O-GDM) or maternal T1DM (O-T1DM) and two control groups of mothers without diabetes in pregnancy: offspring of women with normal oral glucose tolerance test (OGTT) in pregnancy (O-NoGDM) but with risk factors for developing GDM and phenotypically similar to the women who did develop GDM and a control group of offspring of healthy mothers representing the background population (O-BP). The subjects in the cohort have been examined twice: at mean age 22.0 (Clausen et al. 2008, 2009; Kelstrup et al. 2012, 2013, 2015, 2016a) and 30.6 years (Kelstrup et al. 2016b). At the first follow-up ($N = 597$), all four groups participated: (1) O-GDM = 168, (2) O-T1DM = 153, (3) O-NoGDM = 139, and (4) O-BP = 128. In the second follow-up, offspring exposed to diabetes (O-GDM and O-T1DM) and one control group (O-BP) participated, with a total of 206 subjects (O-GDM = 82, O-T1DM = 67, and O-BP = 57).

14.2   RISK OF OBESITY

A major adverse outcome in the field of intrauterine programming due to maternal hyperglycemia is the development of obesity in the offspring. Several studies have explored the association between diabetes in pregnancy and risk of obesity mainly in childhood (Boney et al. 2005; HAPO Study Cooperative Research Group 2009; Lawlor et al. 2010, 2011; Zhu et al. 2016; Krishnaveni et al. 2005, 2010; Uebel et al. 2014; Patel et al. 2012; Kubo et al. 2014; Lindsay et al. 2010; Dabelea et al. 2000, 2008; Malcolm et al. 2006; Manderson et al. 2002; Vaarasmaki et al. 2009). Fewer studies have been performed in offspring reaching teenage or adulthood. Included in these are studies of Pima Indians from Arizona, a group with a specific genotype predisposing to T2DM, with a prevalence of overweight and T2DM of 70% at the age of 25 years. Due to the specific genotype of this population, comparison with other studies must be made carefully (Dabelea et al. 2000; Pettitt et al. 1993).

Using register-based research and the unique system of a personal identity (ID) number, it has been possible to trace offspring beyond childhood in Denmark. One of the studies examined male adult offspring at the time of conscription exposed to maternal diabetes in pregnancy and found the rejection rate higher due to adiposity (Malcolm et al. 2006). The association was most pronounced if the mother had GDM, weaker if the mother had T1DM (Nielsen et al. 2012). The Danish multicenter study EPIgenetic, genetic and environmental effects on COgnitive and Metabolic functions in offspring of mothers with type 1 diabetes (EPICOM) characterized Caucasian teenagers (mean age 16.7, range 13.0–19.8) born to mothers with T1DM ($N = 278$) and controls ($N = 303$) (Vlachova et al. 2015). The maternal data were prospectively reported during pregnancy to a central database under the Danish Diabetes Association (Jensen et al. 2004). The authors found higher body mass index (BMI) standard deviation (SD) score in exposed offspring, including after adjustment for maternal prepregnancy BMI (Vlachova et al. 2015). In line with this, we found in the Copenhagen cohort (first follow-up, offspring aged 18–27 years) the following prevalence of overweight (BMI ≥ 25 kg/m^2): O-GDM, 40%; O-NoGDM, 30%; O-T1DM, 41%; O-BP, 24%. In adjusted analyses, the risk of overweight was significantly higher in both groups exposed to diabetes in pregnancy, O-GDM (odds ratio [OR] 1.79 [confidence interval or CI 95% 1.00–3.24]) and O-T1DM (OR 2.27 [1.30–3.98]), compared with O-BP (Clausen et al. 2009).

14.3 RISK OF TYPE 2 DIABETES

An essential issue in the field of diabetes in pregnancy is the offspring risk of developing diabetes, and this has been addressed in different ways in several studies, with a 2-hour 75-g OGTT being the most frequent test to examine glucose metabolism (Metzger 2007; Dabelea et al. 2000; Krishnaveni et al. 2005; Malcolm et al. 2006; Wroblewska-Seniuk et al. 2009; Holder et al. 2014; Weiss et al. 2000). Two studies in offspring of women with T1DM have been performed with different results. The EPICOM study (N = 581) found significantly elevated fasting plasma glucose (Vlachova et al. 2015), while this was not confirmed in another study including only 44 subjects (Holder et al. 2014).

The adult offspring participating in the Copenhagen cohort underwent OGTT at both first and second follow-up, and the results of the tests were evaluated according to World Health Organization (WHO) criteria (Alberti and Zimmet 1998), with a focus on the development of prediabetes (defined as impaired fasting glucose [IFG] or impaired glucose tolerance [IGT]) and T2DM. At the first follow-up in our cohort of adult offspring (mean age 22.0 years, N = 597), the prevalence of T2DM/prediabetes was O-GDM, 21%; O-T1DM, 11%; and O-NoGDM, 12% compared to O-BP, 4%. During OGTT, O-GDM had higher fasting and 2-hour plasma glucose than O-BP, while O-T1DM had higher 2-hour plasma glucose than O-BP. The adjusted ORs for T2DM/prediabetes were markedly increased in O-GDM (OR 7.76 [95% CI 2.58–23.39]) and to a lesser extent in O-T1DM (4.02 [1.31–12.33]) compared with O-BP. Furthermore, a positive association between maternal glucose level and offspring risk of T2DM/prediabetes was found (Clausen et al. 2008).

In the second follow-up of the adult offspring (mean age 30.6 years, N = 206), the prevalence of T2DM/prediabetes was O-GDM, 12% and O-T1DM, 12% compared to O-BP, 5%; however, these expected trends were not statistically different. During the OGTT, both groups exposed to maternal diabetes (O-GDM and O-T1DM) had significantly higher 2-hour plasma glucose than O-BP but similar fasting values. Furthermore, O-GDM had higher plasma glucose at 30 minutes during OGTT than O-BP (Kelstrup et al. 2016). With regard to the slightly different findings between our two follow-up studies, this is most likely due to a positive selection of participants to our second follow-up as in general the healthiest and leanest subjects accepted our reinvitation. Moreover, only 45% participated in the second follow-up, reducing the statistical power of our study.

14.4 CARDIOVASCULAR MARKERS AND METABOLIC SYNDROME

Various cardiovascular risk factors have been evaluated with main findings of increased systolic blood pressure, increased total cholesterol and low-density lipoprotein

(LDL), decreased high-density lipoprotein (HDL) cholesterol, and increased waist circumference in children of women with diabetes during pregnancy. A study in older children (age 6–13 years) found the same tendency, although no discrimination was made between the type of maternal diabetes as the offspring were pooled in one group ($N = 99$, pregnancies complicated with GDM [$N = 91$] or T1DM [$N = 8$]) when compared with the control group ($N = 422$) (West et al. 2011). The offspring exposed to intrauterine hyperglycemia had significantly increased levels of circulating cellular adhesion molecules (E-selectin, vascular cell adhesion molecule 1 [VCAM-1]), leptin, BMI, waist circumference, and systolic blood pressure, while adiponectin was decreased. Statistically, adjustment for maternal pre-pregnancy BMI was done, and only E-selectin, VCAM-1, and waist circumference remained significantly higher in exposed children (West et al. 2011). Similar findings were reported in another study in offspring of the same age (5–11 years) born to women with T1DM ($N = 61$) in comparison with controls ($N = 57$). Furthermore, the cardiovascular risk factors cholesterol (total and LDL), insulin-like growth factor-1 (IGF-1), and plasminogen activator inhibitor-1 (PAI-1) were also elevated in the exposed offspring (Manderson et al. 2002). A systematic review and meta-analysis confirmed the association between higher systolic blood pressure in the offspring of diabetic mothers and in controls (Aceti et al. 2012).

The EPICOM study (offspring mean age 16.7) found, in adjusted analyses, systolic blood pressure to be the only significant cardiovascular risk factor (Vlachova et al. 2015).

Despite many studies thoroughly examining the children for various cardiovascular risk factors and biomarkers, only one study included all components of the metabolic syndrome and found increased risk in 6–11-year-old offspring of women with GDM (Boney et al. 2005). The risk of the metabolic syndrome (Alberti et al. 2006) from the first follow-up of the cohort of adult offspring (mean age 22.0) was significantly higher in O-GDM, adjusted OR (4.12 [1.69–10.06]) and O-NoGDM (2.74 [1.08–6.97]), as well as in O-T1DM (2.59 [1.04–6.45]) compared with O-BP (Clausen et al. 2009). Moreover, a positive association between maternal glucose levels in pregnancy and the risk of the metabolic syndrome was found. In the second follow-up of the cohort (30.6 years), significantly elevated diastolic blood pressure was found in O-GDM. For both O-GDM and O-T1DM, plasma levels of triglyceride and lipoproteins were similar to those of unexposed offspring (Kelstrup et al. 2016).

14.5 INFLAMMATION

Low-grade inflammation has been reported to be involved in obesity and to precede and predict the development of T2DM, and has been associated with the development of cardiovascular diseases (Pradhan et al. 2001; Donath and Shoelson 2011; Shoelson et al. 2007).

Levels of various biomarkers representing low-grade inflammation in offspring of pregnancies complicated with diabetes have been investigated. The spectrum of biomarkers is broad and most studies have been performed in umbilical cord blood from newborns or placenta (Cross et al. 2010; Lindegaard et al. 2008; Nelson et al. 2007).

A British group has performed a study in offspring of women with T1DM in pregnancy reaching adulthood (aged 16–23 years) ($N = 21$) in comparisons with controls ($N = 23$) (Cross et al. 2009). Various metabolic outcomes were investigated including interleukin 6 (IL-6) and high-sensitivity C-reactive protein (hs-CRP) levels, but no differences were found between offspring exposed to maternal T1DM and controls. The inflammatory markers IL-6, hs-CRP, and YKL-40 have been investigated in our cohort of adult offspring at the first follow-up. We did not find any differences for all three markers between O-GDM ($N = 168$) and O-T1DM ($N = 160$) compared with the control groups O-NoGDM ($N = 141$) and O-BP ($N = 128$). At the second follow-up, only hs-CRP was analyzed and no difference was found between exposed and unexposed offspring.

14.6 INSULIN FUNCTION

Insulin is essential in glucose metabolism, and a larger number of studies have investigated the insulin function in offspring of women with diabetes in pregnancy (Krishnaveni et al. 2010; Vaarasmaki et al. 2009; Wroblewska-Seniuk et al. 2009; Holder et al. 2014; Weiss et al. 2000; Keely et al. 2008; Boerschmann et al. 2010; Buinauskiene et al. 2004; Bush et al. 2011; Pirkola et al. 2008; Hunter et al. 2004; Plagemann et al. 1997; Salbe et al. 2007). The literature is diverse concerning differences in offspring ages, type of maternal diabetes, type of test for glucose tolerance, types of measurements or index representing insulin sensitivity and secretion, and whether both sensitivity and secretion are reported or only one trait. The majority of the studies are performed in children; only a few studies have examined insulin secretion and sensitivity in adult offspring of women with diabetes (Sobngwi et al. 2003; Gautier et al. 2001). A central study in this field compared 15 adult (22–24 years old) offspring of mothers with T1DM with a control group of 16 participants of the same age with a family history of paternal T1DM. Both groups were without a family history of T2DM and had similar human leukocyte antigen - antigen D related (HLA-DR) and DR4 distribution, but there was no information regarding ethnicity. The authors found that intrauterine exposure to hyperglycemia was associated with a defect in insulin secretion but not with adiposity or insulin resistance in the offspring (Sobngwi et al. 2003). Another study was in adult offspring of Pima origin as part of a larger study focusing on the effect of early onset of parental diabetes in 104 subjects aged 22–27 years with normal glucose tolerance. The authors aimed to further explore if this was worsened by intrauterine exposure to diabetes and made a substudy in eight male offspring, who were metabolically evaluated by hyperinsulinemic–euglycemic clamp. The overall conclusion was that offspring of parents with early onset of diabetes had lower insulin secretion and this was worsened by exposure to an intrauterine diabetic environment (Gautier et al. 2001).

Studies in younger diabetes-exposed Caucasian offspring suggest that the primary abnormality is insulin resistance (Plagemann et al. 1997). However, comparison of the studies might be difficult due to differences in offspring age: young adults versus children. One study found that maternal gestational glucose concentration was inversely associated with the offspring's insulin sensitivity and positively associated with β-cell response (Bush et al. 2011).

Insulin sensitivity and insulin response were investigated in the Copenhagen cohort of adult offspring in the first follow-up examination (Kelstrup et al. 2013). Based on OGTT values of insulin and glucose, different indices of insulin sensitivity, insulin release, and disposition index were calculated. Disposition index is an estimate of insulin release taking prevailing insulin sensitivity into account. Both offspring of mothers with GDM ($N = 167$) and with T1DM ($N = 153$) had reduced insulin sensitivity. No differences were found for absolute insulin secretion, but the disposition index was significantly reduced in both groups exposed to intrauterine hyperglycemia. No associations to maternal blood glucose values during pregnancy were found and when including variables of maternal prepregnancy overweight, offspring birth weight, and adult offspring BMI in the analyses, the results did not change.

Similar indices of insulin sensitivity and secretion were used in two other studies: a study from the United States, including obese adolescents of mothers with GDM (Holder et al. 2014), and the EPICOM study, including teenagers of mothers with T1DM (Vlachova et al. 2015). The American study included 255 obese children (mean age 12 years) of mixed ethnicity, exposed to maternal GDM ($N = 45$) or nonexposed offspring of normoglycemic mothers ($N = 210$). The offspring were all obese and normoglycemic at inclusion and the authors aimed to investigate how exposure to maternal GDM *in utero* would affect the children's glucose tolerance over time. After 2.8 years of follow-up and based on OGTT-derived indices, no differences were found in absolute insulin sensitivity or secretion, but the authors found a reduced disposition index in offspring of mothers with GDM compared to controls (Holder et al. 2014).

In the EPICOM study, offspring exposed to maternal T1DM presented both reduced insulin sensitivity and relative insulin secretion deficiency at age 13–18 years compared with controls (Vlachova et al. 2015).

14.7   INCRETIN HORMONES AND GLUCAGON

The incretin hormones glucagon-like peptide-1 (GLP-1) and glucose-dependent insulinotropic peptide (GIP) are released from the gut in response to the oral intake of glucose and stimulate the pancreatic β-cells to release insulin, which in healthy persons may account for up to 70% of postprandial insulin secretion (Nauck et al. 1986). In patients with T2DM, the incretin effect is impaired and contributes to only 20–35% of the insulin response after oral intake of glucose (Ahren et al. 2013; Holst et al. 2009).

So far, two studies have investigated the incretin function in offspring of women with diabetes in pregnancy. The first study was in prepubertal children aged 5–10 years born by mothers with GDM, and evaluated the postprandial response of gut hormones (peptide YY [PYY], GLP-1, and ghrelin) (Chandler-Laney et al. 2014). The participants ($N = 42$) underwent a liquid meal challenge, and a suppressed response of GLP-1 (incremental area under the curve [AUC]) was found in GDM-exposed offspring, independent of greater adiposity. The authors concluded that fetal exposure to maternal GDM might alter the activity of the gut hormones, which may influence satiety and thereby contribute to the increased risk of obesity.

The second study was performed at the first follow-up in the Copenhagen cohort of adult offspring (18–27 years) born to women with either GDM or T1DM (Clausen et al. 2009). The level of the two incretin hormones GLP-1 and GIP was evaluated during OGTT, and we found that GLP-1 levels in the fasting state were significantly lower in both O-GDM and O-T1DM compared to O-BP. During the OGTT (at 30 and 120 minutes), the levels of GLP-1 did not differ significantly between the groups, and also GIP levels were similar between the two groups exposed to maternal diabetes in utero and the control groups both in the fasting state and during the OGTT (Kelstrup et al. 2015). Maternal blood glucose levels in pregnancy were not associated with the levels of GLP-1 and GIP in the adult offspring.

Glucagon is produced by the α-cell of the pancreas and has the opposite effect to insulin. Glucagon levels are elevated in fasting condition, and an early trait in the pathogenesis of T2DM is increased levels of glucagon (Dunning and Gerich 2007; Faerch et al. 2016; Wewer Albrechtsen et al. 2016; Reaven et al. 1987). In the Copenhagen cohort, increasing maternal blood glucose levels during OGTT in pregnancy (mothers with GDM) were associated with reduced postprandial suppression of glucagon in the adult offspring (O-GDM) (Kelstrup et al. 2015). Besides this study, levels of glucagon in offspring from pregnancies complicated by maternal diabetes have not been evaluated.

14.8 EPIGENETIC STUDIES

Epigenetic studies in both human and animal offspring exposed to intrauterine hyperglycemia have been performed, so far all except one study in offspring of women with GDM, and mainly in tissue from newborns (cord blood and/or placenta) (Bouchard et al. 2012; Xie et al. 2015; El et al. 2013; Houde et al. 2013; Houde et al. 2014; Quilter et al. 2014; Ruchat et al. 2013) or children (age 8–12 years, peripheral blood mononuclear cells) (West et al. 2013). A cross-sectional study has investigated the level of peroxisome proliferator-activated receptor-γ coactivator-1α (PPARCG1A) in placenta and cord blood from mothers with GDM in comparison with placentas from women without diabetes in pregnancy. PPARGC1A is a potent, versatile regulator of gene expression in eukaryotic cells. PPARGC1A is highly expressed in mitochondria-enriched tissues and proposed to play a substantial role in pathways controlling glucose homeostasis (Patti 2004; Soyal et al. 2006). The authors found that the maternal blood glucose level during OGTT in 24–28 weeks of gestation was positively correlated with placental DNA methylation and negatively correlated with cord blood DNA methylation of the PPARGC1A promoter in a CpG site-specific manner. In a subanalysis in the GDM group alone, the placental CpG site-specific methylation of the PPARGC1A promoter was correlated with maternal blood glucose level 2 hours during the OGTT (Xie et al. 2015).

The epigenetic profile of PPARGC1A in insulin-sensitive tissue (skeletal muscle and subcutaneous adipose tissue) has been investigated in the second follow-up in the Copenhagen cohort of adult offspring of women with diabetes in pregnancy (Kelstrup et al. 2016). Reduced gene expression of PPARGC1A was found in skeletal muscle from O-GDM in comparison with O-BP. No differences were found in adipose tissue and no differences were found in levels of methylation in either skeletal or adipose tissue. Regarding O-T1DM, no differences were found in both level of PPARGC1A gene expression and DNA methylation in comparison with O-BP in both skeletal and adipose tissue (Kelstrup et al. 2016).

Different causes may influence the results: other factors in relation to maternal health during pregnancy than solely maternal hyperglycemia might have affected the programming effect. This assumption was based on the negative findings between offspring exposed to maternal T1DM and the control group. O-T1DM was exposed to the worst hyperglycemia compared to O-GDM, as the T1DM mothers were having an absolute lack of endogenous insulin production, thereby being totally dependent on exogenous insulin substitution, while GDM mothers were affected by a milder pregnancy-related diabetes only treated by diet. If only maternal hyperglycemia was inducing epigenetic changes in the offspring, then the largest differences were expected to be found in O-T1DM. The main factor with an impact in pregnancy besides maternal hyperglycemia could be maternal obesity, as 35% of the GDM mothers were overweight (BMI ≥ 25 kg/m^2) in contrast to only 8% of T1DM mothers.

Other mechanisms than intrauterine programming reflected as epigenetic alterations may influence the regulation of *PPARGC1A* expression in adult age: both environmental exposures, especially personal lifestyle, and also genetic predisposition. Women with GDM have an increased risk up to 50% of developing T2DM later in life, with a high association to common genetic variants of T2DM (Lauenborg et al. 2009). It is highly likely that a proportion of these genetic variants will be transmitted to their offspring, thereby contributing to the prediabetic abnormalities in the following generations.

14.9   PERSPECTIVES

A summary of research in the field of intrauterine programming due to maternal diabetes has been given in this chapter. During nearly 70 years, diabetes in pregnancy has been the topic of diverse research from practical clinical issues regarding the health of the pregnant women and their newborn to basic science exploring the developmental mechanisms influencing the long-term perspective. The actuality is ever lasting due to the steep rise in obesity and T2DM worldwide.

The prevailing theory in the field is the "hypothesis of fuel-mediated teratogenesis" as proposed by N. Freinkel in 1980 (Freinkel 1980). However, many questions in the area of developmental programming of metabolic disease remain unanswered. Studies within the field have just started exploring mechanistic explanations to supplement the well-described epidemiological associations between exposure to maternal diabetes and later risk of adverse metabolic health in the offspring. The different epidemiological studies in offspring of varying age show a tendency of increased risk of obesity, impaired glucose mechanism, and pathophysiological traits toward T2DM. However, direct comparison of the studies should be performed with care due to mixed populations studied in terms of offspring age, ethnicity, and type of maternal diabetes. It is possible to separate the influence of environmental and genetics factors in intergenerational animal models to study long-term effects of intrauterine exposure to hyperglycemia in contrast to human studies where multiple factors influence a life perspective. In long-term follow-up human studies confounding will undoubtedly influence the results and conclusions and interpretation should be made carefully. Furthermore, the complex pathophysiology of T2DM is a challenge. The diverse genetic component contributing to the development of the disease together with strong environmental exposures in terms of modern sedentary lifestyle and high-caloric food intake as well as gene–environment interactions all need to be addressed.

The evolving concept of epigenetics provides a conceptual framework of how exposures are transformed into altered phenotype. In the case of maternal diabetes, it is possible that metabolic and nutritional factors in the intrauterine environment can modify ongoing DNA methylation and histone modifications and thereby change gene expression in the offspring. Until now the molecular mechanisms possibly driving this are still unknown and only relatively few studies in epigenetics have been performed so far.

Hopefully, continued follow-up studies of the offspring participating in the hyperglycemia and adverse pregnancy outcome (HAPO) cohort (Metzger et al. 2008; HAPO Study Cooperative Research Group 2008; Lowe et al. 2012; Pettitt et al. 2010; Catalano et al. 2012) and from two randomized controlled trials in GDM treatment will be performed to investigate the long-term effect of maternal treatment on the offspring (Malcolm et al. 2006; Landon et al. 2015).

REFERENCES

Aceti, A, Santhakumaran, S, Logan, KM, Philipps, LH, Prior, E, Gale, C, Hyde, MJ, Modi, N. The diabetic pregnancy and offspring blood pressure in childhood: A systematic review and meta-analysis. *Diabetologia* 55:3114–3127, 2012.

Ahren, B. Incretin dysfunction in type 2 diabetes: Clinical impact and future perspectives. *Diabetes Metab* 39:195–201, 2013.

Alberti, KG, Zimmet, P, Shaw, J. Metabolic syndrome—A new world-wide definition. A Consensus Statement from the International Diabetes Federation. *Diabet Med* 23: 469–480, 2006.

Alberti, KG, Zimmet, PZ. Definition, diagnosis and classification of diabetes mellitus and its complications. Part 1: Diagnosis and classification of diabetes mellitus provisional report of a WHO consultation. *Diabet Med* 15:539–553, 1998.

Boerschmann, H, Pfluger, M, Henneberger, L, Ziegler, AG, Hummel, S. Prevalence and predictors of overweight and insulin resistance in offspring of mothers with gestational diabetes mellitus. *Diabetes Care* 33:1845–1849, 2010.

Boney, CM, Verma, A, Tucker, R, Vohr, BR. Metabolic syndrome in childhood: Association with birth weight, maternal obesity, and gestational diabetes mellitus. *Pediatrics* 115:e290–e296, 2005.

Bouchard, L, Hivert, MF, Guay, SP, St-Pierre, J, Perron, P, Brisson, D. Placental adiponectin gene DNA methylation levels are associated with mothers' blood glucose concentration. *Diabetes* 61:1272–1280, 2012.

Buinauskiene, J, Baliutaviciene, D, Zalinkevicius, R. Glucose tolerance of 2- to 5-yr-old offspring of diabetic mothers. *Pediatr Diabetes* 5:143–146, 2004.

Bush, NC, Chandler-Laney, PC, Rouse, DJ, Granger, WM, Oster, RA, Gower, BA. Higher maternal gestational glucose concentration is associated with lower offspring insulin sensitivity and altered beta-cell function. *J Clin Endocrinol Metab* 96:E803–E809, 2011.

Catalano, PM, McIntyre, HD, Cruickshank, JK, McCance, DR, Dyer, AR, Metzger, BE, Lowe, LP, Trimble, ER, Coustan, DR, Hadden, DR, Persson, B, Hod, M, Oats, JJ. The hyperglycemia and adverse pregnancy outcome study: Associations of GDM and obesity with pregnancy outcomes. *Diabetes Care* 35:780–786, 2012.

Chandler-Laney, PC, Bush, NC, Rouse, DJ, Mancuso, MS, Gower, BA. Gut hormone activity of children born to women with and without gestational diabetes. *Pediatr Obes* 9:53–62, 2014.

Clausen, TD, Mathiesen, ER, Hansen, T, Pedersen, O, Jensen, DM, Lauenborg, J, Damm, P. High prevalence of type 2 diabetes and pre-diabetes in adult offspring of women with gestational diabetes mellitus or type 1 diabetes: The role of intrauterine hyperglycemia. *Diabetes Care* 31:340–346, 2008.

Clausen, TD, Mathiesen, ER, Hansen, T, Pedersen, O, Jensen, DM, Lauenborg, J, Schmidt, L, Damm, P. Overweight and the metabolic syndrome in adult offspring of women with diet-treated gestational diabetes mellitus or type 1 diabetes. *J Clin Endocrinol Metab* 94:2464–2470, 2009.

Cross, JA, Brennan, C, Gray, T, Temple, RC, Dozio, N, Hughes, JC, Levell, NJ, Murphy, H, Fowler, D, Hughes, DA, Sampson, MJ. Absence of telomere shortening and oxidative DNA damage in the young adult offspring of women with pre-gestational type 1 diabetes. *Diabetologia* 52:226–234, 2009.

Cross, JA, Temple, RC, Hughes, JC, Dozio, NC, Brennan, C, Stanley, K, Murphy, HR, Fowler, D, Hughes, DA, Sampson, MJ. Cord blood telomere length, telomerase activity and inflammatory markers in pregnancies in women with diabetes or gestational diabetes. *Diabet Med* 27:1264–1270, 2010.

Dabelea, D, Crume, T. Maternal environment and the transgenerational cycle of obesity and diabetes. *Diabetes* 60:1849–1855, 2011.

Dabelea, D, Hanson, RL, Lindsay, RS, Pettitt, DJ, Imperatore, G, Gabir, MM, Roumain, J, Bennett, PH, Knowler, WC. Intrauterine exposure to diabetes conveys risks for type 2 diabetes and obesity: A study of discordant sibships. *Diabetes* 49:2208–2211, 2000.

Dabelea, D, Mayer-Davis, EJ, Lamichhane, AP, D'Agostino, RB, Jr., Liese, AD, Vehik, KS, Narayan, KM, Zeitler, P, Hamman, RF. Association of intrauterine exposure to maternal diabetes and obesity with type 2 diabetes in youth: The SEARCH Case-Control Study. *Diabetes Care* 31:1422–1426, 2008.

Donath, MY, Shoelson, SE. Type 2 diabetes as an inflammatory disease. *Nat Rev Immunol* 11:98–107, 2011.

Dunning, BE, Gerich, JE. The role of alpha-cell dysregulation in fasting and postprandial hyperglycemia in type 2 diabetes and therapeutic implications. *Endocr Rev* 28:253–283, 2007.

El, HN, Pliushch, G, Schneider, E, Dittrich, M, Muller, T, Korenkov, M, Aretz, M, Zechner, U, Lehnen, H, Haaf, T. Metabolic programming of MEST DNA methylation by intrauterine exposure to gestational diabetes mellitus. *Diabetes* 62:1320–1328, 2013.

Faerch, K, Vistisen, D, Pacini, G, Torekov, SS, Johansen, NB, Witte, DR, Jonsson, A, Pedersen, O, Hansen, T, Lauritzen, T, Jorgensen, ME, Ahren, B, Holst, JJ. Insulin resistance is accompanied by increased fasting glucagon and delayed glucagon suppression in individuals with normal and impaired glucose regulation. *Diabetes* 2016.

Freinkel, N. Banting Lecture 1980. Of pregnancy and progeny. *Diabetes* 29:1023–1035, 1980.

Gautier, JF, Wilson, C, Weyer, C, Mott, D, Knowler, WC, Cavaghan, M, Polonsky, KS, Bogardus, C, Pratley, RE. Low acute insulin secretory responses in adult offspring of people with early onset type 2 diabetes. *Diabetes* 50:1828–1833, 2001.

HAPO Study Cooperative Research Group. Hyperglycemia and Adverse Pregnancy Outcome (HAPO) Study: Associations with neonatal anthropometrics. *Diabetes* 58:453–459, 2009.

Holder, T, Giannini, C, Santoro, N, Pierpont, B, Shaw, M, Duran, E, Caprio, S, Weiss, R. A low disposition index in adolescent offspring of mothers with gestational diabetes: A risk marker for the development of impaired glucose tolerance in youth. *Diabetologia* 57:2413–2420, 2014.

Holst, JJ, Vilsboll, T, Deacon, CF. The incretin system and its role in type 2 diabetes mellitus. *Mol Cell Endocrinol* 297:127–136, 2009.

Houde, AA, Guay, SP, Desgagne, V, Hivert, MF, Baillargeon, JP, St-Pierre, J, Perron, P, Gaudet, D, Brisson, D, Bouchard, L. Adaptations of placental and cord blood ABCA1 DNA methylation profile to maternal metabolic status. *Epigenetics* 8:1289–1302, 2013.

Houde, AA, St-Pierre, J, Hivert, MF, Baillargeon, JP, Perron, P, Gaudet, D, Brisson, D, Bouchard, L. Placental lipoprotein lipase DNA methylation levels are associated with gestational diabetes mellitus and maternal and cord blood lipid profiles. *J Dev Orig Health Dis* 5:132–141, 2014.

Hunter, WA, Cundy, T, Rabone, D, Hofman, PL, Harris, M, Regan, F, Robinson, E, Cutfield, WS. Insulin sensitivity in the offspring of women with type 1 and type 2 diabetes. *Diabetes Care* 27:1148–1152, 2004.

Jensen, DM, Damm, P, Moelsted-Pedersen, L, Ovesen, P, Westergaard, JG, Moeller, M, Beck-Nielsen, H. Outcomes in type 1 diabetic pregnancies: A nationwide, population-based study. *Diabetes Care* 27:2819–2823, 2004.

Keely, EJ, Malcolm, JC, Hadjiyannakis, S, Gaboury, I, Lough, G, Lawson, ML. Prevalence of metabolic markers of insulin resistance in offspring of gestational diabetes pregnancies. *Pediatr Diabetes* 9:53–59, 2008.

Kelstrup, L, Clausen, TD, Mathiesen, ER, Hansen, T, Damm, P. Low-grade inflammation in young adults exposed to intrauterine hyperglycemia. *Diabetes Res Clin Pract* 97:322–330, 2012.

Kelstrup, L, Clausen, TD, Mathiesen, ER, Hansen, T, Holst, JJ, Damm, P. Incretin and glucagon levels in adult offspring exposed to maternal diabetes in pregnancy. *J Clin Endocrinol Metab* 100:jc2014–3978, 2015

Kelstrup, L, Damm, P, Mathiesen, ER, Hansen, T, Vaag, AA, Pedersen, O, Clausen, TD. Insulin resistance and impaired pancreatic beta-cell function in adult offspring of women with diabetes in pregnancy. *J Clin Endocrinol Metab* 98:3793–3801, 2013.

Kelstrup, L, Dejgaard, TF, Clausen, TD, Mathiesen, ER, Hansen, T, Vestergaard, H, Damm, P. Levels of the inflammation marker YKL-40 in young adults exposed to intrauterine hyperglycemia. *Diabetes Res Clin Pract* 114:50–54, 2016a.

Kelstrup, L, Hjort, L, Houshmand-Oeregaard, A, Clausen, TD, Hansen, NS, Broholm, C, Borch-Johnsen, L, Mathiesen, ER, Vaag, AA, Damm, P. Gene expression and DNA methylation of PPARGC1A in Muscle and Adipose Tissue from Adult Offspring of Women with Diabetes in Pregnancy. *Diabetes* 65:2900–2910, 2016b.

Krishnaveni, GV, Hill, JC, Leary, SD, Veena, SR, Saperia, J, Saroja, A, Karat, SC, Fall, CH. Anthropometry, glucose tolerance, and insulin concentrations in Indian children: Relationships to maternal glucose and insulin concentrations during pregnancy. *Diabetes Care* 28:2919–2925, 2005.

Krishnaveni, GV, Veena, SR, Hill, JC, Kehoe, S, Karat, SC, Fall, CH. Intrauterine exposure to maternal diabetes is associated with higher adiposity and insulin resistance and clustering of cardiovascular risk markers in Indian children. *Diabetes Care* 33:402–404, 2010.

Kubo, A, Ferrara, A, Windham, GC, Greenspan, LC, Deardorff, J, Hiatt, RA, Quesenberry, CP, Jr., Laurent, C, Mirabedi, AS, Kushi, LH. Maternal hyperglycemia during pregnancy predicts adiposity of the offspring. *Diabetes Care* 37:2996–3002, 2014.

Landon, MB, Rice, MM, Varner, MW, Casey, BM, Reddy, UM, Wapner, RJ, Rouse, DJ, Biggio, JR, Jr., Thorp, JM, Chien, EK, Saade, G, Peaceman, AM, Blackwell, SC, VanDorsten, JP. Mild gestational diabetes mellitus and long-term child health. *Diabetes Care* 38:445–452, 2015.

Lauenborg, J, Grarup, N, Damm, P, Borch-Johnsen, K, Jorgensen, T, Pedersen, O, Hansen, T. Common type 2 diabetes risk gene variants associate with gestational diabetes. *J Clin Endocrinol Metab* 94:145–150, 2009.

Lawlor, DA, Fraser, A, Lindsay, RS, Ness, A, Dabelea, D, Catalano, P, Davey, SG, Sattar, N, Nelson, SM. Association of existing diabetes, gestational diabetes and glycosuria in pregnancy with macrosomia and offspring body mass index, waist and fat mass in later childhood: Findings from a prospective pregnancy cohort. *Diabetologia* 53:89–97, 2010.

Lawlor, DA, Lichtenstein, P, Langstrom, N. Association of maternal diabetes mellitus in pregnancy with offspring adiposity into early adulthood: Sibling study in a prospective cohort of 280,866 men from 248,293 families. *Circulation* 123:258–265, 2011.

Lindegaard, ML, Svarrer, EM, Damm, P, Mathiesen, ER, Nielsen, LB. Increased LDL cholesterol and CRP in infants of mothers with type 1 diabetes. *Diabetes Metab Res Rev* 24:465–471, 2008.

Lindsay, RS, Nelson, SM, Walker, JD, Greene, SA, Milne, G, Sattar, N, Pearson, DW. Programming of adiposity in offspring of mothers with type 1 diabetes at age 7 years. *Diabetes Care* 33:1080–1085, 2010.

Lowe, LP, Metzger, BE, Dyer, AR, Lowe, J, McCance, DR, Lappin, TR, Trimble, ER, Coustan, DR, Hadden, DR, Hod, M, Oats, JJ, Persson, B. Hyperglycemia and Adverse Pregnancy Outcome (HAPO) Study: Associations of maternal A1C and glucose with pregnancy outcomes. *Diabetes Care* 35:574–580, 2012.

Malcolm, JC, Lawson, ML, Gaboury, I, Lough, G, Keely, E. Glucose tolerance of offspring of mother with gestational diabetes mellitus in a low-risk population. *Diabet Med* 23:565–570, 2006.

Manderson, JG, Mullan, B, Patterson, CC, Hadden, DR, Traub, AI, McCance, DR. Cardiovascular and metabolic abnormalities in the offspring of diabetic pregnancy. *Diabetologia* 45:991–996, 2002.

Metzger, BE, Lowe, LP, Dyer, AR, Trimble, ER, Chaovarindr, U, Coustan, DR, Hadden, DR, McCance, DR, Hod, M, McIntyre, HD, Oats, JJ, Persson, B, Rogers, MS, Sacks, DA. Hyperglycemia and adverse pregnancy outcomes. *N Engl J Med* 358:1991–2002, 2008.

Metzger, BE. Long-term outcomes in mothers diagnosed with gestational diabetes mellitus and their offspring. *Clin Obstet Gynecol* 50:972–979, 2007.

Nauck, MA, Homberger, E, Siegel, EG, Allen, RC, Eaton, RP, Ebert, R, Creutzfeldt, W. Incretin effects of increasing glucose loads in man calculated from venous insulin and C-peptide responses. *J Clin Endocrinol Metab* 63:492–498, 1986.

Nelson, SM, Sattar, N, Freeman, DJ, Walker, JD, Lindsay, RS. Inflammation and endothelial activation is evident at birth in offspring of mothers with type 1 diabetes. *Diabetes* 56:2697–2704, 2007.

Nielsen, GL, Dethlefsen, C, Lundbye-Christensen, S, Pedersen, JF, Molsted-Pedersen, L, Gillman, MW. Adiposity in 277 young adult male offspring of women with diabetes compared with controls: A Danish population-based cohort study. *Acta Obstet Gynecol Scand* 91:838–843, 2012.

Patel, S, Fraser, A, Davey, SG, Lindsay, RS, Sattar, N, Nelson, SM, Lawlor, DA. Associations of gestational diabetes, existing diabetes, and glycosuria with offspring obesity and cardiometabolic outcomes. *Diabetes Care* 35:63–71, 2012.

Patti, ME. Gene expression in humans with diabetes and prediabetes: What have we learned about diabetes pathophysiology? *Curr Opin Clin Nutr Metab Care* 7:383–390, 2004.

Pettitt, DJ, McKenna, S, McLaughlin, C, Patterson, CC, Hadden, DR, McCance, DR. Maternal glucose at 28 weeks of gestation is not associated with obesity in 2-year-old offspring: The Belfast Hyperglycemia and Adverse Pregnancy Outcome (HAPO) family study. *Diabetes Care* 33:1219–1223, 2010.

Pettitt, DJ, Nelson, RG, Saad, MF, Bennett, PH, Knowler, WC. Diabetes and obesity in the offspring of Pima Indian women with diabetes during pregnancy. *Diabetes Care* 16:310–314, 1993.

Pirkola, J, Vaarasmaki, M, Leinonen, E, Bloigu, A, Veijola, R, Tossavainen, P, Knip, M, Tapanainen, P. Maternal type 1 and gestational diabetes: Postnatal differences in insulin secretion in offspring at preschool age. *Pediatr Diabetes* 9:583–589, 2008.

Plagemann, A, Harder, T, Kohlhoff, R, Rohde, W, Dorner, G. Glucose tolerance and insulin secretion in children of mothers with pregestational IDDM or gestational diabetes. *Diabetologia* 40:1094–1100, 1997.

Pradhan, AD, Manson, JE, Rifai, N, Buring, JE, Ridker, PM. C-reactive protein, interleukin 6, and risk of developing type 2 diabetes mellitus. *JAMA* 286:327–334, 2001.

Quilter, CR, Cooper, WN, Cliffe, KM, Skinner, BM, Prentice, PM, Nelson, L, Bauer, J, Ong, KK, Constancia, M, Lowe, WL, Affara, NA, Dunger, DB. Impact on offspring methylation patterns of maternal gestational diabetes mellitus and intrauterine growth restraint suggest common genes and pathways linked to subsequent type 2 diabetes risk. *FASEB J* 28:4868–4879, 2014.

Reaven, GM, Chen, YD, Golay, A, Swislocki, AL, Jaspan, JB. Documentation of hyperglucagonemia throughout the day in nonobese and obese patients with noninsulin-dependent diabetes mellitus. *J Clin Endocrinol Metab* 64:106–110, 1987.

Ruchat, SM, Hivert, MF, Bouchard, L. Epigenetic programming of obesity and diabetes by in utero exposure to gestational diabetes mellitus. *Nutr Rev* 71 Suppl 1:S88–S94, 2013.

Salbe, AD, Lindsay, RS, Collins, CB, Tataranni, PA, Krakoff, J, Bunt, JC. Comparison of plasma insulin levels after a mixed-meal challenge in children with and without intrauterine exposure to diabetes. *J Clin Endocrinol Metab* 92:624–628, 2007.

Shoelson, SE, Herrero, L, Naaz, A. Obesity, inflammation, and insulin resistance. *Gastroenterology* 132:2169–2180, 2007.

Sobngwi, E, Boudou, P, Mauvais-Jarvis, F, Leblanc, H, Velho, G, Vexiau, P, Porcher, R, Hadjadj, S, Pratley, R, Tataranni, PA, Calvo, F, Gautier, JF. Effect of a diabetic environment in utero on predisposition to type 2 diabetes. *Lancet* 361:1861–1865, 2003

Soyal, S, Krempler, F, Oberkofler, H, Patsch, W. PGC-1alpha: A potent transcriptional cofactor involved in the pathogenesis of type 2 diabetes. *Diabetologia* 49:1477–1488, 2006.

Uebel, K, Pusch, K, Gedrich, K, Schneider, KT, Hauner, H, Bader, BL. Effect of maternal obesity with and without gestational diabetes on offspring subcutaneous and preperitoneal adipose tissue development from birth up to year-1. *BMC Pregnancy Childbirth* 14:138, 2014.

Vaarasmaki, M, Pouta, A, Elliot, P, Tapanainen, P, Sovio, U, Ruokonen, A, Hartikainen, AL, McCarthy, M, Jarvelin, MR. Adolescent manifestations of metabolic syndrome among children born to women with gestational diabetes in a general-population birth cohort. *Am J Epidemiol* 169:1209–1215, 2009.

Vlachova, Z, Bytoft, B, Knorr, S, Clausen, TD, Jensen, RB, Mathiesen, ER, Hojlund, K, Ovesen, P, Beck-Nielsen, H, Gravholt, CH, Damm, P, Jensen, DM. Increased metabolic risk in adolescent offspring of mothers with type 1 diabetes: The EPICOM study. *Diabetologia* 58:1454–1463, 2015.

Weiss, PA, Scholz, HS, Haas, J, Tamussino, KF, Seissler, J, Borkenstein, MH. Long-term follow-up of infants of mothers with type 1 diabetes: Evidence for hereditary and nonhereditary transmission of diabetes and precursors. *Diabetes Care* 23:905–911, 2000.

West, NA, Crume, TL, Maligie, MA, Dabelea, D. Cardiovascular risk factors in children exposed to maternal diabetes in utero. *Diabetologia* 54:504–507, 2011.

West, NA, Kechris, K, Dabelea, D. Exposure to maternal diabetes in utero and DNA methylation patterns in the offspring. *Immunometabolism* 1:1–9, 2013.

Wewer Albrechtsen, NJ, Kuhre, RE, Pedersen, J, Knop, FK, Holst, JJ. The biology of glucagon and the consequences of hyperglucagonemia. *Biomark Med* 2016.

Wroblewska-Seniuk, K, Wender-Ozegowska, E, Szczapa, J. Long-term effects of diabetes during pregnancy on the offspring. *Pediatr Diabetes* 10:432–440, 2009.

Xie, X, Gao, H, Zeng, W, Chen, S, Feng, L, Deng, D, Qiao, FY, Liao, L, McCormick, K, Ning, Q, Luo, X. Placental DNA methylation of peroxisome-proliferator-activated receptor-gamma co-activator-1alpha promoter is associated with maternal gestational glucose level. *Clin Sci* 129:385–394, 2015.

Zhu, Y, Olsen, SF, Mendola, P, Yeung, EH, Vaag, A, Bowers, K, Liu, A, Bao, W, Li, S, Madsen, C, Grunnet, LG, Granstrom, C, Hansen, S, Martin, K, Chavarro, JE, Hu, FB, Langhoff-Roos, J, Damm, P, Zhang, C. Growth and obesity through the first 7 y of life in association with levels of maternal glycemia during pregnancy: A prospective cohort study. *Am J Clin Nutr* 103:794–800, 2016.

15 Mother–Child Microbiomes

Andreas Friis Pihl, Cilius Esmann Fonvig, Oluf Pedersen, Jens-Christian Holm, and Torben Hansen

CONTENTS

15.1 INTRODUCTION

The microbiota living in the human gut has received tremendous attention within the last decade. A broad spectrum of high-prevalence pediatric diseases has been associated with alterations in gut microbiota (presented here in order of total number of publications on PubMed with the most prevalent diseases first): overweight and metabolism, *Clostridium difficile* infection, irritable bowel syndrome, inflammatory bowel disease (IBD), allergy, necrotizing enterocolitis, gut–brain axis disorders (e.g., autism, neurodevelopment, depression), malnutrition, celiac disease, asthma, and colic. Major scientific contributions with regard to microbiota have been published within the field of overweight/obesity and metabolism. This chapter focuses on the intestinal microbiota and its association with metabolic dysfunctions and pediatric overweight as well as elucidates recent research regarding the acquisition and development of the gut microbiota pre-, peri-, and postnatally and, furthermore, seeks to clarify the suggested potential factors influencing the gut microbiota in pregnancy and in the first period of life.

Childhood and adolescent overweight and obesity are of major concern in regards to global public health and economy. The prevalence of childhood overweight and obesity has seemed to stabilize (Brown et al. 2015), but recent studies have shown that the incidence of severe childhood obesity has continued to rise (Skinner et al. 2016), predominantly in high-risk populations (Brown et al. 2015). Furthermore, children with obesity suffer from a long list of obesity-related complications (Han et al. 2010). The cause of overweight and obesity is multifaceted where environmental factors are interacting with a genetic susceptibility. The microbiota has recently been attributed an important role in the development of childhood overweight and obesity, where both obesity and type 2 diabetes mellitus (T2DM) have been associated with significant changes in the gut microbiota composition and function (Ley et al. 2006; Qin et al. 2012; Turnbaugh et al. 2009). Since the gut microbiota may potentially be altered by pre-, pro- and antibiotics, it is possible that the microbiota can offer a novel and beneficial prevention and treatment of childhood overweight and obesity.

The microbiome is the collective genome of all the microorganisms (including bacterial, archaean, fungal, protozoan, and viral species) living upon or within the individual (e.g., the skin, urogenital, or intestines). The majority of research regarding childhood obesity and health has focused on the gut bacterial microbiome but the virome (the collective viral genome) receives increasing attention (Columpsi et al. 2016). It has been argued that in a human being, the gut microbiota outnumbers the total human cells by a factor of ten, but recent research finds the ratio to be approximately 1:1 (Sender et al. 2016). Furthermore, through an updated microbiome gene catalog, almost 10,000,000 microbial genes have been identified, and thereby it outnumbers the human genome (existing of around 22,000 genes) by nearly three orders of magnitude (Li et al. 2014).

Of the 30 known bacterial phyla (see Figure 15.1), the Firmicutes and Bacteroidetes phylae are predominant and account for more than 90% of the bacteria in the distal intestine (Qin et al. 2010). The vast number of bacteria in the human gut is mutualistic (i.e. living in symbiosis with the host) and in this symbiosis the bacteria contribute to the fermentation of dietary fibers and vitamin synthesis, and furthermore, the bacteria have been associated with various immune, nerve, and endocrine functions (Carvalho et al. 2013). The gut bacteria are mainly anaerobic and thus difficult to cultivate, but within the era of new genome sequencing techniques it is now possible, at least at draft genome level, to get both quantitative and genetic information of the recently unknown intestinal bacteria (Qin et al. 2010; Carvalho et al. 2013).

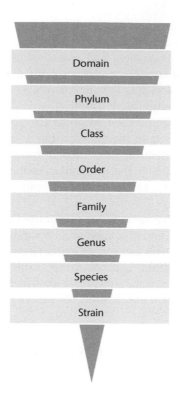

FIGURE 15.1 Biologic taxonomic classification.

15.2 THE TRANSITION OF MATERNAL GUT MICROBIOTA DURING PREGNANCY

During pregnancy, various well-known maternal physiological changes occur and recent data are now suggesting that the maternal intestinal microbiota changes as well. In general, it seems that the microbial count increases (Collado et al. 2008) and the microbiome becomes more diverse (Koren et al. 2012) from the first to the third trimester. During the first trimester, the microbiome is similar overall when compared to nonpregnant healthy women and girls from a young age (Koren et al. 2012). The transfer of third trimester microbiota from pregnant women to germ-free mice induces greater adiposity and inflammation compared with a first trimester transplant from the same women (Koren et al. 2012). Despite the significant change in quantity and composition during pregnancy, the maternal gut microbiota remains stable during the perinatal period and the following 1–6 months postnatally (J4; Carrothers et al. 2015).

A range of modifiable (e.g., diet, pre-, pro-, and antibiotics, tobacco, substance use/abuse, stress, depression, infections) and nonmodifiable (e.g., genetic) factors are known to affect the human microbiome (Dunlop et al. 2015). These factors also affect the maternal microbiome during pregnancy and lactation and may thereby potentially modify the acquisition of the fetal and neonate gut microbiome associated with health and thus potentially disease.

Prepregnancy maternal overweight and excess weight gain during pregnancy cause a dysbiosis in the gut microbiota, distinctly different from the normal weight pregnant woman, but the associating specific microbiota composition change is discussed (Gohir et al. 2014; Collado et al. 2008).

Maternal antibiotic administration prior to parturition has been shown to affect not only the microbiota in the neonate, but also the structural and functional development of the offspring's gut in both rats (Fåk et al. 2008) and pigs (Arnal et al. 2014). Interestingly, the neonatal microbiota composition seems to respond to maternal probiotic administration in both animal and human studies (Gohir et al. 2014).

Maternal prenatal stress has recently been associated with significant changes in the neonatal gut microbiota toward a microbiota composition associated with obesity, that is, high proteobacteria and low bifidobacteria counts and low lactic acid bacterial concentrations (Zijlmans et al. 2015), and furthermore, it is suggested in a murine model that maternal prenatal stress has a long-lasting effect on the gut microbiota composition and health of the offspring (Golubeva et al. 2015).

15.3 THE ESTABLISHMENT AND DEVELOPMENT OF GUT MICROBIOTA

Recent studies challenge the notion that the fetal and intrauterine environment is sterile, because traces of microbes and perhaps even living microbiota have been found in the placenta, fetal membranes, amniotic fluid, umbilical cord blood, and meconium (Jiménez et al. 2005; Gohir et al. 2014). It has been suggested that this vertical transmission is reflecting the maternal intestinal changes during pregnancy (Luoto et al. 2013). Human studies have yet to prove if the vertical transmission includes live bacteria, but a rodent study suggests that live bacteria may be transmitted from the mother to the fetus (Mueller et al. 2015). Both the fetal and the placental immune physiology may be modulated by maternal probiotic supplementation two weeks prior to elective cesarean section (Rautava et al. 2012).

The gut microbiota composition of the newborn is unstable, low in diversity, and readily affected by multiple factors, but after the first 3 years in life it becomes comparable with the adult "mature" gut microbiome, which is relatively stable until the 70th year (Dominguez-Bello et al. 2011). There are still differences in the microbiota of the child compared to that of the adult, and it seems that there is a gradual transition toward the mature adult microbiome during growth and development (Agans et al. 2011). The mature adult gut microbiota exhibits a high individual specificity at the taxon level (Turnbaugh et al. 2009). Despite these significant interpersonal variations, a "core microbiome" has been suggested to exist. This accounts for approximately half of the functional microbiomes, and this is suggested to catalyze certain metabolic functions, as adults with comparable gut microbiota profiles exhibit comparable metabolic profiles (Turnbaugh et al. 2009).

15.4 MODULATING FACTORS OF THE EARLY LIFE GUT MICROBIOTA

The establishment of the gut microbiome takes place during birth and within the first months of life, and in the following we present multiple factors that are suggested to induce these early changes in the gut microbiota (Figure 15.2).

15.4.1 PRENATAL

Maternal antibiotic treatment during the second or third trimester has been associated with a 84% higher risk of childhood obesity at age 7 years as opposed to unexposed children (Mueller et al. 2014), hereby indicating that maternal use of antibiotics has long-term consequences on body composition of the offspring (Mueller et al. 2015). Another study reported that prenatal antibiotic exposure combined with a birth weight lower than 3,500 g increased the risk of overweight at age 7–16 years, but not obesity and children with a birth weight greater than 3,500 g had a reduced risk of developing overweight at 7–16 years of age (Mor et al. 2015). Furthermore, a proportional correlation between the number of prenatal antibiotic treatments and development of overweight in school age was described (Mor et al. 2015).

15.4.2 THE HOST GENOME

The human host genome affects the gut microbiota, but the direct effect of the human genome is difficult to elucidate because the gut microbiota is affected by various potent environmental factors (Carmody et al. 2015) that have the ability to overwhelm the interpersonal differences in the microbiome (David et al. 2014). Human adult twins show greater interpersonal similarity in their gut microbiota compared to unrelated individuals (Turnbaugh et al. 2009), and furthermore, the gut microbiome of monozygotic twins is more comparable than dizygotic twins (Goodrich et al. 2014). A recent study with 2,731 individuals demonstrated how the human genes seem to control certain bacterial taxa and that the involved human genes are part of diet sensing, metabolism, and the immune system (Goodrich et al. 2016).

In a murine model, where specific immune regulatory genes are knocked out, it is possible to indirectly change the gut microbiota and thus induce metabolic

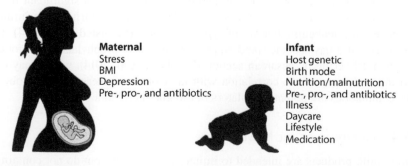

Maternal
Stress
BMI
Depression
Pre-, pro-, and antibiotics

Infant
Host genetic
Birth mode
Nutrition/malnutrition
Pre-, pro-, and antibiotics
Illness
Daycare
Lifestyle
Medication

FIGURE 15.2 Factors suggested to affect fetal and infant gut microbiota.

dysfunctions, including increased body weight, adiposity, glucose intolerance, and insulin resistance (Revelo et al. 2014). Despite the distorting effects of environmental factors, a recent study reported a clear association between the host genotype and the gut microbiome showing that specific bacteria families and phyla are more heritable than others, while others (primarily Bacteroidetes) are more sensitive to dietary changes (Goodrich et al. 2014). A recent genome-wide association study attempted to overcome the influence of environmental factors on the gut microbiota, by studying groups who lived and ate communally (Davenport et al. 2015). Despite a small sample size ($n = 184$), the study revealed at least eight bacterial taxa that were significantly related to human genetic variation, for example, an association between the bacterial genus *Akkermansia* and a genetic variant near the phospholipase D1 (PLD1) gene, which is a gene previously linked with body mass index (BMI) (Davenport et al. 2015). The underlying mechanisms by which the host genes affect the microbiota composition and function remain unclear (Benson et al. 2010), although immune modulation, metabolism, and energy regulation are proposed as possible pathways (Davenport et al. 2015).

15.4.3 BIRTH MODE

The primary bacterial inoculation starts at birth where birth mode (vaginally versus cesarean section) is an important factor. Vaginally delivered babies are primarily inoculated by maternal vaginal, fecal, and cutaneous bacteria and subsequently from the surrounding environment. Conversely, infants born by cesarean section show lower microbial diversity (Grönlund et al. 1999; Jakobsson et al. 2014; Salminen et al. 2004) and less resemblance to their mothers' gut microbiota compared to vaginally delivered infants (Bäckhed et al. 2015). It has been recently suggested that infants born by cesarean section are exposed to the microbes contained in the dust in the operating room (Shin et al. 2015). It has been debated whether birth mode influences later onset of weight gain, and three recent meta-analyses conclude that there is a moderate to strong correlation between cesarean delivery and weight gain and obesity in childhood, adolescence, and adulthood (Li et al. 2013; Darmasseelane et al. 2014; Kuhle et al. 2015); one of the meta-analyses estimated that cesarean delivered infants have a 33% greater risk of developing childhood obesity (Darmasseelane et al. 2014). A large retrospective study recently analyzed the correlation between cesarean section and chronic immune disorders, and reported a significant higher risk of asthma, systemic connective tissue disorders, juvenile arthritis, IBD, immune deficiencies, and leukemia, but not of type 1 diabetes (Sevelsted et al. 2014). It is noteworthy that it has become standard procedure to give prophylactic antibiotic to all women delivering by cesarean section (Sevelsted et al. 2014), which may confound the evaluation of the correlation with later onset of overweight and obesity because antibiotics are potent modulators of the gut microbiota.

15.4.4 NUTRITION OF THE NEWBORN

Formula milk products are intended to imitate human milk, but do not contain all the same ingredients. Formulas do not contain antibodies, and furthermore, the ingredient composition in formulas is static, whereas the composition of breast milk is changing during a single breastfeed (Hassiotou et al. 2013b) and over the whole lactating period (Hassiotou et al. 2013a; Neville et al. 1991). On the other hand, formula holds a potential to add health-promoting vitamins and pre- and probiotics (Vandenplas et al. 2015). It is well established that human breast milk and formula both influence the human gut microbiota and thus affect the host metabolism both short and long term. Breast milk contains many bioactive molecules including antibodies (predominantly IgA), which is suggested to affect the gut microbiota composition in both mice (Rogier et al. 2014) and human infants (Kaetzel 2014), and further a murine model demonstrated that early exposure to breast milk–derived IgA resulted in gut microbiota changes both short and long term (Rogier et al. 2014). The antibodies further protect the child from infections, and because it is suggested that illness can modify the gut microbiota composition, this is another indirect way that the breast milk possibly affects the gut microbiota (Koenig et al. 2011).

Breastfed infants have a more stable and uniform gut microbiota compared with formula-fed infants, which is proposed to be caused by the natural contents of pre- and probiotics in human breast milk (Mueller et al. 2015). A meta-analysis including 11 studies found that formula-fed infants exhibit a marginally higher fat mass at 12 months of age (Gale et al. 2012).

Breastfeeding is proposed to protect against later onset of childhood overweight and obesity and a recent meta-analysis covering 10 studies found that breastfeeding significantly decreased the risk of developing overweight in childhood by 15%; the results on the duration of breastfeeding were inconclusive (Weng et al. 2012). Conversely, several studies found no significant obesity-protective effect of breastfeeding (Kaplan and Walker 2012), but proposed major predictors for childhood obesity to be maternal pre-pregnancy overweight, high infant birth weight, and rapid weight gain during the first year of life (Weng et al. 2012). Recently, it has been suggested that breast milk, in contrast to formula feeding, enhances the gut microbiota plasticity and thereby eases the transition into solid foods (Thompson et al. 2015).

It seems evident that the diet is determining the microbiota composition and function independently of the host phenotype (Carmody et al. 2015; David et al. 2014; Hildebrandt et al. 2009). Diet alterations are reflected by a shift in the gut microbiota composition within 24–48 hours in both mice (Carmody et al. 2015) and human adults (David et al. 2014), and these diet-induced microbiota dynamics in adults are shown to be reversible (David et al. 2014; Carmody et al. 2015).

A pioneering study from 2006 reported that adults on a fat- or carbohydrate restricted low-calorie diet showed significant changes in the gut microbiota composition where the Bacteroidetes/Firmicutes ratio increased (Ley et al. 2006). Thus, the diet is a potent modulator of the gut microbiota composition, and the greatest gut microbiota transformation is seen with the introduction of solid foods (Bergström et al. 2014), but it seems that the cessation of breastfeeding rather than the introduction of solid food is the main factor in the maturation of the infant gut microbiome (Bäckhed et al. 2015).

Malnutrition has also been associated with the gut microbiota. A recent study demonstrated a gut microbiota dysbiosis accompanying malnutrition and showed that severe acute malnutrition is associated with a depletion of anaerobic and methanogenic prokaryotes (Million et al. 2016). Furthermore, studies have shown that moderate and severe acute malnutrition is linked with persisting immaturity of the gut microbiota and a small prospective study further found that growth stunted children are enriched in inflammogenic bacterial taxa compared to nonstunted children (Dinh et al. 2016).

15.4.5 PROBIOTICS

Probiotics are live, nonpathogenic microorganisms that are believed to exert a healthy benefit on the host when administered in sufficient amounts. Most probiotic studies in pediatric research have been conducted with different strains of *Bifidobacterium* and *Lactobacillus* (Chassard et al. 2014). Different species of these two genera have been reported to both increase (Angelakis et al. 2013) and decrease (Kadooka et al. 2010; Simon et al. 2015) body weight and fat mass, and hence it seems relevant that future studies focus on the effect of specific bacterial strains or communities instead of the overall genera.

Probiotic supplements to adult humans and mice have been reported to decrease body weight, adipose tissue mass, leptin, and cholesterol concentrations, and further to improve insulin and glucagon-like peptide-1 (GLP-1) secretion (Kadooka et al. 2010; Simon et al. 2015; Balasubramanian 2015). The vast majority of literature on the health beneficial effects of probiotics on body mass and metabolism originates from adult and animal studies (Balasubramanian 2015), although it has been proposed that probiotic supplements are the most potent contributor to later-onset obesity in the neonate and infant population (Luoto et al. 2013; Kalliomäki et al. 2008). Nevertheless, two recent studies with 120 and 113 children and a follow-up time of 8 and 10 years, respectively, assessed the effects of two different *Lactobacillus* strains administered in the first year of life and found no significant association with the development of obesity or metabolic derangement at follow-up in school age (Luoto et al. 2010; Stenlund et al. 2015). One of these studies found a tendency, although nonsignificant, that the examined probiotic restrained excessive weight gain during the first year of life (Luoto et al. 2010). A large multicenter prospective follow-up study demonstrated that probiotic supplementation within the first 27 days of life reduced the risk of islet autoimmunity in children with the highest genetic risk of T1DM (Uusitalo et al. 2016).

15.4.6 PREBIOTICS

Prebiotics are food ingredients and a class of dietary fibers that, among other characteristics, selectively stimulate the occurrence or activity of one or more gut microbial species. Prebiotics are nondigestible by the human intestinal enzymes, but fermentable by the gut microbiota to which they supply energy and thus stimulate their growth. Both inulin and galacto-oligosaccharides are well-studied prebiotics that are both reported to increase the fecal *Bifidobacterium* and *Lactobacillus* count in infants (Staelens et al. 2011; Schmelzle et al. 2003). A high bifidobacterial concentration in infancy seems important because it has been associated with protection against later-onset obesity (Kalliomäki et al. 2008).

The use of prebiotic supplementation in formulas is common, and specific prebiotic supplements in infancy have been associated with changes in the stool pattern (Ashley et al. 2012), stool consistency, and bacterial composition (Mugambi et al. 2012) resembling the pattern of the breastfed infants (Staelens et al. 2011; Vandenplas et al. 2015). Young adolescents who receive a daily supplementation of prebiotic, that is, oligofructose and long-chained inulin, for 1 year have been reported to have a significantly smaller increase in BMI and total fat mass compared with a control group (Abrams 2007). Furthermore, a murine model with oligofructose supplementation verified the bifidogenic effect (the increase of *Bifidobacterium*) and demonstrated a normalization of the metabolic endotoxemia and the inflammatory response associated with a high-fat diet (Cani et al. 2007a).

The specific antiobese effect of prebiotics is still not elucidated, but there is a strong tendency indicating that prebiotics potentially can prevent and treat obesity. Furthermore, it is notable that prebiotics are nondigestible and often replace sugar or fat and they may potentially contribute to a lower dietary energy intake (Cherbut 2002); it is suggested, in adult studies, that prebiotics increase satiety and thus reduce the energy intake (Cani et al. 2006).

15.4.7 ANTIBIOTICS

Antibiotics appear to potently affect the gut microbiota in the 0–4-year-old child (Jernberg et al. 2010), and antibiotic exposure may cause gut microbiota dysbiosis in the fetus and infant when administered to the mother or the infant pre-, peri-, and postpartum (Mueller et al. 2015). The overall antibiotic dispensing rates among children declined from 2000 to 2010 in the United States and reached a new plateau in 2010. Despite the decline in outpatient antibiotic prescription rates over the past decade, the use of antibiotics is still immense, and by 2010, outpatient children under the age of 2 years received approximately one to two antibiotic prescriptions per person-year (Vaz et al. 2014), and the highest rates of antibiotic use in the pediatric population are occurring in children under two years of age, which seems to be the most vulnerable group (Vaz et al. 2014). Prenatal maternal antibiotic exposure may disrupt the development of the intestinal microbiota of the infant via the circulation in the placenta, and the gut microbiota of the newborn can either be directly affected by antibiotic administration or indirectly by maternal antibiotic use that modulates the microbiome in the breast milk, and hence the gut microbiota of the breastfed (Mueller et al. 2014).

Early antibiotic exposure seems correlated with later-onset overweight and obesity, and it has been reported that antibiotic exposure within the first year of life increases the risk of preadolescent overweight and central adiposity among boys (Azad et al. 2014). It seems that the first 6 months of life is a critical period for seeding the gut microbiome and thus defining body mass. The critical window (within the first 6 months of life) for antibiotic exposure is consistent in several studies, and interestingly, antibiotic exposure from the 6th to the 23rd month is not correlated with an increased body mass later in life (Trasande et al. 2012). One study found that antibiotic exposure during the critical window increased the risk of overweight at age 7 years if the mother was normal weight and decreased the risk if the mother was overweight (Ajslev et al. 2011). A recent murine model suggested that antibiotics exert their systemic effects via alterations in the intestinal permeability, and that these changes depend on the antibiotics class (Tulstrup et al. 2015). In accordance, a human adult study found that long-term treatment with vancomycin was associated with the development of obesity, while amoxicillin showed no association (Hartstra et al. 2014). A recent retrospective study found that the use of macrolides at age 2–7 years were associated with a long-lasting shift in the intestinal microbiota and metabolism, while penicillins had a weaker impact (Korpela et al. 2016).

It has been recently suggested that the effects of antibiotics on the gut microbiota are cumulative in an individual (Blaser 2016), and a recent study found that the number of antibiotic exposures before the age of 2 years was positively associated with the risk of being overweight at age 4 (Scott et al. 2016). By administering subtherapeutic long-term dosage of antibiotics (chlortetracycline and penicillin) to young mice, it is possible to induce significant gut-microbiota changes and obesity (Cho et al. 2012), and long-term penicillin dosage to mice has been shown to enhance the effect of high-fat, diet-induced obesity and cause long-term metabolic effects even after cessation of the treatment, suggesting that the bacterial composition in early life participates in metabolic programming (Cox et al. 2014).

It has been proposed that the future antibiotic treatment should, ideally, precisely eliminate pathogenic microbiota instead of carpet bombing the gut microbiota with broad-spectrum antibiotics, which would minimize the so-called collateral damage that the antibiotics seem to exert on the commensal gut microbiota.

15.4.8 LIFESTYLE AND OTHER ENVIRONMENTAL FACTORS

Some additional factors have been reported to significantly influence the gut microbiota of the child; the association of these factors with childhood obesity is not yet clarified, but will be mentioned in the following. Siblings have been reported to have a distinct different gut microbiota compared to infants without siblings (Penders et al. 2006), and furthermore the composition of the gut microbiota has been reported to exert geographical differences (Rodriguez et al. 2015).

A recent small study (with nine healthy infants) found that children attending out-of-home daycare had a significantly higher gut microbial diversity compared to infants cared for in their own home, independently of feeding patterns (Thompson et al. 2015). This association has yet to be verified by other larger studies. Furthermore, illness has been linked with changes in the gut microbiota (Koenig et al. 2011). It is notable that these above-mentioned factors should be included in the statistical analysis of forthcoming studies to avoid confounded results.

In a recent human study in 784 adults with T2DM, it was found that the most widely used antidiabetic drug, metformin, led to gut microbiota dysbiosis (Forslund et al. 2015). It was suggested that the antimicrobial effect of metformin, which affects the short-chain fatty acid (SCFA) metabolism, is the primary determining factor of the drug's efficacy on the host metabolism (Blaser 2016). Thus, medication is another confounding factor that future research must focus upon to clarify these associations.

15.5 GUT MICROBIOTA AND HOST METABOLISM

The commensal colonic bacteria exhibit various functions important to both themselves and their host. The bacterial fermentation of indigestible dietary fibers produces SCFAs, primarily acetate, butyrate, and propionate, which are then absorbed and thus provide energy to the intestinal epithelium or enter the circulation are used as a part of the *de novo* synthesis to glucose and lipids (Carvalho et al. 2013) (Figure 15.3). Thus, bacteria are extracting energy from otherwise nondigestible carbohydrates, and are thereby contributing to a positive energy balance in the host. It is suggested that the obese gut microbiota is extracting more energy from the ingested food compared to lean individuals, as shown by the fact that obese adults have higher cecal SCFA and lower fecal SCFA concentration than their lean counterparts (Nieuwdorp et al. 2014).

The different SCFAs are affecting the host in various ways; both propionate and butyrate have been reported to exert antiobese effects in mice (Lin et al. 2012), and acetate has recently been shown to promote metabolic syndrome in rodents (Perry et al. 2016). Therefore, it seems relevant that recent studies focus on the specific SCFAs, instead of the group as a whole. The SCFAs are involved in other roles as well: several G-protein–coupled receptors on intestinal enteroendocrine cells have been identified as endogenous receptors for SCFAs (Poul et al. 2003) producing glucose-dependent insulinotropic polypeptide (GIP) and GLP-1. GIP and GLP-1 are incretin hormones regulating glucose control, metabolism, and food intake by release of several other hormones, and a rodent study demonstrated that butyrate and propionate, but not acetate, induce the release of gut hormones and reduce food intake (Lin et al. 2012). The same authors demonstrated that SCFA administration to mice protected against diet-induced obesity and insulin resistance (Lin et al. 2012). Consequently, gut bacteria may indirectly stimulate the hypothalamic appetite regulation through the secretion of GLP-1 and the hormone peptide tyrosine tyrosine (PYY) (Lin et al. 2012; Carvalho et al. 2013). Although a large body of literature demonstrates that the gut-bacteria-produced SCFAs induce GLP-1 secretion, a novel report demonstrated that germ-free mice, low in SCFA, had a three times higher plasma GLP-1 concentration than their conventionally raised counterparts, which indicates that the exact mechanisms are not yet understood (Pais et al. 2015). It has been reported that a selective microbiota shift can control and increase the endogenous GLP-2 secretion and thereby improve the gut epithelial barrier and then exert an antiobese effect (Cani et al. 2009). An impaired intestinal barrier and immune function have in several studies been suggested to be a causal factor in the development of the metabolic syndrome (Cox et al. 2014; Cani et al. 2008). MyD88 gene knockout mice, involving Toll-like receptors, which are the major pathogen recognition receptors, are protected against diet-induced obesity, diabetes, and inflammation, suggesting that the intestinal immune system acts as a sensor regulating the host metabolism according to the diet (Everard et al. 2014).

The bile acid circulation system is another pathway by which the gut microbiota may affect the host metabolism, and it is suggested that they do so by deconjugation of bile salts and dehydroxylation of primary bile acids to secondary ones (Kootte et al. 2012), and the gut microbiota furthermore seems to influence the lipolysis and fatty acid oxidation (Carvalho et al. 2013). It was demonstrated that the bile acid concentration in the small intestine of germ-free rats was increased threefold compared to their conventionally raised counterparts and that the germ-free mice had a 25% greater absorption of dietary cholesterol (Wostmann 1973).

Lipopolysaccharides (LPS), also known as endotoxins, are a part of the outer membrane of Gram-negative bacteria, which elicit a strong immune response in animals. When the Gram-negative bacteria decay, LPS are translocated into intestinal capillaries, transported by chylomicrons, causing systemic inflammation and insulin resistance, especially in the liver, muscle, and adipose tissue (Figure 15.3) (Piya et al. 2013). In mice, it is demonstrated that the circulating bacterial LPS can partly explain the metabolic endotoxemia associated with feeding on a high-fat diet (Piya et al. 2013), and that endotoxemia in mice increases body weight, body fat, liver fat, and other cardiovascular and diabetic risk factors (Cani et al. 2007b). Human adult studies have shown that increased serum concentrations of LPS are associated with increased food intake (Nieuwdorp et al. 2014) and the development of insulin resistance (Hartstra et al. 2014).

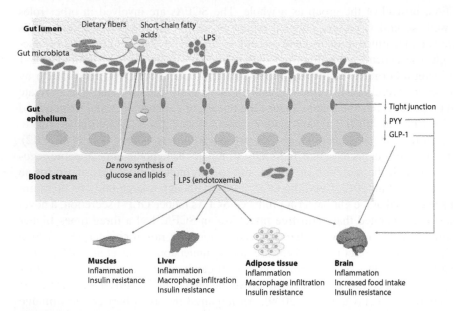

FIGURE 15.3 Suggested ways that the gut microbiota is affecting the human metabolism. This figure presents two potential pathways that the gut microbiota can affect the body weight and metabolism in overweight and obese individuals. (1) The gut microbiota ferments indigestible dietary fibers to short-chain fatty acids (SCFAs), which may be metabolized by the gut epithelium or be part of the *de novo* synthesis of glucose and lipids. (2) Due to an increased gut permeability caused by weakness in the *tight junctions*, lipopolysaccharides (LPS) from the membrane of the Gram-negative bacteria are able to enter the circulation (i.e., endotoxemia) and hereby potentially cause immunological responses, inflammation, macrophage infiltration, and insulin resistance in several tissues including muscle, liver, and adipose tissue. Insulin resistance and a decreased expression of anorectic hormones (including GLP-1 and PYY) on hypothalamus stimulate food intake.

Blood and internal organs are thought to be sterile but novel ultramicroscopic studies demonstrate that a great many bacteria that are difficult to cultivate exist in blood and inside erythrocytes and that this dormant microbiome might play a role in different inflammatory diseases (Potgieter et al. 2015). Furthermore, it has been discovered that internal human tissue (liver, adipose tissue, and blood) also has a distinct microbiome and this "tissue microbiota hypothesis" may be a potential pathway whereby the gut microbiota affects the host's metabolic homeostasis (Burcelin et al. 2013). Researchers recently optimized a 16S metagenomics sequencing technique that will make it possible to catalog the different bacterial DNA species in various tissues (Lluch et al. 2015). The intestinal epithelial permeability increases following gut microbiota dysbiosis (Luoto et al. 2013) and a high-fat diet (Cani et al. 2008) will amplify the bacterial translocation and the gathering of the tissue microbiota and endotoxemia. Furthermore, it is demonstrated that "the blood microbiota" is an independent biomarker of the risk of diabetes and abdominal adiposity, but not obesity in the general population (Amar et al. 2011).

It seems evident that a cornerstone in the pathway by which the gut microbiota is affecting the human metabolism is by modulation of the innate and adaptive immune system. A recent study in mice proposed that the cross talk between the small intestine mucosal microbiota and the corresponding adaptive immune response regulates the metabolic state where subcutaneous injection of ileum microbial extracts prevented hyperglycemia and insulin resistance (Pomié et al. 2016).

15.6 GUT MICROBIOTA AND OBESITY

Germ-free mice inoculated with feces from conventionally raised adult mice resulted in a 60% increase in body fat content and the development of insulin resistance within 14 days, despite a lower food intake, thereby indicating the important role of the gut microbiota in the host's metabolism (Bäckhed et al. 2004). It is evident that overweight and obesity are associated with a gut microbiota dysbiosis, but the specific shift in microbial composition of the obese phenotype is not clearly understood (Kaplan and Walker 2012). On a phylum level, studies in both mice (Ley et al. 2005) and adults (Ley et al. 2006) suggest that obesity is associated with an improvement in the Firmicutes/Bacteroidetes ratio, but the inverse relation has been reported as well (Le Chatelier et al. 2013).

On a genera level, one study found that a high intestinal bifidobacterial (belonging to the Actinobacterium phylum) count protected against later-onset obesity and that a high number of *Staphylococcus aureus* predicted later-onset obesity (Kalliomäki et al. 2008).

A recent study examined the effect of transplanting feces from adult twins discordant for obesity to germ-free mice and found that the increase in adipose mass of mice that received a fecal transplant from an obese twin was significantly greater than the increase in animals receiving gut microbiota from the lean twin (Ridaura et al. 2013). Furthermore, the authors demonstrated that cohousing the obese and lean mice prevented an increased adipose phenotype due to the coprophagic nature of the mice (Ridaura et al. 2013).

Obese adults have been reported to have a lower gut microbiota diversity compared to normal-weight adults (Turnbaugh et al. 2009). This was confirmed in a large study where individuals with low bacterial richness were characterized by more overall adiposity, insulin resistance, dyslipidemia, and proinflammation (Le Chatelier et al. 2013). The increased inflammation associated with low bacterial richness has been linked to a lower activity in the butyrate-producing bacteria, an increased production of hydrogen sulfide, and a reduced capability for management of oxidative stress (Ursell et al. 2014). An increased production of the SCFA butyrate may induce beneficial metabolic effects, including a prevention of the metabolic endotoxemia and IBD (Hartstra et al. 2014). Bacteria belonging to the Firmicutes phylum are the primary butyrate producers, but nine other bacterial phyla have also been reported to potentially produce butyrate as an end product of the fermentation (Vital et al. 2014). Oral supplements with butyrate have been reported to reverse the intestinal inflammation seen in IBD and thus hold the potential to inhibit the inflammation associated with obesity (Hartstra et al. 2014). Conversely, it has been demonstrated that an increase in BMI at age 9–18 months is positively correlated with the prevalence of some butyrate-producing bacteria and negatively correlated with the prevalence of Enterobacteriaceae (Bergström et al. 2014).

Despite the discrepancy in elucidating the specific phylum-level microbiota shift associated with overweight, some distinct bacterial genera hold great potential. Obese schoolchildren have a higher count of *Escherichia coli* and a lower count of bifidobacteria compared to nonobese children (Gao et al. 2015), and it is suggested that a higher count of *Bifidobacterium* in both infancy (Kalliomäki et al. 2008) and adulthood (Angelakis and Armougom 2012) protects against obesity.

The gut microbiota holds potential as an epigenetic regulator, and when Firmicutes is the dominant group, the changes in the epigenetic methylations are associated with an increased risk of cardiovascular disease via altering lipid metabolism, obesity, and inflammation (Kumar et al. 2014).

15.7   BACTERIOTHERAPY

The allogenic transplantation of feces from one human to another has been termed fecal microbiota transplantation (FMT), but researchers argue that this term is an impediment for the potential acceptance of treatment and they suggest the name gut microbiota transplantation (GMT) instead (Jayasinghe et al. 2016). GMT has been used as a treatment for diarrhea for more than a thousand years (Jayasinghe et al. 2016) and is still part of the treatment of relapsing and treatment-refractory *Clostridium difficile* colitis, with a success rate of about 90% (Khan et al. 2014). Even though there are several murine studies, the existing literature elucidating the effectiveness of GMT on obesity and diabetes in humans has been limited to a single pilot study so far (Jayasinghe et al. 2016). The study demonstrated that 6 weeks of nasoduodenal GMT infusions, from lean adults to adults with metabolic syndrome, resulted in a significant 75% increase in insulin sensitivity and fasting plasma lipid concentrations (Vrieze et al. 2012), although the long-term effects (including body weight and composition) of these transplantations were not elucidated. One study evaluated the bacterial intestinal microbiome of 145 European women with either normal, impaired, or diabetic glucose control, and with these data they created a mathematical model that identified T2DM with high accuracy (Karlsson et al. 2013). In fact, they demonstrated that the model was better at predicting the later onset of T2DM than other obvious factors such as BMI (Khan et al. 2014; Karlsson et al. 2013). This may contribute to the development of new strategies in predicting and thereby preventing childhood obesity. A recent review concludes that the effectiveness of GMT in the treatment of adult obesity is inconclusive (Jayasinghe et al. 2016), and it is still unknown whether GMT or daily supplementation of an anaerobic capsule containing a complex bacterial ecosystem will have a therapeutic effect. At present, there are two registered trials evaluating the potential role of GMT in the treatment of obesity (Jayasinghe et al. 2016).

15.8 CONCLUSION

The gut microbiota is influenced by a variety of factors including the host genetics, delivery method, diet, age, infections, environment, and the use of pre-, pro-, and antibiotics. These factors can lead to an imbalance in the composition and function of the gut microbiota seen in childhood obesity and are hypothesized to be involved in many phases of the obesity pathogenesis. Multiple factors are affecting the gut microbiota in various ways and to avoid confounding factors, future studies must take these parameters into consideration to deliver more accurate results.

Recent high-throughput metagenomic sequencing techniques, and related bio-informatics analyses, have improved the possibility of exploring the relationship between gut microbiota at species and even at strain resolution levels and multiple diseases—including childhood obesity. Such correlation studies need to be elaborated by a series of mechanistic studies in animals and in various *in vitro* systems. New insights in the complex microbial ecosystem in the gut of both healthy and overweight children are important in new clinical intervention studies that may alter and benefit the gut microbiota and thus contribute to the prevention and treatment of childhood onset obesity.

The mechanisms by which the gut microbiota are affecting the host metabolism are complex and not yet comprehensively understood, although many different pathways have been suggested. It seems evident that obesity and metabolic dysfunction are associated with high concentrations of acetate-producing bacteria and a decreased concentration/or activity of both propionate- and butyrate-producing bacteria. Novel studies should focus on the specific SCFAs to elucidate this correlation.

The greatest impacts upon the natural variation of the neonatal microbiome seem to be early antibiotic exposure, cesarean section, and formula feeding. The increased prevalence of these three factors may indicate an important challenge to tackle childhood obesity, and further research elucidating the health potential within the gut microbiota is called upon. Future antibiotic treatment—especially to children under the age of 6 months—should be prescribed with the highest possible accuracy and care to target the pathogenic bacteria instead of the broad spectrum antibiotics affecting the entire gut microbiota, which are often prescribed in daily clinical pediatric practice.

REFERENCES

Abrams, S A. 2007. Effect of prebiotic supplementation and calcium intake on body mass index. *Journal of Pediatrics* 151: 293–298.

Agans, R, L Rigsbee, H Kenche, S Michail, H J Khamis, and O Paliy. 2011. Distal gut microbiota of adolescent children is different from that of adults. *FEMS Microbiology Ecology* 77 (2): 404–412.

Ajslev, T A, C S Andersen, M Gamborg, T I A Sørensen, and T Jess. 2011. Childhood overweight after establishment of the gut microbiota: The role of delivery mode, pre-pregnancy weight and early administration of antibiotics. *International Journal of Obesity* 35 (4): 522–529.

Amar, J, M Serino, C Lange, C Chabo, J Iacovoni, S Mondot, P Lepage et al. 2011. Involvement of tissue bacteria in the onset of diabetes in humans: Evidence for a concept. *Diabetologia* 54 (12): 3055–3061.

Angelakis, E, and F Armougom. 2012. The relationship between gut microbiota and weight gain in humans. Future Microbiology 7: 91–109.

Angelakis, E, V Merhej, and Didier Raoult. 2013. Related actions of probiotics and antibiotics on gut microbiota and weight modification. *Lancet Infectious Diseases* 13 (10): 889–899.

Arnal, M E, J Zhang, S Messori, P Bosi, H Smidt, and J P Lalls. 2014. Early changes in microbial colonization selectively modulate intestinal enzymes, but not inducible heat shock proteins in young adult swine. *PLoS One* 9 (2).

Ashley, C, W H Johnston, C L Harris, S I Stolz, J L Wampler, and C L Berseth. 2012. Growth and tolerance of infants fed formula supplemented with polydextrose (PDX) and/or galactooligosaccharides (GOS): Double-blind, randomized, controlled trial. *Nutrition Journal* 11: 1–10.

Azad, M B, S L Bridgman, A B Becker, and A L Kozyrskyj. 2014. Infant antibiotic exposure and the development of childhood overweight and central adiposity. *International Journal of Obesity* 38 (10): 1–35.

Balasubramanian, H. 2015. Early probiotics to prevent childhood metabolic syndrome: A systematic review. *World Journal of Methodology* 5 (3): 157.

Benson, A K, S A Kelly, R Legge, F Ma, S Jen, J Kim, M Zhang et al. 2010. Individuality in gut microbiota composition is a complex polygenic trait shaped by multiple environmental and host genetic factors. *Proceedings of the National Academy of Sciences of the United States of America* 107 (44): 18933–18938.

Bergström, A, T H Skov, M I Bahl, H M Roager, L B Christensen, K T Ejlerskov, C Mølgaard et al. 2014. Establishment of intestinal microbiota during early life: A longitudinal, explorative study of a large cohort of Danish infants. *Applied and Environmental Microbiology* 80 (9): 2889–2900.

Blaser, M J. 2016. Antibiotic use and its consequences for the normal microbiome. *Science* 352 (6285): 544–545.

Brown, C L, E E Halvorson, G M Cohen, S Lazorick, and J A Skelton. 2015. Addressing childhood obesity: Opportunities for prevention. *Pediatric Clinics of North America* 62 (5): 1241–1261.

Burcelin, R, M Serino, C Chabo, L Garidou, C Pomié, M Courtney, J Amar et al. 2013. Metagenome and metabolism: The tissue microbiota hypothesis. *Diabetes, Obesity and Metabolism* 15 (S3): 61–70.

Bäckhed, F, H Ding, T Wang, L V Hooper, G Y Koh, A Nagy, C F Semenkovich et al. 2004. The gut microbiota as an environmental factor that regulates fat storage. *Proceedings of the National Academy of Sciences of the United States of America* 101 (44): 15718–15723.

Bäckhed, F, J Roswall, Y Peng, Q Feng, H Jia, P Kovatcheva-Datchary, Y Li et al. 2015. Dynamics and stabilization of the human gut microbiome in the first year of life. *Cell Host Microbe* 17 (5): *690-703*.

Cani, P D, J Amar, M A Iglesias, M Poggi, C Knauf, D Bastelica, A M Neyrinck et al. 2007b. Metabolic endotoxemia initiates obesity and insulin resistance. *Diabetes* 56 (7): 1761–1772.

Cani, P D, R Bibiloni, C Knauf, A M Neyrinck, and N M Delzenne. 2008. Changes in gut microbiota control metabolic diet–induced obesity and diabetes in mice. *Diabetes* 57 (6): 1470–1481.

Cani, P D, E Joly, Y Horsmans, and N M Delzenne. 2006. Oligofructose promotes satiety in healthy human: A pilot study. *European Journal of Clinical Nutrition* 60 (5): 567–572.

Cani, P D, A M Neyrinck, F Fava, C Knauf, R G Burcelin, K M Tuohy, G R Gibson et al. 2007a. Selective increases of bifidobacteria in gut microflora improve high-fat-diet-induced diabetes in mice through a mechanism associated with endotoxaemia. *Diabetologia* 50 (11): 2374–2383.

Cani, P D, S Possemiers, T Van de Wiele, Y Guiot, A Everard, O Rottier, L Geurts et al. 2009. Changes in gut microbiota control inflammation in obese mice through a mechanism involving GLP-2-driven improvement of gut permeability. *Gut* 58 (8): 1091–1103.

Carmody, R N, G K Gerber, J M Luevano, D M Gatti, L Somes, K L Svenson, and P J Turnbaugh. 2015. Diet dominates host genotype in shaping the murine gut microbiota. *Cell Host & Microbe* 17 (1): 72–84.

Carrothers, J M, M A York, S L Brooker, K A Lackey, J E Williams, B Shafii, W J Price et al. 2015. Fecal microbial community structure is stable over time and related to variation in macronutrient and micronutrient intakes in lactating women. *Journal of Nutrition* 145 (C): 2379–2388.

Carvalho, B M, M Jose, and A Saad. 2013. Review article: Influence of gut microbiota on subclinical inflammation and insulin resistance. *Mediators of Inflammation* 2013: 1–13.

Chassard, C, T de Wouters, and C Lacroix. 2014. Probiotics tailored to the infant: A window of opportunity. *Current Opinion in Biotechnology* 26: 141–147.

Cherbut, C. 2002. Inulin and oligofructose in the dietary fibre concept. *British Journal of Nutrition* 87 (Suppl 2): S159–S162.

Cho, I, S Yamanishi, L Cox, B A Methé, J Zavadil, K Li, Z Gao et al. 2012. Antibiotics in early life alter the murine colonic microbiome and adiposity. *Nature* 488 (7413): 621–626.

Collado, M C, E Isolauri, K Laitinen, and S Salminen. 2008. Distinct composition of gut microbiota during pregnancy in overweight and normal-weight women. *American Journal of Clinical Nutrition* 88 (4): 894–899.

Columpsi, P, P Sacchi, V Zuccaro, S Cima, C Sarda, M Mariani, A Gori et al. 2016. Beyond the gut bacterial microbiota: The gut virome. *Journal of Medical Virology* 30 (12): 4799–4804.

Cox, L M, S Yamanishi, J Sohn, A V Alekseyenko, J M Leung, I Cho, S G Kim et al. 2014. Altering the intestinal microbiota during a critical developmental window has lasting metabolic consequences. *Cell* 158: 705–721.

Darmasseelane, K, M J Hyde, S Santhakumaran, C Gale, and N Modi. 2014. Mode of delivery and offspring body mass index, overweight and obesity in adult life: A systematic review and meta-analysis. *PLoS One* 9 (2): e87896.

Davenport, E R, D A Cusanovich, K Michelini, and L B Barreiro. 2015. Genome-wide association studies of the human gut microbiota. *PLoS One* 10 (11).

David, L A, C F Maurice, R N Carmody, D B Gootenberg, J E Button, B E Wolfe, A V Ling et al. 2014. Diet rapidly and reproducibly alters the human gut microbiome. *Nature* 505 (7484): 559–563.

Dinh, D M, B Ramadass, D Kattula, R Sarkar, P Braunstein, A Tai, C A Wanke et al. 2016. Longitudinal analysis of the intestinal microbiota in persistently stunted young children in South India. *PLoS One* 11 (5): e0155405.

Dominguez-Bello, M G, M J Blaser, R E Ley, and R Knight. 2011. Development of the human gastrointestinal microbiota and insights from high-throughput sequencing. *Gastroenterology* 140 (6): 1713–1719.

Dunlop, A L, J G Mulle, E P Ferranti, S Edwards, A B Dunn, and E J Corwin. 2015. Maternal microbiome and pregnancy outcomes that impact infant health: A review. *Advances in Neonatal Care:* 15 (6): 377–385.

Everard, A, L Geurts, R Caesar, H M Van, S Matamoros, T Duparc, R G Denis et al. 2014. Intestinal epithelial MyD88 is a sensor switching host metabolism towards obesity according to nutritional status. *Nature Communications* 5 (2041-1723 (Electronic)): 5648.

Forslund, K, F Hildebrand, T Nielsen, G Falony, E Le Chatelier, S Sunagawa, E Prifti et al. 2015. Disentangling type 2 diabetes and metformin treatment signatures in the human gut microbiota. *Nature* 528 (7581): 262–266.

Fåk, F, S Ahrné, G Molin, B Jeppsson, and B Weström. 2008. Microbial manipulation of the rat dam changes bacterial colonization and alters properties of the gut in her offspring. *American Journal of Physiology. Gastrointestinal and Liver Physiology* 294 (1): G148–G154.

Gale, C, K M Logan, S Santhakumaran, J R C Parkinson, M J Hyde, and N Modi. 2012. Effect of breastfeeding compared with formula feeding on infant body composition: A systematic review and meta-analysis. *American Journal of Clinical Nutrition* 95 (3): 656–669.

Gao, X, R Jia, L Xie, L Kuang, L Feng, and C Wan. 2015. Obesity in school-aged children and its correlation with gut E.coli and bifidobacteria: A case–control study. *BMC Pediatrics* 15 (1): 64.

Gohir, W, E M Ratcliffe, D M Sloboda, and B Sciences. 2014. Of the bugs that shape us: Maternal obesity, the gut microbiome, and long-term disease risk. *Pediatric Research* 77 (1): 196–204.

Golubeva, A V, S Crampton, L Desbonnet, D Edge, O O'Sullivan, K W Lomasney, A V Zhdanov et al. 2015. Prenatal stress-induced alterations in major physiological systems correlate with gut microbiota composition in adulthood. *Psychoneuroendocrinology* 60: 58–74.

Goodrich, J K, E R Davenport, M Beaumont, J T Bell, A G Clark, and R E Ley. 2016. Genetic determinants of the gut microbiome in UK twins correspondence. *Cell Host and Microbe* 19 (5): 731–743.

Goodrich, J K, J L Waters, A C Poole, J L Sutter, O Koren, R Blekhman, M Beaumont et al. 2014. Human genetics shape the gut microbiome. *Cell* 159 (4): 789–799.

Grönlund, M M, O P Lehtonen, E Eerola, and P Kero. 1999. Fecal microflora in healthy infants born by different methods of delivery: Permanent changes in intestinal flora after cesarean delivery. *Journal of Pediatric Gastroenterology and Nutrition* 28 (1): 19–25.

Han, J C, D A Lawlor, and S Y Kimm. 2010. Childhood obesity. *Lancet* 375 (9727): 1737–1748.

Hartstra, A V, K E C Bouter, F Bäckhed, and M Nieuwdorp. 2014. Insights into the role of the microbiome in obesity and type 2 diabetes. *Diabetes Care* 38 (January): 159–165.

Hassiotou, F, A R Hepworth, P Metzger, C T Lai, N Trengove, P E Hartmann, and L Filgueira. 2013a. Maternal and infant infections stimulate a rapid leukocyte response in breast milk. *Clinical & Translational Immunology* 2 (4).

Hassiotou, F, A R Hepworth, T M Williams, A J Twigger, S Perrella, C T Lai, L Filgueira et al. 2013b. Breastmilk cell and fat contents respond similarly to removal of breastmilk by the infant. *PLoS One* 8 (11): e78232.

Hildebrandt, M A, C Hoffmann, S A Sherrill Mix, S A Keilbaugh, M Hamady, Y-Y Chen, R Knight et al. 2009. High-fat diet determines the composition of the murine gut microbiome independently of obesity. *Gastroenterology* 137 (5): 1712–1716.

Jakobsson, H E, T R Abrahamsson, M C Jenmalm, K Harris, C Quince, C Jernberg, B Björkstén et al. 2014. Decreased gut microbiota diversity, delayed Bacteroidetes colonisation and reduced Th1 responses in infants delivered by caesarean section. *Gut* 63 (4): 559–566.

Jayasinghe, T N, V Chiavaroli, D J Holland, W S Cutfield, and J M O'Sullivan. 2016. The new era of treatment for obesity and metabolic disorders: Evidence and expectations for gut microbiome transplantation. *Frontiers in Cellular and Infection Microbiology* 6 (February): 1–11.

Jernberg, C, S Löfmark, C Edlund, and J K Jansson. 2010. Long-term impacts of antibiotic exposure on the human intestinal microbiota. *Microbiology* 156 (Pt 11): 3216–3223.

Jiménez, E, L Fernández, M L Marín, R Martín, J M Odriozola, C Nueno-Palop, A Narbad et al. 2005. Isolation of commensal bacteria from umbilical cord blood of healthy neonates born by cesarean section. *Current Microbiology* 51 (4): 270–274.

Jost, T C Lacroix, C Braegger, and C Chassard. 2014. Stability of the maternal gut microbiota during late pregnancy and early lactation. *Current Microbiology* 68 (4): 419–427.

Kadooka, Y, M Sato, K Imaizumi, A Ogawa, K Ikuyama, Y Akai, M Okano et al. 2010. Regulation of abdominal aadiposity by probiotics (Lactobacillus gasseri SBT2055) in adults with obese tendencies in a randomized controlled trial. *European Journal of Clinical Nutrition* 64 (6): 636–643.

Kaetzel, C S. 2014. Cooperativity among secretory IgA, the polymeric immunoglobulin receptor, and the gut microbiota promotes host-microbial mutualism. *Immunology Letters* 162 (2): 10–21.

Kalliomäki, M, M C Collado, S Salminen, and E Isolauri. 2008. Early differences in fecal microbiota composition in children may predict overweight. *American Journal of Clinical Nutrition* 87 (3): 534–538.

Kaplan, J L, and W A Walker. 2012. Early gut colonization and subsequent obesity risk. *Current Opinion in Clinical Nutrition and Metabolic Care* 15 (3): 278–284.

Karlsson, F H, V Tremaroli, I Nookaew, G Bergström, C J Behre, B Fagerberg et al. 2013. Gut metagenome in European women with normal, impaired and diabetic glucose control. *Nature* 498 (7452): 99–103.

Karlsson Videhult, F, Öhlund, I,Stenlund, H, O Hernell, and C E West. 2015. Probiotics during weaning: A follow-up study on effects on body composition and metabolic markers at school age. *European Journal of Nutrition* 54 (3): 355–363.

Khan, M T, M Nieuwdorp, and F Bäckhed. 2014. Microbial modulation of insulin sensitivity. *Cell Metabolism* 20: 753–760.

Koenig, J E, A Spor, N Scalfone, A D Fricker, J Stombaugh, R Knight, L T Angenent et al. 2011. Succession of microbial consortia in the developing infant gut microbiome. *Proceedings of the National Academy of Sciences of the United States of America* 108 (Suppl 1): 4578–4585.

Kootte, R S, A Vrieze, F Holleman, G M Dallinga-Thie, E G Zoetendal, W M de Vos, A K Groen et al. 2012. The therapeutic potential of manipulating gut microbiota in obesity and type 2 diabetes mellitus. *Diabetes, Obesity & Metabolism* 14 (2): 112–120.

Koren, O, J K Goodrich, T C Cullender, A Spor, K Laitinen, H K Bäckhed, A Gonzalez et al. 2012. SI-host remodeling of the gut microbiome and metabolic changes during pregnancy. *Cell* 150 (3): 470–480.

Korpela, K, A Salonen, L J Virta, R A Kekkonen, K Forslund, P Bork, and W M De Vos. 2016. Intestinal microbiome is related to lifetime antibiotic use in Finnish pre-school children. *Nature Communications* 7: 1–8.

Kuhle, S, O S Tong, and C G Woolcott. 2015. Association between caesarean section and childhood obesity: A systematic review and meta-analysis. *Obesity Reviews* 16 (4): 295–303.

Kumar, H, R Lund, A Laiho, K Lundelin, R E Ley, E Isolauri, and S Salminen. 2014. Gut microbiota as an epigenetic regulator: Pilot study based on whole-genome methylation analysis. *mBio* 5 (6): 1–4.

Le Chatelier, E, T Nielsen, J Qin, E Prifti, F Hildebrand, G Falony, M Almeida et al. 2013. Richness of human gut microbiome correlates with metabolic markers. *Nature* 500 (7464): 541–546.

Ley, R E, F Bäckhed, P Turnbaugh, C A Lozupone, R D Knight, and J I Gordon. 2005. Obesity alters gut microbial ecology. *Proceedings of the National Academy of Sciences of the United States of America* 102 (31): 11070–11075.

Ley, R E, P J Turnbaugh, S Klein, and J I Gordon. 2006. Microbial ecology: Human gut microbes associated with obesity. *Nature* 444 (7122): 1022–1023.

Li, J, H Jia, X Cai, H Zhong, Q Feng, S Sunagawa, M Arumugam et al. 2014. An integrated catalog of reference genes in the human gut microbiome. *Nature Biotechnology* advance on (8): 834–841.

Li, H-T, Y-R Zhou, and J-M Liu. 2013. The impact of cesarean section on offspring overweight and obesity: A systematic review and meta-analysis. *International Journal of Obesity* 37 (7): 893–899.

Lin, H V, A Frassetto, E J Kowalik, A R Nawrocki, M M Lu, J R Kosinski, J A Hubert et al. 2012. Butyrate and propionate protect against diet-induced obesity and regulate gut hormones via free fatty acid receptor 3-independent mechanisms. *PLoS One* 7 (4): 1–9.

Lluch, J, F Servant, S Païssé, C Valle, S Valière, C Kuchly, G Vilchez et al. 2015. The characterization of novel tissue microbiota using an optimized 16S metagenomic sequencing pipeline. *PLoS One* 10 (11): 1–22.

Luoto, R, M C Collado, S Salminen, and E Isolauri. 2013. Reshaping the gut microbiota at an early age: Functional impact on obesity risk? *Annals of Nutrition and Metabolism* 63 (suppl 2): 17–26.

Luoto, R, M Kalliomäki, K Laitinen, and E Isolauri. 2010. The impact of perinatal probiotic intervention on the development of overweight and obesity: Follow-up study from birth to 10 years. *International Journal of Obesity* 34 (10): 1531–1537.

Million, M, M T Alou, S Khelaifia, D Bachar, J-C Lagier, N Dione, S Brah et al. 2016. Increased gut redox and depletion of anaerobic and methanogenic prokaryotes in severe acute malnutrition. *Scientific Reports* 6 (October 2015): 26051.

Mor, A, S Antonsen, J Kahlert, V Holsteen, S Jørgensen, J Holm-Pedersen, H T Sørensen, O Pedersen, and V Ehrenstein. 2015. Prenatal exposure to systemic antibacterials and overweight and obesity in Danish schoolchildren: A prevalence study. *International Journal of Obesity* 39 (10): 1450–1455.

Mueller, N T, E Bakacs, J Combellick, Z Grigoryan, and M G Dominguez-Bello. 2015. The infant microbiome development: Mom matters. *Trends in Molecular Medicine* 21 (2): 109–117.

Mueller, N T, R Whyatt, L Hoepner, S Oberfield, M G Dominguez-Bello, E M Widen, A Hassoun et al. 2014. Prenatal exposure to antibiotics, cesarean section and risk of childhood obesity. *International Journal of Obesity*, 39 (4): 665–670.

Mugambi, M N, A Musekiwa, M Lombard, T Young, and R Blaauw. 2012. Synbiotics, probiotics or prebiotics in infant formula for full term infants: A systematic review. *Nutrition Journal* 11: 81

Neville, M C, J C Allen, P C Archer, C E Casey, J Seacat, R P Keller, V Lutes et al. 1991. Studies in human lactation: Milk volume and nutrient composition during weaning and lactogenesis. *American Journal of Clinical Nutrition* 54 (1): 81–92.

Nieuwdorp, M, P W Gilijamse, N Pai, and L M Kaplan. 2014. Role of the microbiome in energy regulation and metabolism. *Gastroenterology* 146 (6): 1525–1533.

Pais, R, F M Gribble, and F Reimann. 2015. Stimulation of incretin secreting cells. *TherapeuticAdvances in Endocrinology and Metabolism* 7 (1) 24–42.

Penders, J, C Thijs, C Vink, F F Stelma, B Snijders, I Kummeling, P A van den Brandt et al. 2006. Factors influencing the composition of the intestinal microbiota in early infancy. *Pediatrics* 118 (2): 511–521.

Perry, R J, L Peng, N A Barry, G W Cline, D Zhang, R L Cardone, K F Petersen et al. 2016. Acetate mediates a microbiome–brain–β-cell axis to promote metabolic syndrome. *Nature* 534 (7606): 213–217.

Piya, M K, A L Harte, and P G McTernan. 2013. Metabolic endotoxaemia: Is it more than just a gut feeling? *Current Opinion in Lipidology* 24 (1): 78–85.

Pomié, C, V Blasco-Baque, P Klopp, S Nicolas, A Waget, P Loubières, V Azalbert et al. 2016. Triggering the adaptive immune system with commensal gut bacteria protects against insulin resistance and dysglycemia. *Molecular Metabolism* 5 (6): 1–12.

Potgieter, M, J Bester, D B Kell, and E Pretorius. 2015. The dormant blood microbiome in chronic, inflammatory diseases. *FEMS Microbiology Reviews* 39 (4): 567–591.

Poul, E L, C Loison, S Struyf, J-Y Springael, V Lannoy, M-E Decobecq, S Brezillon et al. 2003. Functional characterization of human receptors for short chain fatty acids and their role in polymorphonuclear cell activation. *Journal of Biological Chemistry* 278 (28): 25481–25489.

Qin, J, R Li, J Raes, M Arumugam, K S Burgdorf, C Manichanh, T Nielsen et al. 2010. A human gut microbial gene catalogue established by metagenomic sequencing. *Nature* 464 (7285): 59–65.

Qin, J, Y Li, Z Cai, S Li, J Zhu, F Zhang, S Liang et al. 2012. A metagenome-wide association study of gut microbiota in type 2 diabetes. *Nature* 490 (7418): 55–60.

Rautava, S, M C Collado, S Salminen, and E Isolauri. 2012. Probiotics modulate host-microbe interaction in the placenta and fetal gut: A randomized, double-blind, placebo-controlled trial. *Neonatology* 102 (3): 178–184.

Revelo, X S, S Tsai, H Lei, H Luck, M Ghazarian, H Tsui, S Y Shi et al. 2014. Perforin is a novel immune regulator of obesity related insulin resistance. *Diabetes* 64 (January): 90–103.

Ridaura, V K, J J Faith, F E Rey, J Cheng, A E Duncan, A L Kau, N W Griffin et al. 2013. Gut microbiota from twins discordant for obesity modulate metabolism in mice. *Science* 341 (6150): 1241214.

Rodriguez, J M, K Murphy, C Stanton, R P Ross, O I Kober, N Juge, E Avershina et al. 2015. The composition of the gut microbiota throughout life, with an emphasis on early life. *Microbial Ecology Health Disease* 26: 26050.

Rogier, E W, A L Frantz, M E C Bruno, L Wedlund, D A Cohen, A J Stromberg, and C S Kaetzel. 2014. Lessons from mother: Long-term impact of antibodies in breast milk on the gut microbiota and intestinal immune system of breastfed offspring. *Gut Microbes* 5 (5): 663–668.

Salminen, S, G R Gibson, A L McCartney, and E Isolauri. 2004. Influence of mode of delivery on gut microbiota composition in seven year old children. *Gut* 53 (9): 1388–1389.

Schmelzle, H, S Wirth, H Skopnik, M Radke, J Knol, H-M Böckler, A Brönstrup et al. 2003. Randomized double-blind study of the nutritional efficacy and bifidogenicity of a new infant formula containing partially hydrolyzed protein, a high beta-palmitic acid level, and nondigestible oligosaccharides. *Journal of Pediatric Gastroenterology Nutrition* 36(3): 343–351.

Scott, F I, D B Horton, R Mamtani, K Haynes, D S Goldberg, D Y Lee, and J D Lewis. 2016. Administration of antibiotics to children before age 2 years increases risk for childhood obesity. *Gastroenterology* 151(1): 120–129.

Sender, R, S Fuchs, and R Milo. 2016. Are we really vastly outnumbered? Revisiting the ratio of bacterial to host cells in humans. *Cell* 164 (3): 337–340.

Sevelsted, A, J Stokholm, K Bonnelykke, and H Bisgaard. 2014. Cesarean section and chronic immune disorders—Editorial comment. *Pediatrics* 135 (1): e92–e98.

Shin, H, Z Pei, K A Martinez, J I Rivera-Vinas, K Mendez, H Cavallin, and M G Dominguez-Bello. 2015. The first microbial environment of infants born by C-section: The operating room microbes. *Microbiome* 3 (1): 59.

Simon, M-C, K Strassburger, B Nowotny, H Kolb, P Nowotny, V Burkart, F Zivehe et al. 2015. Intake of *Lactobacillus reuteri* improves incretin and insulin secretion in glucose tolerant humans: A proof of concept. *Diabetes Care* 38 (10): 1827–1834.

Skinner, A C, E M Perrin, and J A Skelton. 2016. Prevalence of obesity and severe obesity in US children, 1999–2014. *Obesity* 24 (5): 1116–1123.

Thompson, A L, A Monteagudo-Mera, M B Cadenas, M L Lampl, and M A Azcarate-Peril. 2015. Milk- and solid-feeding practices and daycare attendance are associated with differences in bacterial diversity, predominant communities, and metabolic and immune function of the infant gut microbiome. *Frontiers in Cellular and Infection Microbiology* 5 (February): 3.

Trasande, L, J Blustein, M Liu, E Corwin, L M Cox, and M J Blaser. 2012. Infant antibiotic exposures and early-life body mass. *Nature Biotechnology* 37 (1): 16–23.

Tulstrup, M V-L, E G Christensen, V Carvalho, C Linninge, S Ahrné, O Højberg, T R Licht et al. 2015. Antibiotic treatment affects intestinal permeability and gut microbial composition in Wistar rats dependent on antibiotic class. *PLoS One* 10 (12): e0144854.

Turnbaugh, P J, M Hamady, T Yatsunenko, B L Cantarel, A Duncan, R E Ley, M L Sogin et al. 2009. A core gut microbiome in obese and lean twins. *Nature* 457 (7228): 480–484.

Ursell, L K, H J Haiser, W V Treuren, N Garg, L Reddivari, J Vanamala, P C Dorrestein et al. 2014. The intestinal metabolome: An intersection between microbiota and host. *Gastroenterology* 146 (6): 1470–1476.

Uusitalo, U, X Liu, J Yang, C A Aronsson, S Hummel, M Butterworth, Å Lernmark et al. 2016. Association of early exposure of probiotics and islet autoimmunity in the TEDDY study. *JAMA Pediatrics* 170 (1): 20–28.

Vandenplas, Y, E D Greef, and G Veereman. 2015. Prebiotics in infant formula. *Gut Microbes* 5 (6): 681–687.

Vaz, L E, K P Kleinman, M A Raebel, J D Nordin, M D Lakoma, M M Dutta-linn, J A Finkelstein et al. 2014. Recent trends in outpatient antibiotic use in children. *Pediatrics* 133 (3): 375–385.

Veereman-Wauters, G Staelens, S, Van de Broek, H K Plaskie, F Wesling, L C Roger, A L Mccartney, and P Assam. 2011. Physiological and bifidogenic effects of prebiotic supplements in infant formulae. *Journal of Pediatric Gastroenterology Nutrition* 52 (6): 763–771.

Vital, M, A C Howe, and J M Tiedje. 2014. Revealing the bacterial butyrate synthesis pathways by analyzing (meta)genomic data. *mBio* 5 (2): 1–11.

Vrieze, A A, E E Van Nood, F F Holleman, J J Salojärvi, R S R S Kootte, J F W M J F Bartelsman, G M G M Dallinga-Thie et al. 2012. Transfer of intestinal microbiota from lean donors increases insulin sensitivity in individuals with metabolic syndrome. *Gastroenterology* 143 (4): 913–919e7.

Weng, S F, S A Redsell, J A Swift, M Yang, and C P Glazebrook. 2012. Systematic review and meta-analyses of risk factors for childhood overweight identifiable during infancy. *Archives of Disease in Childhood* 97 (12): 1019–1026.

Wostmann, B S. 1973. Intestinal bile acids and cholesterol absorption in the germfree rat. *Journal of Nutrition* 103 (7): 982–990.

Zijlmans, M A C, K Korpela, J M Riksen-Walraven, W M de Vos, and C de Weerth. 2015. Maternal prenatal stress is associated with the infant intestinal microbiota. *Psychoneuroendocrinology* 53: 233–245.

Section V

Epigenetic Mechanisms of Early Programming

16 Early Life Nutrition and Metabolic Programming: Epigenetic Phenomenon

Mina Desai and Michael G. Ross

CONTENTS

16.1 INTRODUCTION

The premise that the nutritional environment during developmental periods can influence the risk of propensity for adult obesity and its associated metabolic abnormalities (metabolic syndrome) is the basis of the "developmental programming" concept. Epigenetic phenomenon is one of the critical underlying mechanisms that link early nutrition and metabolic programming. Essentially, the epigenome-mediated programmed changes in metabolism, gene expression, and phenotype occur via nongenomic (i.e., DNA methylation, histone modifications, noncoding RNA [ncRNA]) rather than the genomic (DNA sequence) influence. The effects of epigenetic–nutrition interaction on growth, changes in cellular make-up, and gene expression are generally apparent early in life, whereas the effects on metabolic dysfunction including phenotype (e.g., obesity, insulin resistance, hypertension) are manifested later in life. Remarkably, not only the programmed effects but the epigenomic changes may persist despite optimal postnatal nutrition. This suggests that the epigenetic changes in response to early nutrition retain "memory" to yield phenotypes and ensure their stability throughout the lifespan. Nonetheless, evidence that the epigenome is malleable during developmental periods offers novel opportunities for early detection and prevention strategies for programmed metabolic syndrome. In this chapter, we discuss the evidence in human and animal studies for the nutrition-mediated epigenomic mechanisms in programmed obesity and metabolic syndrome.

16.2   EPIDEMIC OF OBESITY AND METABOLIC SYNDROME

The continuing increase in prevalence of obesity presents a challenging public health crisis, contributing to significant morbidity and mortality throughout the world (Seidell 2005). Obesity is central to the development of metabolic syndrome, which includes a cluster of metabolic abnormalities comprised of insulin resistance, elevated triglycerides, hypertension, and atherosclerosis (Reilly and Rader 2003). Among U.S. adults, 69% of U.S. adults are overweight (body mass index [BMI] 25–<30 kg/m²), and 36% of males and 40% of females are obese (BMI ≥ 30 kg/m²) (Flegal et al. 2016). In parallel with this, 35% of adults and 50% of those aged 60 years or older exhibit metabolic syndrome, a concerning incidence given the aging U.S. population (Aguilar et al. 2015). Of equal concern, there is a marked and continuing increase in the prevalence of obesity (~30%) and gestational diabetes among pregnant women. Not only do women begin pregnancy at a higher BMI, but women also gain excess gestational weight (Rooney and Schauberger 2002), both of which are associated with high birth weight newborns as well as a risk factor for offspring childhood obesity. Consistent with this, there is a 25% increase in the incidence of high birth weight babies during the past decade and childhood obesity rates approach 20% (Ogden et al. 2016). More importantly, among the obese children, 29% exhibit metabolic syndrome (Friend et al. 2013), a feature that in the past was seen only in middle-aged individuals.

Obesity is often attributed to a Western-style, high-fat diet combined with decreased activity levels. While there is little doubt that these factors are strong determinants of obesity, the strategy of dieting combined with exercise has often not yielded effective long-term outcome. This may be partly because the propensity for obesity and metabolic syndrome may begin *in utero* as a result of early exposure to an adverse nutritional environment, including both undernutrition and relative over-nutrition. There is compelling evidence for this, as discussed below.

16.3   EARLY NUTRITION AND METABOLIC PROGRAMMING

Nutrition undoubtedly plays an important role in health and disease. Its role during development is emphasized by the beneficial effects seen as a result of maternal nutritional supplementation, especially during pregnancy. For example, maternal iodine and folate supplementation prevent iodine deficiency-induced cretinism and spina bifida, respectively. Similarly, maternal polymorphic genes involved in folate metabolism are associated with abnormalities including cleft palate defects, heart defects, or intrauterine growth restriction (Antony 2007). In addition to facilitating the conversion of homocysteine to methionine, the functional mechanism for folate likely involves epigenetic effects as folate generates the principal methyl donor (S-adenosyl methionine) that participates in the methylation of DNA and histones. As described below, DNA methylation, particularly in promoter regions, serves to silence the transcription of genes.

The premise that suboptimal nutrition during pregnancy could permanently change growth and metabolism of the offspring was provided by the pioneer collective work of McCance and Widdowson, and Winick and Nobel (Widdowson and McCance 1975; Winick and Noble 1966). Barker expanded this fundamental concept and proposed that adult disease such as cardiovascular disease, diabetes, hypertension, and lipid abnormalities may have its origin during the developmental period (Hales and Barker 2001). The supportive evidence for the "Barker hypothesis" initially came from epidemiologic studies that demonstrated an association between birth weight, a proximate measure for *in utero* growth and development, and adult diseases. Earlier studies focused on low birth weight infants that develop in a state of relative maternal "undernutrition." In particular, the Dutch famine cohort showed that offspring of mothers exposed to the famine during the early pregnancy had lower birth weights, though paradoxically a higher incidence of obesity than the general population (Lumey 1992). In particular, low birth weight newborns with rapid catch-up growth during infancy had the highest risk of adult obesity and metabolic syndrome (Monteiro and Victora 2005). Recent studies have focused on the effect of maternal overnutrition and have shown similar adverse effects on the offspring health. Thus, there is in fact an increased risk of adult obesity at both the low and high ends of birth weight (Pettitt and Jovanovic 2001). The association between suboptimal maternal nutrition and risk of offspring metabolic syndrome has been largely replicated worldwide in various ethnic groups, ages, men, and women. To understand the mechanistic basis of developmental programming health and disease, several animal models of maternal nutritional manipulation have been established. Essentially, the results from animal studies replicate the human findings (Desai et al. 2007; Howie et al. 2013; Lane 2014).

In general, the programming effects that are evident early in life are usually subtle effects on altered growth and gene expression (Desai et al. 2015). The majority of the programmed effects that influence health and manifest as disease (obesity, insulin resistance, hypertension, lipid abnormalities) are deferred and expressed at a later age (Ross and Desai 2013; Zambrano and Nathanielsz 2013). This raises the question as to how the memory of early events is stored and later expressed, despite continuous cellular replication and replacement. This may in part be explained through epigenetic regulation of gene expression, which involves the modification of the genome without altering the DNA sequence itself (Figure 16.1) as discussed below.

Another milestone of the programming effects was the delineation of "critical periods" that essentially demonstrated that the cellular effects of early nutrition were dependent upon the phase of growth of the animal at the time of suboptimal nutritional exposure. Very early exposure in life may irreversibly impact cell division, differentiation, and organ growth, whereas later in life, it may impact cell composition and cell size (Widdowson and McCance 1975; Winick and Noble 1965). Furthermore, the earlier the exposure, the less likely is the recovery after the insult is discontinued. Thus, suboptimal supply of nutrients during prenatal and perhaps postnatal life may also interfere with stem cell proliferation and differentiation

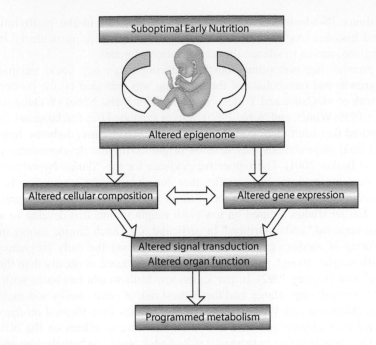

FIGURE 16.1 Early nutrition, epigenome, and programmed metabolism. Early nutrition interacts with the epigenome to alter (a) cellular proliferation and/or differentiation and ultimately cell types, (b) gene expression, and (c) organ structure and function. These individually or collectively impact metabolism.

and ultimately influence the lineage commitment, cellular composition, and organ structure and function. In the past decade, many epigenetic regulatory mechanisms have been shown to play a large role in the timing and determination of stem cell lineages.

16.4   EPIGENETICS

16.4.1   EMBRYONIC STEM CELLS

Embryonic stem cells can self-renew to increase the stem cell pool and differentiate to generate specialized cell types of tissues/organs through epigenetic mechanisms (Leeb and Wutz 2012; Wutz 2013). During differentiation, precise characteristics and identity are acquired by the cells for the specific assigned functional role (Figure 16.2). Once differentiated, it is essential for the cells to maintain their gene expression patterns for optimal function and prevention of adverse outcome. It is thought that "epigenetic memory" allows cells to maintain their identity, even when exposed to extracellular environments. The cellular inheritance is regulated by three major epigenetic regulators that include DNA methylation, histone modifications, and microRNA (miRNA) that together impact chromatin remodeling and ultimately gene expression (Figure 16.3).

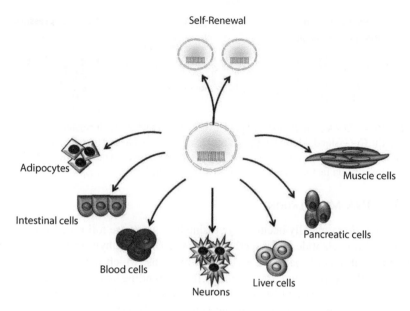

FIGURE 16.2   Stem cells can self-renew or differentiate to specific cell types that give rise to brain, pancreatic, liver, intestinal, pancreatic, muscle, or adipose cells.

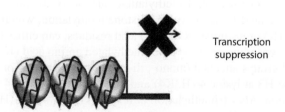

FIGURE 16.3   Epigenetic regulation of gene expression. Chromatin consists of DNA packaged around histones. Packaging of chromatin into an open (euchromatic) state activates gene expression and a closed (heterochromatic) state suppresses it.

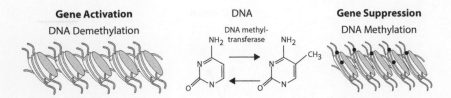

FIGURE 16.4 DNA methylation and gene expression. DNA methyltransferase adds methyl groups to the CpG island. Methylation renders DNA inaccessible and thereby suppresses gene expression. Methyl groups can be passively or actively removed which renders DNA accessible to transcription factors that activate gene expression.

16.4.2 DNA METHYLATION

DNA methylation typically occurs on cytosine bases that are followed by a guanine, termed CpG dinucleotides. The methylation by a DNA methyltransferase (DNMT) leads to recruitment of methyl-CpG binding proteins, which induce transcriptional silencing both by blocking transcription factor binding and by recruiting transcriptional corepressors or histone-modifying complexes. Increased methylation is associated with transcriptional silencing (Figure 16.4). DNA methylation is highly dynamic during embryogenesis. Following fertilization and prior to implantation, DNA is hypomethylated and thereafter there is a progressive increase in DNA methylation that leads to differentiation and organogenesis (Clarke 1992). With aging, the reverse process occurs marked by a global loss of DNA methylation. It is during embryogenesis and early postnatal life that DNA methylation patterns are fundamentally established, and are imperative for silencing of specific gene regions, such as imprinted genes and repetitive nucleic acid sequences.

16.4.3 HISTONE MODIFICATIONS

Histone modifications represent an additional mechanism of regulating gene expression. Chromatin consists of DNA packaged around histones, and open chromatin (euchromatic) represents activation of gene expression, whereas a closed (heterochromatic) state is associated with gene silencing. Posttranslational modifications of histone tails can alter histone interaction with DNA and recruit proteins (e.g., transcriptional factors) that alter chromatin conformation. These modifications that commonly involve methylation/demethylation and acetylation/deacetylation are mediated by histone-modifying enzymes. Histone methylation, which typically takes place on lysine (K) or arginine (R) amino acid residues, can either repress or activate transcription depending on the type of methylated amino acid (K or R) and the number of methyl groups attached (mono-, di-, or trimethylation). For example, methylation of histone H3 at lysine 4 (H3K4) and arginine of H3 and H4 results in transcriptional activation. Also, trimethylation of histone H3 at lysine 4 (H3K4me3) is associated with active gene transcription, whereas dimethylation of histone H3 at lysine 9 (H3K9me2) is associated with transcriptional silencing. Unlike the complexity of methylation-mediated effects, acetylation potentiates and deacetylation suppresses gene expression (Cosgrove 2007) (Figure 16.5).

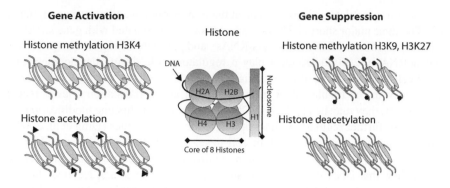

FIGURE 16.5 Histone modifications and gene expression. Chromatin consists of DNA packaged around histones. Posttranslational modifications of histone tails involve methylation/demethylation and acetylation/deacetylation. Histone methylation can repress or activate transcription depending on which amino acid is methylated and the number of methyl groups added. Methylation at lysine 4 (H3K4) is associated with active gene transcription whereas at lysine 9 and 27 (H3K9, H3K27) is associated with transcriptional silencing. In contrast, acetylation potentiates and deacetylation suppresses gene expression.

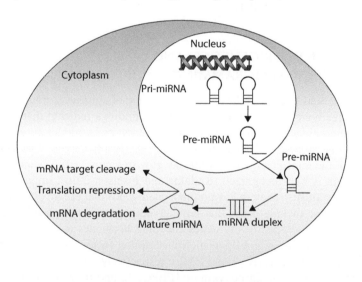

FIGURE 16.6 Synthesis of microRNA (miRNA). miRNA genes are transcribed as large primary transcripts (pri-miRNA) and processed to form precursor microRNA (pre-miRNA). This is subsequently transported to the cytoplasm where pre-miRNA is further processed to form a mature microRNA of approximately 22 nucleotides. The mature miRNA is then incorporated into a ribonuclear particle to form the RNA-induced silencing complex, which mediates gene silencing.

16.4.4 Noncoding RNAs

ncRNAs also participate in the epigenetic regulation of gene transcription (Bayoumi et al. 2016). ncRNAs are transcribed from DNA but are not translated into proteins and function to regulate gene expression at the transcriptional and posttranscriptional level. The three major short ncRNAs (<30 nucleotides) associated with gene silencing are miRNAs, short inhibitory RNAs (siRNAs), and piwi-interacting RNAs (piRNAs). Long ncRNAs (>200 nucleotides) play a regulatory role during development and exhibit cell type-specific expression (Figure 16.6). While these ncRNAs are usually associated with the regulation of gene expression at the translational level, recent work suggests they may be involved in DNA methylation and histone modifications as well, thereby further regulating transcription of their target genes (Ding et al. 2009).

To summarize, during early stem cell development, the epigenome undergoes global remodeling that determines and maintains lineage commitment of stem cells. Studies show that DNA methylation is susceptible to intrinsic and extrinsic factors making it a prime candidate as the basis for fetal programming. Abnormal DNA methylation, histone modification, and altered miRNA are associated with inappropriate gene silencing or activation, and such changes in epigenetic marks are associated with several human diseases (e.g., cancers, neurological disorders, inflammation, and obesity). As methylation involves the supply and enzymatic transfer of methyl groups, it is plausible that early nutritional (e.g., methyl donors), hormonal, or other metabolic cues alter the timing and direction of methylation patterns during development (Burdge et al. 2011).

16.5 NUTRITION, EPIGENETICS, AND METABOLIC PROGRAMMING

Animal and limited human studies provide evidence of epigenetic-mediated mechanisms for metabolic abnormalities. Overall, the findings indicate that nutritional and environmental factors can interact with the genotype by modulating epigenetic markings in the somatic cells and thus impacting the phenotype. The epigenetic modulation of the imprinted gene insulin-like growth factor 2 (*IGF2*) and its impact on body weight is well recognized (Kadakia and Josefson 2016). Importantly, epigenetic changes are also seen in key nonimprinted genes that are involved in energy metabolism. These include genes that regulate adipogenesis, glucose homeostasis, and insulin signaling. Specifically genes encoding hormones (e.g., leptin), nuclear receptors (e.g., adipogenic and lipogenic transcription factors peroxisome proliferator-activated receptor [PPAR]γ and PPARα, respectively), gluconeogenic enzymes (e.g., phosphoenolpyruvate carboxykinase [PEPCK]), and transmembrane proteins (e.g., uncoupling protein 1 [UCP1]) (Milagro et al. 2009; Noer et al. 2007; Fujiki et al. 2009; Sullivan et al. 2007) are susceptible to epigenetic modulation.

16.5.1 HUMAN STUDIES

Human studies have used blood and biopsy samples (muscle, adipose tissue) to show changes in DNA methylation, histone modification, and miRNA and in some cases have related these changes to obesity and diabetes. A study of monozygous twins clearly demonstrates the environmental influence on the regulation of gene expression wherein the offspring exhibits divergent DNA methylation and histone acetylation patterns despite a similar genotype (Fraga et al. 2005). In this study, lymphocyte and muscle biopsy samples were obtained from 3- to 74-year-old Spanish monozygotic twins (monochorionic and dichorionic) to address the discordance (anthropomorphic features and susceptibility to disease) seen in monozygous twins. Global and locus-specific DNA methylation and histone acetylation revealed that the older, but not younger, twins exhibited differences in their epigenetic markings and their gene-expression profile. These findings suggest that later life environments may alter the epigenome.

Other studies further demonstrate that changes in global DNA methylation, specific histone methylation (H3K4 and H3K9), or certain miRNAs are positively associated with BMI (Jufvas et al. 2013; Ortega et al. 2010). Obese and lean humans have distinct DNA methylation levels in certain genes and expression of miRNAs as demonstrated in tissue (subcutaneous adipose) as well as cultured preadipocytes and mature adipocytes. Furthermore, the expression pattern of miRNAs in human adipose tissue was associated not only with obesity but also parameters of glucose metabolism (Ortega et al. 2010). With regard to histone modification, the degree of specific histone lysine methylation (di- and trimethylation of K4) differed in overweight individuals with and without type 2 diabetes. Using primary human adipocytes, this study revealed lower levels of K4 dimethylation in overweight nondiabetic and higher levels of K4 trimethylation in overweight diabetic compared with normalweight individuals (Jufvas et al. 2013).

With respect to programming effects as a result of maternal nutritional exposures, both pregnancy under- and overnutrition reduced DNA methylation of the imprinted *IGF2* gene in the offspring. The findings of maternal undernutrition exposure effects came from the study on the Dutch famine (1944–1945) cohort. In this study, prenatally famine-exposed 60-year-old adults exhibited hypomethylation of whole-blood *IGF2* gene, and hypermethylation of two obesity-related nonimprinted genes (*TNF*, leptin) compared with their unexposed, same-sex siblings. This association was specific for periconceptional exposure, reinforcing that the early developmental period is crucial for establishing and maintaining epigenetic marks (Heijmans et al. 2008; Tobi et al. 2009). More recently, parental obesity and specifically paternal obesity were associated with *IGF2* hypomethylation in umbilical cord blood leukocytes of newborns (Soubry et al. 2013). Specific maternal characteristics, including gestational weight gain and gestational diabetes, have also been associated with signature DNA methylation in cord blood and increased placental leptin gene methylation, respectively (Morales et al. 2014; Bouchard et al. 2010). Furthermore, maternal carbohydrate intake in early pregnancy was associated with the umbilical cord methylation levels of the nuclear receptor gene, retinoid X receptor-α, which heterodimers with the adipogenic transcription factor PPARγ, as well as with adiposity in later childhood (Godfrey et al. 2011). Human newborn studies are generally limited to determination of umbilical blood leukocytes or placental tissue epigenetic assessments, which may not parallel organ-specific cellular changes.

16.5.2 Animal Studies

Animal studies provide further evidence implicating epigenetic mechanisms in the regulation of genes involved in appetite, adipogenesis, and lipid/glucose metabolism.

Notably, nutrition interacts with the epigenome to influence gene expression. The classic study on *agouti* mouse undoubtedly shows the effects of diet on methylation status and phenotype of the animal. In agouti mice, the normally methylated agouti gene results in mice that are thin with a brown coat color. Conversely, unmethylated agouti gene results in mice that are obese and diabetic with yellow coat color. Despite identical genotype of the "fat yellow mice" and "skinny brown mice," the phenotype is different due to epigenetic changes. Importantly, these methylation patterns are transmittable across generations (Morgan et al. 1999). However, supplementation of methyl-rich diet during "yellow mice" pregnancy prevents obesity and shifts the phenotype to that of "skinny brown mice" (Waterland et al. 2007). These results illustrate the interaction between nutrition and the epigenome and offer opportunities for potential intervention.

In addition to influencing the general phenotype, nutrition–epigenome interaction is evident at the level of specific genes. For example, plasma levels of leptin, a satiety hormone produced by adipocytes, can be modulated by diet via epigenetic mechanisms. In retroperitoneal adipocytes of rats fed a high-fat diet, there was increased methylation of leptin gene promoter that was associated with lower circulating leptin levels, suggesting that leptin methylation affects leptin gene expression (Milagro et al. 2009). Similarly, studies link histone modifications (methylation and acetylation) and miRNA to the regulation of the principal adipogenic transcription factor (PPAR) and its target genes, resulting in obesity, hyperphagia, and hyperlipidemia. Likewise, the increased hepatic gluconeogenesis seen in rats fed a high-calorie diet was attributed to increased mRNA levels of rate-limiting gluconeogenic enzyme *Pepck* as a result of hypomethylated *Pepck* gene (Burdge et al. 2011).

Beyond the gene–metabolic effects, evidence shows the influence of epigenetics on gene–cellular development. For example, adipocyte differentiation and induction of adipogenic transcription factors (PPARγ, CCAAT-enhancer-binding protein [C/EBPα]) are regulated by histone lysine methylation (H3K4) and acetylation (AcH3). Increase in histone trimethylation (H3K4me3) and acetylation (AcH3K9/K14) coincides with upregulation of PPARγ and C/EBPα and terminal adipocyte differentiation. Therefore, untimely increase in H3K4me3 and AcH3K9/K14 is likely to cause early induction of adipogenic genes with resultant premature adipocyte differentiation leading to obesity (Musri and Parrizas 2012).

Equally important is the supportive evidence implicating epigenetic–nutrition influence on cell lineage fate. For example, maternal obesity/high-fat diet in mice resulted in increased expression of a key transcription factor responsible for adipogenic lineage commitment (Zinc finger protein [Zfp423]) during fetal development. Consistent with this, the repressive histone methylation (H3K27me3) was lower in the Zfp423 promoter of fetal tissues from maternal obese mice (Yang et al. 2013). Similarly, another study showed decreased DNA methylation of CpG sites and CpG island (CGI) shores (regions immediately flanking CpG islands) with increased mRNA expression of proadipogenic factors (*Zfp423* and *C/EBP-β*) in 3-week-old rat offspring from obese pregnancies (Borengasser et al. 2013). Thus, nutrition–epigenetic phenomena can influence cell lineage, cellular composition of tissue/organ, gene expression, metabolism, and ultimately the phenotype.

Surprisingly, despite the evidence from the aforementioned studies, the role of enzymes mediating DNA methylation in the development of obesity is at best perplexing. For instance, the studies on DNMT knockout mice do not support its role in obesity. Mice with genetically increased or decreased levels of DNMT1 and DNMT3b (maintenance enzymes) do not gain weight or have increased adiposity (Kamei et al. 2010). Further compounding the issue are the findings that obese mice do exhibit increased DNMT3a (*de novo*) in white adipose tissue, though the transgenic mice with adipose tissue specific overexpression of DNMT3a do not show increased body weight or adiposity (Kamei et al. 2010). It is, however, reassuring that in contrast to the role of DNMT, there is robust evidence that supports the role of specific histone methyl transferases in regulation of adipogenesis. Mice with loss of function of the H3K9-specific demethylase, JmjC domain-containing histone demethylase 2A (Jhdm2a), are obese and hyperlipidemic (Tateishi et al. 2009; Inagaki et al. 2009). In contrast, mice with mutations in the histone H3, lysine 4 methyltransferase MLL3 exhibit reduced adipogenesis and are protected from high-fat diet induced obesity (Lee et al. 2008), indicating lysine-specific effects. Although more studies are needed to understand the role of DNMT in obesity, it may be that histone deacetylases that serve specialized functions and have tissue-specific expression are major contributors rather than ubiquitous DNMT.

Overall, epigenetic phenomena are evident in the programming effects of maternal nutritional status prior to and during pregnancy and lactation (under- and overnutrition) on the development of offspring metabolic syndrome (Ganu et al. 2012). It is remarkable that despite normal nutrition of the offspring, there is persistent long-term change not only in gene expression but also in DNA methylation, histone modification, and miRNA. This is evident in genes regulating growth (Tosh et al. 2010), adipogenesis (Desai et al. 2015), brain appetite/satiety, and reward pathways (Plagemann et al. 2009; Vucetic et al. 2010) and glucose homeostasis (Raychaudhuri et al. 2008). More importantly, epigenetic changes can be inherited (Jimenez-Chillaron et al. 2016). We now know that DNA methylation is not completely erased during very early development or gametogenesis (Fan and Zhang 2009). As such, some methylated sites survive and are replicated every time a cell divides and the DNA is passed along with associated histones. These markings can then be copied every time the cell divides, influencing gene expression throughout life. Studies suggest that epigenetic phenomenon due to early nutritional exposures can be transmitted via germ-line modifications (Barres and Zierath 2011) or can be inherited mitotically in somatic cells (Skinner 2011).

In general, both human and animal studies provide support for epigenetic-mediated programmed metabolic syndrome resulting from early nutritional exposures and suggest that epigenetic variation of nonimprinted genes may be a major contributing factor. The subtle differences between human and animal findings, including genetically modified mice, may partly be attributed to certain factors, such as sampling tissue (umbilical blood versus specific tissue/cells), period, and duration of exposure (periconceptual, fetal, or neonatal) and in the case of humans, lifestyle. The modification of epigenetic changes with postnatal environmental alterations, as well as with age alone, raises the possibility of a "double-hit" mechanism responsible for the ultimate manifestation of programmed phenotypes and thus, optimistically, therapeutic or lifestyle approaches to prevent the "second hit."

16.6 CONCLUSIONS

The fundamental concept of nutrition–epigenome interaction on programming metabolism is supported by compelling evidence from both human and animal studies. Nonetheless, what is not clear and remains to be established is (1) the cause and effect of epigenetic modifications on relevant phenotypes; (2) whether single analysis of one specific tissue is an accurate assessment of the epigenetic profile of putative, alternative cell types; and more importantly (3) whether the epigenetic changes are modifiable or reversible. For the latter, there is evidence that some of the pregnancy-related nutritional effects on offspring gene expression and metabolism including the phenotype can be manipulated during the postnatal nursing period (Desai et al. 2005, 2007). It is likely that there is a critical "window" during which the epigenome is responsive and this may provide an opportunity to reverse the effects of metabolic programming.

REFERENCES

Aguilar M, Bhuket T, Torres S, Liu B, Wong RJ. Prevalence of the metabolic syndrome in the United States, 2003–2012. *JAMA* 2015 May 19;313(19):1973–4.

Antony AC. In utero physiology: Role of folic acid in nutrient delivery and fetal development. *Am J Clin Nutr* 2007 Feb;85(2):598S-603S.

Barres R, Zierath JR. DNA methylation in metabolic disorders. *Am J Clin Nutr* 2011 Apr;93(4):897S-900.

Bayoumi AS, Sayed A, Broskova Z, Teoh JP, Wilson J, Su H, et al. Crosstalk between long noncoding RNAs and microRNAs in health and disease. *Int J Mol Sci* 2016;17(3):356.

Borengasser SJ, Zhong Y, Kang P, Lindsey F, Ronis MJ, Badger TM, et al. Maternal obesity enhances white adipose tissue differentiation and alters genome-scale DNA methylation in male rat offspring. *Endocrinol* 2013 Nov;154(11):4113–25.

Bouchard L, Thibault S, Guay SP, Santure M, Monpetit A, St-Pierre J, et al. Leptin gene epigenetic adaptation to impaired glucose metabolism during pregnancy. *Diabetes Care* 2010 Nov;33(11):2436–41.

Burdge GC, Hoile SP, Uller T, Thomas NA, Gluckman PD, Hanson MA, et al. Progressive, transgenerational changes in offspring phenotype and epigenotype following nutritional transition. *PLoS One* 2011;6(11):e28282.

Clarke HJ. Nuclear and chromatin composition of mammalian gametes and early embryos. *Biochem Cell Biol* 1992 Oct;70(10–11):856–66.

Cosgrove MS. Histone proteomics and the epigenetic regulation of nucleosome mobility. *Expert Rev Proteomics* 2007 Aug;4(4):465–78.

Desai M, Babu J, Ross MG. Programmed metabolic syndrome: Prenatal undernutrition and postweaning overnutrition. *Am J Physiol Regul Integr Comp Physiol* 2007 Dec;293(6):R2306–R2314.

Desai M, Gayle D, Babu J, Ross MG. Programmed obesity in intrauterine growth-restricted newborns: Modulation by newborn nutrition. *Am J Physiol Regul Integr Comp Physiol* 2005 Jan;288(1):R91–R96.

Desai M, Gayle D, Babu J, Ross MG. The timing of nutrient restriction during rat pregnancy/lactation alters metabolic syndrome phenotype. *Am J Obstet Gynecol* 2007 Jun; 196(6):555–7.

Desai M, Jellyman JK, Han G, Lane RH, Ross MG. Programmed regulation of rat offspring adipogenic transcription factor (PPARgamma) by maternal nutrition. *J Dev Orig Health Dis* 2015 Dec;6(6):530–8.

Ding XC, Weiler J, Grosshans H. Regulating the regulators: Mechanisms controlling the maturation of microRNAs. *Trends Biotechnol* 2009 Jan;27(1):27–36.

Fan S, Zhang X. CpG island methylation pattern in different human tissues and its correlation with gene expression. *Biochem Biophys Res Commun* 2009 Jun 12;383(4):421–5.

Flegal KM, Kruszon-Moran D, Carroll MD, Fryar CD, Ogden CL. Trends in obesity among adults in the United States, 2005 to 2014. *JAMA* 2016 Jun 7;315(21):2284–91.

Fraga MF, Ballestar E, Paz MF, Ropero S, Setien F, Ballestar ML, et al. Epigenetic differences arise during the lifetime of monozygotic twins. *Proc Natl Acad Sci USA* 2005 Jul 26;102(30):10604–9.

Friend A, Craig L, Turner S. The prevalence of metabolic syndrome in children: A systematic review of the literature. *Metab Syndr Relat Disord* 2013 Apr;11(2):71–80.

Fujiki K, Kano F, Shiota K, Murata M. Expression of the peroxisome proliferator activated receptor gamma gene is repressed by DNA methylation in visceral adipose tissue of mouse models of diabetes. *BMC Biol* 2009;7:38.

Ganu RS, Harris RA, Collins K, Aagaard KM. Maternal diet: A modulator for epigenomic regulation during development in nonhuman primates and humans. *Int J Obes Suppl* 2012 Dec;2(Suppl 2):S14–S18.

Godfrey KM, Sheppard A, Gluckman PD, Lillycrop KA, Burdge GC, McLean C, et al. Epigenetic gene promoter methylation at birth is associated with child's later adiposity. *Diabetes* 2011 May;60(5):1528–34.

Hales CN, Barker DJ. The thrifty phenotype hypothesis. *Br Med Bull* 2001;60:5–20.

Heijmans BT, Tobi EW, Stein AD, Putter H, Blauw GJ, Susser ES, et al. Persistent epigenetic differences associated with prenatal exposure to famine in humans. *Proc Natl Acad Sci USA* 2008 Nov 4;105(44):17046–9.

Howie GJ, Sloboda DM, Reynolds CM, Vickers MH. Timing of maternal exposure to a high fat diet and development of obesity and hyperinsulinemia in male rat offspring: Same metabolic phenotype, different developmental pathways? *J Nutr Metab* 2013;2013:517384.

Inagaki T, Tachibana M, Magoori K, Kudo H, Tanaka T, Okamura M, et al. Obesity and metabolic syndrome in histone demethylase JHDM2a-deficient mice. *Genes Cells* 2009 Aug;14(8):991–1001.

Jimenez-Chillaron JC, Ramon-Krauel M, Ribo S, Diaz R. Transgenerational epigenetic inheritance of diabetes risk as a consequence of early nutritional imbalances. *Proc Nutr Soc* 2016 Feb;75(1):78–89.

Jufvas A, Sjodin S, Lundqvist K, Amin R, Vener AV, Stralfors P. Global differences in specific histone H3 methylation are associated with overweight and type 2 diabetes. *Clin Epigenetics* 2013;5(1):15.

Kadakia R, Josefson J. The relationship of insulin-like growth factor 2 to fetal growth and adiposity. *Horm Res Paediatr* 2016;85(2):75–82.

Kamei Y, Suganami T, Ehara T, Kanai S, Hayashi K, Yamamoto Y, et al. Increased expression of DNA methyltransferase 3a in obese adipose tissue: Studies with transgenic mice. *Obesity* 2010 Feb;18(2):314–21.

Lane RH. Fetal programming, epigenetics, and adult onset disease. *Clin Perinatol* 2014 Dec;41(4):815–31.

Lee J, Saha PK, Yang QH, Lee S, Park JY, Suh Y, et al. Targeted inactivation of MLL3 histone H3-Lys-4 methyltransferase activity in the mouse reveals vital roles for MLL3 in adipogenesis. *Proc Natl Acad Sci USA* 2008 Dec 9;105(49):19229–34.

Leeb M, Wutz A. Establishment of epigenetic patterns in development. *Chromosoma* 2012 Jun;121(3):251–62.

Lumey LH. Decreased birthweights in infants after maternal in utero exposure to the Dutch famine of 1944–1945. *Paediatr Perinat Epidemiol* 1992 Apr;6(2):240–53.

Milagro FI, Campion J, Garcia-Diaz DF, Goyenechea E, Paternain L, Martinez JA. High fat diet-induced obesity modifies the methylation pattern of leptin promoter in rats. *J Physiol Biochem* 2009 Mar;65(1):1–9.

Monteiro PO, Victora CG. Rapid growth in infancy and childhood and obesity in later life— A systematic review. *Obes Rev* 2005 May;6(2):143–54.

Morales E, Groom A, Lawlor DA, Relton CL. DNA methylation signatures in cord blood associated with maternal gestational weight gain: Results from the ALSPAC cohort. *BMC Res Notes* 2014;7:278.

Morgan HD, Sutherland HG, Martin DI, Whitelaw E. Epigenetic inheritance at the agouti locus in the mouse. *Nat Genet* 1999 Nov;23(3):314–8.

Musri MM, Parrizas M. Epigenetic regulation of adipogenesis. *Curr Opin Clin Nutr Metab Care* 2012 Jul;15(4):342–9.

Noer A, Boquest AC, Collas P. Dynamics of adipogenic promoter DNA methylation during clonal culture of human adipose stem cells to senescence. *BMC Cell Biol* 2007;8:18.

Ogden CL, Carroll MD, Lawman HG, Fryar CD, Kruszon-Moran D, Kit BK, et al. Trends in obesity prevalence among children and adolescents in the United States, 1988–1994 through 2013–2014. *JAMA* 2016 Jun 7;315(21):2292–9.

Ortega FJ, Moreno-Navarrete JM, Pardo G, Sabater M, Hummel M, Ferrer A, et al. MiRNA expression profile of human subcutaneous adipose and during adipocyte differentiation. *PLoS One* 2010;5(2):e9022.

Pettitt DJ, Jovanovic L. Birth weight as a predictor of type 2 diabetes mellitus: The U-shaped curve. *Curr Diab Rep* 2001 Aug;1(1):78–81.

Plagemann A, Harder T, Brunn M, Harder A, Roepke K, Wittrock-Staar M, et al. Hypothalamic proopiomelanocortin promoter methylation becomes altered by early overfeeding: An epigenetic model of obesity and the metabolic syndrome. *J Physiol* 2009 Oct 15;587(Pt 20):4963–76.

Raychaudhuri N, Raychaudhuri S, Thamotharan M, Devaskar SU. Histone code modifications repress glucose transporter 4 expression in the intrauterine growth-restricted offspring. *J Biol Chem* 2008 May 16;283(20):13611–26.

Reilly MP, Rader DJ. The metabolic syndrome: More than the sum of its parts? *Circulation* 2003 Sep 30;108(13):1546–51.

Rooney BL, Schauberger CW. Excess pregnancy weight gain and long-term obesity: One decade later. *Obstet Gynecol* 2002 Aug;100(2):245–52.

Ross MG, Desai M. Developmental programming of offspring obesity, adipogenesis, and appetite. *Clin Obstet Gynecol* 2013 Sep;56(3):529–36.

Seidell JC. Epidemiology of obesity. *Semin Vasc Med* 2005 Feb;5(1):3–14.

Skinner MK. Environmental epigenetic transgenerational inheritance and somatic epigenetic mitotic stability. *Epigenetics* 2011 Jul;6(7):838–42.

Soubry A, Schildkraut JM, Murtha A, Wang F, Huang Z, Bernal A, et al. Paternal obesity is associated with IGF2 hypomethylation in newborns: Results from a Newborn Epigenetics Study (NEST) cohort. *BMC Med* 2013;11:29.

Sullivan KE, Reddy AB, Dietzmann K, Suriano AR, Kocieda VP, Stewart M, et al. Epigenetic regulation of tumor necrosis factor alpha. *Mol Cell Biol* 2007 Jul;27(14):5147–60.

Tateishi K, Okada Y, Kallin EM, Zhang Y. Role of Jhdm2a in regulating metabolic gene expression and obesity resistance. *Nature* 2009 Apr 9;458(7239):757–61.

Tobi EW, Lumey LH, Talens RP, Kremer D, Putter H, Stein AD, et al. DNA methylation differences after exposure to prenatal famine are common and timing and sex-specific. *Hum Mol Genet* 2009 Nov 1;18(21):4046–53.

Tosh DN, Fu Q, Callaway CW, McKnight RA, McMillen IC, Ross MG, et al. Epigenetics of programmed obesity: Alteration in IUGR rat hepatic IGF1 mRNA expression and histone structure in rapid vs. delayed postnatal catch-up growth. *Am J Physiol Gastrointest Liver Physiol* 2010 Nov;299(5):G1023–G1029.

Vucetic Z, Kimmel J, Totoki K, Hollenbeck E, Reyes TM. Maternal high-fat diet alters methylation and gene expression of dopamine and opioid-related genes. *Endocrinol* 2010 Oct;151(10):4756–64.

Waterland RA, Travisano M, Tahiliani KG. Diet-induced hypermethylation at agouti viable yellow is not inherited transgenerationally through the female. *FASEB J* 2007 Oct;21(12):3380–5.

Widdowson EM, McCance RA. A review: New thoughts on growth. *Pediatr Res* 1975 Mar;9(3):154–6.

Winick M, Noble A. Cellular response in rats during malnutrition at various ages. *J Nutr* 1966 Jul;89(3):300–6.

Winick M, Noble A. Quantitative changes in DNA, RNA, and protein during prenatal and postnatal growth in the rat. *Dev Biol* 1965 Dec;12(3):451–66.

Wutz A. Epigenetic regulation of stem cells: The role of chromatin in cell differentiation. *Adv Exp Med Biol* 2013;786:307–28.

Yang QY, Liang JF, Rogers CJ, Zhao JX, Zhu MJ, Du M. Maternal obesity induces epigenetic modifications to facilitate Zfp423 expression and enhance adipogenic differentiation in fetal mice. *Diabetes* 2013 Nov;62(11):3727–35.

Zambrano E, Nathanielsz PW. Mechanisms by which maternal obesity programs offspring for obesity: Evidence from animal studies. *Nutr Rev* 2013 Oct;71(Suppl 1):S42–S54.

Vucetic Z, Kimmel J, Totoki K, Hollenbeck E, Reyes TM. Maternal high-fat diet alters methylation and gene expression of dopamine and reward-related genes. Endocrinology 2010 Oct;151(10):4756-64.

Waterland RA, Travisano M, Tahiliani KG. Diet-induced hypermethylation at agouti viable yellow is not inherited transgenerationally through the female. FASEB J 2007 Oct;21(12):3380-5.

Waddington CH, McGrath RA. A review: New thoughts on genetic coding. Sci 1957 May;4(3):175-6.

Waterland RA, Jirtle RL. Early nutrition, epigenetic changes at transposons and imprinted genes, and enhanced susceptibility to adult chronic diseases. Nutr 2004 Jan;20(1):63-8.

Waterland RA, Jirtle RL. Transposable elements: targets for early nutritional effects on epigenetic gene regulation. Mol Cell Biol 2003 Aug;23(15):5293-300.

Wu Q, Suzuki M. Parental obesity and overweight affect the body-fat accumulation in the offspring: the possible effect of a high-fat diet through epigenetic inheritance. Obes Rev 2006 Aug;7(2):201-8.

Yang QY, Liang JF, Rogers CJ, Zhao JX, Zhu MJ, Du M. Maternal obesity induces epigenetic modifications to facilitate Zfp423 expression and enhance adipogenic differentiation in fetal mice. Diabetes 2013 Nov;62(11):3727-35.

Zimmerman E, Haberland PW. Methods used to video the natural course of obesity: programming of study. J Perinatal Neonatal 2011 Oct;41 Suppl 1):S48-S50.

17 Epigenetics, Telomeres, MicroRNA, and System Biology in Fetal Programming

Silvia Sookoian, Mariana Tellechea,
Maria S. Landa, and Carlos J. Pirola

CONTENTS

17.1 INTRODUCTION

A large body of epidemiological evidence has consistently shown that impaired intrauterine growth is associated with adult metabolic and cardiovascular disorders (CVDs), including coronary heart disease, type 2 diabetes (T2D), and insulin resistance (IR) (Curhan et al. 1996; Forsen et al. 1999; Harder et al. 2007; Osmond et al. 1993). These disorders cluster in the metabolic syndrome (MS), also known as cardiometabolic syndrome or "Syndrome X," of which the presence of IR in various tissues was initially regarded as the underlying factor. Indeed, IR has been regarded as the main link between all disorders grouped in the MS (Reaven 1998), including T2D, dyslipidemia, central obesity, arterial hypertension, prothrombotic and proinflammatory states, polycystic ovary, and nonalcoholic fatty liver disease (NAFLD). From the perspective of the clinical importance, the MS has two important features that include its global prevalence that is increasing dramatically and its strong association with CVD. It is widely accepted that IR results from a complex interaction between the gene variants and the environment (Sookoian and Pirola 2007, 2011). For example, environmental factors such as decreased physical activity, increasing nutrient availability, and overfeeding play an important role in the development of metabolic disorders associated with IR, and they are widely recognized as responsible for the modern epidemic of MS and its related phenotypes. However, no environmental factors or genes by themselves explain the pathophysiology of IR and MS. This is partly explained by environmental factors operating at different levels and their influence is even more significant in a genetically predisposed ground, but so far the gene variants associated with the various components of MS together account for a very small portion variability of each phenotype (Sookoian and Pirola 2007, 2011). Therefore, it is reasonable to speculate that the interaction between genes and environment is a strong modifier of the IR state and this interaction is modulated by epigenetic mechanisms.

In this chapter, we integrate genomic, molecular, and physiological data by systems biology to explore the interplay between the underlying genetic and epigenetic mechanisms involved in fetal metabolic programming and its association with adult disease. We also contrast the hypothesis that abnormal nutrient availability during the fetal period is associated with different biological processes depending on fetus exposure to a maternal protein/nutrient restriction or an overnutrition/high-fat maternal environment.

Moreover, we discuss whether fetal metabolic programming is controlled by metabolically active target tissues, such as the liver, or on the contrary, is modulated by central neural pathways involved in appetite and energy balance regulation, such as the hypothalamus. In addition, we introduce the concept of "fetal mitochondrial programming" of adult chronic diseases.

Finally, we show new data about the role of chromatin remodeling and illustrate areas of future research that remain poorly explored, such as the role or microRNAs (miRNA) in the regulation of fetal metabolic programming.

17.2 A BRIEF INTRODUCTION TO EPIGENETIC MODIFICATIONS

The notion of epigenetics is important in understanding the pathogenesis of IR and is supported not only by biological plausibility as it refers to changes in the DNA that are potentially modifiable by the environment, nutritional status, and any intervention, but also because epigenetic modifications regulate gene transcription and chromosome organization (Jaenisch and Bird 2003). In fact, an epigenetic factor is defined as any chromatin modification that alters the ability of a gene to be expressed independently of the DNA sequence; this issue has been reviewed elsewhere (Jaenisch and Bird 2003; Sookoian and Pirola 2012). Furthermore, epigenetic modifications are highly dynamic and are able to function in a "tissue-specific manner."

Currently, there are several well-known epigenetic changes. For example, methylation of cytosine (C) at position 5 (5-methylcytosine), usually when preceding a guanosine (G), is a very common epigenetic modification, but methylation of other nucleotides has also been observed, with *N*6-methyladenine a new and important form of DNA modification in mouse embryonic stem cells (Wu et al. 2016). About 5% of the cytosines are methylated, and almost 50–60% of genes have very rich regions called "CpG" islands but in fact, they are mostly unmethylated and located in promoters. During fetal development and in adult life, some normal somatic cells (and also cancer cells) show changes associated with DNA methylation induced by environmental stimuli. 5-hydroxymethylcytosine (5-hmC) is an epigenetic modification whose role in the pathogenesis of complex diseases remains unexplored, although 5-hmC appears to play a role in DNA demethylation and is prevalent in the mitochondrial genome. The ten-eleven translocation (TET) family of proteins is responsible for catalyzing the conversion of 5-methylcytosine to 5-hmC.

Epigenetic modifications are also posttranslational changes in histones, octameric proteins around which DNA is lining. These modifications are involved in how dense chromatin is condensed. In fact, histone methylation at specific amino acid residues, such as lysine (Lys, K), in histone N-terminal tails is an important modification defining chromatin state; methylations at H3 lysine 4 (H3K4) and lysine 36 (H3K36) appear to be signals of chromatin activation, whereas methylation of H3K9 and H3K27 seems to be related to chromatin condensation.

A brief overview of the main characteristics of epigenetic modifications is mentioned in Table 17.1; a more comprehensive review has been reported elsewhere (Turner 2002).

17.3 EPIGENETIC CHANGES AND THEIR IMPACT ON INTRAUTERINE GROWTH AND METABOLIC PROGRAMMING

A growing body of evidence supports the notion that epigenetic alterations, such as DNA methylation and histone modifications, mediate phenomena such as genomic imprinting, which may also contribute to metabolic programming (Patel and Srinivasan 2002; Sookoian et al. 2013).

Perhaps the most important consequence of metabolic programming is the transmission of the phenotype from mother to offspring and even across generations (Patel and Srinivasan 2002).

This observation has a direct impact on public health as epidemiological data indicate that impaired fetal growth is directly related to metabolic and CVDs of the adult (Barker 1995, 2001; Curhan et al. 1996; Harder et al. 2007).

The concept of fetal metabolic programming can be defined as a permanent change in the metabolism of newborns exposed to an adverse intrauterine environment, which continues to be expressed throughout their life even without the original stimulus. This premise has been well documented in rodents (Armitage et al. 2004; Patel and Srinivasan 2002) in which a dietary intervention in pregnancy with donors of methyl groups or precursors involved in the metabolism of methyl groups (diets rich in methionine, choline, vitamin B12, or folate) can alter the phenotype of the progeny by modifying the transcription of the agouti gene, whose protein inhibits

TABLE 17.1
Epigenetic Modifications: A Brief Summary

Type of Epigenetic Modification	Main Results and Impact
1. DNA methylation	
Methylation of CpG-rich regions or CpG islands	Modulates gene transcription
The regions are usually more than 500 base pairs	• Methylation of CpG islands in the
GpC content >55%	promoter region is mostly associated with
Located in the promoter regions and the end of the 5'	the silencing of gene expression
region. Types of promoters: rich and poor in CpG islands	• The CpG dinucleotide methylation
Methylated sites are distributed globally by 80% of	located in the coding sequence of the
the region's CpGs	gene is weakly associated with gene
The enzymes involved in this process are DNA	silencing
methyltransferase (DNMT) DNMT1, DNMT3a,	
DNMT3b, and DNMT2, and accessory proteins such	
as DNMT3L	
Stable in somatic cells but modifiable by	
environmental factors	
Methylation levels can show a great interindividual	
heterogeneity	
Different tissues are able to show local differences in	
DNA methylation	
2. Posttranslational modifications of histones	
Modifications:	
- Acetylation, methylation, ubiquitination,	Involved in *de novo* DNA methylation
sumoylation, and lysine residues	• Histone acetylation: associated with more
- The phosphorylation serine residues	open chromatin and transcriptional
- The methylation arginines	activation
- Frequently changes in the lysines of the N terminal	• Hypo of histones: associated with
of histones: methylation of histone H3 in Lys9	condensed chromatin structure and
(H3–K9) or Lys27 (H3–K27), which is associated	repression of gene transcription
with gene silencing and methylation or histone	
acetylation Lys4 H3 (H3–K4) or acetylation of H3 at	
Lys27 (H3–K27); associate transcriptional activation	
The enzymes involved in these processes:	HATs can be divided into several families,
- Histone acetyltransferases (HATs)	including PCAF/Gcn5, p300/CBP, MYST,
- Histone deacetylases (HDACs)	SRC, TAFII250, HAT1, and families of ATF-2
- Histone methyltransferases	• HDACs are classified into four groups
Methyl-binding domain protein MECP2	(I–IV)

Note: ATF-2, activating transcription factor 2; CBP, CREB-binding protein; HAT, histone acetyl transferase; MECP2, methyl-CpG binding domain 2; MYST, MYST/Esa1-associated factor 6; PCAF,
glycine acetyl transferase 2b; SRC, SRC-proto-oncogene, non receptor tyrosine kinase; TAF,
TATA box binding protein-associated factor.

the action of melanocyte stimulating hormone alpha (α-MSH) on its receptors MC1R
and MC4R with an effect not only on the coat color but also on the energy balance

(Wolff et al. 1998). But, few human studies have examined the interaction between an adverse effect on the environment within the uterus and epigenetic modifications as a potential mechanism for explaining the later development of MS-related diseases.

The strongest point about the influence of the prenatal environment in DNA methylation came from epigenetic studies examining people who were exposed to famine during gestation, such as the Dutch famine at the end of World War II, which affected the western part of the Netherlands in the period 1944–1945 (Heijmans et al. 2009). For example, Heijmans et al. evaluated 60 individuals subjected to this famine and showed that those who were exposed prenatally to the Dutch famine had, six decades later, less DNA methylation in the gene encoding the insulin-like growth factor type 2 (*IGF2*), compared with the unexposed population, including same-sex siblings (Heijmans et al. 2008).

In fact, Heijmans and his group showed that exposure to starvation during the periconceptional period was associated with a 5.2% lower DNA methylation in the *IGF2* promoter (Heijmans et al. 2008). *IGF2* encodes a member of a family of growth factors related to insulin, which are involved in organismal development and growth.

To further explore the relationship between prenatal caloric deficiency (as low as 500 kcal/day) and DNA methylation, Tobi and colleagues studied a series of families, exploring the state of methylation in 15 candidate genes involved in metabolic and cardiovascular diseases (Tobi et al. 2009, 2011). They found that six of these genes showed significant differences in DNA methylation after exposure to famine during the periconceptional period, such as insulin-insulin-like growth factor 2 read-through product (*INSIGF*), GNAS-antisense RNA 1 (*GNASAS*), maternally expressed 3 (*MEG3*), interleukin 10 (*IL10*), leptin (*LEP*), and ATP-binding cassette family A member 1 (ABCA1) (Tobi et al. 2009, 2011).

Similarly, children born with either low body weight (Curhan et al. 1996) (small for gestational age [SGA]) or high body weight (large for gestational age [LGA]) (Boney et al. 2005) have an increased risk of developing metabolic diseases and complications (Roseboom et al. 2001a,b).

This association between birth weight (BW) and chronic diseases also demonstrates the concept of the aforementioned metabolic programming. In fact, the epidemiological evidence on the relationship between abnormal fetal growth and adult disease has been replicated around the world (Osmond et al. 1993; Stein et al. 1996). This concept illustrates the importance of *in utero* nutrition and suggests the induction of epigenetic marks, which are able to reprogram the metabolic machinery of the offspring. A summary of these concepts is plotted in Figure 17.1.

17.4   DNA METHYLATION AND EPIGENETIC CHANGES MIGHT CONNECT BOTH EXTREMES OF ABNORMAL FETAL GROWTH (SGA AND LGA) WITH METABOLIC PROGRAMMING

We have reported that both extremes of neonatal BW are associated with decreased umbilical cord mitochondrial DNA content (Gemma et al. 2006). Hence, we examined the DNA methylation status of promoters of master genes that control both the number of copies of mitochondrial DNA—such as transcription factor A, mitochondrial (*TFAM*)—or mitochondrial function, adaptive thermogenesis, metabolism of

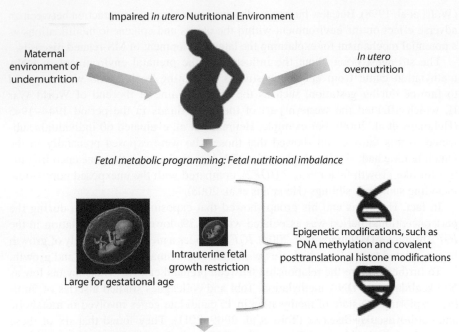

FIGURE 17.1 A summary diagram about the complex metabolic networks that modulate fetal metabolic programming. This picture summarizes the putative molecular mechanisms linking impaired nutrient availability during the fetal period with adult chronic diseases, such as metabolic and cardiovascular disorders (CVDs), including coronary heart disease, type 2 diabetes (T2D), and insulin resistance (IR). The figure illustrates the concept that fetuses adapt to an inadequate supply of nutrients (under- or overnutrition) by changing their physiology and metabolism, in particular, by modulating the metabolic transcriptional program of target tissues. Epigenetic modifications, such as DNA methylation and covalent posttranslational histone modifications, provide a molecular explanation of how these complex metabolic networks coordinately influence fetal metabolic programming.

glucose, and fat oxidation in muscle and adipose tissue, and gluconeogenesis in the liver—such as the gene called peroxisome proliferator-activated receptor gamma, coactivator 1 alpha (*PPARGC1A*) and adipogenesis and insulin signaling, such as peroxisome proliferator-activated receptor gamma (*PPARG*), in the umbilical cords of newborn babies between extremes of abnormal fetal growth, namely SGA and LGA. We also evaluated the relationship between promoter methylation status of these genes and the characteristics of mothers. Interestingly, we observed a positive correlation between methylation of one of these genes, *PPARGC1A*, and body mass index (BMI) suggesting a possible role of methylation in the metabolic programming of the fetus (Gemma et al. 2009). In addition, a novel aspect of our report is the evaluation of epigenetic marks on the DNA of the umbilical cord, which is a crucial link between the mother and fetus during pregnancy (Gemma et al. 2009). Interestingly, in a recent study, the fetal placenta shows a significant degree of partial methylated areas along the entire genome, in potentially modifiable zones strongly associated with changes in gene expression (Schroeder et al. 2013).

The evidence shows that the maternal environment alters fetal growth and also suggests the concept of "parental effect" defined as the effect on the phenotype of offspring, which is determined by the environment and the genotype inherited from parents (Youngson and Whitelaw 2008). The clearest example of this concept is the influence of maternal environment in the development of adiposity of the fetus, which shows that mothers with low BW are more likely to give birth to babies with low weight and overweight women are more likely to give birth to larger babies like our group and others have shown (Gemma et al. 2006; Knight et al. 2005). In our case, we note that pregestational BMI of the mother is associated with the weight of their children; babies of low BW had thin mothers (BMI: 21.4 ± 0.7) and LGA babies had mothers who were overweight (BMI: 26.7 ± 1.4) compared with babies with adequate weight for gestational age (BMI: 23.0 ± 0.7, $p < .003$). Moreover, the weight of newborns can be predicted from the weight of older brothers (Gemma et al. 2009).

At this point, it should be noted that these alterations of mitochondrial DNA and its association with promoter methylation of *PPARGC1A* could be replicated in adolescents and adults with MS (Gemma et al. 2010; Gianotti et al. 2008; Sookoian et al. 2010).

17.5   INTRAUTERINE ENVIRONMENT AND FETAL PROGRAMMING: NUTRITION VS. MALNUTRITION— DO THEY SHARE THE SAME BIOLOGICAL PATHWAYS?

The first epidemiological studies show that fetal malnutrition during pregnancy was associated with increased mortality due to ischemic heart disease in adulthood and increased risk of diseases grouped in the MS (Forsen et al. 1999). Interestingly, a meta-analysis that included 14 studies and a total of 132,180 people showed that low BW (<2500 g) and high BW (>4000 g) were associated with an increased risk of T2D in Harder et al. (2007). However, whether a maternal–fetal programming environment in obesity involves the same mechanisms that maternal malnutrition is unknown.

Therefore, we asked whether biological processes and pathways of disease in these two fetal opposite environments are similar or, conversely, if they differ significantly. To answer this question, we use bioinformatic tools such as the web resource ToppGene Suite (http://toppgene.cchmc.org, Cincinnati, OH). Interestingly, the analysis showed that the regions of the genome associated with intrauterine growth restriction were integrated into several functional pathways and biological processes that differ significantly from those reported for fetal growth in an environment of high maternal fat diet (Sookoian et al. 2013).

For example, biological processes associated with intrauterine growth restriction are mainly enriched by mechanisms of gene transcription and regulation of chromatin and DNA structure (Sookoian et al. 2013). Conversely, if the prediction of biological processes related to a maternal obesogenic environment during pregnancy is mainly associated with cellular control mechanisms of glucose, lipid, and lipoprotein metabolism and hormonal activity (Sookoian et al. 2013).

This analysis also showed a fundamental role of the liver in the metabolic fetal programming, which could explain the strong association between the severity of

NAFLD and atherosclerosis as recently demonstrated (Sookoian et al. 2010, 2012; Sookoian and Pirola 2008, 2011).

In conclusion, it appears that intrauterine growth restriction is most likely associated with the induction of persistent changes in tissue structure and function primarily regulated by growth factors. By contrast, an obesogenic maternal environment seems to be associated with metabolic reprogramming of glucose and lipid metabolism (Sookoian et al. 2013).

17.6 FETAL PROGRAMMING OF METABOLICALLY ACTIVE TISSUES: COMMON MOLECULAR PATHWAYS OR SPECIFIC TISSUE METABOLIC IMPRINTING

The thrifty phenotype hypothesis proposed that fetal adaptations to poor *in utero* nutrition lead to permanent changes in metabolism of insulin and glucose (Hales and Barker 2001).

Therefore, it is reasonable to then speculate that metabolically active tissues, such as the liver, are key participants in fetal metabolic programming (Burgueno et al. 2010, 2013a,b; Camm et al. 2011; George et al. 2012). Conversely, it is also postulated that fetal metabolic programming is regulated centrally in the hypothalamus by proopiomelanocortin (POMC) and neuropeptide Y (NPY) genes, which are themselves regulated by leptin (LEP), thereby controlling the energy balance and appetite (Begum et al. 2012; Chen et al. 2008).

To explore how strong the evidence is for each theory, we used modern bioinformatics tools, such as systems biology and text mining tools (Barbosa-Silva et al. 2011) to provide an answer to the question of whether metabolic reprogramming is centrally regulated or on the contrary, imprinted in peripheral tissues (Sookoian et al. 2013). We observed that "liver metabolic programming" involves large networks of genes and proteins that are not necessarily limited to insulin-related pathways. Evidence from human studies showed in fact that hypoxia-inducible factor 1 (HIF1α and HIF1β, alias aryl hydrocarbon receptor nuclear translocator [ARNT]), nuclear receptors (NR1H2, alias liver X receptor), and signal transducer and activator of transcription (STAT) are critical determinants of genetic susceptibility to NAFLD, MS-related phenotypes, and regulation of the hepatic mitochondrial function (Burgueno et al. 2012; Carabelli et al. 2011; Sookoian et al. 2008). Furthermore, SERPINE1 (inhibitor of plasminogen activator or PAI-1), involved in CVD risk and the MS (Rosselli et al. 2009; Sookoian and Pirola 2011) also integrates the predicted nodes.

Supporting the biologically plausibility of the above-mentioned observations, our group showed that high-fat diet during pregnancy is associated with an altered *PPARGC1A* gene expression pattern in the liver and that predisposes offspring to develop IR- and MS-related phenotypes in later life. Interestingly, these changes differ in offspring of different sex, affecting more males than females. Then, sexual dimorphism in metabolic reprogramming (Burgueno et al. 2010, 2013a) might also explain differences in prevalence and incidence of MS in adult populations around the world and so it deserves to be further explored.

At the same time, we have shown that "metabolic liver imprinting" may be associated with the number of copies of mitochondrial DNA (Burgueno et al. 2010, 2013a).

At this point, it is worth mentioning that mitochondria are unique cell organelles containing their own DNA that self-replicate and encode for some essential genes of the respiratory chain (oxidative phosphorylation chain [OXPHOS]). However, mitochondria do not possess DNA repair capacity or coating of DNA by histones, hence rendering mitochondrial DNA vulnerable to mutagenic stimuli. Then, the concept of "mitochondrial programming" despite unexplored is remarkable as there is proved evidence from human studies that epigenetic mechanisms operate on mitochondrial function and critically modulate IR and MS-related phenotypes by altering not only the nuclear but also the mitochondrial genome (Pirola et al. 2013; Sookoian et al. 2010). Indeed, the new concept of "mitocondrial epigenetics" is emerging. Unfortunately, there is no evidence that epigenetic marks on mitochondrial DNA play a role in fetal reprogramming.

By using a text mining tool (Barbosa-Silva et al. 2011) and using the keywords "fetal programming or BW or SGA or LGA and hypothalamus," we discovered more than 130 studies and recovered 228 co-occurrences (Sookoian et al. 2013). The analysis of the interaction between the terms showed four central axes centered on POMC, leptin, insulin receptor substrate 1 (IRS1), possibly involved in the ontogeny of pituitary gonadotrophin (PROP1), and SLC7A5 (a transporter involved in cellular uptake of amino acids, particularly arginine, and also the precursor of nitric oxide [NO], a powerful vasodilator with multiple cardiovascular and metabolic functions). Two notable results were also found in the search for liver programming that are noteworthy. One of them was related to the gene CLOCK, a master regulator of the circadian function, which was associated with MS in humans (Sookoian et al. 2007, 2008). The second closely related to the SLC7A5 node, the thyrotropin-releasing hormone (TRH) gene that our group has previously associated with essential hypertension, obesity-associated hypertension, and weight control in humans and rodents, respectively (Burgueno et al. 2007; Garcia et al. 1997, 2002; Landa et al. 2007, 2008).

Interestingly, Torrens et al. (2008) described that hypertension induced in rat offspring by maternal protein restriction can be transferred to the next generation. Recently, Jia et al. (2015) reported that a pharmacological intervention with valproic acid (or valproate, VPA), which inhibits histone deacetylases (HDACs), could impart transgenerational effects by altering DNA and histone methylation. Taking into account that VPA can modulate gene expression through epigenetic alterations, we studied the role of VPA in the regulation of the diencephalic pre-TRH (dTRH) gene expression and its effect on the pathogenesis of hypertension. We treated 7-week-old male spontaneously hypertensive rats (SHRs) and their normotensive controls, Wistar–Kyoto (WKY) rats with VPA (700 mg/kg body weight/day), and vehicle during 10 weeks; blood pressure (BP) was recorded weekly. As expected, BP and dTRH expression were increased in vehicle-treated SHR vs. WKY and VPA attenuated these differences without any effect on the WKY strain. As hypothesized, changes in BP were paired with alterations in the dTRH messenger RNA (mRNA) expression and DNA methylation of dTRH promoter. Indeed, we found a significant 62% reduction in the abundance of dTRH-mRNA of the VPA-treated SHR group compared with the control SHR group. The decreasing effect of HDAC inhibition on TRH-mRNA abundance was confirmed *in vitro* by primary neuron culture using trichostatin A. Another group of male and female SHR and WKY was treated with VPA as mentioned. After 2 weeks of the treatment interruption, rats were mated. Even when offspring born from VPA-treated parents did not receive VPA ever, we observed that changes in BP, dTRH expression, and methylation status of the dTRH promoter in offspring were similar to those observed in VPA-treated adults, reinforcing the concept of a transgenerational inheritance. Thus, these results suggest that TRH modulation by epigenetic mechanisms may affect BP and could be inherited by the next generation in SHR (personal communication). Our findings open the intriguing possibility of a putative therapeutic intervention before the generation at high risk are born.

Unfortunately, there is scarce information about the role of histone modifications and changes in fetal chromatin structure and human metabolic programming. Therefore, we have started to explore patterns of histone methylation across the promoter of *PPARGC1A* (from −320 to −700 bp from the transcription start site) and *TFAM* (from −512 to −930 bp from the transcription start site) in newborns exposed to different prenatal environments. For that end, DNA from chromatin with and without enrichment in specific histone modifications by chromatin inmmunoprecipitation (CHIP) from the cell nuclei of umbilical cord was extracted. We evaluated 50 newborns, including 16 with appropriate weight for gestational age and 34 representing both extremes of abnormal fetal growth: SGA ($n = 17$) and LGA ($n = 17$). We used antibodies specific for modified H3, such as H3K4Me3 and H3K9Me3 (Active Motif, Carlsbad, CA). Specific gene abundance was evaluated by real-time quantitative PCR (qPCR). Interestingly, we observed that H3K4Me3-related *TFAM* promoter levels, which represent a 10% of input DNA, are associated with BW (Wilks: 0.60, $p < .014$) independently of mothers BMI and fetal homocysteine levels despite the fact that H3K4Me3-related *TFAM* promoter levels correlated with fetal homocysteine levels (Pearson R: 0.31, $p < .03$) (Sookoian et al. 2013). It is worth noting that homocysteine is a modifiable CVD risk factor. Interestingly, plasma homocysteine of the neonate, although positively correlated with mother plasma homocysteine (Spearman R: 0.51, $p < .001$), was 50% higher in neonates than in mothers ($p < .001$) and was inversely correlated with neonate plasma folic acid (Spearman R: −0.35, $p < .002$), indicating that the methyl group metabolism is central to the fetus and can be regulated by folate supplementation. This phenomenon seems to also affect chromatin around circadian rhythm genes because H3K9Me3-related *CLOCK* promoter negatively correlated with newborn folic acid levels (Spearman R: -0.35, $p < .037$). The process of histone methylation in K seems to be general because this affects most of the circadian rhythm genes simultaneously. For instance, H3K4Me3 around period circadian clock 1 (PER1), CLOCK, and aryl hydrocarbon receptor nuclear translocator-like protein 1 (BMAL) promoters are highly correlated (R: 0.7, $p < .0000005$ and R: 0.7, $p < .00002$, respectively). Finally, this process seems to be modulated by the homozygosity for the more replicated obesity-associated risk allele of the fat mass and obesity associated (FTO), the rs9930506 A, as we reported for the PPARGC1A (PGC1A) promoter (Gemma et al. 2009).

17.7 TELOMERE LENGTH AND FETAL PROGRAMMING

It has been recently suggested that telomere length (TL) may, at least in part, underlie the fetal origin of the susceptibility for complex, common adverse health disorders in adult life (Barnes and Ozanne 2011; Demerath et al. 2004).

Telomeres consist of DNA repeat sequences and associated proteins that cap the end of eukaryotic chromosomes and maintain chromosomal stability. In telomerase-negative cells, telomeres shorten at each cell division and when telomeres are shortened beyond a critical length, cells are triggered into replicative senescence, resulting in cell cycle arrest and phenotypic and functional alterations (Demerath et al. 2004; von 2002). Telomere shortening at cell division is also highly dependent on oxidative DNA damage (von 2002).

TL is a function of the initial (newborn) setting and the subsequent attrition rate over time (Aviv 2012). Despite the fact that variation in TL among individuals is to a large extent genetically determined, heritability accounts for only a small proportion of the variance in TL throughout lifespan (Aviv 2012; Prescott et al. 2011), thereby highlighting the potential importance of the intrauterine environment in the establishment of TL at birth (Entringer et al. 2012). TL differs widely at birth between babies and variation among newborns is as wide as variation in TL among adults, suggesting that variation in TL among adults is in large part attributed to determinants (genetic and environmental) that start exerting their effect *in utero* (Okuda et al. 2002). Many, but not all, studies have found an association between exposure to suboptimal or adverse conditions in intrauterine life and subsequent shorter offspring TL (Entringer et al. 2012).

Low BW seems not to be associated with shorter leukocyte TL at birth (Akkad et al. 2006; Friedrich et al. 2001; Tellechea et al. 2015) or in adulthood (de Rooij et al. 2015; Kajantie et al. 2012). Nonetheless, rural Bangladeshi children who were born with low BW had shorter leukocyte TL than children who had a normal BW (Raqib et al. 2007), but a paradoxical finding of longer telomeres in men born after intrauterine growth retardation (IUGR) was also reported (Laganovic et al. 2014). Interestingly, LGA babies have shorter leukocyte telomeres in comparison with small babies (Tellechea et al. 2015).

Telomeres in the placenta are found to be shorter in pregnancies complicated with IUGR and importantly the expression/activity of telomerase is lower in the IUGR placentas (Biron-Shental et al. 2010; Davy et al. 2009). Because shortened telomeres are associated with cellular senescence, these observations may suggest that antenatal shortening would have significant effects on health and disease susceptibility later in life, although the design of this studies prevents against any further speculation about adult health outcomes of the babies. Follow-up may validate telomere dynamics as indicators of future health risk. Young adults who presented perinatal complications at birth exhibited shorter leukocyte TL (Shalev et al. 2014).

Evidence from animal studies linking intrauterine adversity with subsequent shorter telomeres provides further biological plausibility for this relationship. Protein restriction during pregnancy followed by postnatal catch-up growth has produced a shortening of TL in pancreatic islets, kidneys, and aorta in rats (Fyhrquist et al. 2013; Tarry-Adkins et al. 2008, 2009), and experimentally induced fetal growth restriction in rodents has shown to produce telomere attrition in the kidneys (Jennings et al. 1999).

Surprisingly, leukocyte TL and the percentage of short telomeres at age 68 years did not differ between those exposed to famine during early gestation and those unexposed during gestation (de Rooij et al. 2015). On the other hand, a recent study has linked maternal nutritional status in pregnancy with subsequent TL in the newborn. Maternal total folate concentration in early pregnancy was associated with cord blood TL (Entringer et al. 2015).

A number of studies looked at the effects of hypertension during pregnancy or preeclampsia on fetal, placental, and newborn TL. Biron-Shental et al. have provided evidence that TL is shorter in preeclampsia and preeclampsia plus IUGR placentae (Biron-Shental et al. 2010). Likewise, leukocyte TL at birth is associated not only with arterial BP of mothers during pregnancy but also with the history of arterial hypertension in previous pregnancies (Tellechea et al. 2015). However, a study has reported no shorter TL in fetuses of mothers complicated with preeclampsia or gestational hypertension (Xu et al. 2014).

TL was found to be shortened in fetuses of women with gestational diabetes compared with fetuses of normal pregnant women (Xu et al. 2014). Furthermore, the activity of telomerase was higher in cord blood mononuclear cells of type 1 diabetes and gestational diabetes pregnancies, although with no differences in cord blood TL (Cross et al. 2010). Combined, these observations provide some evidence for a role of a senescent phenotype characterized by telomere shortening in diabetic pregnancies; however, young adult offspring of women with pregestational type 1 diabetes were indistinguishable from controls without this maternal history in terms of TL abnormalities (Cross et al. 2009).

Maternal stress seems to be a critical factor in the modulation of TL. The offspring of mothers who experienced maternal psychosocial stress have shorter cord blood telomeres than the offspring of mothers who experienced lower levels of stress during gestation (Entringer et al. 2013; Marchetto et al. 2016). Remarkably, maternal psychosocial stress exposure during pregnancy is also associated with shorter leukocyte TL in offspring in adult life (Entringer et al. 2011). Besides, it is established that stressful life events occur more frequently in individuals of lower socioeconomic status (SES), and the association between SES and leukocyte TL has also been addressed (Kajantie et al. 2012; de Rooij et al. 2015).

Additionally, shortened umbilical cord TL at birth (Salihu et al. 2015) and shortened salivary TL in children (Theall et al. 2013) were found when assessing the relationship between exposure to prenatal tobacco and postnatal TL.

To summarize, shortened telomeres or reduced telomerase production, or both, have been linked to several aging-associated diseases, including, but not limited to, CVD, hypertension, atherosclerosis, heart failure, and T2D. Some findings support the so-called telomere hypothesis of CVD implying that shorter telomeres are a primary, heritable abnormality causally leading to an increased risk of CVD (Brouilette et al. 2008; Fyhrquist et al. 2013). To some extent, these findings are confirmed in other cohorts (Dei et al. 2013; Salpea et al. 2008; Willeit et al. 2010; Wong et al. 2011). Nevertheless, data from the Asklepios Study do not support that subjects with a family history of CVD had shorter telomeres, although it should be noted that the family history of CVD in this study was only self-reported (De et al. 2012). Additional carefully designed studies are required to determine whether TL is causally involved in the development of CVD, and if so, what the underlying mechanism is.

The question remains as to whether suboptimal or adverse conditions during intrauterine development can produce variations in TL, thereby potentially setting up a long-term trajectory at birth that defines or contributes to individual susceptibility to disease in adulthood. There is a need for well-designed, large, prospective, and longitudinal human studies to unveil the mechanisms underlying prenatal programming of TL.

17.8 NONCODING RNAs AS NOVEL REGULATORS OF GENE EXPRESSION: miRNAs AS INDUCERS OF EPIGENETIC MARKS

Finally, unexplored mechanisms of gene expression regulation, such as miRNAs, small noncoding RNAs involved in transcriptional and posttranscriptional gene regulation, represent attractive candidates in the modulation of fetal programming. miRNAs exert their biologic functions after binding (in a sequence-specific manner) to the 3′-untranslated region (UTR) of mRNA targets, facilitating mRNA degradation or translational inhibition, although a few exceptions have been reported about the putative binding of miRNAs to 5′UTR with the upregulation of gene expression (Pirola et al. 2015a).

There are isolated but interesting reports about programmed changes in miRNA expression linking early-life nutrition to adult disease. Among the few, Ferland-McCollough showed that miRNA-483-3p is upregulated in adipose tissue in low birth weight adult humans and prediabetic adult rats exposed to suboptimal nutrition in early life (Ferland-McCollough et al. 2012). Another human study showed that the expression of miRNA-16 and miRNA-21 were markedly reduced in SGA infants (Maccani et al. 2011). In addition, an experimental study observed that maternal obesity was associated with fetal muscle miRNA let-7g expression, thereby influencing intramuscular adipogenesis (Yan et al. 2013).

Therefore, we performed a gene network analysis using the web server application Topplcluster (http://toppcluster.cchmc.org/) for the comparative enrichment of the candidate gene list shown in Supplementary Table 17.1 of the reference (Sookoian et al. 2013) and miRNAs prediction. Interestingly, among them the miRNA34a shows a novel regulator of Smad4/transforming growth factor beta (TGFβ) signaling (Genovese et al. 2012) associated with the transcriptional regulation of the nicotinamide adenine dinucleotide (NAD)-dependent deacetylase or SIRTUIN 1 (Yamakuchi 2012), which regulates stress response pathways and metabolism.

Interestingly, a search by text mining (Barbosa-Silva et al. 2011) with the terms "miRNAs AND fetal programming" rendered a series of loci with a great similarity to those already mentioned including metabolic (insulin [INS], insulin receptor [INSR], AKT serine/threonine kinase 1 [AKT1]-2), apoptotic BCL2-associated X (BAX), and IGF1-2 nodes, ranking among the top, DNA methyltransferase (DNMT) and RNASEN, also known as DROSHA, an important RNAse III involved in the full length nuclear precursor of microRNAs (primiRNA) maturation (Jinek and Doudna 2009) (Figure 17.2).

17.9 CONCLUSIONS AND PROSPECTS

We have reviewed the epigenetic mechanisms by which covalent modifications of DNA and histones may participate in fetal metabolic programming, thus playing a crucial role in the pathogenesis of chronic adult diseases. 5-hmC and the TET family of proteins responsible for catalyzing the conversion of 5-methylcytosine to 5-hmC have emerged as a new epigenetic factor. We have recently demonstrated that epigenetic editing by 5-hmC, which appears to be prevalent in the mitochondrial genome,

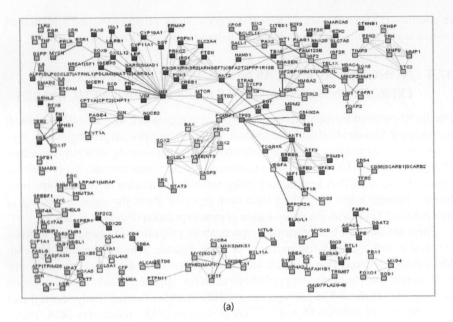

(a)

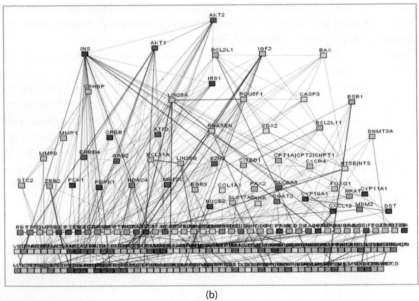

(b)

FIGURE 17.2 Graphic illustrations of gene/protein co-occurrence and their relatedness to biological concepts with the search query "fetal programming AND miRNA." Prediction was performed by PESCADOR (available at http://cbdm.mdc-berlin.de/tools/pescador/), a web-based tool to assist large-scale integration text mining of biointeractions extracted from MEDLINE abstracts (Barbosa-Silva et al. 2011). The graphs (panel a, network of genes with similar functions; panel b, hierarchical-ordered nodes) were constructed using the free available program MEDUSA, which is a Java application for visualizing and manipulating graphs of interaction (www.bork.embl.de/medusa). (From Hooper and Bork 2005.)

and the genetic variation in TET genes might be novel mechanisms through which NAFLD-associated molecular traits could be explained (Pirola et al. 2015b).

It is important to emphasize that epigenetic marks are potentially reversible by environmental factors and modifiable by medical intervention. This aspect is relevant when intervening on maternal health care periconceptionally and during pregnancy. A clear example is the recommendation to increase folic acid intake during pregnancy; by a mechanism not completely elucidated, it is effective in preventing neural tube defects in newborns. Other interventions tested in rodents with supplements of other vitamins and minerals such as Zn and others (Wolff et al. 1998) should be investigated more deeply in humans to prove their beneficial effects and lack of adverse effects. The last aspect to be considered is whether the investigations must be directed at the entire genome or candidate genes. The cost effectiveness suggests that they would be better directed to certain genes already associated with fetal reprogramming as was mentioned and that were recently analyzed more thoroughly (Sookoian et al. 2013). A similar approach using systems biology could be applied to specific pregnancy complications such as gestational diabetes or preeclampsia.

ACKNOWLEDGMENTS

This study was partially supported by grants PICT 2010-0441, PICT2014-1816, and PICT2014-0442 (Agencia Nacional de Promoción Científica y Tecnológica).

REFERENCES

Akkad, A., Hastings, R., Konje, J. C. et al. Telomere length in small-for-gestational-age babies, *BJOG*. 113, no. 3 (2006): 318–23.

Armitage, J. A., Khan, I. Y., Taylor, P. D., Nathanielsz, P. W., and Poston, L. Developmental programming of the metabolic syndrome by maternal nutritional imbalance: How strong is the evidence from experimental models in mammals? *J Physiol*. 561, Pt 2 (2004): 355–77.

Aviv, A. Genetics of leukocyte telomere length and its role in atherosclerosis, *Mutat Res*. 730, no. 1–2 (2012): 68–74.

Barbosa-Silva, A., Fontaine, J. F., Donnard, E. R. et al. PESCADOR, a web-based tool to assist text-mining of biointeractions extracted from PubMed queries, *BMC Bioinformatics*. 12, (2011): 435.

Barker, D. J. Intrauterine programming of adult disease, *Mol Med Today*. 1, no. 9 (1995): 418–23.

Barker, D. J. A new model for the origins of chronic disease, *Med Health Care Philos*. 4, no. 1 (2001): 31–5.

Barnes, S. K. and Ozanne, S. E. Pathways linking the early environment to long-term health and lifespan, *Prog Biophys Mol Biol*. 106, no. 1 (2011): 323–36.

Begum, G., Stevens, A., Smith, E. B. et al. Epigenetic changes in fetal hypothalamic energy regulating pathways are associated with maternal undernutrition and twinning, *FASEB J*. 26, no. 4 (2012): 1694–703.

Biron-Shental, T., Sukenik, Halevy R., Goldberg-Bittman, L. et al. Telomeres are shorter in placental trophoblasts of pregnancies complicated with intrauterine growth restriction (IUGR), *Early Hum Dev*. 86, no. 7 (2010): 451–6.

Boney, C. M., Verma, A., Tucker, R., and Vohr, B. R. Metabolic syndrome in childhood: Association with birth weight, maternal obesity, and gestational diabetes mellitus, *Pediatrics*. 115, no. 3 (2005): e290–e96.

Brouilette, S. W., Whittaker, A., Stevens, S. E. et al. Telomere length is shorter in healthy offspring of subjects with coronary artery disease: Support for the telomere hypothesis, *Heart.* 94, no. 4 (2008): 422–5.

Burgueno, A. L., Cabrerizo, R., Gonzales, M. N., Sookoian, S., and Pirola, C. J. Maternal high-fat intake during pregnancy programs metabolic-syndrome-related phenotypes through liver mitochondrial DNA copy number and transcriptional activity of liver PPARGC1A, *J Nutr Biochem.* 24 (2013a): 6–13.

Burgueno, A. L., Carabelli, J., Sookoian, S., and Pirola, C. J. The impact of maternal high-fat feeding on liver and abdominal fat accumulation in adult offspring under a long-term high-fat diet, *Hepatology.* 51, no. 6 (2010): 2234–5.

Burgueno, A. L., Fernandez, Gianotti T., Gonzales, Mansilla N., Pirola, C. J., and Sookoian, S. Cardiovascular disease is associated with high fat diet-induced liver damage and upregulation of hepatic expression of hypoxia-inducible factor 1 alpha in a rat model, *Clin Sci.* 124, no 1 (2013b): 53–63.

Burgueno, A. L., Landa, M. S., Schuman, M. L. et al. Association between diencephalic thyroliberin and arterial blood pressure in agouti-yellow and Ob/Ob mice may be mediated by leptin, *Metabolism.* 56, no. 10 (2007): 1439–43.

Camm, E. J., Martin-Gronert, M. S., Wright, N. L. et al. Prenatal hypoxia independent of undernutrition promotes molecular markers of insulin resistance in adult offspring, *FASEB J.* 25, no. 1 (2011): 420–7.

Carabelli, J., Burgueno, A. L., Rosselli, M. S. et al. High fat diet-induced liver steatosis promotes an increase in liver mitochondrial biogenesis in response to hypoxia, *J Cell Mol Med.* 15, no. 6 (2011): 1329–38.

Chen, H., Simar, D., Lambert, K., Mercier, J., and Morris, M. J. Maternal and postnatal overnutrition differentially impact appetite regulators and fuel metabolism, *Endocrinology.* 149, no. 11 (2008): 5348–56.

Cross, J. A., Brennan, C., Gray, T. et al. Absence of telomere shortening and oxidative DNA damage in the young adult offspring of women with pre-gestational type 1 diabetes, *Diabetologia.* 52, no. 2 (2009): 226–34.

Cross, J. A., Temple, R. C., Hughes, J. C. et al. Cord blood telomere length, telomerase activity and inflammatory markers in pregnancies in women with diabetes or gestational diabetes, *Diabet Med.* 27, no. 11 (2010): 1264–70.

Curhan, G. C., Willett, W. C., Rimm, E. B. et al. Birth weight and adult hypertension, diabetes mellitus, and obesity in US men, *Circulation.* 94, no. 12 (1996): 3246–50.

Davy, P., Nagata, M., Bullard, P., Fogelson, N. S., and Allsopp, R. Fetal growth restriction is associated with accelerated telomere shortening and increased expression of cell senescence markers in the placenta, *Placenta.* 30, no. 6 (2009): 539–42.

de Rooij, S. R., van Pelt, A. M., Ozanne, S. E. et al. Prenatal undernutrition and leukocyte telomere length in late adulthood: The Dutch famine birth cohort study, *Am J Clin Nutr.* 102, no. 3 (2015): 655–60.

De, M. T., Van Daele, C. M., De Buyzere, M. L. et al. No shorter telomeres in subjects with a family history of cardiovascular disease in the Asklepios study, *Arterioscler Thromb Vasc Biol.* 32, no. 12 (2012): 3076–81.

Dei, C. A., Spigoni, V., Franzini, L. et al. Lower endothelial progenitor cell number, family history of cardiovascular disease and reduced HDL-cholesterol levels are associated with shorter leukocyte telomere length in healthy young adults, *Nutr Metab Cardiovasc Dis.* 23, no. 3 (2013): 272–8.

Demerath, E. W., Cameron, N., Gillman, M. W., Towne, B., and Siervogel, R. M. Telomeres and telomerase in the fetal origins of cardiovascular disease: A review, *Hum Biol.* 76, no. 1 (2004): 127–46.

Entringer, S., Buss, C., and Wadhwa, P. D. Prenatal stress, telomere biology, and fetal programming of health and disease risk, *Sci Signal.* 5, no. 248 (2012): t12.

Entringer, S., Epel, E. S., Kumsta, R. et al. Stress exposure in intrauterine life is associated with shorter telomere length in young adulthood, *Proc Natl Acad Sci USA*. 108, no. 33 (2011): E513–E8.

Entringer, S., Epel, E. S., Lin, J. et al. Maternal folate concentration in early pregnancy and newborn telomere length, *Ann Nutr Metab*. 66, no. 4 (2015): 202–8.

Entringer, S., Epel, E. S., Lin, J. et al. Maternal psychosocial stress during pregnancy is associated with newborn leukocyte telomere length, *Am J Obstet Gynecol*. 208, no. 2 (2013): 134–7.

Ferland-McCollough, D., Fernandez-Twinn, D. S., Cannell, I. G. et al. Programming of adipose tissue miR-483-3p and GDF-3 expression by maternal diet in type 2 diabetes, *Cell Death Differ*. 19, no. 6 (2012): 1003–12.

Forsen, T., Eriksson, J. G., Tuomilehto, J., Osmond, C., and Barker, D. J. Growth in utero and during childhood among women who develop coronary heart disease: Longitudinal study, *BMJ*. 319, no. 7222 (1999): 1403–7.

Friedrich, U., Schwab, M., Griese, E. U., Fritz, P., and Klotz, U. Telomeres in neonates: New insights in fetal hematopoiesis, *Pediatr Res*. 49, no. 2 (2001): 252–6.

Fyhrquist, F., Saijonmaa, O., and Strandberg, T. The roles of senescence and telomere shortening in cardiovascular disease, *Nat Rev Cardiol*. 10, no. 5 (2013): 274–83.

Garcia, S. I., Landa, M. S., Porto, P. I. et al. Thyrotropin-releasing hormone decreases leptin and mediates the leptin-induced pressor effect, *Hypertension*. 39, no. 2 Pt 2 (2002): 491–5.

Garcia, S. I., Porto, P. I., Alvarez, A. L. et al. Central overexpression of the TRH precursor gene induces hypertension in rats: Antisense reversal, *Hypertension*. 30, no. 3 Pt 2 (1997): 759–66.

Gemma, C., Sookoian, S., Alvarinas, J. et al. Mitochondrial DNA depletion in small- and large-for-gestational-age newborns, *Obesity*. 14, no. 12 (2006): 2193–9.

Gemma, C., Sookoian, S., Alvarinas, J. et al. Maternal pregestational BMI is associated with methylation of the PPARGC1A promoter in newborns, *Obesity*. 17, no. 5 (2009): 1032–9.

Gemma, C., Sookoian, S., Dieuzeide, G. et al. Methylation of TFAM gene promoter in peripheral white blood cells is associated with insulin resistance in adolescents, *Mol Genet Metab*. 100, no. 1 (2010): 83–7.

Genovese, G., Ergun, A., Shukla, S. A. et al. MicroRNA regulatory network inference identifies MiR-34a as a novel regulator of TGF beta signaling in GBM, Cancer Discov. 2, (2012): 736–49.

George, L. A., Zhang, L., Tuersunjiang, N. et al. Early maternal undernutrition programs increased feed intake, altered glucose metabolism and insulin secretion, and liver function in aged female offspring, *Am J Physiol Regul Integr Comp Physiol*. 302, no. 7 (2012): R795–R804.

Gianotti, T. F., Sookoian, S., Dieuzeide, G. et al. A decreased mitochondrial DNA content is related to insulin resistance in adolescents, *Obesity*. 16, no. 7 (2008): 1591–5.

Hales, C. N. and Barker, D. J. The thrifty phenotype hypothesis, *Br Med Bull*. 60 (2001): 5–20.

Harder, T., Rodekamp, E., Schellong, K., Dudenhausen, J. W., and Plagemann, A. Birth weight and subsequent risk of type 2 diabetes: A meta-analysis, *Am J Epidemiol*. 165, no. 8 (2007): 849–57.

Heijmans, B. T., Tobi, E. W., Lumey, L. H., and Slagboom, P. E. The epigenome: Archive of the prenatal environment, *Epigenetics*. 4, no. 8 (2009): 526–31.

Heijmans, B. T., Tobi, E. W., Stein, A. D. et al. Persistent epigenetic differences associated with prenatal exposure to famine in humans, *Proc Natl Acad Sci USA*. 105, no. 44 (2008): 17046–9.

Hooper, S. D. and Bork, P., Medusa: A simple tool for interaction graph analysis, *Bioinformatics*. 21, no. 24 (2005): 4432–3.

Jaenisch, R. and Bird, A. Epigenetic regulation of gene expression: How the genome integrates intrinsic and environmental signals, *Nat Genet*. 33 Suppl (2003): 245–54.

Jennings, B. J., Ozanne, S. E., Dorling, M. W., and Hales, C. N. Early growth determines longevity in male rats and may be related to telomere shortening in the kidney, *FEBS Lett.* 448, no. 1 (1999): 4–8.

Jia, H., Morris, C. D., Williams, R. M., Loring, J. F., and Thomas, E. A. HDAC inhibition imparts beneficial transgenerational effects in Huntington's disease mice via altered DNA and histone methylation, *Proc Natl Acad Sci USA.* 112, no. 1 (2015): E56–E64.

Jinek, M. and Doudna, J. A. A three-dimensional view of the molecular machinery of RNA interference, *Nature.* 457, no. 7228 (2009): 405–12.

Kajantie, E., Pietilainen, K. H., Wehkalampi, K. et al. No association between body size at birth and leucocyte telomere length in adult life—Evidence from three cohort studies, *Int J Epidemiol.* 41, no. 5 (2012): 1400–8.

Knight, B., Shields, B. M., Turner, M. et al. Evidence of genetic regulation of fetal longitudinal growth, *Early Hum Dev.* 81, no. 10 (2005): 823–31.

Laganovic, M., Bendix, L., Rubelj, I. et al. Reduced telomere length is not associated with early signs of vascular aging in young men born after intrauterine growth restriction: A paradox? *J Hypertens.* 32, no. 8 (2014): 1613–9.

Landa, M. S., Garcia, S. I., Schuman, M. L. et al. Knocking down the diencephalic thyrotropin-releasing hormone precursor gene normalizes obesity-induced hypertension in the rat, *Am J Physiol Endocrinol Metab.* 292, no. 5 (2007): E1388–E1394.

Landa, M. S., Garcia, S. I., Schuman, M. L. et al. Thyrotropin-releasing hormone precursor gene knocking down impedes melanocortin-induced hypertension in rats, *Hypertension.* 52, no. 2 (2008): e8.

Maccani, M. A., Padbury, J. F., and Marsit, C. J. MiR-16 and MiR-21 Expression in the placenta is associated with fetal growth, *PLoS One.* 6, no. 6 (2011): e21210.

Marchetto, N. M., Glynn, R. A., Ferry, M. L. et al. Prenatal stress and newborn telomere length, *Am J Obstet Gynecol.* 215, no. 1 (2016): 1–8.

Okuda, K., Bardeguez, A., Gardner, J. P. et al. Telomere length in the newborn, *Pediatr Res.* 52, no. 3 (2002): 377–81.

Osmond, C., Barker, D. J., Winter, P. D., Fall, C. H., and Simmonds, S. J. Early growth and death from cardiovascular disease in women, *BMJ.* 307, no. 6918 (1993): 1519–24.

Patel, M. S. and Srinivasan, M. Metabolic programming: Causes and consequences, *J Biol Chem.* 277, no. 3 (2002): 1629–32.

Pirola, C. J., Fernandez Gianotti T., Castano, G. O. et al. Circulating microRNA signature in non-alcoholic fatty liver disease: From serum non-coding RNAs to liver histology and disease pathogenesis, *Gut.* 64, no. 5 (2015a): 800–12.

Pirola, C. J., Gianotti T. F., Burgueno, A. L. et al. Epigenetic modification of liver mitochondrial DNA is associated with histological severity of nonalcoholic fatty liver disease, *Gut.* 62, no 9 (2013):1356–1363.

Pirola, C. J., Scian, R., Gianotti, T. F. et al. Epigenetic modifications in the biology of non-alcoholic fatty liver disease: The role of DNA hydroxymethylation and TET proteins, *Medicine.* 94, no. 36 (2015b): e1480.

Prescott, J., Kraft, P., Chasman, D. I. et al. Genome-wide association study of relative telomere length, *PLoS One.* 6, no. 5 (2011): e19635.

Raqib, R., Alam, D. S., Sarker, P. et al. Low birth weight is associated with altered immune function in rural Bangladeshi children: A birth cohort study, *Am J Clin Nutr.* 85, no. 3 (2007): 845–52.

Reaven, G. M. Hypothesis: Muscle insulin resistance is the ("not-so") thrifty genotype, *Diabetologia.* 41, no. 4 (1998): 482–4.

Roseboom, T. J., van der Meulen, J. H., Ravelli, A. C. et al. Effects of prenatal exposure to the Dutch famine on adult disease in later life: An overview, *Mol Cell Endocrinol.* 185, no. 1–2 (2001a): 93–8.

Roseboom, T. J., van der Meulen, J. H., van Montfrans, G. A. et al. Maternal nutrition during gestation and blood pressure in later life, *J Hypertens.* 19, no. 1 (2001b): 29–34.

Rosselli, M. S., Burgueno, A. L., Carabelli, J. et al. Losartan reduces liver expression of plasminogen activator inhibitor-1 (PAI-1) in a high fat-induced rat nonalcoholic fatty liver disease model, *Atherosclerosis.* 206, no. 1 (2009): 119–26.

Salihu, H. M., Pradhan, A., King, L. et al. Impact of intrauterine tobacco exposure on fetal telomere length, *Am J Obstet Gynecol.* 212, no. 2 (2015): 205–8.

Salpea, K. D., Nicaud, V., Tiret, L. et al. The association of telomere length with paternal history of premature myocardial infarction in the European Atherosclerosis Research Study II, *J Mol Med.* 86, no. 7 (2008): 815–24.

Schroeder, D. I., Blair, J. D., Lott, P. et al. The human placenta methylome, *Proc Natl Acad Sci USA.* 110, no. 15 (2013): 6037–42.

Shalev, I., Caspi, A., Ambler, A. et al. Perinatal complications and aging indicators by midlife, *Pediatrics.* 134, no. 5 (2014): e1315–e1323.

Sookoian, S., Castano, G., Gemma, C. et al. Common genetic variations in CLOCK transcription factor are associated with nonalcoholic fatty liver disease, *World J Gastroenterol.* 13, no. 31 (2007): 4242–8.

Sookoian, S., Castano, G., Gianotti, T. F. et al. Genetic variants in STAT3 are associated with nonalcoholic fatty liver disease, *Cytokine.* 44, no. 1 (2008): 201–6.

Sookoian, S., Castano, G. O., Burgueno, A. L. et al. Circulating levels and hepatic expression of molecular mediators of atherosclerosis in nonalcoholic fatty liver disease, *Atherosclerosis.* 209, no. 2 (2010): 585–91.

Sookoian, S., Castano, G. O., and Pirola, C. J. Cardiovascular phenotype of nonalcoholic fatty liver disease: Hanging the paradigm about the role of distant toxic fat accumulation on vascular disease, *Hepatology.* 56, no. 3 (2012): 1185–6.

Sookoian, S., Gemma, C., Gianotti, T. F. et al. Genetic variants of clock transcription factor are associated with individual susceptibility to obesity, *Am J Clin Nutr.* 87, no. 6 (2008): 1606–15.

Sookoian, S., Gianotti, T. F., Burgueno, A. L. et al. Fetal metabolic programming and epigenetic modifications: A systems biology approach, *Pediatr Res.* 73, no. 4–2 (2013): 531–42.

Sookoian, S. and Pirola, C. J. Genetics of the cardiometabolic syndrome: New insights and therapeutic implications, *Ther Adv Cardiovasc Dis.* 1, no. 1 (2007): 37–47.

Sookoian, S. and Pirola, C. J. Non-alcoholic fatty liver disease is strongly associated with carotid atherosclerosis: A systematic review, *J Hepatol.* 49, no. 4 (2008): 600–7.

Sookoian, S. and Pirola, C. J. Metabolic syndrome: From the genetics to the pathophysiology, *Curr Hypertens Rep.* 13, no. 2 (2011): 149–57.

Sookoian, S. and Pirola, C. J. Targeting the renin-Angiotensin system: Potential beneficial effects of the angiotensin II receptor blockers in patients with nonalcoholic steatohepatitis, *Hepatology.* 54, no. 6 (2011): 2276–7.

Sookoian, S. and Pirola, C. J. DNA methylation and hepatic insulin resistance and steatosis, *Curr Opin Clin Nutr Metab Care* 15, no. 4 (2012): 350–6.

Sookoian, S., Rosselli, M. S., Gemma, C. et al. Epigenetic regulation of insulin resistance in nonalcoholic fatty liver disease: Impact of liver methylation of the peroxisome proliferator-activated receptor gamma coactivator 1alpha promoter, *Hepatology.* 52, no. 6 (2010): 1992–2000.

Stein, C. E., Fall, C. H., Kumaran, K. et al. Fetal growth and coronary heart disease in South India, *Lancet.* 348, no. 9037 (1996): 1269–73.

Tarry-Adkins, J. L., Chen, J. H., Smith, N. S. et al. Poor maternal nutrition followed by accelerated postnatal growth leads to telomere shortening and increased markers of cell senescence in rat islets, *FASEB J.* 23, no. 5 (2009): 1521–8.

Tarry-Adkins, J. L., Martin-Gronert, M. S., Chen, J. H. et al. Maternal diet influences DNA damage, aortic telomere length, oxidative stress, and antioxidant defense capacity in rats, *FASEB J.* 22, no. 6 (2008): 2037–44.

Tellechea, M., Gianotti, T. F., Alvarinas, J. et al. Telomere length in the two extremes of abnormal fetal growth and the programming effect of maternal arterial hypertension, *Sci Rep.* 5 (2015): 7869.

Theall, K. P., McKasson, S., Mabile, E. et al. Early hits and long-term consequences: Tracking the lasting impact of prenatal smoke exposure on telomere length in children, *Am J Public Health* 103 Suppl 1 (2013): S133–S135.

Tobi, E. W., Heijmans, B. T., Kremer, D. et al. DNA methylation of IGF2, GNASAS, INSIGF and LEP and being born small for gestational age, *Epigenetics.* 6, no. 2 (2011): 171–6.

Tobi, E. W., Lumey, L. H., Talens, R. P. et al. DNA methylation differences after exposure to prenatal famine are common and timing- and sex-specific, *Hum Mol Genet.* 18, no. 21 (2009): 4046–53.

Torrens, C., Poston, L., and Hanson, M. A. Transmission of raised blood pressure and endothelial dysfunction to the F2 generation induced by maternal protein restriction in the F0, in the absence of dietary challenge in the F1 generation, *Br J Nutr.* 100, no. 4 (2008): 760–6.

Turner, B. M. Cellular memory and the histone code, *Cell.* 111, no. 3 (2002): 285–91.

von, Zglinicki T. Oxidative stress shortens telomeres, *Trends Biochem Sci.* 27, no. 7 (2002): 339–44.

Willeit, P., Willeit, J., Brandstatter, A. et al. Cellular aging reflected by leukocyte telomere length predicts advanced atherosclerosis and cardiovascular disease risk, *Arterioscler Thromb Vasc Biol.* 30, no. 8 (2010): 1649–56.

Wolff, G. L., Kodell, R. L., Moore, S. R. et al. Maternal epigenetics and methyl supplements affect agouti gene expression in Avy/a mice, *FASEB J.* 12, no. 11 (1998): 949–57.

Wong, L. S., Huzen, J., de Boer, R. A. et al. Telomere length of circulating leukocyte subpopulations and buccal cells in patients with ischemic heart failure and their offspring, *PLoS One.* 6, no. 8 (2011): e23118.

Wu, T. P., Wang, T., Seetin, M. G. et al. DNA methylation on N-adenine in mammalian embryonic stem cells, *Nature.* 532, no. 7599 (2016): 329–333.

Xu, J., Ye, J., Wu, Y. et al. Reduced fetal telomere length in gestational diabetes, *PLoS One.* 9, no. 1 (2014): e86161.

Yamakuchi, M. MicroRNA regulation of SIRT1, *Front Physiol.* 3 (2012): 68.

Yan, X., Huang, Y., Zhao, J. X. et al. Maternal obesity downregulates microRNA let-7g expression, a possible mechanism for enhanced adipogenesis during ovine fetal skeletal muscle development, *Int J Obes.* 37, no. 4 (2013): 568–575.

Youngson, N. A. and Whitelaw, E. Transgenerational epigenetic effects, *Annu Rev Genomics Hum Genet.* 9 (2008): 233–57.

18 Paternal Programming and Multigenerational Transmission

Josep C. Jimenez-Chillaron

CONTENTS

Riddle: A man is looking at a photograph of someone. His friend asks who it is. The man replies, "Brothers and sisters, I have none. But that man's father is my father's son." Who is in the photograph?*

---

*Answer: The man's son.
Source: https://www.brainbashers.com/showanswer.asp?ref=ZAUI

18.1 INTRODUCTION

18.1.1 ÖVERKALIX

Överkalix is a remote small municipality located in northeastern Sweden, near the Finnish border. It is now a pleasant beautiful village in which the economy is based on tourism and small businesses. However, in the 19th century, agriculture was the main economic activity and life was much harder than nowadays. The reason is that Överkalix is just below the Arctic Circle and it experiences abrupt temperature differences between the warm short summers and the very long and cold winters. During the winters, the roads were closed and the village remained isolated from the rest of the country. Therefore, the population relied on stored food supplies. Due to these extreme climate conditions, the village suffered recurrent periods of poor agricultural production. Hence, during the years of food shortage, the population, was under nutritional deprivation. These periods of deprivation were followed by periods of abundance when even large families (15 members or more) had enough food to cover their necessities.

The other interesting piece of information related to Överkalix is that the parish archives from the Swedish and Finnish communities were extremely accurate and document birth dates, longevity, and causes of death over a period spanning more than a hundred years (from 1890 to present). Since the mobility of the population was relatively reduced, it is possible to track specific pedigrees covering over three generations. Thus, the so-called Överkalix cohort is a three-generation pedigree, formed by a birth cohort and two additional historical cohorts (Pembrey et al. 2006). Men and women that were born in the years 1890, 1905, and 1920 form the birth cohort. A research team linked the parish registries with the detailed historical records, which document the harvests and food supply for every year season. Hence, they could determine the nutritional status of the parental generation (F0) based on the estimate of food availability for each year (Figure 18.1). Thereafter, they matched F0 access to food during different stages of development and the health of their children and grandchildren (Bygren et al. 2001; Pembrey et al. 2006). Their results were astonishing: there was a positive association between grand-paternal food availability during childhood and mortality rate in the grand-offspring, F2 (Figure 18.1b) (Bygren et al. 2001; Kaati et al. 2002). Specifically, poor availability of food experienced by the grandfathers was associated with extended grandchild lifespan. In contrast, a surfeit of food during the same period reduced longevity in the grand-offspring. Strikingly, such grand-paternal effects were time specific: the prepubertal period, which is around 10 years of age in men, was the only one during which food availability had a significant association with grandchild life spans (Bygren et al. 2001; Bygren 2013). Moreover, these transgenerational effects appeared to be sex specific (Pembrey et al. 2006). That is, grand-paternal food supply (F0) was associated with cardiovascular and diabetic mortality rate of their grandsons (F2), when passed through their fathers (F1). Likewise, grand-maternal nutrient availability influenced the granddaughters' mortality rate.

Combined, the data from the Överkalix cohort clearly state that paternal and grand-paternal life history may have an impact on health in future generations in

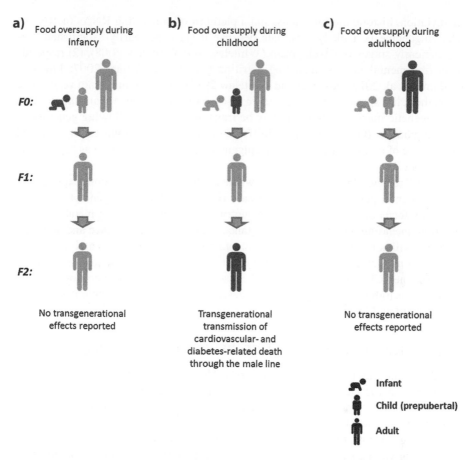

a) Food oversupply during infancy

b) Food oversupply during childhood

c) Food oversupply during adulthood

FO:

F1:

F2:

No transgenerational effects reported

Transgenerational transmission of cardiovascular- and diabetes-related death through the male line

No transgenerational effects reported

Infant

Child (prepubertal)

Adult

FIGURE 18.1 Influence of grandparental nutritional status in the next generations.

human populations. This study was among the first to provide "proof-of-principle that a male-line transgenerational response system exists in humans" (Pembrey et al. 2006). The transgenerational effects described here do not constitute an isolated discovery. Similar effects have been described in other human cohorts (for review, see Jimenez-Chillaron 2014, Roseboom and Painter 2014).

18.1.2 Nongenomic Inheritance

What are the potential mechanisms that lead to transgenerational inheritance of complex traits in response to dietary factors (or environmental cues in general)? In human cohorts, such as the Överkalix, in which many different families are involved and an environmental trigger impinges the phenotypes, the role of genetic variants is supposed to play a marginal role. Instead, it has been proposed that nongenomic mechanisms, such as epigenetic mechanisms, might convey such transgenerational inheritance of complex traits (Gluckman et al. 2007). They include DNA methylation, histone modifications, and a plethora of noncoding RNAs (ncRNAs). The epigenome is a likely candidate because it (1) is primarily established during the early stages of development (Whitelaw and Whitelaw 2008), (2) responds to environmental factors, including nutrition (Jirtle and Skinner 2007; Jiménez-Chillarón et al. 2012; Daxinger and Whitelaw 2012), and (3) can remain very stable throughout life spans. In this chapter we discuss recent evidence that supports that the epigenetic marks might eventually be transmitted to the following generations via the gametes (Gluckman et al. 2007). Consequently, environmentally induced inheritance of complex traits through epigenetic marks is referred to as "epigenetic inheritance."

We will review illustrative examples where environmental conditions experienced by the parental generation increase disease risk in the following generation(s). We primarily focus on examples relating to nutrition and inheritance of metabolic dysfunction, including obesity, insulin resistance, and glucose intolerance and diabetes. Here, we will not consider other environmental factors such as toxins and endocrine-disrupting molecules, which have been described in other specific articles (Dietert 2014; Jiménez-Chillarón et al. 2015). Likewise, we focus on transgenerational effects in mammals (other model organisms are described elsewhere, see Jablonka and Raz 2009; Heard and Martienssen 2014).

18.2   EPIGENETIC INHERITANCE: REVISITING THE DOGMA

Epigenetic inheritance in mammals has recently received enormous attention. The reason is that the current dogma in the biological sciences states that epigenetic mechanisms do not play a role in mediating the inheritance of traits between generations (Bonduriansky 2012). In principle, epigenetic inheritance presupposes that, like genetic variants, the epigenetic variants (or marks) are transmitted from parents to offspring via the gametes (i.e., sperm and oocytes). However, the vast majority of epigenetic marks in the gametes are erased and reset during the processes of gametogenesis and the first postzygotic divisions. This process is known as epigenetic reprogramming. In fact, epigenetic reprogramming of the gametes is precisely aimed to avoid the transfer of environmental, nongenetic, information from one generation to another.

However, recent evidence from human cohorts, such as the Överkalix cohort, and animal models challenge this paradigm and suggest that epigenetic mechanisms might indeed contribute to the inheritance of complex traits (Susiarjo and Bartolomei 2014; Einstein 2014). Studying epigenetic mechanisms in humans is extremely challenging. The reason is that, in addition to the genome and the epigenome, parents can influence their progeny through additional factors, including behavior, culture, and/or maintenance of particular environments (Jablonka and Lamb 2005). These factors might be transmitted and play an essential role for the development of phenotypes in the offspring. For example, nutritional habits are passed from parents to offspring through cultural transmission. Accordingly, it is proposed that the transmission of cooking traditions (i.e., high fats) may underlie a great deal of the prevalence of obesity and its associated comorbidities in Western societies.

Experimental models may help to understand whether the epigenome really plays a role in the transmission of complex traits across generations. In this regard, there are two experimental paradigms that provide strong evidence of epigenetic inheritance: (1) paternal effects and (2) *in vitro* fertilization (IVF) (Figure 18.2).

18.2.1 PATERNAL EFFECTS

"Paternal effects" refer to the situation in which the offspring's phenotype is influenced by the paternal life history. As described previously, in humans, paternal legacy is mediated by the complex interplay of the genome, the epigenome, culture, and behavior. Use of experimental models, such as rats and mice, can minimize these confounding mechanisms. Accordingly, in these models, the sires can be removed from the cage upon pregnancy of the dam. Thus, paternal metabolism and behavior no longer contribute to the offspring's phenotype. Indeed, in these experimental paradigms, the inheritance of traits via the paternal lineage occurs primarily through the information contained in the gametes: the genome and the epigenome (Figure 18.2a). Therefore, the inheritance of acquired phenotypes can be attributed, in part, to epigenetic mechanisms (Ferguson-Smith and Patti 2011; Rando 2012). Here, we will not consider examples describing maternal effects because, like in humans, inheritance of information through the maternal lineage is very complex: transfer of phenotypic information is based on the interplay of several mechanisms, including genetics, epigenetics, mitochondrial DNA transfer, the *in utero* environment, and maternal physiology (Figure 18.2b) (Jablonka and Lamb 2005; Aerts and Van Assche 2006; Zambrano et al. 2006; Benyshek et al. 2006; Burdge et al. 2011; King et al. 2013).

There are now many examples in which environmental factors, including nutrition (Jimenez-Chillaron et al. 2016), lifestyle (Barrès and Zierath 2016), or behavior (Gapp et al. 2014), influence offspring phenotype. As stated elsewhere, here we will focus on those examples where the paternal diet influences diabetes risk in the offspring.

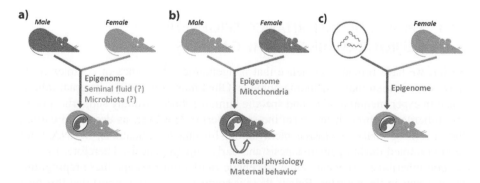

FIGURE 18.2 Experimental paradigms showing evidence of epigenetic inheritance.

18.2.2 *IN VITRO* FERTILIZATION

Natural fecundation cannot completely rule out that additional factors, other than the genome and the epigenome contained in the sperm, might play a role in transferring information across generations. For example, it has been proposed that the paternal microbiota or elements contained in the seminal fluid might have an impact on offspring phenotypes (Figure 18.2a) (Rando and Simmons 2015). IVF stands as a powerful tool to directly explore the role of the gametes (i.e., genome and epigenome) excluding the confounding influence of other factors (Figure 18.2c) (Watson and Rakoczy 2016).

For example, in a recent study, oocytes from control females were fertilized with sperm from males previously fed with a high-fat diet (HFD; Huypens et al. 2016). The *in vitro*-derived embryos were then transferred into surrogate females on a control chow diet. Remarkably, the female offspring derived from the HFD-exposed spermatozoa had higher prevalence of obesity than offspring from control gametes. These data strongly suggest that the metabolic effects observed in the offspring are mediated by epigenetic factors contained in the gametes.

To note, IVF experiments also allow the study of epigenetic inheritance through the maternal lineage (i.e., oocytes). Accordingly, oocytes of nutritionally challenged females were fertilized with sperm from control males and the two-cell embryos transferred into control females (Padmanabhan et al. 2013; Sasson et al. 2015; Huypens et al. 2016). Offspring from HFD-derived oocytes displayed several metabolic anomalies. These experiments suggest that oocyte-derived epigenetic factors, modulated by nutritional cues, also play a major role in the inheritance of metabolic phenotypes via the maternal germline.

IVF techniques are challenging and, so far, there are not many studies reporting this approach. Also, this technique has some critiques, including the fact that the manipulations associated to the IVF itself can induce epigenetic modifications; there are potential biases during the process of oocyte selection. In the next section, we primarily review those studies that (1) focus on *paternal inheritance* and (2) have analyzed the *epigenome of the gametes* (spermatozoa) in response to environmental cues (Table 18.1).

18.3 EPIGENETIC INHERITANCE: EPIGENETIC REPROGRAMMING IN THE GAMETES

So far, we have provided evidence that nongenomic inheritance of complex traits may occur in mammals, including humans (Gluckman et al. 2007). Paternal inheritance in experimental models and specific human cohorts strongly supports epigenetic inheritance through the germline (i.e., sperm). However, as described earlier, the epigenetic marks (cytosine methylation, histone modifications, ncRNAs) are reprogrammed during gametogenesis and early embryogenesis. Therefore, for epigenetic inheritance to occur, some epigenetic marks must escape these reprogramming events in the gametes. Below, there is some evidence to support that this may actually happen.

TABLE 18.1

Studies Reporting an Association between Paternal Inheritance and Epigenetic Modifications in the Sperm

1. DNA Methylation

Dietary Challenge	Transgenerational Phenotype	Gametic Marks	References
Intrauterine caloric restriction	Exposed males: Glucose intolerance, obesity Offspring: Glucose intolerance	• Over 100 regions showed changes in Cytosine methylation in the sperm of founder males. • These methylation marks where NOT inherited into somatic tissues of offspring. • However, the expression of several genes associated to the differentially methylated regions was de-regulated.	Radford et al. 2014
Intrauterine caloric restriction	Exposed males: Glucose intolerance, obesity Offspring: Glucose intolerance	• DNA methylation of the Lxra gene was altered in the sperm of challenged founder males. • This methyl-mark was also found in the embryonic and adult liver of the offspring.	Martinez et al. 2014
Intrauterine hyperglycemia	Exposed males: Impaired insulin secretion and glucose intolerance. Offspring: Same phenotype tan founder males.	• The IGF2/H19 imprinted region was hypermethylated, and expression reduced, in islet cells of founder males and their offspring. • Expression of IGF2/H19 was also reduced in the sperm of challenged mice. • Nevertheless DNA methylation has not been studied/ reported in the sperm of this model.	Ding et al. 2012
High fat diet	Exposed males: Obesity and glucose intolerance. Offspring: Moderate glucose intolerance in female offspring and grand-offspring of high-fat fed male founders.	• 18 methyl-marks were altered in the sperm of founder males and their progeny. • Of them 3 genes were also differentially expressed in WAT and EDL muscle (Slc3a2, Tbrg4 and Usp11) of the offspring.	Castro Barbosa et al. 2016
Low-protein diet	Offspring: Up-regulation of genes involved in lipid biosynthesis in the liver.	• Sperm of founder males showed modest changes in cytosine methylation at the global scale. • At the single locus level, an upstream region of the Ppara was hypermethylated, and the expression of the gene reduced, in the liver of the offspring.	Carone et al. 2011
Paternal pre-diabetes	Exposed males: Increased body weight and obesity, insulin resistance and glucose intolerance. Offspring: Glucose intolerance and insulin resistance.	• More than 8,000 regions were differentially methylated in the sperm of founder males. • A large fraction of these differentially methylated cytosines (30%) were also differentially methylated in islet cells of the offspring. • Only 2 of them (Pik3ca, Pik3r1) were differentially expressed in islet cells.	Wei et al. 2014

(Continued)

TABLE 18.1 (Continued)
Studies Reporting an Association between Paternal Inheritance and Epigenetic Modifications in the Sperm

2. Noncoding RNAs

Dietary Challenge	Transgenerational Phenotype	miRNAs	References
High fat diet	Exposed males: Obesity and glucose intolerance. Offspring: Moderate glucose intolerance in female offspring and grand-offspring of high-fat fed male founders.	• 15 miRNAs were differentially expressed in the sperm of two consecutive generations. • Of them, only Let-7c was also differentially expressed in somatic tissues of the offspring (liver, WAT, EDL muscle). • Many target genes of let-7c were altered at the mRNA and protein level in WAT.	Castro Barbosa et al. 2016
High fat diet	Exposed mice: Obesity. Importantly, in this model obese founder mice did not develop insulin resistance and glucose intolerance. Offspring: Obesity and insulin resistance.	• 23 miRNAs were altered in the testes of founder males. • 4 of them were also altered in the sperm: miR-133-3p, miR-196a-5p, miR-205-5p and miR-340-5p. • Up to 50 direct targets of these miRNAs were differentially expressed in the testes of founder males. • It has not been studied/reported whether these miRNAs also regulate the expression of the target genes in somatic tissues of the offspring.	Fullston et al. 2013

Dietary Challenge	Transgenerational Phenotype	Transfer RNA (tRNA)–Derived Fragments (tRFs)	References
Low-protein diet	Offspring: Up-regulation of genes involved in lipid and cholesterol biosynthesis in the liver.	• 5' fragments of tRNA-Gly-CCC, TCC and GCC; tRF-Lys-CTT and tRF-his-GTG were significantly increased in sperm of the founder males. • Paternal tRNA-Gly-CCC de-regulated the expression of genes involved in embryonic development of the offspring. • It is unknown whether this specific tRF also influences offspring metabolism.	Sharma et al. 2016
High fat diet	Exposed males: Obesity, glucose intolerance and insulin resistance. Offspring: Glucose intolerance and insulin resistance.	• Microinjection of the tRF fraction from the sperm of HFD-fed mice into naïve oocytes recapitulated some metabolic abnormalities in the offspring.	Chen et al. 2016

18.3.1 CYTOSINE METHYLATION

Some methyl-cytosine marks can actually resist either the germline and/or the postzygotic reprogramming events. One well-known example occurs during parental imprinting (Bartolomei et al. 1993). Imprinted genes are a small group of genes which expression depends on the parental origin of the allele (Allis et al. 2007). The selective activation/repression of the parental alleles is accomplished by specific epigenetic marks, primarily DNA methylation. Importantly, the regions that control the imprinting can survive the epigenetic resetting of the early zygote (Daxinger and Whitelaw 2012). Therefore, imprinting provides proof-of-principle that there exists a few methyl-cytosines that can be inherited and maintained in the next-generation offspring.

Aside from imprinted genes, other *loci* also escape the developmental reprogramming. A series of studies have systematically mapped DNA methylation dynamics in germ cells during the process of gametogenesis. They confirmed that more than 90% of the genome was almost completely demethylated during gametogenesis. However, a significant fraction of the genome retained a substantial DNA methylation during this process (Lane et al. 2003; Hajkova et al. 2008; Popp et al. 2010; Borgel et al. 2010; Hackett et al. 2013; Hackett and Surani 2013; Seisenberger et al. 2012). These regions included predominantly intracisternal-A particles (IAPs) of transposons. The transposon activity of these IAPs is actually inactivated through hypermethylation. Hence, it is proposed that the maintenance of IAP hypermethylation during gametogenesis is aimed to prevent transposition and, therefore, new mutations that might compromise embryonic development.

Finally, in addition to these transposable elements, a few hundred CpG islands also showed variable degrees of stable methylation (>40% methylation) during the reprogramming of the primordial germ cells. It has been proposed that they could be "potential carriers of epigenetic inheritance" (Seisenberger et al. 2012). However, it has not been studied whether these regions are actually modifiable in response to environmental challenges and later truly influence offspring' phenotype.

Combined, these studies provide evidence that a small fraction of methyl-cytosines, including imprinting control regions, IAPs, and a group of CpG islands, resist the process of reprogramming and can be transmitted to the offspring.

18.3.2 HISTONE MODIFICATIONS

In the mature sperm, the vast majority of histones are replaced by protamines. However, a small fraction of the genome (2–4% in mice; 10% in humans) retains some histones within nucleosomes (Hammoud et al. 2009; Brykczynska et al. 2010). Furthermore, a few paternal nucleosomes were actually found in the nucleus of the zygote after fertilization (van der Heijden et al. 2006, 2008). Finally, the histones that integrate these nucleosomes may carry covalent modifications (H3K4me or H3K27me3), which might contribute to maintain transcriptional memory.

In sum, these data provide evidence that at least a few histone marks might (1) survive developmental reprogramming and (2) act as carriers of environmentally acquired epigenetic information across generations. As yet, the function of these specific sperm nucleosomes is not fully characterized.

18.3.3 NONCODING RNAs

A plethora of ncRNAs have been recently included as part of the epigenetic machinery. Indeed, despite the fact that the sperm is transcriptionally inactive, it contains a whole set of RNAs, including messenger RNA (mRNA), long ncRNA, microRNA (miRNA), PIWI interacting RNA (piRNA), endogenous interfering RNA, and transfer RNA (tRNA)-derived fragments (TRFs) (Krawetz 2005; Casas and Vavouri 2014). The biological function for some of them is still unclear, but they might play an important role during early embryogenesis and could therefore constitute an additional layer of epigenetic information (Casas and Vavouri 2014). Some functional evidence that miRNAs, piRNAs, and TRFs might carry epigenetic information across generations has been provided.

For example, paternal miRNAs may mediate transgenerational epigenetic inheritance at a specific locus (the *Kit* locus) in mice (Rassoulzadegan et al. 2006, 2007). Likewise, it was shown that dietary challenges, such as high-fat feeding, may change the abundance and composition of miRNAs in the spermatozoa of mice (Grandjean et al. 2015). Furthermore, it was proven that the microinjection of specific miRNAs into control oocytes recapitulated the obese-related phenotypes in the offspring (see next section for further details).

On the other hand, the piRNAs are expressed primarily in the gonads, being most abundant in the testes (Gan et al. 2011). The piRNAs contribute to the establishment of parental imprints and epigenetic silencing of retrotransposons (Watanabe et al. 2011; Kuramochi-Miyagawa et al. 2008). Therefore, it has been proposed that piRNAs are involved in the establishment of epigenetic marks during the process of reprogramming in germ cells and could act as carriers of information across generations (Daxinger and Whitelaw 2012; Ashe et al. 2012).

Finally, TRFs are also particularly abundant in the gametes. Strikingly, two recent articles reported that TRF expression in sperm is affected by paternal diets (HFD and low protein diet, respectively) in mice (Chen et al. 2016; Sharma et al. 2016). Similar to the miRNA experiments, when microinjected into naïve oocytes, these species were able to recapitulate some features of the obese-diabetic paternal phenotypes in the offspring.

In summary, there is evidence to support that some epigenetic marks can survive the reprogramming events that occur during gametogenesis and the first postzygotic divisions. The question now is whether these "resilient" epigenetic marks are (1) modifiable in response to dietary challenges and (2) can influence offspring phenotype.

In the following section, we summarize those studies that strongly support the idea of transgenerational epigenetic inheritance of diabetes risk. They fulfill the conditions that we have so far described in this review: (1) paternal inheritance of diabetes in which (2) the epigenome has been analyzed in the sperm (Table 18.1).

18.4 EPIGENETIC INHERITANCE OF METABOLIC DYSFUNCTION: EXPERIMENTAL MODELS

18.4.1 DNA METHYLATION

There are now multiple examples in which the paternal diet influences offspring phenotypes and has an impact on the sperm methylome. The nutritional challenges include (1) *in utero* malnutrition, (2) HFD, (3) low protein diet, and (4) cytosine deprivation. Also, the effects mediated by paternal prediabetes (i.e., hyperglycemia) will be discussed here.

18.4.1.1 Intrauterine Undernutrition

In utero calorie restriction in mice (50%) results in intrauterine growth restriction (IUGR) and low birth weight (Jimenez-Chillaron et al. 2005, 2006). IUGR male mice developed obesity and glucose intolerance with aging. Strikingly, the offspring of the nutritionally challenged male mice also developed glucose intolerance as adults (Jimenez-Chillaron et al. 2009). Paternal transmission of disease risk strongly suggests epigenetic inheritance via the gametes.

Two independent studies have shown that *in utero* undernutrition modified patterns of DNA methylation in the mature spermatozoa of the dietary-challenged males (Martínez et al. 2014; Radford et al. 2014). At the global scale (MedIP-Seq), more than 100 regions showed changes in DNA methylation (Radford et al. 2014). However, these methylation marks did not persist in the fetal tissues (liver and brain) of the following generation (F2), thus questioning the role of DNA methylation in mediating transmission of phenotypes in this model. Nevertheless, the expression of some target genes that lay in the vicinity of the methylation marks were differentially expressed in somatic tissues of the F2 generation. In agreement, Martinez et al. reported that paternal intrauterine malnutrition influenced the expression of 256 genes in the livers of second-generation offspring (Martínez et al. 2014). Many of them were involved in regulating lipid metabolism. Among them, the transcription factor *Lxra* was significantly reduced in the liver of the F2 mice. The methylation of a canonical CpG island mapping within the first exon and the first intron of the gene was significantly reduced. The important finding was that the same pattern was already present in the mature sperm of the progenitors (i.e., IUGR-F1 males). Even more, the methylation of *Lxra* was also reduced in the fetal liver of the offspring, strongly suggesting that changes in methylation are inherited and do not appear secondarily as mice develop metabolic abnormalities. In sum, this work was among the first to show a line of continuity of a given epigenetic mark in two consecutive generations that (1) strongly suggests epigenetic inheritance and (2) may explain, in part, offspring metabolic phenotypes (Einstein 2014).

Together, these studies confirm that *in utero* malnutrition influences the sperm methylome at the global scale. However, the vast majority of changes were not subsequently inherited into the offspring, with *Lxra* a likely exception. These data strongly suggest that at least a small fraction of the nutritionally induced changes of DNA methylation in sperm might contribute to the following generation.

18.4.1.2 Intrauterine Hyperglycemia (Maternal Diabetes)

In humans, gestational diabetes is strongly associated with a higher risk of obesity and diabetes in the offspring (Aerts and Van Assche 2006). In mice, gestational diabetes impairs insulin secretion and glucose tolerance in the offspring, F1 (Ding et al. 2012). Impaired β-cell function was attributed, in part, to the reduced expression of two imprinted genes: insulin-like growth factor 2 (IGF-2) and H19 (*Igf2/ H19*). Their expression negatively correlated with the level of methylation of a specific Imprinted Control Region of this locus. Furthermore, the diabetic phenotypes were transmitted to the following generation through the paternal lineage. The offspring of males previously exposed to *in utero* hyperglycemia also showed impaired glucose-stimulated insulin secretion and glucose intolerance. Again, impaired β-cell function was associated to hypermethylation of the imprinted control region and reduced expression of *Igf2/H19* genes. These data strongly suggest epigenetic inheritance of specific DNA methylation marks from one generation to the next via the spermatozoa. Intriguingly, the expression of these two imprinted genes was significantly reduced in the sperm of the founder males. Unfortunately, the methylation status of the Imprinted Control Region in sperm was not reported. Therefore, although the data are suggestive of epigenetic inheritance, at this moment we cannot ascertain whether DNA methylation (or other factors) truly plays a role in this model.

18.4.1.3 HFD (Paternal Obesity)

Paternal chronic high-fat feeding in rats and mice strongly influences the risk of developing metabolic abnormalities in the offspring (Fullston et al. 2013; Ng et al. 2010, de Castro Barbosa et al. 2016). However, the role of HFD in reprogramming the epigenome (DNA methylation) has only been recently addressed.

First, it has been shown that high-fat feeding resulted in the reprogramming of DNA methylation in spermatozoa (de Castro Barbosa et al. 2016). Furthermore, up to 18 methyl-marks were altered in the sperm of the founder males (F0) and their progeny (F1), which strongly supports epigenetic inheritance. Next, the transcriptome of liver, white adipose tissue (WAT), and extensor digitorum longus (EDL) muscle was compared with the methylation profile of the F0 and F1 males. Similar to the reported data for the IUGR models, only three genes appeared differentially expressed in concordance with the methylation data. The authors concluded that there exists a "modest link, if any, between differential methylation of paternal sperm and the gene expression signature in somatic tissues of adult offspring" (Castro Barbosa et al. 2016).

Transgenerational inheritance of metabolic dysfunction mediated by HF-fed males might be due to the diet itself and/or other obesity-related signals. To address this issue, Fullston et al. treated adult male mice with an HFD containing a relatively moderate amount of calories from fat (21%) (Fullston et al. 2013). This diet-induced obesity in founder F0 mice in the absence of additional components of the metabolic syndrome, such as insulin resistance, dyslipidemia, or impaired β-cell function. This dietary intervention induced metabolic abnormalities in the offspring (F1) and the grand-offspring (F2) of HFD-fed males (F0). Therefore, paternal impaired glucose homeostasis or diabetes was not a prerequisite for passing ancestral phenotypes to the offspring.

18.4.1.4 Paternal Low Protein Diet

Like in the previous paradigms, paternal low protein feeding in founder males (F0) resulted in the upregulation of genes involved in lipid biosynthesis in the livers of the offspring (F1) (Carone et al. 2010). Furthermore, the liver from F1 offspring showed modest changes in global DNA methylation. At the single *locus* level, the cytosine methylation of an intergenic region upstream of the gene encoding the peroxisome proliferator-activated receptor alpha (*Ppara*) was significantly increased by 30%. Indeed, *Ppara* is a key transcription factor that regulates lipid oxidation and that could explain, in part, the deregulation of fat and cholesterol biosynthesis. However, the methylation of the *Ppara locus* was unaltered in the sperm of the F0 low protein-fed mice. Furthermore, at the global scale (MedIP-Seq) DNA methylation was largely similar in the spermatozoa of low protein fed and control mice. Thus, in agreement with previous models, the authors concluded that the sperm methylome is modifiable in response to dietary factors, but the small reported differences question whether it is the likely carrier of epigenetic information between generations.

18.4.1.5 Paternal Prediabetes

Finally, we will review an example where paternal inheritance of diabetes risk is not associated to nutritional challenges but to diabetes risk itself. Wei et al. developed a model of prediabetes by treating mice with an HFD and low doses of streptozotocin (Wei et al. 2014). The purpose of this combination is that, in rodents, HFD induces obesity and insulin resistance but not diabetes because the β-cells are able to secrete enough insulin to maintain glycemia.

As expected, founder males exposed to HFD and streptozotocin developed increased body weight, increased adiposity, insulin resistance, and glucose intolerance due to β-cell failure. Next, the offspring of the prediabetic males also developed glucose intolerance and insulin resistance. Four hundred and two genes were differentially expressed in islet cells of the offspring of the prediabetic males. In parallel, more than 8000 regions (including 5'-UTR, 3'-UTR, coding sequences, and intronic regions) were differentially methylated in the islets from the offspring. Once again, and as described in the previous models, the correlation between the transcriptome and the methylome was minimal: only three genes, the phosphatidylinositol 3-kinase subunits (*Pik3ca* and *Pik3r1*) and the protein tyrosine phosphatase nonreceptor type 1 gene (*Ptpn1*) were significantly altered. To note, these three genes regulate insulin signaling and their deregulation might contribute to impaired β-cell function.

The key question was, again, whether these epigenetic signatures were inherited from the prediabetic founder mice. In fact, paternal prediabetes substantially altered DNA methylation patterns in the spermatozoa. Therefore, this model shows again that the sperm epigenome is largely sensitive to environmental cues. Strikingly, a substantial fraction of the methylome overlapped between the sperm of F0 mice and the islet cells of F1 mice (around 30%). The most remarkable finding is that the methylation of two of the previous candidates, *Pik3ca* and *Pik3r1*, was also altered in the sperm of the prediabetic mice. Furthermore, the methylation of these two targets was also altered (increased) in embryonic day 3.5 blastocysts from the founder prediabetic mice.

In summary, this study provides the strongest evidence to support the epigenetic inheritance of diabetes risk via DNA methylation in mammals. First, the authors show a line of continuity for many epigenetic marks across two generations. Second, at least two of the marks that show "across generations continuity" may actually play an important role in offspring phenotype.

18.4.2 Noncoding RNAs

It has been argued that ncRNAs might be likely carriers of information across generations (Daxinger and Whitelaw 2012). The reason is that, as stated previously, (1) the mammalian sperm carries a high complexity and abundance of ncRNAs and (2) sperm ncRNAs may influence gene expression of the fertilized egg and, thus, impact the appropriate development of the embryo.

18.4.2.1 miRNAs

It has been shown that paternal obesity/paternal high-fat feeding altered the expression of miRNAs in the sperm of rats and mice (Fullston et al. 2013; Grandjean et al. 2015). It is proposed that these environmentally induced changes in sperm microRNAs might influence oocyte gene expression.

For example, in one study, HFD remodeled the expression of miRNAs in the sperm of the F0 high-fat fed rats and their offspring, F1 (de Castro Barbosa et al. 2016). Up to 15 miRNAs were differentially expressed in both generations. From them, only let-7c was also detected in somatic tissues of adult offspring, including the liver, the gonadal adipose tissue, and EDL muscle. This effect appeared to be highly specific because other members of the let-7 family did not change in response to the paternal dietary challenge. Importantly, the expression of many predicted targets of let-7c was altered at the mRNA and protein level in the WAT. Together, these data strongly suggest that "let-7c contributes to the changes in WAT phenotype in response to HFD feeding in founders" (de Castro Barbosa et al. 2016). Although the potential role of let-7c in mediating transgenerational effects is inferred, it is not known whether the altered expression of let-7c in WAT is truly inherited or whether it is secondarily altered in response to other signals. Also, it is really unlikely that a single miRNA mediates such complex effects in this model. Therefore, either additional miRNAs and/or other epigenetic molecules contribute to the inheritance of complex traits in this model.

In another work, paternal obesity elicited transgenerational transmission of obesity and insulin resistance in the offspring and grand offspring (Fullston et al. 2013). In agreement with the previous study, it was found that HFD altered the expression of 23 miRNAs in the testes of founder mice. Furthermore, four of them were also altered in the spermatozoa of the HFD-fed males: miR-133b-3p, miR-196a-p5, miR-205–5p, and miR-340–5p. To assess their potential impact, the transcriptome was assessed in the testes of founder mice. Among the differentially expressed genes, 50 transcripts were direct targets of these four miRNAs. Furthermore, 28 of them were downregulated as might be expected in response to the upregulation of the miRNAs. Finally, these 50 targets converge on pathways enriched for "metabolic disease, cell death, production of reactive oxygen species (ROS), DNA replication, nuclear factor kappa B (NF-κB) signaling, p53 signaling, recombination and repair, and embryonic development." In sum, this work strongly suggests that HFD reprograms sperm miRNAs that can indeed modulate "embryonic development and provide a mechanism for paternal transmission of obesity and metabolic abnormalities in the next generation" (Fullston et al. 2013).

Finally, direct experimental proof that the miRNAs may carry epigenetic information across generations has been provided by transferring miRNAs into naïve zygotes (Grandjean et al. 2015). Grandjean et al. found that 13 miRNAs were differentially expressed in the testes of high-fat fed founder males. Among them, miR-19b and miR-29a were the two most abundant deregulated miRNAs in testes and sperm. Next, the authors injected these miRNAs separately into fertilized one-cell embryos. miR-19b-microinjected embryos, but not miR-29a embryos, developed obesity when adults. However, miR-19b did not fully recapitulate the phenotypes that were induced by HFD. In any case, this is among the first studies to provide evidence that a specific miRNA may reprogram the zygote, which, in turn, may lead to the development of several pathologies in the adult. Like in the previous work, although a single miRNA may partially recapitulate some metabolic phenotypes in the offspring, it is unlikely that a single miRNA is responsible for the inheritance of such complex traits. Additionally, even more, if we consider that through the microinjections, thousands of RNA molecules are transferred that can additionally cause unspecific phenotypic effects.

18.4.2.2 tRNA-Derived Fragments

TRFs have recently joined the list of molecules potentially carrying epigenetic information across generations. They are small ncRNAs ranging between 28 and 34 nucleotides. Similar to the previously described paradigms, low protein diets and HFDs altered the expression of TRFs in the sperm of mice (Sharma et al. 2016; Chen et al. 2016).

In the low protein models, a few TRFs species showed a significant increase in the spermatozoa of HFD-fed founder mice: 5' fragments of tRNA-Gly-CCC, TCC, and GCC; TRF-Lys-CTT; and TRF-His-GTG (Sharma et al. 2016). The question was whether these paternal TRFs might influence offspring phenotype. Strikingly, tRNA-Gly-GCC regulated the expression of several mRNAs that are driven by the MurineEndogenous Retrovirus (MERVL). MERVL-target genes might affect embryonic growth potential or placental size/function, hence influencing offspring metabolism secondary to altered embryonic development. Finally, it was shown that antisense oligonucleotides for the tRNA-Gly-GCC induced similar deregulation of the expression of MERVL targets in stem cells, zygotes, and two-cell preimplantation embryos. Combined, these data strongly support that paternal diet can (1) influence sperm TRF biogenesis and that (2) sperm TRFs have the potential to regulate embryo RNA expression. Nevertheless, it is not known whether this particular tRNA or the combination of them can actually influence offspring metabolism later in life.

The direct role of TRFs in mediating transmission of complex traits was further assessed in an intergenerational HFD paradigm (Chen et al. 2016). First, the authors isolated different fractions of small RNAs in the spermatozoa of high-fat fed male mice: fractions containing 15–30 nt (which include miRNAs and piRNAs), the fractions sizing 30–40 nt (which contains the TRFs), and the fractions containing RNAs >40 nt. Next, they injected the different fractions into naïve oocytes and found that the fraction of RNAs sizing 30–40 nt had metabolic effects in the offspring. In contrast, the other fractions had no metabolic effects in the offspring. These data strongly suggest that TRFs are necessary mediators for transferring information across generations. Furthermore, the microinjections of TRFs from HFD sires into eight-cell embryos and blastocysts resulted in the deregulation of many genes involved in metabolic regulation pathways and other essential cellular processes (e.g., protein transport and localization). It is argued, again, that these early embryo transcriptional changes might cause profound downstream effects that result in reprogramed gene expression in the adult tissues of the F_1 offspring, hence leading to metabolic disorder (Chen et al. 2016).

However, it cannot completely be excluded that other RNA species ranging 30–40 nt in size may also play a role. In agreement with this possibility, single microinjections of TRFs did not recapitulate the phenotypes in the offspring.

18.4.2.3 piRNAs

Other small ncRNAs have been proposed to carry epigenetic information across generations. For example, piRNAs may induce transgenerational inheritance of complex traits in lower organisms (Casas and Vavouri 2014). Although no evidence has been provided in mammals, it has to be noted that paternal diet, including HFD, may actually influence the expression of a huge amount of piRNAs in the testes (Grandjean et al. 2015) and mature sperm (de Castro Barbosa et al. 2016; Chen et al. 2016). As mentioned, their role in offspring metabolism has not been assessed. Interestingly, Chen et al. conducted microinjections of small ncRNAs of small size 15–30 nt. In fact, this fraction includes mostly miRNAs and piRNAs. As expected, microinjection of the purified fraction from HFD males resulted in embryo lethality, suggesting an essential role in early embryo development. The diluted fraction (20×), though, had no detectable effects in the F1 embryos. While the authors suggested that this fraction has no transgenerational effects, it might be possible that different concentrations might result in metabolic effects, without compromising embryo viability. Therefore, the potential role of other RNA species, including piRNAs or long-ncRNAs, remains an open question.

18.5 CONCLUSION

There is ample evidence to support that environmental cues, including many dietary challenges such as *in utero* malnutrition, HFD, low protein diet, hyperglycemia, etc., may modify the epigenome of the gametes. The epigenetic marks that are susceptible to such nutritional signals include DNA methylation, histone modifications, and several ncRNAs. These epigenetic variants might influence offspring phenotype if (1) they survive the epigenetic reprogramming events occurring during gametogenesis and embryogenesis and (2) are able to influence, directly or indirectly, the expression of target genes in the somatic tissues of the offspring.

Specifically, it has been shown that intrauterine malnutrition, low protein diets, and HFDs cause dramatic changes in the methylome of the gametes. However, most of them are not transferred to the following generation offspring. Only a few isolated methyl-marks show a line of continuity across generations and influence the expression of the target genes. Some of these targets are transcription factors that might explain, in part, the inherited phenotypes. However, it is generally accepted that these isolated candidates cannot fully explain the whole intricacy associated to the inheritance of complex metabolic traits. Therefore, other molecular driver(s) might play a role in transmitting information across generations.

In agreement, it has been shown that both paternal nucleosomes and some small ncRNAs may (1) be modified by nutritional cues, (2) survive the developmental reprogramming, and (3) be transmitted into the zygote. Similar to the cytosine methylation, many miRNAs, piRNAs, and TRFs were altered in the sperm of nutritionally challenged rodents. However, only a few specific miRNAs were altered in the sperm of founder males and somatic tissues of the offspring. miRNAs have a wide regulatory capacity because they can interact with several hundred target genes. Therefore, a few miRNAs might be able to act as carriers of transgenerational information in response to environmental factors. Similarly, TRFs and piRNAs might also induce a wide range of effects in the offspring. Nevertheless, this idea deserves further experimental support. Finally, it has to be noted that paternally inherited RNAs are rapidly degraded in the embryo (after the first divisions). Therefore, their impact on adult metabolic phenotypes should propagate through their impact on gene expression and/or other components of the epigenetic machinery (DNA methylation and histones). They might act secondarily as a means to maintain and propagate the original signals inherited from the sperm. As yet, the potential signaling pathways and mechanisms involved during the very early stages of development remain a black box.

To conclude, recent literature shows that ancestral environments can be passed from parents to offspring through nongenomic mechanisms. There is enough data from animal models to support that epigenetic mechanisms may mediate, in part, such effects. It is unclear which epigenetic mark(s) is primarily responsible for the epigenetic inheritance of complex traits. But a likely scenario is that the inheritance of diabetes risk might be mediated by the interplay between all of them that coordinately transfer environmental information from one generation to another.

REFERENCES

Aerts, L., and F. A. Van Assche. 2006. Animal evidence for the transgenerational development of diabetes mellitus. *Int J Biochem Cell Biol* 38 (5–6):894–903.

Allis, C. D., T. Jenuwein, and D. Reinberg. 2007. *Epigenetics*: New York, NY: Cold Spring Harbor Laboratory Press.

Ashe, A., A. Sapetschnig, E. M. Weick, J. Mitchell, M. P. Bagijn, A. C. Cording, A. L. Doebley, L. D. Goldstein, N. J. Lehrbach, J. Le Pen, G. Pintacuda, A. Sakaguchi, P. Sarkies, S. Ahmed, and E. A. Miska. 2012. piRNAs can trigger a multigenerational epigenetic memory in the germline of C. elegans. *Cell* 150 (1):88–99.

Barrès, R., and J. R. Zierath. 2016. The role of diet and exercise in the transgenerational epigenetic landscape of T2DM. *Nat Rev Endocrinol* 12 (8):441–51.

Bartolomei, M. S., A. L. Webber, M. E. Brunkow, and S. M. Tilghman. 1993. Epigenetic mechanisms underlying the imprinting of the mouse H19 gene. *Genes Dev* 7 (9):1663–73.

Benyshek, D. C., C. S. Johnston, and J. F. Martin. 2006. Glucose metabolism is altered in the adequately-nourished grand-offspring (F3 generation) of rats malnourished during gestation and perinatal life. *Diabetologia* 49 (5):1117–9.

Bondurianky, R. 2012. Rethinking heredity, again. *Trends Ecol Evol* 27 (6):330–6.

Borgel, J., S. Guibert, Y. Li, H. Chiba, D. Schübeler, H. Sasaki, T. Forné, and M. Weber. 2010. Targets and dynamics of promoter DNA methylation during early mouse development. *Nat Genet* 42 (12):1093–100.

Brykczynska, U., M. Hisano, S. Erkek, L. Ramos, E. J. Oakeley, T. C. Roloff, C. Beisel, D. Schübeler, M. B. Stadler, and A. H. Peters. 2010. Repressive and active histone methylation mark distinct promoters in human and mouse spermatozoa. *Nat Struct Mol Biol* 17 (6):679–87.

Burdge, G. C., S. P. Hoile, T. Uller, N. A. Thomas, P. D. Gluckman, M. A. Hanson, and K. A. Lillycrop. 2011. Progressive, transgenerational changes in offspring phenotype and epigenotype following nutritional transition. *PLoS One* 6 (11):e28282.

Bygren, L. O. 2013. Intergenerational health responses to adverse and enriched environments. *Annu Rev Public Health* 34:49–60.

Bygren, L. O., G. Kaati, and S. Edvinsson. 2001. Longevity determined by paternal ancestors' nutrition during their slow growth period. *Acta Biotheor* 49 (1):53–9.

Carone, B. R., L. Fauquier, N. Habib, J. M. Shea, C. E. Hart, R. Li, C. Bock, C. Li, H. Gu, P. D. Zamore, A. Meissner, Z. Weng, H. A. Hofmann, N. Friedman, and O. J. Rando. 2010. Paternally induced transgenerational environmental reprogramming of metabolic gene expression in mammals. *Cell* 143 (7):1084–96.

Casas, E., and T. Vavouri. 2014. Sperm epigenomics: Challenges and opportunities. *Front Genet* 5:330.

Chen, Q., M. Yan, Z. Cao, X. Li, Y. Zhang, J. Shi, G. H. Feng, H. Peng, X. Zhang, J. Qian, E. Duan, Q. Zhai, and Q. Zhou. 2016. Sperm tsRNAs contribute to intergenerational inheritance of an acquired metabolic disorder. *Science* 351 (6271):397–400.

Daxinger, L., and E. Whitelaw. 2012. Understanding transgenerational epigenetic inheritance via the gametes in mammals. *Nat Rev Genet* 13 (3):153–62.

de Castro Barbosa, T., L. R. Ingerslev, P. S. Alm, S. Versteyhe, J. Massart, M. Rasmussen, I. Donkin, R. Sjögren, J. M. Mudry, L. Vetterli, S. Gupta, A. Krook, J. R. Zierath, and R. Barrès. 2016. High-fat diet reprograms the epigenome of rat spermatozoa and transgenerationally affects metabolism of the offspring. *Mol Metab* 5 (3):184–97.

Dietert, R. R. 2014. Transgenerational epigenetics of endocrine-disrupting chemicals. In *Transgenerational Epigenetics: Evidence and Debate*, edited by T. Tollefsbol, 239–254. Amsterdam: Elsevier.

Ding, G. L., F. F. Wang, J. Shu, S. Tian, Y. Jiang, D. Zhang, N. Wang, Q. Luo, Y. Zhang, F. Jin, P. C. Leung, J. Z. Sheng, and H. F. Huang. 2012. Transgenerational glucose intolerance with Igf2/H19 epigenetic alterations in mouse islet induced by intrauterine hyperglycemia. *Diabetes* 61 (5):1133–42.

Einstein, F. H. 2014. Multigenerational effects of maternal undernutrition. *Cell Metab* 19 (6):893–4.

Ferguson-Smith, A. C., and M. E. Patti. 2011. You are what your dad ate. *Cell Metab* 13 (2):115–7.

Fullston, T., E. M. Ohlsson Teague, N. O. Palmer, M. J. DeBlasio, M. Mitchell, M. Corbett, C. G. Print, J. A. Owens, and M. Lane. 2013. Paternal obesity initiates metabolic disturbances in two generations of mice with incomplete penetrance to the F2 generation and alters the transcriptional profile of testis and sperm microRNA content. *FASEB J* 27 (10):4226–43.

Gan, H., X. Lin, Z. Zhang, W. Zhang, S. Liao, L. Wang, and C. Han. 2011. piRNA profiling during specific stages of mouse spermatogenesis. *RNA* 17 (7):1191–203.

Gapp, K., L. von Ziegler, R. Y. Tweedie-Cullen, and I. M. Mansuy. 2014. Early life epigenetic programming and transmission of stress-induced traits in mammals: How and when can environmental factors influence traits and their transgenerational inheritance? *Bioessays* 36 (5):491–502.

Gluckman, P. D., M. A. Hanson, and A. S. Beedle. 2007. Non-genomic transgenerational inheritance of disease risk. *Bioessays* 29 (2):145–54.

Grandjean, V., S. Fourré, D. A. De Abreu, M. A. Derieppe, J. J. Remy, and M. Rassoulzadegan. 2015. RNA-mediated paternal heredity of diet-induced obesity and metabolic disorders. *Sci Rep* 5:18193.

Hackett, J. A., R. Sengupta, J. J. Zylicz, K. Murakami, C. Lee, T. A. Down, and M. A. Surani. 2013. Germline DNA demethylation dynamics and imprint erasure through 5-hydroxymethylcytosine. *Science* 339 (6118):448–52.

Hackett, J. A., and M. A. Surani. 2013. Beyond DNA: Programming and inheritance of parental methylomes. *Cell* 153 (4):737–9.

Hajkova, P., K. Ancelin, T. Waldmann, N. Lacoste, U. C. Lange, F. Cesari, C. Lee, G. Almouzni, R. Schneider, and M. A. Surani. 2008. Chromatin dynamics during epigenetic reprogramming in the mouse germ line. *Nature* 452 (7189):877–81.

Hammoud, S. S., D. A. Nix, H. Zhang, J. Purwar, D. T. Carrell, and B. R. Cairns. 2009. Distinctive chromatin in human sperm packages genes for embryo development. *Nature* 460 (7254):473–8. doi:10.1038/nature08162.

Heard, E., and R. A. Martienssen. 2014. Transgenerational epigenetic inheritance: Myths and mechanisms. *Cell* 157 (1):95–109.

Huypens, P., S. Sass, M. Wu, D. Dyckhoff, M. Tschöp, F. Theis, S. Marschall, M. Hrabě de Angelis, and J. Beckers. 2016. Epigenetic germline inheritance of diet-induced obesity and insulin resistance. *Nat Genet* 48 (5):497–9.

Jablonka, E., and G. Raz. 2009. Transgenerational epigenetic inheritance: Prevalence, mechanisms, and implications for the study of heredity and evolution. *Q Rev Biol* 84 (2):131–76.

Jablonka, E., and M. J. Lamb. 2005. *Evolution in Four Dimensions. Genetic, Epigenetic, Behavioral and Symbolic Variation in the History of Life.* Cambridge, MA: MIT Press.

Jimenez-Chillaron, J. C., M. Hernandez-Valencia, A. Lightner, R. R. Faucette, C. Reamer, R. Przybyla, S. Ruest, K. Barry, J. P. Otis, and M. E. Patti. 2006. Reductions in caloric intake and early postnatal growth prevent glucose intolerance and obesity associated with low birthweight. *Diabetologia* 49 (8):1974–84.

Jimenez-Chillaron, J. C., M. Hernandez-Valencia, C. Reamer, S. Fisher, A. Joszi, M. Hirshman, A. Oge, S. Walrond, R. Przybyla, C. Boozer, L. J. Goodyear, and M. E. Patti. 2005. Beta-cell secretory dysfunction in the pathogenesis of low birth weight-associated diabetes: a murine model. *Diabetes* 54 (3):702–11.

Jimenez-Chillaron, J. C., E. Isganaitis, M. Charalambous, S. Gesta, T. Pentinat-Pelegrin, R. R. Faucette, J. P. Otis, A. Chow, R. Diaz, A. Ferguson-Smith, and M. E. Patti. 2009. Intergenerational transmission of glucose intolerance and obesity by in utero undernutrition in mice. *Diabetes* 58 (2):460–8.

Jimenez-Chillaron, J. C., M. Ramon-Krauel, S. Ribo, and R. Diaz. 2016. Transgenerational epigenetic inheritance of diabetes risk as a consequence of early nutritional imbalances. *Proc Nutr Soc* 75 (1):78–89.

Jimenez-Chillaron, J. C, R. Diaz, M. Ramon-Krauel, and S. Ribo. 2014. Transgenerational epigenetic inheritance of type 2 diabetes. In *Transgenerational Epigenetics. Evidence and Debate*, edited by T Tollefsbol, 281–301. Academic Press. Elsevier.

Jiménez-Chillarón, J. C., R. Díaz, D. Martínez, T. Pentinat, M. Ramón-Krauel, S. Ribó, and T. Plösch. 2012. The role of nutrition on epigenetic modifications and their implications on health. *Biochimie* 94 (11):2242–63.

Jiménez-Chillarón, J. C., M. J. Nijland, A. A. Ascensão, V. A. Sardão, J. Magalhães, M. J. Hitchler, F. E. Domann, and P. J. Oliveira. 2015. Back to the future: Transgenerational transmission of xenobiotic-induced epigenetic remodeling. *Epigenetics* 10 (4):259–73.

Jirtle, R. L., and M. K. Skinner. 2007. Environmental epigenomics and disease susceptibility. *Nat Rev Genet* 8 (4):253–62.

Kaati, G., L. O. Bygren, and S. Edvinsson. 2002. Cardiovascular and diabetes mortality determined by nutrition during parents' and grandparents' slow growth period. *Eur J Hum Genet* 10 (11):682–8.

King, V., R. S. Dakin, L. Liu, P. W. Hadoke, B. R. Walker, J. R. Seckl, J. E. Norman, and A. J. Drake. 2013. Maternal obesity has little effect on the immediate offspring but impacts on the next generation. *Endocrinology* 154 (7):2514–24.

Krawetz, S. A. 2005. Paternal contribution: New insights and future challenges. *Nat Rev Genet* 6 (8):633–42.

Kuramochi-Miyagawa, S., T. Watanabe, K. Gotoh, Y. Totoki, A. Toyoda, M. Ikawa, N. Asada, K. Kojima, Y. Yamaguchi, T. W. Ijiri, K. Hata, E. Li, Y. Matsuda, T. Kimura, M. Okabe, Y. Sakaki, H. Sasaki, and T. Nakano. 2008. DNA methylation of retrotransposon genes is regulated by Piwi family members MILI and MIWI2 in murine fetal testes. *Genes Dev* 22 (7):908–17.

Lane, N., W. Dean, S. Erhardt, P. Hajkova, A. Surani, J. Walter, and W. Reik. 2003. Resistance of IAPs to methylation reprogramming may provide a mechanism for epigenetic inheritance in the mouse. *Genesis* 35 (2):88–93.

Martínez, D., T. Pentinat, S. Ribó, C. Daviaud, V. W. Bloks, J. Cebrià, N. Villalmanzo, S. G. Kalko, M. Ramón-Krauel, R. Díaz, T. Plösch, J. Tost, and J. C. Jiménez-Chillarón. 2014. In utero undernutrition in male mice programs liver lipid metabolism in the second-generation offspring involving altered Lxra DNA methylation. *Cell Metab* 19 (6):941–51.

Ng, S. F., R. C. Lin, D. R. Laybutt, R. Barres, J. A. Owens, and M. J. Morris. 2010. Chronic high-fat diet in fathers programs β-cell dysfunction in female rat offspring. *Nature* 467 (7318):963–6.

Padmanabhan, N., D. Jia, C. Geary-Joo, X. Wu, A. C. Ferguson-Smith, E. Fung, M. C. Bieda, F. F. Snyder, R. A. Gravel, J. C. Cross, and E. D. Watson. 2013. Mutation in folate metabolism causes epigenetic instability and transgenerational effects on development. *Cell* 155 (1):81–93.

Pembrey, M. E., L. O. Bygren, G. Kaati, S. Edvinsson, K. Northstone, M. Sjöström, J. Golding, and ALSPAC Study Team. 2006. Sex-specific, male-line transgenerational responses in humans. *Eur J Hum Genet* 14 (2):159–66.

Popp, C., W. Dean, S. Feng, S. J. Cokus, S. Andrews, M. Pellegrini, S. E. Jacobsen, and W. Reik. 2010. Genome-wide erasure of DNA methylation in mouse primordial germ cells is affected by AID deficiency. *Nature* 463 (7284):1101–5.

Radford, E. J., M. Ito, H. Shi, J. A. Corish, K. Yamazawa, E. Isganaitis, S. Seisenberger, T. A. Hore, W. Reik, S. Erkek, A. H. Peters, M. E. Patti, and A. C. Ferguson-Smith. 2014. In utero effects. In utero undernourishment perturbs the adult sperm methylome and intergenerational metabolism. *Science* 345 (6198):1255903.

Rando, O. J. 2012. Daddy issues: Paternal effects on phenotype. *Cell* 151 (4):702–8.

Rando, O. J., and R. A. Simmons. 2015. I'm eating for two: Parental dietary effects on offspring metabolism. *Cell* 161 (1):93–105.

Rassoulzadegan, M., V. Grandjean, P. Gounon, and F. Cuzin. 2007. Inheritance of an epigenetic change in the mouse: A new role for RNA. *Biochem Soc Trans* 35 (Pt 3):623–5.

Rassoulzadegan, M., V. Grandjean, P. Gounon, S. Vincent, I. Gillot, and F. Cuzin. 2006. RNA-mediated non-Mendelian inheritance of an epigenetic change in the mouse. *Nature* 441 (7092):469–74.

Roseboom, T., and R. Painter. 2014. Epidemiology of epigenetic inheritance. In *Transgenerational Epigenetics: Evidence and Debate*, edited by T. Tollefsbol, 59–66. Amsterdam: Elsevier.

Sasson, I. E., A. P. Vitins, M. A. Mainigi, K. H. Moley, and R. A. Simmons. 2015. Pregestational vs gestational exposure to maternal obesity differentially programs the offspring in mice. *Diabetologia* 58 (3):615–24.

Seisenberger, S., S. Andrews, F. Krueger, J. Arand, J. Walter, F. Santos, C. Popp, B. Thienpont, W. Dean, and W. Reik. 2012. The dynamics of genome-wide DNA methylation reprogramming in mouse primordial germ cells. *Mol Cell* 48 (6):849–62.

Sharma, U., C. C. Conine, J. M. Shea, A. Boskovic, A. G. Derr, X. Y. Bing, C. Belleannee, A. Kucukural, R. W. Serra, F. Sun, L. Song, B. R. Carone, E. P. Ricci, X. Z. Li, L. Fauquier, M. J. Moore, R. Sullivan, C. C. Mello, M. Garber, and O. J. Rando. 2016. Biogenesis and function of tRNA fragments during sperm maturation and fertilization in mammals. *Science* 351 (6271):391–6.

Susiarjo, M., and M. S. Bartolomei. 2014. Epigenetics. You are what you eat, but what about your DNA? *Science* 345 (6198):733–4.

van der Heijden, G. W., A. A. Derijck, L. Ramos, M. Giele, J. van der Vlag, and P. de Boer. 2006. Transmission of modified nucleosomes from the mouse male germline to the zygote and subsequent remodeling of paternal chromatin. *Dev Biol* 298 (2):458–69.

van der Heijden, G. W., L. Ramos, E. B. Baart, I. M. van den Berg, A. A. Derijck, J. van der Vlag, E. Martini, and P. de Boer. 2008. Sperm-derived histones contribute to zygotic chromatin in humans. *BMC Dev Biol* 8:34.

Watson, E. D., and J. Rakoczy. 2016. Fat eggs shape offspring health. *Nat Genet* 48 (5):478–9.

Watanabe, T., S. Tomizawa, K. Mitsuya, Y. Totoki, Y. Yamamoto, S. Kuramochi-Miyagawa, N. Iida, Y. Hoki, P. J. Murphy, A. Toyoda, K. Gotoh, H. Hiura, T. Arima, A. Fujiyama, T. Sado, T. Shibata, T. Nakano, H. Lin, K. Ichiyanagi, P. D. Soloway, and H. Sasaki. 2011. Role for piRNAs and noncoding RNA in de novo DNA methylation of the imprinted mouse Rasgrf1 locus. *Science* 332 (6031):848–52.

Wei, Y., C. R. Yang, Y. P. Wei, Z. A. Zhao, Y. Hou, H. Schatten, and Q. Y. Sun. 2014. Paternally induced transgenerational inheritance of susceptibility to diabetes in mammals. *Proc Natl Acad Sci USA* 111 (5):1873–8.

Whitelaw, N. C., and E. Whitelaw. 2008. Transgenerational epigenetic inheritance in health and disease. *Curr Opin Genet Dev* 18 (3):273–9.

Zambrano, E., C. J. Bautista, M. Deás, P. M. Martínez-Samayoa, M. González-Zamorano, H. Ledesma, J. Morales, F. Larrea, and P. W. Nathanielsz. 2006. A low maternal protein diet during pregnancy and lactation has sex- and window of exposure-specific effects on offspring growth and food intake, glucose metabolism and serum leptin in the rat. *J Physiol* 571 (Pt 1):221–30.

Section VI

Interventions

19 Fetal and Early Postnatal Programming of Dyslipidemia and Potential Intervention with Dietary Nutraceuticals

Todd C. Rideout and Jerad H. Dumolt

CONTENTS

19.1 INTRODUCTION

The tremendous impact of cardiovascular diseases (CVDs) on the health and well-being of Americans cannot be overemphasized as it presents major challenges to society on several fronts. First, CVDs including acute myocardial infarction, ischemic heart disease, peripheral vascular disease, high blood pressure, and stroke causally underlie >33% of all U.S. deaths annually (Writing Group et al. 2016). Second, the fiscal burden of CVDs in the United States is staggering with total direct and indirect annual costs estimated to exceed $400 billion. Third, as the leading cause of premature, permanent disability in the United States, CVD has an immeasurable impact on the daily quality of life of Americans by significantly limiting everyday activity, reducing annual incomes, and contributing to depression and an overall low perception of life satisfaction (Writing Group et al. 2016).

Dyslipidemia is recognized as a major preventable risk factor in the pathophysiology of CVD. Adding to the urgency of CVD as a global health issue is the rise in dyslipidemic risk factors among women of child-bearing age due to underlying genetic, disease state, and dietary factors (Kusters et al. 2010). Although not very well recognized in the medical and research community, gestational dyslipidemia is a high-priority health concern for two reasons. First, a treatment dilemma currently exists in the medical community as the use of lipid-lowering medication in dyslipidemic pregnancies is contraindicated due to fears around fetal toxicity. Therefore, limitations in acceptable therapeutic options result in an acknowledged increase in CVD risk for dyslipidemic mothers (Avis et al. 2009). Second, fetal exposure to excessive fat and cholesterol as a result of maternal diet-induced dyslipidemia during pregnancy has been shown to increase fetal plasma cholesterol concentrations and aortic fatty streak formation and predispose adult offspring to diet-induced obesity, hyperlipidemia, and arterial plaque development (Palinski and Napoli 2002; Palinski et al. 2001). This chapter provides an overview of what is currently known regarding the influence of maternal dyslipidemia on lipid metabolism and CVD risk in offspring and examines the safety and efficacy of natural health product supplementation in obese and dyslipidemic pregnancies to protect the fetus from maladaptive early exposure to dyslipidemic CVD risk factors.

19.2 DEFINING MATERNAL DYSLIPIDEMIA

Pregnancy is associated with well-defined adaptive changes in maternal lipid metabolism that ultimately ensures adequate energy and nutrients to support fetal growth and maturation (Wiznitzer et al. 2009). Maternal lipid metabolism during pregnancy can be divided into two phases: a net anabolic phase through the first two trimesters and a net catabolic phase in the third trimester (Douglas et al. 2007; Ramos et al. 2003). The anabolic phase of pregnancy is characterized by an increase in maternal fat deposition that is due to behavioral changes including hyperphagia associated with leptin resistance (Trujillo et al. 2011) and metabolic changes including enhanced insulin sensitivity and increased circulating levels of steroid hormones such as estrogen and progesterone that stimulate *de novo* lipogenesis and fat deposition when the energy demands of the fetus are low. Alternatively, the catabolic phase of pregnancy corresponds to the time of maximal fetal energy demands and growth and is characterized by an underlying metabolic shift that provides growth substrates to the fetus through a reduction in maternal insulin sensitivity that increases adipose tissue lipolysis, peripheral fat oxidation, and gluconeogenesis from glycerol (Herrera et al. 2006).

These maternal changes in lipid metabolism, particularly during late pregnancy, give rise to a normal physiological state of hyperlipidemia that peaks immediately prior to delivery and is characterized by transient elevations in circulating blood lipids including total cholesterol (total-C, ~25–50%), low-density lipoprotein cholesterol (LDL-C, ~70%), high-density lipoprotein cholesterol (HDL-C, ~40%), and triglycerides (TG, 200–400%) (Phan and Toth 2014; Wiznitzer et al. 2009; Huda et al. 2009). Although not sufficiency characterized, pregnancy is also associated with changes in lipoprotein particle profile as demonstrated by an increase in large very LDL (VLDL) particle numbers due to enhanced hepatic VLDL production and cholesterol-ester transfer protein activity (Alvarez et al. 1996). Previous work also suggests that there is a shift toward a smaller, denser LDL subclass distribution during pregnancy (Sattar et al. 1997; Hubel et al. 1998).

However, as detailed below, a growing body of literature suggests that excessive maternal hyperlipidemia during pregnancy can adversely program fetal lipid metabolism predisposing offspring to increased CVD risk as adults. Compared with other maternal factors such as hyperglycemia and obesity, overt maternal dyslipidemia during pregnancy has received relatively little research attention (Mendelson et al. 2016), likely due to the fact that routine lipid blood work during pregnancy is not emphasized due to the "normal" transient hyperlipidemic state during observed pregnancy.

Several underlying prepregnancy and pregnancy conditions predispose a mother to excessive increases in blood lipids during pregnancy. Prepregnancy factors include conditions that contribute to a preexisting dyslipidemic state prior to pregnancy such as poor nutrition and lifestyle factors, obesity, and underlying genetic causes of dyslipidemia such as familial hypercholesterolemia (FH). In these pregnancies, the mother may exhibit a higher absolute peak in blood lipid concentrations throughout pregnancy due to an elevated baseline value (Leiva et al. 2013).

Also, a number of pathological complications encountered during pregnancy, including glucose intolerance (Retnakaran et al. 2011), gestational diabetes (Rizzo et al. 2008), polycystic ovary syndrome (Kim and Choi 2013), and preeclampsia (Harville et al. 2011), are associated with excessive dyslipidemia that may increase CVD risk for both mother and fetus. Although the precise incidence of excessive maternal dyslipidemia during pregnancy is not known, it is thought to be relatively high given the alarming increase in dyslipidemia among women of childbearing age (Leiva et al. 2013). According to the National Health and Nutrition Examination Survey (NHANES), ~25% of women of child-bearing age have unhealthy LDL-C and ~22% have unhealthy TG concentrations (Laz et al. 2013). Moreover, additional data from the NHANES report that among women of child-bearing age (aged 18–44), 2.4% have diabetes, 2.9% have chronic kidney disease, and 57.6% are either overweight or obese, all conditions that are associated with a specific dyslipidemic profile (Wild et al. 2016). At such a high prevalence, obesity is particularly of concern as previous work suggests that obese women have higher mean levels of TG, total-C, and LDL-C in pregnancy compared with their lean counterparts (Farias et al. 2016); this is further associated with an atherogenic LDL subfraction phenotype (Meyer et al. 2013) and increased VLDL production (Zambrano et al. 2016).

19.3 ASSOCIATIONS BETWEEN MATERNAL AND OFFSPRING LIPID STATUS

Although not consistently observed (Narverud et al. 2015), previous prospective studies have reported that maternal lipid concentrations in childhood (Narverud et al. 2015), adulthood (Marcovecchio et al. 2012), in the prepregnancy period (Mendelson et al. 2016), and throughout gestation (Narverud et al. 2015; Morrison et al. 2013) are reflective of offspring lipid concentrations in the neonatal, adolescent, and adult periods. Elevated newborn lipid concentrations may be particularly problematic as newborn cholesterol concentrations have been shown to be predictive of CVD risk in adulthood (Webber et al. 1991; Porkka et al. 1994; Juhola et al. 2011). The strength of the correlation is likely dependent on the extent of maternal dyslipidemia and the period during which potential associations are examined (prepregnancy, different gestational periods, etc.). For example, Napoli et al. (1997) reported that fetal cholesterol concentrations before the sixth month of gestation were strongly correlated with maternal cholesterol, but this association was not evident in fetuses 6 months or older (Napoli et al. 1997). Perhaps unexpectedly, maternal cholesterol levels in prepregnancy (Gademan et al. 2014), early pregnancy (Daraki et al. 2015), and at term (Romejko-Wolniewicz et al. 2014) have been shown to be associated with childhood (4–12 years of age) body mass index (BMI) and adiposity status after adjustments for various covariates including maternal prepregnancy BMI. These associations may be more reflective of an overall derangement in maternal lipid metabolism that predisposes the fetus to an obese phenotype rather than hypercholesterolemia per se. Finally, a number of association studies have reported that excessive maternal cholesterol and TG during pregnancy have been associated with preterm delivery and low birth weight (Maymunah et al. 2014; Catov et al. 2007; Magnussen et al. 2011).

19.4   MATERNAL DYSLIPIDEMIA AFFECTS FETAL LIPID METABOLISM

Most of the basis for the association between maternal and offspring lipid status is thought to be due to maladaptive programming of lipid metabolic and regulatory pathways from exposure to excessive dyslipidemia during early development, either during gestation or perhaps in the neonatal period (Figure 19.1). Support for this lipid programming hypothesis can be found in FH cohort studies, suggesting that individuals who inherit FH maternally versus paternally have higher circulating total-C, LDL-C, and ApoB levels as adults (van der Graaf et al. 2010). A series of studies from Palinski and Napoli suggest that *in utero* exposure to excessive cholesterol may program early fatty streak formation in fetuses and influence long-term progression of atherosclerosis. In their investigation of fatty streak formation in aortas from spontaneously aborted fetuses in mothers characterized as normocholesterolemic (175 ± 20 mg/dL), hypercholesterolemic both before and during pregnancy (385 ± 20 mg/dL), or transient hypercholesterolemic only during pregnancy (325 ± 44 mg/dL), they observed significantly more and larger lesions in offspring from mothers with hypercholesterolemia and temporary hypercholesterolemia compared with offspring from mothers with a normal cholesterol range (Napoli et al. 1997). Although arterial fatty streaks have been shown to develop early in life, the clinical significance and manifestation of early fat deposits to the development of advanced unstable plaques has been questioned (McGill et al. 2000). However, in their follow-up autoptic study including 156 children (1–14 years old) examining the evolution of early childhood lesions, the Fate of Early Lesions in Children (FELIC) study results suggested that although fetal fatty streaks may regress after birth, arterial lesions (aortic arch and abdominal aorta) develop "strikingly" faster in children whose mothers were

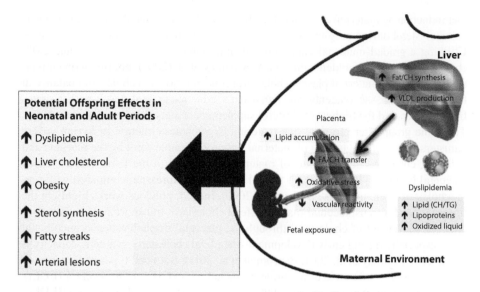

FIGURE 19.1 Potential mechanisms through which excessive maternal dyslipidemia during pregnancy may alter fetal lipid metabolic and regulatory pathways and malprogram lipid metabolism and cardiovascular disease risk in neonates and adults. CH, cholesterol; TG, triglycerides.

hypercholesterolemic during pregnancy (363.88 ± 83.52 mg/dL) versus normocholesterolemic mothers (148.9 ± 62.25 mg/dL) (Napoli et al. 1999).

Additional human work has shown that placental metabolism is distinctly altered in mothers with excessive cholesterol during pregnancy with differential expression of lipid and sterol-regulatory genes (Marseille-Tremblay et al. 2008; Ethier-Chiasson et al. 2007), increased placental oxidative damage and altered arterial vascular reactivity (Liguori et al. 2007), and increased umbilical intima/media ratio with reduced endothelial nitric oxide synthase activity (Leiva et al. 2013).

Although excessive *in utero* cholesterol exposure is thought to directly impact fetal lipid metabolism, there is also suggestion that postnatal cholesterol intake may affect neonatal cholesterol metabolism; however, the long-term implications for offspring CVD risk as adults are not clear. Due to higher cholesterol concentrations in human breast milk compared with commercial formulas, breast-fed infants have been shown to have enhanced circulating cholesterol concentrations than formula-fed infants (Wong et al. 1993; Bayley et al. 1998). Furthermore, this difference in cholesterol intake has also been shown to modulate cholesterol synthesis, with breast-fed infants (~4 months) demonstrating a lower fractional cholesterol synthesis rate than their formula-fed counterparts (Bayley et al. 1998; Demmers et al. 2005), likely through the well-characterized feedback inhibition of 3-hydroxy-3-methylglutaryl coenzyme-A (HMG-CoA) reductase activity.

Animal models have contributed to a greater understanding of how maternal hypercholesterolemia may impact fetal lipid metabolism. As detailed below, numerous maternal hypercholesterolemic animal models established through genetic susceptibility or diet induction by maternal cholesterol feeding have demonstrated that excessive maternal cholesterol during pregnancy predisposes the fetus to overt hypercholesterolemia. Utilizing a graded maternal cholesterol feeding approach (0.0, 0.12, 0.5, and 2.0% cholesterol) in Syrian golden hamsters, McConihay et al. (2001) reported a linear relationship between maternal plasma cholesterol concentration and cholesterol balance in fetal tissues (yolk sac, placenta, and fetus) and a reduction in fetal sterol synthesis rates from mothers fed the highest cholesterol supplemented diets (McConihay et al. 2001). The same group later reported that maternal hypercholesterolemia in Syrian golden hamsters increased the uptake of maternal lipoprotein-cholesterol by the placenta and yolk sac, enhanced the transport of maternal cholesterol to the fetus, and increased placental Niemann–Pick C1-like 1 (NPC1L1) mRNA expression compared with normocholesterolemic mothers (Burke et al. 2009). Indeed, previous works highlight the importance of a transplacental maternal–fetal cholesterol transport system that regulates the movement of cholesterol through the placental trophoblasts and endothelial cells, especially during early development when fetal cholesterol synthetic capacity is limited (McConihay et al. 2001; Baardman et al. 2013). Both cell types express a variety of cholesterol influx and efflux proteins, including NPC1L1, LDL receptor (LDLr), low-density lipoprotein receptor-related protein 1 (LRP-1), VLDL receptor (VLDLr), scavenger receptor class B type1 (SR-B1), and ATP-binding cassette transporter G5 and G8 (ABCG5/G8) (Baardman et al. 2013).

Animal model studies support the programming of atherosclerotic lesion development and add mechanistic insight into how excessive early cholesterol exposure may influence the susceptibility and development of arterial lesions. The apolipoprotein E (apoE) deficient mouse, which lacks the cell surface apoE lipoprotein receptor, is characterized by overt dyslipidemia and spontaneous arterial lesion development and has been used to examine how maternal hypercholesterolemia may program atherosclerotic predisposition in adult offspring (Moghadasian et al. 2001). Xie et al. (2014) reported that adult male apoE-deficient offspring from dams fed a high cholesterol diet during pregnancy demonstrated an atherogenic blood lipid profile and enhanced atherosclerotic lesion development that was exacerbated upon postnatal high-cholesterol feeding. Additionally, animals exposed to excessive cholesterol in the prenatal and postnatal periods displayed increased aortic expression of matrix metalloproteinase-9, a protease involved in atherogenesis and plaque rupture (Xie et al. 2014). In a similar set of studies using the same mouse model, Alkemade and coworkers reported that *in utero* exposure to atherosclerotic risk factors (hypercholesterolemia, oxidative stress, inflammation) programmed a susceptibility to atherosclerosis in morphologically normal adult blood vessels following lesion induction by constrictive carotid collar placement and that this programming was associated with epigenetic histone modifications in the vasculature (Alkemade et al. 2007, 2010).

19.5   INTERVENTIONS FOR MATERNAL DYSLIPIDEMIA

Despite significant advances in the development of effective lipid-lowering drug therapies for the general population, there is a serious gap in suitable treatment options for women with overt hyperlipidemia during pregnancy. As mentioned previously, due to potential teratogenic effects on the developing fetus, the Food and

Drug Administration (FDA) has contraindicated the use of systemically absorbable lipid-lowering drugs (statins, ezetimibe) in expectant mothers and women trying to conceive (Eapen et al. 2012). This has created a clinical treatment dilemma with an acknowledged increased CVD risk for both mother and offspring in hypercholesterolemic pregnancies in the face of limited therapeutic options. Lifestyle therapies, including both dietary and exercise interventions, are considered first-line defenses in reducing maternal dyslipidemia. However, most women demonstrate a modest and variable response to lifestyle interventions during pregnancy for practical (lack of time, motivation) and physiological (change in appetite, fatigue) reasons (Crozier et al. 2009; Evenson et al. 2004). A promising, yet largely unexplored treatment option may be found through supplementing the maternal diet with lipid-lowering nutraceuticals or dietary supplements. Dietary supplements are defined as health-promoting products, including vitamins, minerals, herbs or other botanicals, amino acids, metabolites, or other dietary substances intended to be taken by mouth (capsule, tablet, liquid) to supplement the diet (Pawar and Grundel 2016). The remainder of this chapter reviews the efficacy and safety of specific lipid-lowering nutraceuticals that have been examined for use during dyslipidemic pregnancies. It should be noted, however, that although there are some reports on the effects of maternal nutraceutical supplementation on offspring lipid parameters at various stages throughout the life cycle, the majority of this work has been conducted without any specific focus on the issue of maternal dyslipidemia. Nevertheless, we chose to include some of these studies in our discussion as they do provide rationale (or lack of in some cases) for their potential utility in dyslipidemic pregnancies. We will focus on three dietary supplements reputed for their lipid-lowering response—dietary fiber, omega-3 fatty acids (n–3 FA), and phytosterols (PS)—as these supplements have been more thoroughly investigated in terms of health response, associated mechanisms, and safety.

19.6 DIETARY FIBER

Although there may be no universally accepted definition, dietary fiber can be broadly defined as dietary carbohydrates (both soluble an insoluble forms) that are resistant to intestinal digestion and absorption an therefore able to enter the large intestine as a fermentable microbial substrate with multiple physiological benefits including lowering blood glucose and cholesterol (Edwards et al. 2015). The cholesterol-lowering (total and LDL-C) effect of soluble fibers including psyllium and guar gum has been extensively reviewed (Rideout et al. 2008; Petchetti et al. 2007) and well substantiated in numerous randomized controlled clinical studies. The lipid-lowering effects of soluble fiber are believed to result from both direct (interference with cholesterol and/or bile acid absorption) and indirect (maintenance of healthy gut microflora and production of short-chain fatty acids [SCFA]) mechanisms (Gunness and Gidley 2010).

Using the Wistar rat model, a previous report (Hallam and Reimer 2013) examined the impact of maternal high-fiber consumption (21.6% w/w composed of oligofructose and inulin) versus high-protein consumption (40% w/w) throughout pregnancy and lactation on offspring adiposity and metabolic control in adult offspring challenged with a high-fat/high-sucrose diet for 8 weeks. Although the maternal metabolic milieu in the prepregnancy or pregnancy periods was not reported, dams consuming the high-fiber diet demonstrated a lower gestational weight gain compared with chow or high-protein-fed mothers. Adult offspring from the high-fiber-fed mothers had lower percent body fat (females only) and lower hepatic TG and plasma nonesterified fatty acids concentrations compared with age-matched females from high-protein-fed mothers. These results suggest that early *in utero* and postnatal exposure to dietary fiber through the maternal diet may program a protective anti-obesity and lipid-lowering response in adult offspring challenged with an unhealthy diet. As dietary fiber is inherently nondigestible, it seems likely that the observed programming responses are related to an indirect exposure, perhaps through the production of SCFA produced by fermentation in the mother's large intestine. However, work by Lin et al. (2014) suggests that the protective effects of dietary fiber during pregnancy may extend beyond SCFA production. Using a high-fat-fed Sprague–Dawley rat model, they reported that maternal dietary fiber supplementation during gestation was more effective in ameliorating maternal and placenta oxidative stress than supplementation of the maternal diet with sodium butyrate, a bioactive SCFA produced through microbial hindgut fermentation. However, it is possible that acetate and propionate, two additional microbial-produced fermentation end products with demonstrated systemic health effects (Koh, De Vadder et al. 2016), may play a role in mediating the observed responses.

Although we are not aware of any human studies that have examined the lipid-modulating effects of maternal dietary fiber supplementation during pregnancy, Dasopoulou et al. (2015) conducted a study to examine the influence of postnatal (from birth to postnatal day 16) fructo-oligosaccharide-enriched formula (0.8 g/100 mL) consumption versus a standard preterm formula without exogenous fiber supplementation in healthy preterm neonates ($n = 167$). They reported a lower body weight and reductions in total and LDL-C in fiber-supplemented neonates compared with those consuming the standard formula. The implications of these early changes in blood cholesterol for long-term blood lipid control are unclear. Given the degree of previous research attention devoted to characterizing the lipid-lowering effects and safety of dietary fibers in the general population, the lack of research pertaining to the potential protective effects of maternal fiber consumption during pregnancy on offspring metabolic outcomes is surprising.

19.7   OMEGA-3 FATTY ACIDS

A number of animal model studies suggest that early n–3 FA exposure (both marine-based and plant-derived) modulates lipid metabolism in neonates and may program favorable lipid and lipoprotein responses in adults, potentially reducing CVD risk (Shomonov-Wagner et al. 2015; Hussain et al. 2013). Joshi et al. (2003) investigated the effectiveness of maternal fish oil supplementation in rescuing metabolic malprogramming of disease risk due to maternal protein deficiency in Wistar rats. Compared with the control chow diet with adequate protein, maternal fish oil supplementation (7 g/100 g) to a protein-deficient diet during pregnancy reduced serum total-C, LDL-C, and TG in adult (6 months) male offspring, suggesting that marine-derived fatty acids may play a protective role in the metabolic programming of fetal adaptation to maternal undernutrition. Additionally, adult offspring from hamster mothers fed a n–3 FA supplemented diet during pregnancy and then fed a postweaning high-fat diet throughout adulthood (16 weeks) demonstrated a reduction in postprandial lipemia and hepatic TG secretion compared with offspring from unsupplemented mothers (Kasbi-Chadli et al. 2014).

However, overall, this protective effect has proved difficult to translate in human studies. Due to a limited capacity of the fetus and neonate to synthesize n–3 FA, long-chain polyunsaturated fatty acid (PUFA) status of the fetus and neonate is highly influenced by maternal consumption (Hanebutt et al. 2008). High-dose daily fish oil (4 g/day) supplementation in mothers during gestation has been shown to enhance the erythrocyte n–3 FA status of both the mother (30 and 37 weeks of gestation) and neonate (6-week postpartum) compared with olive oil-supplemented mothers (Dunstan et al. 2004). Demonstrating that maternal n–3 FA supplementation has direct effects on fetal lipid metabolism, Calabuig-Navarro et al. (2016) reported that term placentas from overweight and obese women supplementing with n–3 FA (eicosapentaenoic acid [EPA] + docosahexaenoic acid [DHA], 2 g/day) throughout pregnancy were characterized by a reduction in total lipid content and altered RNA expression of lipid regulatory genes reflecting a reduced capability to esterify and store fat (Calabuig-Navarro et al. 2016). However, despite these early beneficial effects, longer term studies accessing lipid levels in offspring from n–3 supplemented mothers have shown little benefit. Rytter et al. (2011) reported that male and female adolescent (19 years old, n = 243) offspring exposed *in utero* to n–3 FA (1 g EPA/DHA) from the maternal diet during the third trimester of pregnancy had a similar blood lipid profile (total-C, LDL, HDL, and TG) and lipoprotein (small dense LDL particles) pattern as offspring from mothers supplemented with olive oil (Rytter et al. 2011). Additionally, an early childhood diet (weaning to 5 years of age) designed to provide an n–3 to n-6 ratio of ~1:5 (through diet and tuna oil supplementation) showed no favorable effects in lipid profile in 8-year offspring compared with a control group (Ayer et al. 2009). Therefore, although animal studies suggest that early *in utero* or postnatal n–3 FA exposure may alter offspring lipid metabolism, human studies have so far failed to see this effect. However, beyond surrogate lipid markers of CVD risk, a recent study by Bryant et al. (2015) suggests that adolescent offspring (9 years of age) from mothers consuming oily fish during pregnancy have reduced arterial stiffness reflective of long-term CVD risk protection (Bryant et al. 2015).

19.8 PHYTOSTEROLS

PS are plant-derived sterols that closely resemble mammalian cholesterol in their structure and cellular function. PS, including β-sitosterol, campesterol, and stigmasterol, are a natural component of plant-based foods and can be found in a wide variety of fortified products, including juices and spreads (Berger et al. 2004). PS carry a health claim by the U.S. FDA and are recommended by the National Cholesterol Education Program at a dose of 2 g/day for cholesterol lowering and CVD prevention. Over 50 years of cell culture, animal model, and human clinical investigations have repeatedly demonstrated the ability of PS to reduce cholesterol by up to 15%

by limiting intestinal cholesterol absorption (Abumweis et al. 2008). Beyond LDL-C lowering, research also suggests that PS may reduce blood and tissue triglyceride concentrations, stimulate a nonbiliary route of reverse cholesterol transport, and have antiatherogenic, anti-inflammatory, and antioxidative properties (Theuwissen et al. 2009; Brufau et al. 2011; Devaraj et al. 2011; Mannarino et al. 2009).

A number of preclinical investigations (Waalkens-Berendsen et al. 1999; Whittaker et al. 1999; Ryokkynen et al. 2005) and one clinical investigation (Laitinen et al. 2009) have examined the safety of PS use during pregnancy with no adverse health consequences observed. This strong safety record and proven lipid-lowering efficacy in the general population make PS an intriguing diet-based therapeutic option for the treatment of maternal dyslipidemia.

We have developed and characterized two animal models to examine the safety and utility of maternal PS supplementation during gestation and lactation: a Syrian golden hamster model to investigate the role of diet-induced maternal hypercholesterolemia on offspring CVD risk and an apoE-deficient mouse model to investigate how maternal genetic hypercholesterolemia-modulated offspring lipid responses. Results from both of these animal models suggest that newly weaned pups born to hypercholesterolemic mothers supplemented with PS during pregnancy/lactation are protected against maladaptive increases in blood lipid and lipoprotein biomarkers. Compared with 21-day-old apoE-deficient mouse pups from chow-fed dams, age-matched pups from dams fed a cholesterol-enriched diet displayed increases ($p < .05$) in total-C (+68%), non-HDL-C (+123%), LDL-C (+154%), HDL-C (+30%), total LDL particle number (+216%), and VLDL particle number (+254%). However, supplementing the maternal cholesterol-enriched diet with PS during prepregnancy, gestation, and lactation was effective in preventing dyslipidemic responses in offspring (Rideout et al. 2015). Compared with pups from cholesterol-fed dams, offspring born to PS-fed dams demonstrated reductions ($p < .05$) in total-C (-26%), non-HDL-C (-32%), LDL-C (-29%), and HDL-C (-19%). Furthermore, compared with pups from cholesteol-fed dams, pups from PS-supplemented dams displayed a reduction ($p < .05$) in the number of total LDL particles (-34%) and VLDL particles (-31%). Although maternal cholesterol feeding increased hepatic cholesterol levels in pups compared with pups from chow-fed dams, this response was normalized in offspring from PS-supplemented dams. Results in the Syrian golden hamster model were similar with newly weaned pups from PS-supplemented mothers demonstrating reductions in blood and hepatic cholesterol fractions compared with pups from cholesterol-fed mothers (Liu et al. 2016). Additionally, compared with chow pups, pups from cholesterol-fed dams demonstrated increased protein expression of both the LDLr (~twofold) and HMG-CoAr (~1.8 fold) that was normalized to chow levels in pups from PS-supplemented dams. It is likely that a number of mechanisms may have contributed to these protective effects. First, by reducing hypercholesterolemia in mothers, maternal PS supplementation may have indirectly impeded excessive maternal cholesterol transfer to the offspring *in utero*. Second, early exposure to PS during fetal development and/or through postnatal milk consumption could have directly impacted cholesterol homeostasis in offspring. Maternal PS supplementation during lactation has previously been shown to increase PS concentrations in maternal milk and result in increased circulating PS levels in infants (Mellies et al. 1979). In both models, we detected an increase in serum β-sitosterol concentrations in offspring from PS-fed dams compared with pups from the cholesterol group. Enhanced circulating levels of PS have been shown to directly influence the expression of cholesterol-regulatory genes, possibly by acting as ligands for liver X receptor in the liver and peripheral tissues (Calpe-Berdiel et al. 2008; Plat et al. 2005).

Pups from PS-supplemented mothers developed normally, without any alterations in litter birth weight, sex ratio, or neonatal growth, suggesting that maternal PS supplementation is not associated with adverse health responses in offspring, at least at these whole-body indices. However, on a cautionary note, although maternal PS supplementation protected against hypercholesterolemia in hamster (but not mouse) pups, we also observed an unexpected rise in serum TG compared with pups born to unsupplemented mothers (Liu et al. 2016). The implications of this early increase in serum TG and whether this response causes more permanent adaptations in TG metabolism in adulthood are not clear. Although these results in newly weaned animals are promising, work is ongoing to characterize if the protective cholesterol-lowering effects of PS observed in newly weaned pups will extend into adulthood and whether these changes can program long-term CVD risk protection throughout the life course.

19.9 FUTURE CONSIDERATIONS

Overall, there is relatively little current work examining the malprogramming effects of maternal dyslipidemia on offspring CVD risk compared with other more well-characterized maternal conditions such as gestational diabetes. Although excessive maternal hypercholesterolemia has received some attention, much less is known regarding the impact of overt gestational hypertriglyceridemia due to conditions such as familial chylomicronemia syndromes (Gupta et al. 2014; Montes et al. 1984). Although the early life programming of maternal hypertriglyceridemia as a component of maternal obesity and excessive gestational weight gain is currently a major research focus (Desai et al. 2014), it is difficult to separate the specific effects of dyslipidemia in obese models from that of other contributing obesity-associated metabolic disturbances including insulin resistance, inflammation, and oxidative stress. It is also evident that while there is a fairly large database of preclinical research that has examined the influence of maternal high fat or high carbohydrate feeding on developmental programming of offspring, the majority of this work does not tease out the specific effects of maternal dyslipidemia and, moreover, does not always adequately characterize the maternal metabolic lipid environment throughout the pre- and postnatal periods (Hellgren et al. 2014; Hallam and Reimer 2013).

Finally, from an intervention standpoint, more research is necessary to more fully characterize the impact of other natural health products with lipid-lowering potential, including probiotics (Ishimwe et al. 2015), conjugated linoleic acid (Reynolds et al. 2015), alpha-lipoic acid (Pashaj et al. 2015), and quercetin (Wu et al. 2014) in protecting against the metabolic malprogramming effects of maternal dyslipidemia.

REFERENCES

Abumweis, S. S., R. Barake, and P. J. Jones. 2008. Plant sterols/stanols as cholesterol lowering agents: A meta-analysis of randomized controlled trials. *Food Nutr Res* 52.

Alkemade, F. E., A. C. Gittenberger-de Groot, A. E. Schiel et al. 2007. Intrauterine exposure to maternal atherosclerotic risk factors increases the susceptibility to atherosclerosis in adult life. *Arterioscler Thromb Vasc Biol* 27 (10):2228–35.

Alkemade, F. E., P. van Vliet, P. Henneman et al. 2010. Prenatal exposure to apoE deficiency and postnatal hypercholesterolemia are associated with altered cell-specific lysine methyltransferase and histone methylation patterns in the vasculature. *Am J Pathol* 176 (2):542–8.

Alvarez, J. J., A. Montelongo, A. Iglesias, M. A. Lasuncion, and E. Herrera. 1996. Longitudinal study on lipoprotein profile, high density lipoprotein subclass, and postheparin lipases during gestation in women. *J Lipid Res* 37 (2):299–308.

Avis, H. J., B. A. Hutten, M. T. Twickler et al. 2009. Pregnancy in women suffering from familial hypercholesterolemia: A harmful period for both mother and newborn? *Curr Opin Lipidol* 20 (6):484–90.

Ayer, J. G., J. A. Harmer, W. Xuan, et al. 2009. Dietary supplementation with n-3 polyunsaturated fatty acids in early childhood: Effects on blood pressure and arterial structure and function at age 8 y. *Am J Clin Nutr* 90 (2):438–46.

Baardman, M. E., W. S. Kerstjens-Frederikse, R. M. Berger et al. 2013. The role of maternal-fetal cholesterol transport in early fetal life: Current insights. *Biol Reprod* 88 (1):24.

Bayley, T. M., M. Alasmi, T. Thorkelson et al. 1998. Influence of formula versus breast milk on cholesterol synthesis rates in four-month-old infants. *Pediatr Res* 44 (1):60–7.

Berger, A., P. J. Jones, and S. S. Abumweis. 2004. Plant sterols: Factors affecting their efficacy and safety as functional food ingredients. *Lipids Health Dis* 3:5.

Brufau, G., F. Kuipers, Y. G. Lin, E. A. Trautwein, and A. K. Groen. 2011. A reappraisal of the mechanism by which plant sterols promote neutral sterol loss in mice. *PLoS One* 6 (6): e21576.

Bryant, J., M. Hanson, C. Peebles et al. 2015. Higher oily fish consumption in late pregnancy is associated with reduced aortic stiffness in the child at age 9 years. *Circ Res* 116 (7):1202–5.

Burke, K. T., P. L. Colvin, L. Myatt et al. 2009. Transport of maternal cholesterol to the fetus is affected by maternal plasma cholesterol concentrations in the golden Syrian hamster. *J Lipid Res* 50 (6):1146–55.

Calabuig-Navarro, V., M. Puchowicz, P. Glazebrook et al. 2016. Effect of omega-3 supplementation on placental lipid metabolism in overweight and obese women. *Am J Clin Nutr* 103 (490):1064–72.

Calpe-Berdiel, L., J. C. Escola-Gil, and F. Blanco-Vaca. 2008. New insights into the molecular actions of plant sterols and stanols in cholesterol metabolism. *Atherosclerosis* 203 (1):18–31.

Catov, J. M., L. M. Bodnar, K. E. Kip et al. 2007. Early pregnancy lipid concentrations and spontaneous preterm birth. *Am J Obstet Gynecol* 197 (6):610 e1–7.

Crozier, S. R., S. M. Robinson, K. M. Godfrey, C. Cooper, and H. M. Inskip. 2009. Women's dietary patterns change little from before to during pregnancy. *J Nutr* 139 (10):1956–63.

Daraki, V., V. Georgiou, S. Papavasiliou et al. 2015. Metabolic profile in early pregnancy is associated with offspring adiposity at 4 years of age: The Rhea pregnancy cohort Crete, Greece. *PLoS One* 10 (5):e0126327.

Dasopoulou, M., D. D. Briana, T. Boutsikou et al. 2015. Motilin and gastrin secretion and lipid profile in preterm neonates following prebiotics supplementation: A double-blind randomized controlled study. *JPEN J Parenter Enteral Nutr* 39 (3):359–68.

Demmers, T. A., P. J. Jones, Y. Wang et al. 2005. Effects of early cholesterol intake on cholesterol biosynthesis and plasma lipids among infants until 18 months of age. *Pediatrics* 115 (6):1594–601.

Desai, M., J. K. Jellyman, G. Han et al. 2014. Maternal obesity and high-fat diet program offspring metabolic syndrome. *Am J Obstet Gynecol* 211 (3):237 e1–237 e13.

Devaraj, S., I. Jialal, J. Rockwood, and D. Zak. 2011. Effect of orange juice and beverage with phytosterols on cytokines and PAI-1 activity. *Clin Nutr* 30 (5):668–71.

Douglas, A. J., L. E. Johnstone, and G. Leng. 2007. Neuroendocrine mechanisms of change in food intake during pregnancy: A potential role for brain oxytocin. *Physiol Behav* 91 (4):352–65.

Dunstan, J. A., T. A. Mori, A. Barden et al. 2004. Effects of n-3 polyunsaturated fatty acid supplementation in pregnancy on maternal and fetal erythrocyte fatty acid composition. *Eur J Clin Nutr* 58 (3):429–37.

Eapen, D. J., K. Valiani, S. Reddy, and L. Sperling. 2012. Management of familial hypercholesterolemia during pregnancy: Case series and discussion. *J Clin Lipidol* 6 (1):88–91.

Edwards, C. A., C. Xie, and A. L. Garcia. 2015. Dietary fibre and health in children and adolescents. *Proc Nutr Soc* 74 (3):292–302.

Ethier-Chiasson, M., A. Duchesne, J. C. Forest et al. 2007. Influence of maternal lipid profile on placental protein expression of LDLr and SR-BI. *Biochem Biophys Res Commun* 359 (1):8–14.

Evenson, K. R., D. A. Savitz, and S. L. Huston. 2004. Leisure-time physical activity among pregnant women in the US. *Paediatr Perinat Epidemiol* 18 (6):400–7.

Farias, D. R., A. B. Franco-Sena, A. Vilela et al. 2016. Lipid changes throughout pregnancy according to pre-pregnancy BMI: Results from a prospective cohort. *BJOG* 123 (4):570–8.

Gademan, M. G., M. Vermeulen, A. J. Oostvogels et al. 2014. Maternal prepregancy BMI and lipid profile during early pregnancy are independently associated with offspring's body composition at age 5–6 years: The ABCD study. *PLoS One* 9 (4):e94594.

Gunness, P. and M. J. Gidley. 2010. Mechanisms underlying the cholesterol-lowering properties of soluble dietary fibre polysaccharides. *Food Funct* 1 (2):149–55.

Gupta, N., S. Ahmed, L. Shaffer, P. Cavens, and J. Blankstein. 2014. Severe hypertriglyceridemia induced pancreatitis in pregnancy. *Case Rep Obstet Gynecol* 2014:485493.

Hallam, M. C. and R. A. Reimer. 2013. A maternal high-protein diet predisposes female offspring to increased fat mass in adulthood whereas a prebiotic fibre diet decreases fat mass in rats. *Br J Nutr* 110 (9):1732–41.

Hanebutt, F. L., H. Demmelmair, B. Schiessl, E. Larque, and B. Koletzko. 2008. Long-chain polyunsaturated fatty acid (LC-PUFA) transfer across the placenta. *Clin Nutr* 27 (5):685–93.

Harville, E. W., J. S. Viikari, and O. T. Raitakari. 2011. Preconception cardiovascular risk factors and pregnancy outcome. *Epidemiology* 22 (5):724–30.

Hellgren, L. I., R. I. Jensen, M. S. Waterstradt, B. Quistorff, and L. Lauritzen. 2014. Acute and perinatal programming effects of a fat-rich diet on rat muscle mitochondrial function and hepatic lipid accumulation. *Acta Obstet Gynecol Scand* 93 (11):1170–80.

Herrera, E., E. Amusquivar, I. Lopez-Soldado, and H. Ortega. 2006. Maternal lipid metabolism and placental lipid transfer. *Horm Res* 65 (3 Suppl):59–64.

Hubel, C. A., Y. Shakir, M. J. Gallaher, M. K. McLaughlin, and J. M. Roberts. 1998. Low-density lipoprotein particle size decreases during normal pregnancy in association with triglyceride increases. *J Soc Gynecol Investig* 5 (5):244–50.

Huda, S. S., N. Sattar, and D. J. Freeman. 2009. Lipoprotein metabolism and vascular complications in pregnancy. *Clinical Lipidology* 4 (1):91–102.

Hussain, A., I. Nookaew, S. Khoomrung et al. 2013. A maternal diet of fatty fish reduces body fat of offspring compared with a maternal diet of beef and a post-weaning diet of fish improves insulin sensitivity and lipid profile in adult C57BL/6 male mice. *Acta Physiol* 209 (3):220–34.

Ishimwe, N., E. B. Daliri, B. H. Lee, F. Fang, and G. Du. 2015. The perspective on cholesterol-lowering mechanisms of probiotics. *Mol Nutr Food Res* 59 (1):94–105.

Joshi, S., S. Rao, A. Golwilkar, M. Patwardhan, and R. Bhonde. 2003. Fish oil supplementation of rats during pregnancy reduces adult disease risks in their offspring. *J Nutr* 133 (10):3170–4.

Juhola, J., C. G. Magnussen, J. S. Viikari et al. 2011. Tracking of serum lipid levels, blood pressure, and body mass index from childhood to adulthood: The Cardiovascular Risk in Young Finns Study. *J Pediatr* 159 (4):584–90.

Kasbi-Chadli, F., C. Y. Boquien, G. Simard et al. 2014. Maternal supplementation with n-3 long chain polyunsaturated fatty acids during perinatal period alleviates the metabolic syndrome disturbances in adult hamster pups fed a high-fat diet after weaning. *J Nutr Biochem* 25 (7):726–33.

Kim, J. J. and Y. M. Choi. 2013. Dyslipidemia in women with polycystic ovary syndrome. *Obstet Gynecol Sci* 56 (3):137–42.

Koh, A., F. De Vadder, P. Kovatcheva-Datchary, and F. Backhed. 2016. From Dietary Fiber to Host Physiology: Short-Chain Fatty Acids as Key Bacterial Metabolites. *Cell* 165 (6):1332–45.

Kusters, D. M., S. J. Homsma, B. A. Hutten et al. 2010. Dilemmas in treatment of women with familial hypercholesterolaemia during pregnancy. *Neth J Med* 68 (1):299–303.

Laitinen, K., E. Isolauri, L. Kaipiainen, H. Gylling, and T. A. Miettinen. 2009. Plant stanol ester spreads as components of a balanced diet for pregnant and breast-feeding women: Evaluation of clinical safety. *Br J Nutr* 101 (12):1797–804.

Laz, T. H., M. Rahman, and A. B. Berenson. 2013. Trends in serum lipids and hypertension prevalence among non-pregnant reproductive-age women: United States National Health and Nutrition Examination Survey 1999–2008. *Matern Child Health J* 17 (8):1424–31.

Leiva, A, C. Diez de Medina, E. Guzmán-Gutiérrez et al. 2013. Maternal hypercholesterolemia in gestational diabetes and the association with placental endothelial dysfunction. *In Gestational Diabetes—Causes, Diagnosis and Treatment*, Dr. Luis Sobrevia (Ed.). Rijeka: InTech; 2013:103–134.

Liguori, A., F. P. D'Armiento, A. Palagiano et al. 2007. Effect of gestational hypercholesterolaemia on omental vasoreactivity, placental enzyme activity and transplacental passage of normal and oxidised fatty acids. *BJOG* 114 (12):1547–56.

Lin, Y., Z. F. Fang, L. Q. Che et al. 2014. Use of sodium butyrate as an alternative to dietary fiber: effects on the embryonic development and anti-oxidative capacity of rats. *PLoS One* 9 (5):e97838.

Liu, J., A. Iqbal, A. Raslawsky et al. 2016. Influence of maternal hypercholesterolemia and phytosterol intervention during gestation and lactation on dyslipidemia and hepatic lipid metabolism in offspring of Syrian golden hamsters. *Mol Nutr Food Res* 60 (10):2151–2160.

Magnussen, E. B., L. J. Vatten, K. Myklestad, K. A. Salvesen, and P. R. Romundstad. 2011. Cardiovascular risk factors prior to conception and the length of pregnancy: Population-based cohort study. *Am J Obstet Gynecol* 204 (6):526 e1–8.

Mannarino, E., M. Pirro, C. Cortese et al. 2009. Effects of a phytosterol-enriched dairy product on lipids, sterols and 8-isoprostane in hypercholesterolemic patients: A multicenter Italian study. *Nutr Metab Cardiovasc Dis* 19 (2):84–90.

Marcovecchio, M. L., P. H. Tossavainen, J. J. Heywood, R. N. Dalton, and D. B. Dunger. 2012. An independent effect of parental lipids on the offspring lipid levels in a cohort of adolescents with type 1 diabetes. *Pediatr Diabetes* 13 (6):463–9.

Marseille-Tremblay, C., M. Ethier-Chiasson, J. C. Forest et al. 2008. Impact of maternal circulating cholesterol and gestational diabetes mellitus on lipid metabolism in human term placenta. *Mol Reprod Dev* 75 (6):1054–62.

Maymunah, A. O., O. Kehinde, G. Abidoye, and A. Oluwatosin. 2014. Hypercholesterolaemia in pregnancy as a predictor of adverse pregnancy outcome. *Afr Health Sci* 14 (4):967–73.

McConihay, J. A., P. S. Horn, and L. A. Woollett. 2001. Effect of maternal hypercholesterolemia on fetal sterol metabolism in the Golden Syrian hamster. *J Lipid Res* 42 (7):1111–9.

McGill, H. C., Jr., C. A. McMahan, E. E. Herderick et al. 2000. Origin of atherosclerosis in childhood and adolescence. *Am J Clin Nutr* 72 (5 Suppl):1307S–1315S.

Mellies, M. J., T. T. Ishikawa, P. S. Gartside et al. 1979. Effects of varying maternal dietary fatty acids in lactating women and their infants. *Am J Clin Nutr* 32 (2):299–303.

Mendelson, M. M., A. Lyass, C. J. O'Donnell et al. 2016. Association of maternal prepregnancy dyslipidemia with adult offspring dyslipidemia in excess of anthropometric, lifestyle, and genetic factors in the framingham heart study. *JAMA Cardiology* 1 (1):26–35.

Meyer, B. J., F. M. Stewart, E. A. Brown et al. 2013. Maternal obesity is associated with the formation of small dense LDL and hypoadiponectinemia in the third trimester. *J Clin Endocrinol Metab* 98 (2):643–52.

Moghadasian, M. H., L. B. Nguyen, S. Shefer et al. 2001. Hepatic cholesterol and bile acid synthesis, low-density lipoprotein receptor function, and plasma and fecal sterol levels in mice: Effects of apolipoprotein E deficiency and probucol or phytosterol treatment. *Metabolism* 50 (6):708–14.

Montes, A., C. E. Walden, R. H. Knopp et al. 1984. Physiologic and supraphysiologic increases in lipoprotein lipids and apoproteins in late pregnancy and postpartum. Possible markers for the diagnosis of "prelipemia". *Arteriosclerosis* 4 (4):407–17.

Morrison, K. M., S. S. Anand, S. Yusuf et al. 2013. Maternal and pregnancy related predictors of cardiometabolic traits in newborns. *PLoS One* 8 (2):e55815.

Napoli, C., F. P. D'Armiento, F. P. Mancini et al. 1997. Fatty streak formation occurs in human fetal aortas and is greatly enhanced by maternal hypercholesterolemia. Intimal accumulation of low density lipoprotein and its oxidation precede monocyte recruitment into early atherosclerotic lesions. *J Clin Invest* 100 (11):2680–90.

Napoli, C., C. K. Glass, J. L. Witztum et al. 1999. Influence of maternal hypercholesterolaemia during pregnancy on progression of early atherosclerotic lesions in childhood: Fate of Early Lesions in Children (FELIC) study. *Lancet* 354 (9186):1234–41.

Narverud, I., J. R. van Lennep, J. J. Christensen et al. 2015. Maternal inheritance does not predict cholesterol levels in children with familial hypercholesterolemia. *Atherosclerosis* 243 (1):155–60.

Palinski, W., F. P. D'Armiento, J. L. Witztum et al. 2001. Maternal hypercholesterolemia and treatment during pregnancy influence the long-term progression of atherosclerosis in offspring of rabbits. *Circ Res* 89 (11):991–6.

Palinski, W. and C. Napoli. 2002. The fetal origins of atherosclerosis: Maternal hypercholesterolemia, and cholesterol-lowering or antioxidant treatment during pregnancy influence in utero programming and postnatal susceptibility to atherogenesis. *FASEB J* 16 (11):1348–60.

Pashaj, A., M. Xia, and R. Moreau. 2015. Alpha-lipoic acid as a triglyceride-lowering nutraceutical. *Can J Physiol Pharmacol* 93 (12):1029–41.

Pawar, R. S. and E. Grundel. 2016. Overview of regulation of dietary supplements in the USA and issues of adulteration with phenethylamines (PEAs). *Drug Test Anal*.

Petchetti, L., W. H. Frishman, R. Petrillo, and K. Raju. 2007. Nutriceuticals in cardiovascular disease: Psyllium. *Cardiol Rev* 15 (3):116–22.

Phan, B. A. and P. P. Toth. 2014. Dyslipidemia in women: Etiology and management. *Int J Womens Health* 6:185–94.

Plat, J., J. A. Nichols, and R. P. Mensink. 2005. Plant sterols and stanols: Effects on mixed micellar composition and LXR (target gene) activation. *J Lipid Res* 46 (11):2468–76.

Porkka, K. V., J. S. Viikari, S. Taimela, M. Dahl, and H. K. Akerblom. 1994. Tracking and predictiveness of serum lipid and lipoprotein measurements in childhood: A 12-year follow-up. The Cardiovascular Risk in Young Finns study. *Am J Epidemiol* 140 (12):1096–110.

Ramos, M. P., M. D. Crespo-Solans, S. del Campo, J. Cacho, and E. Herrera. 2003. Fat accumulation in the rat during early pregnancy is modulated by enhanced insulin responsiveness. *Am J Physiol Endocrinol Metab* 285 (2):E318–28.

Retnakaran, R., Y. Qi, M. Sermer et al. 2011. The postpartum cardiovascular risk factor profile of women with isolated hyperglycemia at 1-hour on the oral glucose tolerance test in pregnancy. *Nutr Metab Cardiovasc Dis* 21 (9):706–12.

Reynolds, C. M., S. A. Segovia, X. D. Zhang, C. Gray, and M. H. Vickers. 2015. Conjugated linoleic Acid supplementation during pregnancy and lactation reduces maternal high-fat-diet-induced programming of early-onset puberty and hyperlipidemia in female rat offspring. *Biol Reprod* 92 (2):40.

Rideout, T. C., S. V. Harding, P. J. Jones, and M. Z. Fan. 2008. Guar gum and similar soluble fibers in the regulation of cholesterol metabolism: Current understandings and future research priorities. *Vasc Health Risk Manag* 4 (5):1023–33.

Rideout, T. C., C. Movsesian, Y. T. Tsai et al. 2015. Maternal phytosterol supplementation during pregnancy and lactation modulates lipid and lipoprotein response in offspring of apoE-deficient mice. *J Nutr* 145 (8):1728–34.

Rizzo, M., K. Berneis, A. E. Altinova et al. 2008. Atherogenic lipoprotein phenotype and LDL size and subclasses in women with gestational diabetes. *Diabet Med* 25 (12):1406–11.

Romejko-Wolniewicz, E., Z. Lewandowski, J. Zareba-Szczudlik, and K. Czajkowski. 2014. BMI of the firstborn offspring at age 12 reflects maternal LDL and HDL cholesterol levels at term pregnancy and postpartum. *J Matern Fetal Neonatal Med* 27 (9):914–20.

Ryokkynen, A., U. R. Kayhko, A. M. Mustonen, J. V. Kukkonen, and P. Nieminen. 2005. Multigenerational exposure to phytosterols in the mouse. *Reprod Toxicol* 19 (4):535–40.

Rytter, D., E. B. Schmidt, B. H. Bech et al. 2011. Fish oil supplementation during late pregnancy does not influence plasma lipids or lipoprotein levels in young adult offspring. *Lipids* 46 (12):1091–9.

Sattar, N., I. A. Greer, J. Louden et al. 1997. Lipoprotein subfraction changes in normal pregnancy: Threshold effect of plasma triglyceride on appearance of small, dense low density lipoprotein. *J Clin Endocrinol Metab* 82 (8):2483–91.

Shomonov-Wagner, L., A. Raz, and A. Leikin-Frenkel. 2015. Alpha linolenic acid in maternal diet halts the lipid disarray due to saturated fatty acids in the liver of mice offspring at weaning. *Lipids Health Dis* 14:14.

Theuwissen, E., J. Plat, C. J. van der Kallen, M. M. van Greevenbroek, and R. P. Mensink. 2009. Plant stanol supplementation decreases serum triacylglycerols in subjects with overt hypertriglyceridemia. *Lipids* 44 (12):1131–40.

Trujillo, M. L., C. Spuch, E. Carro, and R. Senaris. 2011. Hyperphagia and central mechanisms for leptin resistance during pregnancy. *Endocrinology* 152 (4):1355–65.

van der Graaf, A., M. N. Vissers, D. Gaudet et al. 2010. Dyslipidemia of mothers with familial hypercholesterolemia deteriorates lipids in adult offspring. *Arterioscler Thromb Vasc Biol* 30 (12):2673–7.

Waalkens-Berendsen, D. H., A. P. Wolterbeek, M. V. Wijnands, M. Richold, and P. A. Hepburn. 1999. Safety evaluation of phytosterol esters. Part 3. Two-generation reproduction study in rats with phytosterol esters—a novel functional food. *Food Chem Toxicol* 37 (7):683–96.

Webber, L. S., S. R. Srinivasan, W. A. Wattigney, and G. S. Berenson. 1991. Tracking of serum lipids and lipoproteins from childhood to adulthood. The Bogalusa Heart Study. *Am J Epidemiol* 133 (9):884–99.

Whittaker, M. H., V. H. Frankos, A. P. Wolterbeek, and D. H. Waalkens-Berendsen. 1999. Two-generation reproductive toxicity study of plant stanol esters in rats. *Regul Toxicol Pharmacol* 29 (2 Pt 1):196–204.

Wild, R., E. A. Weedin, and D. Wilson. 2016. Dyslipidemia in pregnancy. *Endocrinol Metab Clin North Am* 45 (1):55–63.

Wiznitzer, A., A. Mayer, V. Novack et al. 2009. Association of lipid levels during gestation with preeclampsia and gestational diabetes mellitus: A population-based study. *Am J Obstet Gynecol* 201 (5):482 e1–8.

Wong, W. W., D. L. Hachey, W. Insull, A. R. Opekun, and P. D. Klein. 1993. Effect of dietary cholesterol on cholesterol synthesis in breast-fed and formula-fed infants. *J Lipid Res* 34 (8):1403–11.

Writing Group, Members, D. Mozaffarian, E. J. Benjamin et al. 2016. Heart disease and stroke statistics-2016 update: A report from the American Heart Association. *Circulation* 133 (4):e38–60.

Wu, Z., J. Zhao, H. Xu et al. 2014. Maternal quercetin administration during gestation and lactation decrease endoplasmic reticulum stress and related inflammation in the adult offspring of obese female rats. *Eur J Nutr* 53 (8):1669–83.

Xie, C. H., L. Zhang, B. H. Zeng et al. 2014. Hypercholesterolemia in pregnant mice increases the susceptibility to atherosclerosis in adult life. *Vascular* 22 (5):328–35.

Zambrano, E., C. Ibanez, P. M. Martinez-Samayoa et al. 2016. Maternal obesity: Lifelong metabolic outcomes for offspring from poor developmental trajectories during the perinatal period. *Arch Med Res* 47(1):1–12.

20 Role of Taurine in Developmental Programming of Metabolic Disease

Lea H. Larsen and Ole H. Mortensen

CONTENTS

20.1 AN INTRODUCTION TO TAURINE

Taurine (2-aminoethanesulfonic acid) is a semiessential sulfur-containing amino acid and taurine and its derivatives are the only biological sulfonic acids in mammals. Taurine is one of the four common sulfur-containing amino acids, with the others being methionine, cysteine, and homocysteine. However, in contrast to most other amino acids, taurine does not enter into protein synthesis but remains free intracellularly and is traditionally considered an inert molecule without any reactive groups. Taurine is found in large amounts in mammalian tissues (5–50 mM) and plasma (50–100 µM) (Han et al. 2006). Although the functions of taurine are not fully understood, it is thought to be implicated in a number of physiological functions, such as bile acid formation, intracellular osmolyte for volume regulation, mitochondrial transfer RNA (tRNA) conjugation, central nervous system function, cardiac function, retinal function, antioxidation, and reproduction (reviewed in Hansen 2001; Jacobsen and Smith 1968; Huxtable 1992; Lambert et al. 2015).

Taurine is thus not expected to be directly involved in metabolic pathways. Nevertheless, taurine deficiency in the cat results in a marked dysfunction of energy demanding tissues (Sturman 1993), and similar observations are seen in the taurine-transporter (TauT) knockout mouse (Warskulat et al. 2007). The biosynthetic capacity of taurine is low in humans, high in rodents, and completely absent in cats (Hansen 2001) and taurine deficiency in cats results in several severe pathologies such as degeneration of the retina and impaired reproduction, as well as dysfunction of heart and skeletal muscle (Sturman 1993). The liver is the main site for degradation of sulfur-containing amino acids, and therefore also the organ responsible for the main export of taurine via plasma to other tissues. However, enzymes involved in taurine synthesis (e.g., degradation of sulfur-containing amino acids) have been found in many other tissues such as kidney, brain, heart, skeletal muscle, lung, and adipose tissue (Stipanuk 2004; Dominy et al. 2008; Stipanuk et al. 2009) and if taurine synthesis is blocked in the liver, extrahepatic tissues will upregulate their taurine synthesis (Ueki et al. 2012).

Taurine, which was originally isolated from ox bile acid (bos taurus), accounts for approximately 0.1% of the total bodyweight in humans and most mammals (Huxtable 1992). Whole-body and intracellular taurine content is in equilibrium between the rate of *de novo* biosynthesis, kidney reabsorption, taurine transport, and taurine uptake from the diet (primarily meat and seafood) (Lambert 2004; Tappaz 2004; Spitze et al. 2003) and a high taurine intake will lead to taurine excretion in the urine to maintain homeostasis (Chesney et al. 1983). However, it is possible to increase the available taurine pool by a prolonged increased intake as shown, for example, in humans (Brøns et al. 2004). Taurine biosynthesis starts with oxidation of cysteine to cysteine sulfinate by cysteine dioxygenase (CDO) (Sakakibara et al. 1976). Hypotaurine is then produced by decarboxylation of cysteine sulfinate catalyzed by what is believed to be the rate-limiting enzyme cysteine sulfinic acid decarboxylase (CSAD) (de la Rosa and Stipanuk 1985) or by the newly discovered glutamate decarboxylase-like protein 1 (GADL1) (Liu et al. 2012), which is then oxidized to taurine, most likely in a spontaneous reaction (Ueki et al. 2012; Dominy et al. 2007). In a secondary pathway, hypotaurine is synthesized from oxidation of cysteamine (2-aminoethanethiol) by dioxygenase (ADO) (Dominy et al. 2007).

Taurine is transported into cells mainly by its primary transporter, the sodium-dependent TauT (Han et al. 2006), with a secondary transporter, proton-assisted amino acid transporter 1 (PAT1) (Roig-Pérez, Moretó, and Ferrer 2005), playing a minor role as exemplified by the more than 90% reduction in tissue taurine content in TauT$^{-/-}$ mice (Heller-Stilb et al. 2002; Warskulat et al. 2007). Interestingly, a defect in the renal reabsorption of taurine has been reported for the C57BL/6J mouse strain (Harris and Searle 1953), later characterized as a transporter defect (Chesney, Scriver, and Mohyuddin 1976; Mandla, Scriver, and Tenenhouse 1988; Rozen, Scriver, and Mohyuddin 1983). Hence, C57BL/6J mice may be more susceptible to the effects of a taurine-deficient diet and/or taurine supplementation and care should be taken when interpreting studies on taurine performed in C57BL/6J mice, especially regarding interpolation to other mammals.

20.2   TAURINE AND METABOLIC DISEASE

In 1935, Ackermann et al. demonstrated that taurine had a beneficial effect on glucose homeostasis in diabetic patients (Ackermann and Heinsen 1935) and in 1976 taurine was placed in the category of nutrients that play a role in type 2 diabetes and is stimulating for glycogenesis and glycolysis, as it demonstrates an insulin-like activity (Dokshina, Silaeva, and Lartsev 1976).

Several studies have observed that taurine homeostasis is dysregulated in individuals with diabetes. In type 1 diabetic patients, taurine excretion by the kidneys was increased (Mårtensson and Hermansson 1984). In both type 1 and type 2 diabetes patients, taurine plasma concentrations were decreased (De Luca et al. 2001a,b; Franconi et al. 1995). Furthermore, nondiabetic women, who had gestational diabetes during pregnancy, had lower plasma taurine concentrations several years after giving birth, indicating long-term changes in taurine homeostasis despite gestational diabetes recovery (Seghieri et al. 2007). However, the amount of epidemiological studies examining the effect of taurine intervention on glucose homeostasis in prediabetic patients or patients with full born diabetes are limited and better studies are needed. In animals, type 1 diabetes does not seem to alter taurine homeostasis, as taurine plasma concentration was unaffected in streptozotocin-induced type 1 diabetes in rats (Trachtman, Futterweit, and Sturman 1992). In a type 2 diabetes animal model, the Zucker fatty rat, taurine plasma concentration (Wijekoon et al. 2004), and kidney excretion (Williams et al. 2005) were both increased, whereas in the high-fructose-fed rat (another type 2 diabetes model), a decrease in plasma taurine concentration was reported (Nandhini, Thirunavukkarasu, and Anuradha 2005).

In terms of human intervention studies, some studies have reported a positive effect of taurine supplementation on plasma glucose in type 1 diabetes (Elizarova and Nedosugova 1996) as well as an improvement in insulin sensitivity in a lipid infusion model of insulin resistance (Xiao, Giacca, and Lewis 2008), whereas other studies have reported no effect of taurine supplementation on insulin secretion and insulin sensitivity in nondiabetic men (Brøns et al. 2004) as well as no effect on fasting plasma glucose, plasma insulin levels, or HbA1c in type 2 diabetes patients (Chauncey et al. 2003). The same conflicting results with regard to the antidiabetic effect of taurine supplementation are seen in animal models where taurine has been shown to ameliorate type 2 diabetes in both the high-fructose-fed rat (El Mesallamy et al. 2010; Nandhini, Thirunavukkarasu, and Anuradha 2005) and the Otsuka Long–Evans Tokushima Fatty rat (Harada et al. 2004; Nakaya et al. 2000) as well as prevent the high-fat diet-induced increase in body weight and fat mass in mice (Tsuboyama-Kasaoka et al. 2006). On the other hand, no effect of taurine supplementation was observed in the nonobese GK rats (Nishimura et al. 2002). However, taurine has been shown to protect against β-cell destruction, induced by streptozotocin in rodents, indicated by lower plasma glucose (Alvarado-Vásquez et al. 2003; Odetti et al. 2003; Di Leo et al. 2004; Song et al. 2003). A plasma glucose lowering effect of taurine has also been observed in several other type 1 diabetes models in both mice (Lim, Park, and Kim 1998), rats (Gavrovskaya et al. 2008), and rabbits (Tenner, Zhang, and Lombardini 2003).

The effect of taurine supplementation on metabolic disease may be related to a general mitochondrial protective effect (Han et al. 2004; Mulder and Ling 2009; Maechler et al. 2010), by remodeling of pancreatic islets (El Idrissi, Boukarrou, and L'Amoreaux 2009) or by the anti-inflammatory (Schuller-Levis and Park 2003) or chaperone (Ozcan et al. 2006) effects of taurine derivatives, taurine-chloramine, and taurine-conjugated bile acids, respectively.

20.3   TAURINE AND DEVELOPMENT

Taurine is considered an essential amino acid during development, as the endogenous synthesis of taurine is inadequate in the fetus (Hibbard et al. 1990) making the fetus dependent on the maternal taurine supply. Furthermore, animal studies suggest that taurine is a marker of fetal well-being (de Boo and Harding 2007), although excessive taurine intake during gestation may also have detrimental effects later in life for the offspring (Hultman et al. 2007). Human intrauterine growth-restricted (IUGR) fetuses exhibit a decreased plasma taurine content (Cetin et al. 1990; Economides et al. 1989), something which has also been seen in animal models of IUGR (Reusens et al. 1995; Wu et al. 1998), and maternal obesity as well as preeclampsia decrease taurine transport across the placenta (Desforges et al. 2013; Ditchfield et al. 2015). It has been reported that pre- and postnatal tissue development was incomplete in the fetus if maternal diet was taurine insufficient (Aerts and Van Assche 2002; Sturman and Messing 1991; Sturman 1993). High intracellular taurine levels are found specifically in the brain during fetal development as well as in newborns, and taurine is involved in the proliferation of cerebellar cells and necessary for neuron survival (Chen et al. 1998). In humans, a low plasma taurine concentration in the infant has been linked to detrimental mental development (Heird 2004; Wharton et al. 2004), something that has also been observed in animal studies (Sturman 1993). Furthermore, taurine supplementation in mice has shown that the exact timing of taurine supplementation during gestation can influence the learning ability of the offspring, with taurine sufficiency seemingly being most important during the perinatal and early postnatal period (Suge et al. 2007).

Interestingly, taurine deficiency during gestation results in a lower birth weight in cats (Sturman 1991) and rodents (Ejiri et al. 1987). As cats are completely dependent on taurine dietary intake they are good model systems for taurine deficiency, and in fact the result of taurine deficiency is very profound in this species. Thus, offspring of cats reared on a taurine-free diet exhibit profound developmental abnormalities, among these being smaller brain weight and abnormal hind leg development, as well as a degeneration or abnormal development of the retina and visual cortex (Sturman 1991). Furthermore, mice deficient in TauT show a smaller overall size, although no information about birth weight has been reported (Warskulat et al. 2007). TauT knockout mice also show defects in heart and skeletal muscle development (Ito et al. 2008; Warskulat et al. 2004) have decreased exercise capacity and smaller adult body size (Warskulat et al. 2007), as well as chronic liver disease (Warskulat et al. 2006), which may be attributed to mitochondrial defects. In addition to these findings, knock down of TauT caused retinal degeneration complemented by impaired reproductive potential (Heller-Stilb et al. 2002). It is possible that some of the detrimental effects seen in the TauT knockout mouse and to some extent in the cat are due to developmental taurine deficiency and that these may be corrected in adult life with an adequate taurine supply. However, the nature of the TauT knockout mouse and the difficulty in using the cat as an animal model make this difficult to examine. Other animal models, like the recently developed CDO (Ueki et al. 2011) and CSAD (Park et al. 2014) knockout mice where exogenous taurine can be supplied in adult life, may be more suitable for examination of these issues. Overall, these findings indicate that taurine sufficiency is important during development and that taurine and/or TauT deficiency can lead to adverse developmental programming in offspring, although it may be difficult to discriminate between real developmental effects of taurine insufficiency and the effects of a lifelong taurine insufficiency. Furthermore, maternal malnutrition leads to adverse developmental programming in various metabolically active tissues like pancreatic islets, liver, and skeletal muscle (Figure 20.1a), something that is believed to be ameliorated by gestational taurine supplementation (Figure 20.1b).

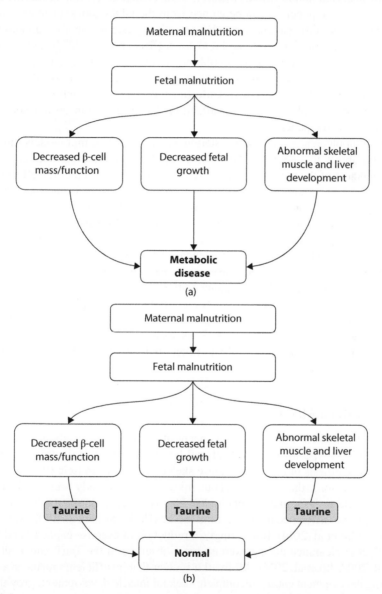

FIGURE 20.1   A depiction of the areas of developmental programming of metabolic disease affected by maternal taurine supplementation. (a) The situation that caused abnormal developmental programming was due to gestational protein restriction. (b) The rescuing effect of taurine on (a) results in normal offspring.

20.3.1 PANCREATIC ISLETS

Although not much research has been done on the effects of taurine insufficiency during gestation on pancreatic function, a lot of studies have focused on the rescuing effect of taurine supplementation during gestation upon adverse fetal programming caused by maternal malnutrition. However, some evidence of a role of taurine in the development of the pancreas can be gained from the CDO knockout mouse, where it was observed that the pancreas may have a unique cysteine metabolism making it susceptible to decreases in cysteine breakdown (Roman et al. 2013). Furthermore, TauT knockout mice are more susceptible to streptozotocin-induced type 1 diabetes (Han et al. 2015) even though they display a higher glucose disposal rate under normal conditions (Ito et al. 2015). Unfortunately, there is a lack of experiments examining the sole role of taurine availability during gestation on developmental programming of the pancreas.

Taurine supplementation during gestation has in several animal models showed a remarkable ability to ameliorate the detrimental effects of maternal malnutrition on the development of the pancreas and on β-cell function, but whether the effect is due to a normalization of taurine levels or other properties of taurine is unclear. Maternal taurine supplementation is as such able to restore normal proliferation and apoptosis as well as vascularization and sensitivity to nitric oxide (NO) and interleukin (IL)-1β of rat islets in a gestational protein restriction model of adverse developmental programming (Boujendar et al. 2002; Boujendar et al. 2003). Furthermore, the gestational protein restriction induced sensitivity of islets toward cytokines and NO was normalized by maternal taurine supplementation (Merezak et al. 2001, 2004). In the context of gestational protein restriction, maternal taurine supplementation seemed to be able to rescue the changes in islet gene expression, which was primarily found to be changes in mitochondrial genes (Reusens et al. 2008) and it was later found that taurine restored both structural and functional changes in the mitochondria of β-cells (Lee et al. 2011).

20.3.2 SKELETAL MUSCLE

In the TauT knockout mice, taurine concentrations decrease to about 1–2% compared with wild-type mice in skeletal and heart muscle. Overall, this indicates a very low biosynthesis of taurine in mouse skeletal and heart muscle (Ito et al. 2008, 2014). Furthermore, the TauT knockout mice had lower body weight, decreased skeletal muscle growth, and morphological abnormalities compared with wild-type mice, despite no difference in overall food intake (Heller-Stilb et al. 2002; Warskulat et al. 2004; Ito et al. 2014). Interestingly, a reduction in exercise capacity and faster blood glucose clearance during exercise were observed in the TauT knockout mice (Ito et al. 2008; Ito et al. 2014). All in all it is clear that insufficient taurine availability during development causes incomplete skeletal muscle development, growth, and exercise ability in adulthood. However, whether or not these changes are solely due to a developmental effect caused by taurine deficiency remains to be examined, but some indirect evidence comes from the observation that taurine treatment seems to increase differentiation of myoblasts into myotubes (Miyazaki et al. 2013).

Taurine supplementation during gestation has been shown to be able to partly rescue the changes in gene expression caused by gestational protein restriction in mice and the genes rescued were primarily related to mitochondrial function (Mortensen et al. 2010). This suggests that the rescuing effect of taurine is not specific to the pancreas, something that may also be important in human development, as a reduced activity of the placental TauTs has been observed in low birth weight babies (Norberg, Powell, and Jansson 1998) as well as in obese mothers and mothers with preeclampsia (Ditchfield et al. 2015; Desforges et al. 2013).

20.3.3 LIVER

Taurine deficiency, as seen in the TauT knockout mouse, results in major hepatic dysfunctions and chronic liver disease due to unspecific hepatitis, liver fibrosis, and inflammation (Warskulat et al. 2006). As with both pancreas and skeletal muscle, the defect also seems to center around a mitochondrial dysfunction as liver mitochondria had a decreased respiratory control ratio (Warskulat et al. 2006). A taurine insufficiency-induced decrease in hepatic mitochondrial function was confirmed in the CDO knockout mouse that exhibited signs of a decreased electron transport chain capacity (Ueki et al. 2011). Interestingly, supplementation of taurine to adult CDO knockout mice did not rescue the phenotype suggesting that at least some of the effects were due to developmental effect caused by a lack of taurine (Ueki et al. 2011). However, no experiments with maternal taurine supplementation of CDO knockout mice have been reported.

Maternal taurine supplementation is able to rescue at least some of the detrimental effects of maternal malnutrition in several models of developmental programming. For example, in gestational protein restriction, maternal taurine supplementation rescued a large part of the changes in gene expression seen in newborn mice (Mortensen et al. 2010). Furthermore, maternal taurine supplementation was able to rescue the resulting offspring phenotype of both maternal obesity and the effect of a maternal high-fructose diet upon markers of inflammation and lipid metabolism in the liver (Li et al. 2013, 2015).

20.3.4 ADIPOSE TISSUE

Some evidence suggests that taurine may also be able to influence adipose tissue and obesity. In the CDO knockout mouse, a high-fat diet challenge resulted in a higher degree of obesity, but again, whether this is due to developmental programming is unknown. However, a study examining the effect of maternal taurine supplementation found that taurine supplementation alone could increase adiposity of the offspring in a gender-specific manner (Hultman et al. 2007) as well as induce insulin resistance.

20.4 TAURINE IN POSTNATAL NUTRITION

Taurine can also be considered an essential amino acid in newborns because the ability to synthesize taurine in newborns is limited and ingestion via lactation is mandatory. Taurine concentration is high in human and rat milk but much lower in (about 10% of human and rat) cow milk (Aerts and Van Assche 2002). Of interest, it should be noted that vegetarians have both lower plasma taurine levels (Laidlaw et al. 1988) and a lower taurine concentration in breast milk (Chesney et al. 1998). The total pool of taurine available is, as in adults, regulated by the kidney in newborns and excess taurine is excreted by the kidneys. However, some evidence suggests that kidney taurine reabsorption may be limited in early life (Chesney et al. 1998; Sturman 1993) making the adequacy of taurine content in breast milk as well as in infant formula even more important. The results of a low taurine intake during early life are so far unknown but from studies examining the main tissue uptake location of taurine supplied during lactation, it can be inferred that a taurine deficiency in early life may affect mainly energy demanding tissues like liver, brain, and muscle (Kuo and Stipanuk 1984; Sturman, Rassin, and Gaull 1977) and studies in adult cats have shown that taurine depletion results in severe cerebellar damage (Lu, Xu, and Sturman 1996).

20.5 CONCLUSIONS

There can be no doubt that taurine is important for correct development programming and the importance of further studying the effects of taurine deficiency as well as taurine supplementation on development is corroborated by observations that vegetarians have decreased taurine plasma levels and also possible tissue levels (Laidlaw et al. 1988; Chesney et al. 1998). Due to societal pressure toward more sustainable food sources (e.g., plant based instead of animal based), we may inadvertently subject more fetuses to a developmental environment low in taurine. The long-term effects of this on metabolic health of the offspring are unknown but simply supplementing all pregnant women with taurine may not be beneficial, as taurine excess during pregnancy also seems to have detrimental effects (Hultman et al. 2007).

REFERENCES

Ackermann, D and H A Heinsen. 1935. Über die physiologische wirkung des asterubins und anderer, zum teil neu dargestellter schwelfelhaltiger guanidinderivate. *Hoppe Seyles Z Physiol Chemie* 235:115–21.

Aerts, L and F A Van Assche. 2002. Taurine and taurine-deficiency in the perinatal period. *Journal of Perinatal Medicine* 30 (4): 281–86. doi:10.1515/JPM.2002.040.

Alvarado-Vásquez, N, P Zamudio, E Cerón, B Vanda, E Zenteno, and G Carvajal-Sandoval. 2003. Effect of glycine in streptozotocin-induced diabetic rats. *Comparative Biochemistry and Physiology. Toxicology & Pharmacology: CBP* 134 (4): 521–27.

Boujendar, S, E Arany, D Hill, C Remacle, and B Reusens. 2003. Taurine supplementation of a low protein diet fed to rat dams normalizes the vascularization of the fetal endocrine pancreas. *Journal of Nutrition* 133 (9): 2820–25.

Boujendar, S, B Reusens, S Merezak, M T Ahn, E Arany, D Hill, and C Remacle. 2002. Taurine supplementation to a low protein diet during foetal and early postnatal life restores a normal proliferation and apoptosis of rat pancreatic islets. *Diabetologia* 45 (6): 856–66.

Brøns, C, C Spohr, H Storgaard, J Dyerberg, and A Vaag. 2004. Effect of taurine treatment on insulin secretion and action, and on serum lipid levels in overweight men with a genetic predisposition for type II diabetes mellitus. *European Journal of Clinical Nutrition* 58 (9): 1239–47. doi:10.1038/sj.ejcn.1601955.

Cetin, I, C Corbetta, L P Sereni, A M Marconi, P Bozzetti, G Pardi, and F C Battaglia. 1990. Umbilical amino acid concentrations in normal and growth-retarded fetuses sampled in utero by cordocentesis. *American Journal of Obstetrics and Gynecology* 162 (1): 253–61.

Chauncey, K B, T E Tenner, J B Lombardini, B G Jones, M L Brooks, R D Warner, R L Davis, and R M Ragain. 2003. The effect of taurine supplementation on patients with type 2 diabetes mellitus. *Advances in Experimental Medicine and Biology* 526:91–6.

Chen, X C, Z L Pan, D S Liu, and X. Han. 1998. Effect of taurine on human fetal neuron cells: Proliferation and differentiation. *Advances in Experimental Medicine and Biology* 442:397–403.

Chesney, R W, N Gusowski, and A L Friedman. 1983. Renal adaptation to altered dietary sulfur amino acid intake occurs at luminal brushborder membrane. *Kidney International* 24 (5): 588–94.

Chesney, R W, R A Helms, M Christensen, A M Budreau, X Han, and J A. Sturman. 1998. The role of taurine in infant nutrition. *Advances in Experimental Medicine and Biology* 442:463–76.

Chesney, R W, C R Scriver, and F Mohyuddin. 1976. Localization of the membrane defect in transepithelial transport of taurine by parallel studies in vivo and in vitro in hypertaurinuric mice. *Journal of Clinical Investigation* 57 (1): 183–93. doi:10.1172/JCI108258.

de Boo, H A and J E Harding. 2007. Taurine as a marker for foetal wellbeing? *Neonatology* 91 (3): 145–54.

de la Rosa, J and M H Stipanuk. 1985. Evidence for a rate-limiting role of cysteinesulfinate decarboxylase activity in taurine biosynthesis in vivo. *Comparative Biochemistry and Physiology. B, Comparative Biochemistry* 81 (3): 565–71.

De Luca, G, P R Calpona, A Caponetti, V Macaione, A Di Benedetto, D Cucinotta, and R M Di Giorgio. 2001a. Preliminary report: Amino acid profile in platelets of diabetic patients. *Metabolism: Clinical and Experimental* 50 (7): 739–41. doi:10.1053/meta.2001.24193.

De Luca, G, P R Calpona, A Caponetti, G Romano, A Di Benedetto, D Cucinotta, and R M Di Giorgio. 2001b. Taurine and osmoregulation: Platelet taurine content, uptake, and release in type 2 diabetic patients. *Metabolism: Clinical and Experimental* 50 (1): 60–4. doi:10.1053/meta.2001.19432.

Desforges, M, A Ditchfield, C R Hirst, C Pegorie, K Martyn-Smith, C P Sibley, and S L Greenwood. 2013. Reduced placental taurine transporter (TauT) activity in pregnancies complicated by pre-eclampsia and maternal obesity. *Advances in Experimental Medicine and Biology* 776:81–91. doi:10.1007/978-1-4614-6093-0_9.

Di Leo, M A S, S A Santini, N Gentiloni Silveri, B Giardina, F Franconi, and G Ghirlanda. 2004. Long-term taurine supplementation reduces mortality rate in streptozotocin-induced diabetic rats. *Amino Acids* 27 (2): 187–91. doi:10.1007/s00726-004-0108-2.

Ditchfield, A M, M Desforges, T A Mills, J D Glazier, M Wareing, K Mynett, C P Sibley, and S L Greenwood. 2015. Maternal obesity is associated with a reduction in placental taurine transporter activity. *International Journal of Obesity* 39 (4): 557–64. doi:10.1038/ijo.2014.212.

Dokshina, G A, T Iu Silaeva, and E I Lartsev. 1976. [Insulin-like effects of taurine]. *Voprosy Meditsinskoĭ Khimii* 22 (4): 503–7.

Dominy, J E, J Hwang, S Guo, L L Hirschberger, S Zhang, and M H Stipanuk. 2008. Synthesis of amino acid cofactor in cysteine dioxygenase is regulated by substrate and represents a novel post-translational regulation of activity. *Journal of Biological Chemistry* 283 (18): 12188–201. doi:10.1074/jbc.M800044200.

Dominy, J E, C R Simmons, L L Hirschberger, J Hwang, R M Coloso, and M H Stipanuk. 2007. Discovery and characterization of a second mammalian thiol dioxygenase, cysteamine dioxygenase. *Journal of Biological Chemistry* 282 (35): 25189–98. doi:10.1074/jbc.M703089200.

Economides, D L, K H Nicolaides, W A Gahl, I Bernardini, and M I Evans. 1989. Plasma amino acids in appropriate- and small-for-gestational-age fetuses. *American Journal of Obstetrics and Gynecology* 161 (5): 1219–27.

Ejiri, K, S Akahori, K Kudo, K Sekiba, and T Ubuka. 1987. Effect of guanidinoethyl sulfonate on taurine concentrations and fetal growth in pregnant rats. *Biology of the Neonate* 51 (4): 234–40.

El Idrissi, A, L Boukarrou, and W L'Amoreaux. 2009. Taurine supplementation and pancreatic remodeling. *Advances in Experimental Medicine and Biology* 643:353–8.

El Mesallamy, H O, E El-Demerdash, L N Hammad, and H M El Magdoub. 2010. Effect of taurine supplementation on hyperhomocysteinemia and markers of oxidative stress in high fructose diet induced insulin resistance. *Diabetology & Metabolic Syndrome* 2: 46. doi:10.1186/1758-5996-2-46.

Elizarova, E P and L V Nedosugova. 1996. First experiments in taurine administration for diabetes mellitus. The effect on erythrocyte membranes. *Advances in Experimental Medicine and Biology* 403:583–8.

Franconi, F, F Bennardini, A Mattana, M Miceli, M Ciuti, M Mian, A Gironi, R Anichini, and G Seghieri. 1995. Plasma and platelet taurine are reduced in subjects with insulin-dependent diabetes mellitus: Effects of taurine supplementation. *American Journal of Clinical Nutrition* 61 (5): 1115–9.

Gavrovskaya, L K, O V Ryzhova, A F Safonova, A K Matveev, and N S Sapronov. 2008. Protective effect of taurine on rats with experimental insulin-dependent diabetes mellitus. *Bulletin of Experimental Biology and Medicine* 146 (2): 226–8.

Han, J, J H Bae, S Y Kim, H Y Lee, B C Jang, I K Lee, C H Cho et al. 2004. Taurine increases glucose sensitivity of UCP2-overexpressing beta-cells by ameliorating mitochondrial metabolism. *American Journal of Physiology. Endocrinology and Metabolism* 287 (5): E1008–18. doi:10.1152/ajpendo.00008.2004.

Han, X, A B Patters, T Ito, J Azuma, S W Schaffer, and R W Chesney. 2015. Knockout of the TauT gene predisposes C57BL/6 mice to streptozotocin-induced diabetic nephropathy. *PLoS One* 10 (1): e0117718. doi:10.1371/journal.pone.0117718.

Han, X, A B Patters, D P Jones, I Zelikovic, and R W Chesney. 2006. The taurine transporter: Mechanisms of regulation. *Acta Physiologica* 187 (1–2): 61–73. doi:APS1573.

Hansen, S H. 2001. The role of taurine in diabetes and the development of diabetic complications. *Diabetes/Metabolism Research and Reviews* 17 (5): 330–46.

Harada, N, C Ninomiya, Y Osako, M Morishima, K Mawatari, A Takahashi, and Y Nakaya. 2004. Taurine alters respiratory gas exchange and nutrient metabolism in type 2 diabetic rats. *Obesity Research* 12 (7): 1077–84. doi:10.1038/oby.2004.135.

Harris, H and A G Searle. 1953. Urinary amino-acids in mice of different genotypes. *Annals of Eugenics* 17 (3): 165–7.

Heird, W C. 2004. Taurine in neonatal nutrition—revisited. *Archives of Disease in Childhood. Fetal and Neonatal Edition* 89 (6): F473–4. doi:10.1136/adc.2004.055095.

Heller-Stilb, B, C van Roeyen, K Rascher, H G Hartwig, A Huth, M W Seeliger, U Warskulat, and D Häussinger. 2002. Disruption of the taurine transporter gene (Taut) leads to retinal degeneration in mice. *FASEB Journal: Official Publication of the Federation of American Societies for Experimental Biology* 16 (2): 231–3. doi:10.1096/fj.01-0691fje.

Hibbard, J U, G Pridjian, P F Whitington, and A H Moawad. 1990. Taurine transport in the in vitro perfused human placenta. *Pediatric Research* 27 (1): 80–4.

Hultman, K, C Alexanderson, L Mannerås, M Sandberg, A Holmäng, and T Jansson. 2007. Maternal taurine supplementation in the late pregnant rat stimulates postnatal growth and induces obesity and insulin resistance in adult offspring. *Journal of Physiology* 579 (Pt 3): 823–33. doi:10.1113/jphysiol.2006.124610.

Huxtable, R J. 1992. Physiological actions of taurine. *Physiological Reviews* 72 (1): 101–63.

Ito, T, Y Kimura, Y Uozumi, M Takai, S Muraoka, T Matsuda, K Ueki et al. 2008. Taurine depletion caused by knocking out the taurine transporter gene leads to cardiomyopathy with cardiac atrophy. *Journal of Molecular and Cellular Cardiology* 44 (5): 927–37. doi:10.1016/j.yjmcc.2008.03.001.

Ito, T, N Yoshikawa, T Inui, N Miyazaki, S W Schaffer, and J Azuma. 2014. Tissue depletion of taurine accelerates skeletal muscle senescence and leads to early death in mice. *PLoS One* 9 (9): e107409. doi:10.1371/journal.pone.0107409.

Ito, T, N Yoshikawa, H Ito, and S W Schaffer. 2015. Impact of taurine depletion on glucose control and insulin secretion in mice. *Journal of Pharmacological Sciences* 129 (1): 59–64. doi:10.1016/j.jphs.2015.08.007.

Ito, T, N Yoshikawa, S W Schaffer, and J Azuma. 2014. Tissue taurine depletion alters metabolic response to exercise and reduces running capacity in mice. *Journal of Amino Acids* 2014: 964680. doi:10.1155/2014/964680.

Jacobsen, J G and L H Smith. 1968. Biochemistry and physiology of taurine and taurine derivatives. *Physiological Reviews* 48 (2): 424–511.

Kuo, S.M and M H Stipanuk. 1984. Changes in cysteine dioxygenase and cysteinesulfinate decarboxylase activities and taurine levels in tissues of pregnant or lactating rat dams and their fetuses or pups. *Biology of the Neonate* 46 (5): 237–48.

Laidlaw, S A, T D Shultz, J T Cecchino, and J D Kopple. 1988. Plasma and urine taurine levels in vegans. *American Journal of Clinical Nutrition* 47 (4): 660–3.

Lambert, I.H, D M Kristensen, J B Holm, and O H Mortensen. 2015. Physiological role of taurine--from organism to organelle. *Acta Physiologica* 213 (1): 191–212. doi:10.1111/apha.12365.

Lambert, I H. 2004. Regulation of the cellular content of the organic osmolyte taurine in mammalian cells. *Neurochemical Research* 29 (1): 27–63.

Lee, Y Y, H J Lee, S S Lee, J S Koh, C J Jin, S H Park, K H Yi, K S Park, and H K Lee. 2011. Taurine supplementation restored the changes in pancreatic islet mitochondria in the fetal protein-malnourished rat. *British Journal of Nutrition* 106 (8): 1198–206. doi:10.1017/S0007114511001632.

Li, M, C M Reynolds, D M Sloboda, C Gray, and M H Vickers. 2015. Maternal taurine supplementation attenuates maternal fructose-induced metabolic and inflammatory dysregulation and partially reverses adverse metabolic programming in offspring. *Journal of Nutritional Biochemistry* 26 (3): 267–76. doi:10.1016/j.jnutbio.2014.10.015.

Li, M, C M Reynolds, D M Sloboda, C Gray, and M H Vickers. 2013. Effects of taurine supplementation on hepatic markers of inflammation and lipid metabolism in mothers and offspring in the setting of maternal obesity. *PLoS One* 8 (10): e76961. doi:10.1371/journal.pone.0076961.

Lim, E, S Park, and H Kim. 1998. Effect of taurine supplementation on the lipid peroxide formation and the activities of glutathione-related enzymes in the liver and islet of type I and II diabetic model mice. *Advances in Experimental Medicine and Biology* 442:99–103.

Liu, P, X Ge, H Ding, H Jiang, B M Christensen, and J Li. 2012. Role of glutamate decarboxylase-like protein 1 (GADL1) in taurine biosynthesis. *Journal of Biological Chemistry* 287 (49): 40898–906. doi:10.1074/jbc.M112.393728.

Lu, P, W Xu, and J A Sturman. 1996. Dietary beta-alanine results in taurine depletion and cerebellar damage in adult cats. *Journal of Neuroscience Research* 43 (1): 112–9. doi:10.1002/jnr.490430115.

Maechler, P, N Li, M Casimir, L Vetterli, F Frigerio, and T Brun. 2010. Role of mitochondria in beta-cell function and dysfunction. *Advances in Experimental Medicine and Biology* 654:193–216. doi:10.1007/978-90-481-3271-3_9.

Mandla, S, C R Scriver, and H S Tenenhouse. 1988. Decreased transport in renal basolateral membrane vesicles from hypertaurinuric mice. *American Journal of Physiology* 255 (1 Pt 2): F88–95.

Mårtensson, J and G Hermansson. 1984. Sulfur amino acid metabolism in juvenile-onset nonketotic and ketotic diabetic patients. *Metabolism: Clinical and Experimental* 33 (5): 425–8.

Merezak, S, A A Hardikar, C S Yajnik, C Remacle, and B Reusens. 2001. Intrauterine low protein diet increases fetal beta-cell sensitivity to NO and IL-1 beta: The protective role of taurine. *Journal of Endocrinology* 171 (2): 299–308.

Merezak, S, B Reusens, A Renard, K Goosse, L Kalbe, M T Ahn, J Tamarit-Rodriguez, and C Remacle. 2004. Effect of maternal low-protein diet and taurine on the vulnerability of adult wistar rat islets to cytokines. *Diabetologia* 47 (4): 669–75.

Miyazaki, T, A Honda, T Ikegami, and Y Matsuzaki. 2013. The role of taurine on skeletal muscle cell differentiation. *Advances in Experimental Medicine and Biology* 776:321–8. doi:10.1007/978-1-4614-6093-0_29.

Mortensen, O H, H L Olsen, L Frandsen, P E Nielsen, F C Nielsen, N Grunnet, and B Quistorff. 2010. Gestational protein restriction in mice has pronounced effects on gene expression in newborn offspring's liver and skeletal muscle; protective effect of taurine. *Pediatric Research* 67 (1): 47–53. doi:10.1203/PDR.0b013e3181c4735c.

Mulder, H and C Ling. 2009. Mitochondrial dysfunction in pancreatic beta-cells in type 2 diabetes. *Molecular and Cellular Endocrinology* 297 (1–2): 34–40. doi:10.1016/j.mce.2008.05.015.

Nakaya, Y, A Minami, N Harada, S Sakamoto, Y Niwa, and M Ohnaka. 2000. Taurine improves insulin sensitivity in the otsuka long-evans tokushima fatty rat, a model of spontaneous type 2 diabetes. *American Journal of Clinical Nutrition* 71 (1): 54–8.

Nandhini, A T A, V Thirunavukkarasu, and C V Anuradha. 2005. Taurine prevents collagen abnormalities in high fructose-fed rats. *Indian Journal of Medical Research* 122 (2): 171–7.

Nishimura, N, C Umeda, H Ona, and H Yokogoshi. 2002. The effect of taurine on plasma cholesterol concentration in genetic type 2 diabetic GK rats. *Journal of Nutritional Science and Vitaminology* 48 (6): 483–90.

Norberg, S, T L Powell, and T Jansson. 1998. Intrauterine growth restriction is associated with a reduced activity of placental taurine transporters. *Pediatric Research* 44 (2): 233–8.

Odetti, P, C Pesce, N Traverso, S Menini, E P Maineri, L Cosso, S Valentini et al. 2003. Comparative trial of N-acetyl-cysteine, taurine, and oxerutin on skin and kidney damage in long-term experimental diabetes. *Diabetes* 52 (2): 499–505.

Ozcan, U, E Yilmaz, L Ozcan, M Furuhashi, E Vaillancourt, R O Smith, C Z Görgün, and G S Hotamisligil. 2006. Chemical chaperones reduce ER stress and restore glucose homeostasis in a mouse model of type 2 diabetes. *Science* 313 (5790): 1137–40.

Park, E, S Y Park, C Dobkin, and G Schuller-Levis. 2014. Development of a novel cysteine sulfinic acid decarboxylase knockout mouse: Dietary taurine reduces neonatal mortality. *Journal of Amino Acids* 2014: 346809. doi:10.1155/2014/346809.

Reusens, B, S Dahri, A Snoech, N Bennis-Taleb, C Remacle, and J J Hoet. 1995. Long-term consequences of diabetes and its complications may have a fetal origin: Experimental and epidemiological evidence. *Nestle Nutrition Workshop Series* 35:187–98.

Reusens, B, T Sparre, L Kalbe, T Bouckenooghe, N Theys, M Kruhøffer, T F Orntoft, J Nerup, and C Remacle. 2008. The intrauterine metabolic environment modulates the gene expression pattern in fetal rat islets: Prevention by maternal taurine supplementation. *Diabetologia* 51 (5): 836–45. doi:10.1007/s00125-008-0956-5.

Roig-Pérez, S, M Moretó, and R Ferrer. 2005. Transepithelial taurine transport in caco-2 cell monolayers. *Journal of Membrane Biology* 204 (2): 85–92. doi:10.1007/s00232-005-0750-y.

Roman, H B, L L Hirschberger, J Krijt, A Valli, V Kožich, and M H Stipanuk. 2013. The cysteine dioxgenase knockout mouse: Altered cysteine metabolism in nonhepatic tissues leads to excess H2S/HS(-) production and evidence of pancreatic and lung toxicity. *Antioxidants & Redox Signaling* 19 (12): 1321–36. doi:10.1089/ars.2012.5010.

Rozen, R, C R Scriver, and F Mohyuddin. 1983. Hypertaurinuria in the C57BL/6J mouse: Altered transport at the renal basolateral membrane. *American Journal of Physiology* 244 (2): F150–5.

Sakakibara, S, K Yamaguchi, Y Hosokawa, N Kohashi, and I Ueda. 1976. Purification and some properties of rat liver cysteine oxidase (cysteine dioxygenase). *Biochimica Et Biophysica Acta* 422 (2): 273–9.

Schuller-Levis, G B, and E Park. 2003. Taurine: New implications for an old amino acid. *FEMS Microbiology Letters* 226 (2): 195–202.

Seghieri, G, F Tesi, L Bianchi, A Loizzo, G Saccomanni, G Ghirlanda, R Anichini, and F Franconi. 2007. Taurine in women with a history of gestational diabetes. *Diabetes Research and Clinical Practice* 76 (2): 187–92. doi:10.1016/j.diabres.2006.08.008.

Song, X D, C Z Chen, B Dong, Y Y Shi, W Zhang, L S Yan, and G A Luo. 2003. [Study on the intervening mechanism of taurine on streptozotocin-induced diabetic cataracts]. *Zhonghua Yan Ke Za Zhi] Chinese Journal of Ophthalmology* 39 (10): 605–9.

Spitze, A R, D L Wong, Q R Rogers, and A J Fascetti. 2003. Taurine concentrations in animal feed ingredients; cooking influences taurine content. *Journal of Animal Physiology and Animal Nutrition* 87 (7–8): 251–62.

Stipanuk, M H, I Ueki, J E Dominy, C R Simmons, and L L Hirschberger. 2009. Cysteine dioxygenase: A robust system for regulation of cellular cysteine levels. *Amino Acids* 37 (1): 55–63. doi:10.1007/s00726-008-0202-y.

Stipanuk, M H. 2004. Role of the liver in regulation of body cysteine and taurine levels: A brief review. *Neurochemical Research* 29 (1): 105–10.

Sturman, J A. 1991. Dietary taurine and feline reproduction and development. *Journal of Nutrition* 121 (Suppl 11): S166–70.

Sturman, J A. 1993. Taurine in development. *Physiological Reviews* 73 (1): 119–47.

Sturman, J A, and J M Messing. 1991. Dietary taurine content and feline reproduction and outcome. *Journal of Nutrition* 121 (8): 1195–203.

Sturman, J A, D K Rassin, and G E Gaull. 1977. Taurine in developing rat brain: Maternal-fetal transfer of [35 S] taurine and its fate in the neonate. *Journal of Neurochemistry* 28 (1): 31–9.

Suge, R, N Hosoe, M Furube, T Yamamoto, A Hirayama, S Hirano, and M Nomura. 2007. Specific timing of taurine supplementation affects learning ability in mice. *Life Sciences* 81 (15): 1228–34. doi:10.1016/j.lfs.2007.08.028.

Tappaz, M L. 2004. Taurine biosynthetic enzymes and taurine transporter: Molecular identification and regulations. *Neurochemical Research* 29 (1): 83–96. doi:14992266.

Tenner, T E, X J Zhang, and J B Lombardini. 2003. Hypoglycemic effects of taurine in the alloxan-treated rabbit, a model for type 1 diabetes. *Advances in Experimental Medicine and Biology* 526:97–104.

Trachtman, H, S Futterweit, and J A Sturman. 1992. Cerebral taurine transport is increased during streptozocin-induced diabetes in rats. *Diabetes* 41 (9): 1130–40.

Tsuboyama-Kasaoka, N, C Shozawa, K Sano, Y Kamei, S Kasaoka, Y Hosokawa, and O Ezaki. 2006. Taurine (2-aminoethanesulfonic acid) deficiency creates a vicious circle promoting obesity. *Endocrinology* 147 (7): 3276–84. doi:10.1210/en.2005-1007.

Ueki, I, H B Roman, L L Hirschberger, C Junior, and M H Stipanuk. 2012. Extrahepatic tissues compensate for loss of hepatic taurine synthesis in mice with liver-specific knockout of cysteine dioxygenase. *American Journal of Physiology. Endocrinology and Metabolism* 302 (10): E1292–9. doi:10.1152/ajpendo.00589.2011.

Ueki, I, H B Roman, A Valli, K Fieselmann, J Lam, R Peters, L L Hirschberger, and M H Stipanuk. 2011. Knockout of the murine cysteine dioxygenase gene results in severe impairment in ability to synthesize taurine and an increased catabolism of cysteine to hydrogen sulfide. *American Journal of Physiology. Endocrinology and Metabolism* 301 (4): E668–84. doi:10.1152/ajpendo.00151.2011.

Warskulat, U, E Borsch, R Reinehr, B Heller-Stilb, I Mönnighoff, D Buchczyk, M Donner et al. 2006. Chronic liver disease is triggered by taurine transporter knockout in the mouse. *FASEB Journal* 20 (3): 574–6. doi:10.1096/fj.05-5016fje.

Warskulat, U, U Flögel, C Jacoby, H G Hartwig, M Thewissen, M W Merx, A Molojavyi, B Heller-Stilb, J Schrader, and D Häussinger. 2004. Taurine transporter knockout depletes muscle taurine levels and results in severe skeletal muscle impairment but leaves cardiac function uncompromised. *FASEB Journal* 18 (3): 577–9. doi:10.1096/fj.03-0496fje.

Warskulat, U, B Heller-Stilb, E Oermann, K Zilles, H Haas, F Lang, and D Häussinger. 2007. Phenotype of the taurine transporter knockout mouse. *Methods in Enzymology* 428:439–58. doi:10.1016/S0076-6879(07)28025-5.

Wharton, B A, R Morley, E B Isaacs, T J Cole, and A Lucas. 2004. Low plasma taurine and later neurodevelopment. *Archives of Disease in Childhood. Fetal and Neonatal Edition* 89 (6): F497–8. doi:10.1136/adc.2003.048389.

Wijekoon, E P, C Skinner, M E Brosnan, and J T Brosnan. 2004. Amino acid metabolism in the zucker diabetic fatty rat: Effects of insulin resistance and of type 2 diabetes. *Canadian Journal of Physiology and Pharmacology* 82 (7): 506–14. doi:10.1139/y04-067.

Williams, R E, E M Lenz, J A Evans, I D Wilson, J H Granger, R S Plumb, and C L Stumpf. 2005. A combined (1)H NMR and HPLC-MS-based metabonomic study of urine from obese (Fa/fa) zucker and normal wistar-derived rats. *Journal of Pharmaceutical and Biomedical Analysis* 38 (3): 465–71. doi:10.1016/j.jpba.2005.01.013.

Wu, G, W G Pond, T Ott, and F W Bazer. 1998. Maternal dietary protein deficiency decreases amino acid concentrations in fetal plasma and allantoic fluid of pigs. *Journal of Nutrition* 128 (5): 894–902.

Xiao, C, A Giacca, and G F Lewis. 2008. Oral taurine but not N-acetylcysteine ameliorates NEFA-induced impairment in insulin sensitivity and beta cell function in obese and overweight, non-diabetic men. *Diabetologia* 51 (1): 139–46.

21 Maternal Obesity: Effects of Dietary and Exercise Interventions to Prevent Adverse Negative Outcomes

Elena Zambrano and
Guadalupe L. Rodríguez-González

CONTENTS

21.1 INTRODUCTION

Human and experimental animal models have shown an association between high maternal body mass index (BMI) and/or gestational weight gain (GWG) and disrupted childhood metabolism and cardiovascular function. There is a relationship between maternal obesity and developmental programing in offspring. Developmental programming is defined as the response to a specific challenge to the mammalian organism during a critical developmental time window that alters the trajectory of development with resulting effects on health that persist throughout life (Zambrano and Nathanielsz 2013). Several mechanisms act together to produce adverse health outcomes problems such as (1) changes in maternal metabolic hormones (Forhead and Fowden 2009; Nakae et al. 2001) (insulin and leptin) as well as steroid hormones (Bispham et al. 2003; Bondesson et al. 2015; Hiort 2013) (androgens, estrogens, and corticosterone) that play a key role in cell differentiation, proliferation, and apoptosis; (2) increase in oxidative stress (Luo et al. 2006) leading to cell damage components like proteins, lipids, and DNA; (3) impaired placental transfer of nutrients from mother to fetus; and (4) epigenetic alterations (Lane 2014; Perera and Herbstman 2011) such as DNA methylation, histone modification, chromatin packing, and microRNA expression that can alter gene expression. The demonstration of the role of these mechanisms in the developmental induction of noncommunicable diseases opens the possibility to develop effective interventions to prevent adverse negative outcomes and guide management in human pregnancy, and focus on promoting healthy lifestyle choices before and during pregnancy as well as during postnatal life to ameliorate maternal and offspring outcomes due to maternal obesity.

21.2 OBESITY

Obesity is the result of chronic positive energy imbalance and is characterized by excess white adipose tissue. As obesity develops, excess energy is stored in adipocytes as triacylglycerol leading to an increase in adipocyte size (hypertrophy); but if the capacity of the adipocytes is not enough to store surplus lipids, the pool of adipocytes increases through hyperplasia (Faust et al. 1978). The excess of lipids causes adipose tissue inflammation (de Ferranti and Mozaffarian 2008), ectopic lipid storage in the liver, muscle, and pancreas, and higher circulation levels in the blood (Faust et al. 1978). These metabolic abnormalities trigger insulin resistance, and insufficient insulin production, which may predispose to type 2 diabetes (de Ferranti and Mozaffarian 2008; Ozcan et al. 2004).

The recent rise in obesity rates is associated with the interaction between genes, physical activity, and changes in dietary habits. However, in women, independent of BMI, pregnancy is also a risk factor for obesity because usually the weight gained in pregnancy is not lost after delivery and women tend to gain more weight in additional pregnancies (Poston 2012). Obesity in pregnancy is associated with miscarriage, fetal congenital anomalies, thromboembolism, gestational diabetes, preeclampsia, dysfunctional labor, postpartum weight retention, stillbirth, and neonatal death (Nathanielsz et al. 2013; Zambrano et al. 2016). Human and experimental animal studies indicate that maternal obesity predisposes offspring to a wide variety of chronic, later life diseases through fetal programming including obesity, dyslipidemia, type 2 diabetes mellitus, and hypertension (Zambrano et al. 2016).

21.3 PREVENTION STRATEGIES

The prevalence of obesity, especially in women of child-bearing age, is a global health concern because it is recognized as a major complication in pregnant women with adverse fetal effects. Therefore, there is a clear need to develop prevention strategies to reduce adverse maternal–fetal outcomes. The World Health Organization (WHO) has identified women of reproductive age as a key group to target in obesity prevention, particularly through limiting weight gain in pregnancy and postpartum weight retention (Organization World Health 2008). Ideally, obese women should lose weight before conception but this goal is quite difficult to achieve. Bariatric surgery is an interventional strategy to reduce the weight of obese women; however, it is expensive and may have potential surgical complications (Catalano and Ehrenberg 2006). Currently, there is much interest to promote maternal weight loss before pregnancy through diet and/or exercise to reduce fetal exposure to an obesogenic maternal environment. The optimal timing and extent to which adverse effects of the maternal metabolic phenotype resulting from maternal obesity and associated high-calorie diets can be prevented and/or possibly reversed by these interventions remain unanswered questions of considerable physiological interest and importance in clinical obstetric management (Nathanielsz 2013). It is important to remember that poor maternal nutrition also programs adverse offspring outcomes (Armitage et al. 2004, 2005, 2008) and sudden and excessive restriction of maternal and fetal nutrient availability may introduce new dangers. Thus, when considering a specific intervention to benefit developmental programming outcomes, a distinction must always be made between interventions designed to prevent negative offspring outcomes and interventions conducted at later stages of an offspring's life to reverse adverse health outcomes. Thus, firm scientific data are needed to guide interventions because clearly prevention is a better strategy than to try to reverse problems.

21.4 NUTRITIONAL INTERVENTIONS

21.4.1 EPIDEMIOLOGICAL STUDIES

During pregnancy, the nutritional requirement is enhanced and women generally attend to this demand by increasing their food intake. However, cultural beliefs, such as "eating for two" may contribute to a caloric intake above the ordinary demands of pregnancy (Carruth and Skinner 1991; Clark and Ogden 1999). According to the Institute of Medicine (IOM) and based on BMI before conception, normal women (BMI: 18.5–24.9) during pregnancy are recommended to gain between 11.4 and 15.9 kg, overweight women (BMI: 25.0–29.9) between 6.8 and 11.4 kg, and obese women (BMI: $\geq$30) between 5.0 and 9.0 kg (Institute of Medicine of National Academies 2009) (Figure 21.1). Currently, in the United Kingdom, 20%–40% of women gain more than the recommended weight during pregnancy (Thangaratinam et al. 2012a). Excessive GWG is associated with postpartum weight retention and maternal health problems like risk of cardiovascular disease (Shah et al. 2008), type 2 diabetes (Hedderson et al. 2010), and obesity (Rooney et al. 2005). For the child, excessive GWG increases birth weight above 4 kg, which is associated with childhood obesity (Rooney et al. 2011; Wrotniak et al. 2008). It has been estimated that the risk of early childhood obesity increases by a factor of 1.08 per kilogram of maternal weight gained during pregnancy (Schack-Nielsen et al. 2010). One of the main environmental factors regulating fetal growth is maternal substrate delivery to the placenta, such as maternal blood glucose levels (McGowan and McAuliffe 2010; Walsh et al. 2011). Maternal diet and particularly the carbohydrate type and content influence maternal blood glucose concentrations. In a recent study, Huang et al. evaluated, in women with type 1 diabetes, the association of prepregnancy BMI and postpartum weight retention with hemoglobin A1c (HbA1c) levels. The authors reported that prepregnancy BMI and postpartum weight retention were positively associated HbA1c during the first postpartum (Huang et al. 2015). A randomized

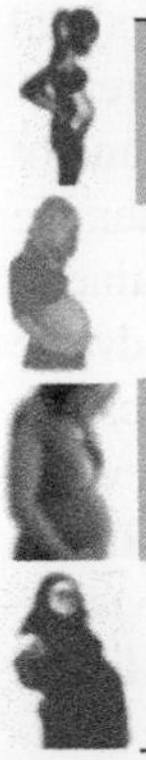

Prepregnancy	BMI (km/m²) (WHO)	Total weight gain range		Rates of weight gain 2nd and 3rd trimester mean (range)	
		kg	lbs	kg/week	lbs/week
Underweight	<18.5	12.5–18	28–40	0.51 (0.44–0.58)	1 (1–1.3)
Normal weight	18.5–24.9	11.5–16	25–35	0.42 (0.35–0.50)	1 (0.8–1)
Overweight	25.0–29–9	7–11.5	15–25	0.28 (0.23–0.33)	0.6 (0.5–0.7)
Obese (includes all classes)	≥30.0	5–9	11–20	0.22 (0.17–0.27)	0.5 (0.4–0.6)

FIGURE 21.1 Recommendations for total and rate of weight gain during pregnancy, by prepregnancy body mass index (BMI). *Note*: Calculations assume a 0.5–2 kg (1.1–4.4 lb) weight gain in the first trimester. (Adapted from the Institute of Medicine of National Academies, *Weight Gain during Pregnancy: Reexamining the Guidelines*, National Academies Press, Washington, DC, 2009.)

controlled trial of a low glycemic index dietary intervention was carried out. Briefly, 800 women were randomized in early pregnancy to receive low glycemic index and healthy eating dietary advice or to receive standard maternity care. Dietary intervention in early pregnancy has a positive influence on maternal glycemic index, food and nutrient intake, and GWG (McGowan et al. 2013). In a study performed in Ireland, women were randomly divided into two groups to receive either a low glycemic index diet or dietary intervention from early pregnancy to term. Neonates whose mothers were on a low glycemic index diet during pregnancy had lower thigh circumference in comparison with the control diet (Donnelly et al. 2015). Also, a low glycemic index diet in pregnant women improves maternal glycemia and reduces infant birth weight (McGowan et al. 2013). In a systematic review involving women of all BMI, it was suggested that dietary intervention is associated with a modest reduction in GWG (Thangaratinam et al. 2012b). In another systematic review, the evidence on dietary and lifestyle interventions to reduce or prevent weight gain of obese pregnant woman was evaluated. By analyzing 30 randomized studies, the authors reported that the reduction in GWG was largest in the dietary intervention group. In addition, in a total of 29 randomized trials, the effects of interventions in pregnancy on obstetric outcomes was also evaluated and the review reported that dietary interventions in pregnancy resulted in a significant decrease in preeclampsia and gestational hypertension and that dietary intervention also resulted in a significant reduction in preterm births and toward a reduction in the incidence of gestational diabetes (Thangaratinam et al. 2012a). Other reviews have tried to summarize the available evidence of maternal obesity interventions (Dodd et al. 2010, 2014; Skouteris et al. 2010); however, the reviews have shown some inconsistent results, which has made it difficult to identify effective strategies to prevent excessive GWG among normal weight and obese women. Birth and neonatal outcomes are less certain (Thangaratinam et al. 2012a, b; Dodd et al. 2014).

Additionally, supplements to a healthy diet during pregnancy are recommended. There is significant scientific evidence to support the requirement for maternal vitamin D sufficiency in pregnancy to ensure normal development of the fetal brain (Lapillonne 2010). There is a greater risk of vitamin D deficiency in obese pregnant women and their children compared with pregnant women with normal BMI (Holick 2007; Bodnar et al. 2007). The effect of long-chain polyunsaturated fatty acids (LC-PUFAs) supplementation has also been evaluated during pregnancy, specifically n–3 (omega-3), which is derived from fish oils and has been shown to exhibit anti-inflammatory effects (Simopoulos 2003). N–3 LC-PUFA supplementation in pregnancy or lactation has a beneficial impact on children's body composition. However, reports of outcomes of omega-3 fatty acids supplementation are controversial. Some studies suggest that high level of fish intake may decrease birth weight, and optimum levels of intake need to be established (Helland et al. 2008). Despite the beneficial effects of supplements, much caution and research are still needed before supplement interventions can be recommended in complicated pregnancies. Maternal obesity and weight gain during pregnancy and lactation influence microbiota composition and activity by affecting microbial diversity in the gut and breast milk. Such changes may be transferred to the offspring during delivery and also during lactation, affecting infant microbial colonization and immune system maturation (Garcia-Mantrana and Collado 2016). Recent scientific advances point to a gut microbiota dysbiosis, with a resulting low-grade inflammation as a contributing element, in obesity and its comorbidities (Isolauri et al. 2015). In a systematic review, the search in online databases of the terms "probiotics," "pregnancy," "maternal outcomes," and "metabolism" showed that the use of probiotics during pregnancy could significantly reduce maternal fasting glucose, incidence of gestational diabetes mellitus, and preeclampsia rates and levels of C-reactive protein. The authors concluded that probiotics could be a safe therapeutic tool for the prevention of pregnancy complications and adverse outcomes related to maternal metabolism (Lindsay et al. 2013). Further studies are needed among those at high risk of metabolic disorders, such as overweight and obese pregnant women (Figure 21.2).

21.4.2 ANIMAL STUDIES

There are many reasons why animal intervention studies are needed. Importantly, animal studies are much more controllable than human clinical interventions, which are the parallel human approach to hypothesis-driven animal research. In addition, a greater depth of mechanistic interrogation is possible resulting from tissue retrieval and multiple testing in animal studies and results are obtained much more quickly to guide management in human pregnancy. Reproducibility and independent confirmation, the indispensable requirements of scientific certainty, are also generally easier to achieve in animal studies (Nathanielsz et al. 2013; Zambrano et al. 2016). Rodents, ewe, and nonhuman primates are the major animal models used for maternal obesity and programming (Figure 21.3). However, reports of experimental interventions

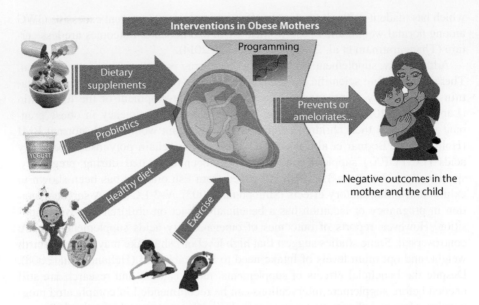

FIGURE 21.2   Types of maternal interventions to prevent the negative effects of programming.

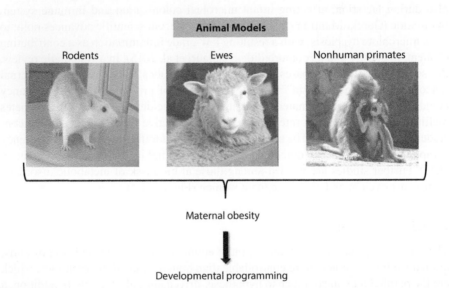

FIGURE 21.3   Animal models frequently used to study how maternal obesity programs development predispose offspring to later life chronic diseases.

in animal models in the setting of obesity are scarce. In a study, female rats aged 3 weeks underwent the following treatments: rats were fed with cafeteria diet over 34 weeks or rats ate cafeteria diet followed by a chow diet (26 and 8 weeks, respectively). Dietary change resulted in energy intake, body weight, visceral adipose tissue, and liver weight and insulin sensitivity similar to the control group (Goularte et al. 2012). These results may help to develop interventions before pregnancy to prevent the adverse outcomes due to maternal obesity in both the mother and the offspring. In the pregnant rat, we have conducted studies on maternal dietary intervention before and during pregnancy and have demonstrated that maternal dietary intervention 1 month before mating and during pregnancy and lactation partially prevents some of the negative biochemical and metabolic parameters observed in offspring from obese mothers (Zambrano et al. 2010). It is of interest that it was not necessary to return maternal weight to control levels for benefit to accrue. This study provides evidence that unwanted developmental programming effects on offspring that result from maternal obesity are at least partially prevented by dietary intervention prior to pregnancy (Nathanielsz et al. 2013; Zambrano et al. 2010). We have also evaluated the effects of maternal high-fat diet and dietary intervention at different periconceptional periods on male offspring anxiety-related behavior, exploration, learning, and motivation. Dietary intervention prevented the increased exploratory behavior displayed by offspring of obese mothers in the open field test. Additionally, dietary intervention restores normal levels of motivation (Rodriguez et al. 2012) (Figure 21.4). In the pregnant ewe fed an obesogenic diet, reduction on dietary intake (from 150% to 100% of the control diet), beginning on day 28 of gestation, was early enough to at least in part prevent some of the negative outcomes in the fetus such as fetal growth, adiposity, and glucose/insulin dynamics (Tuersunjiang et al. 2013). In the sheep, day 28 of gestation is equivalent to around

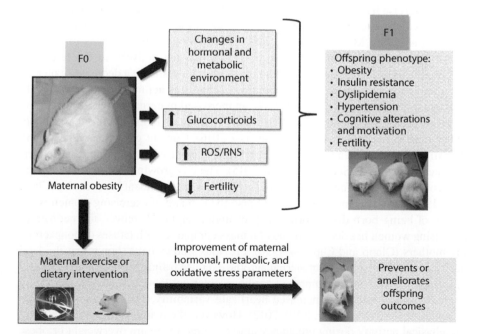

FIGURE 21.4 Programming mechanisms in a rodent model: maternal obesity and intervention effects.

day 50 in human pregnancy, which is about the time when women confirm they are pregnant and early enough to provide overweight/obese women with a dietary intervention if necessary (Nathanielsz et al. 2013). Resveratrol is a stilbenoid (natural phenol) naturally produced by the skin of red grapes (Segovia et al. 2014) and it has gained significant interest because it exerts a variety of pharmacological effects, such as anticancer and anti-inflammatory. Resveratrol also exerts a strong inhibitory effect on production of reactive oxygen species and free radical scavenging properties in many experimental systems (Vega et al. 2016). A recent study assessed the role of resveratrol supplementation during pregnancy in nonhuman primates. Briefly, mothers were fed a Western-style diet (36% fat) with or without resveratrol supplementation. Resveratrol improved placental inflammatory markers, maternal and fetal hepatic triglyceride accumulation, uterine blood flow, and insulin sensitivity. Resveratrol was detected in maternal plasma, demonstrating an ability to cross the placental barrier and exert effects on the fetus (Roberts et al. 2014).

21.5   EXERCISE INTERVENTIONS

21.5.1   Epidemiological Studies

Physical activity is defined as any voluntary movement produced by skeletal muscles that lead to energy expenditure. On the other hand, exercise is defined as a physical activity that is planned, structured, and repetitive whose objective is the improvement and/or maintenance of physical fitness (Caspersen et al. 1985). The effects of aerobic exercise have been long understood. However, the effects of exercise during pregnancy on the fetus and neonate are just beginning to be explored (Clapp 2003; Clapp et al. 1998; May et al. 2010, 2014). The hemodynamic changes of physical activity during pregnancy can cause decreased oxygen delivery to the fetus and potential fetal growth restriction. Although studies have shown a decrease in uterine circulation due to maternal exercise, many mechanisms act to maintain a relatively constant oxygen delivery to the fetus like an increased maternal hematocrit and oxygen transport in the blood, as well as a redistribution of blood flow to the placenta rather than to the uterus (Cid and Gonzalez 2016). Current guidelines recommend that all pregnant women without contraindications engage in ≥30 minutes of moderate-intensity exercise (Seneviratne et al. 2015). There is growing evidence that during maternal exercise the fetus is not at risk of hypoxia or significant bradycardia (Clapp et al. 1995, 2000; Kennelly et al. 2002); also the neonate of exercising women is not at risk of being born disproportionately or underweight. Moreover, the neonate of exercising women has decreased body fat mass compared with fetuses of nonexercising mothers (Clapp and Capeless 1990). Previous studies have shown that the fetal health adapts in response to maternal aerobic exercise training. For example, fetuses of exercising women had improved cardiovascular autonomic control indicated by decreased heart rates and increased heart rate variability (HRV), relative to those of nonexercisers (May et al. 2010, 2012). However, the available literature evaluating physical activity during pregnancy among women who are overweight or obese is more limited and contradictory. In a study conducted, 75 women aged 18–40 years with a BMI ≥ 25 kg/m² and a singleton pregnancy <20 weeks of gestation were randomized in the study (intervention $n = 38$, control $n = 37$). The intervention group participated in a structured home-based moderate-intensity antenatal exercise program utilizing magnetic stationary bicycles from 20 to 35 weeks of gestation. Participants received a written program prescribing frequency and duration of weekly exercises and were provided with heart rate monitors to wear only during all cycling sessions to maintain exercise sessions at moderate intensity (40%–59% VO_2 reserve). Each exercise session included a 5-minute warm-up and cool-down period at low intensity. A total of 67 sessions were prescribed. The authors reported that offspring birth weight and perinatal outcomes were similar between groups. Aerobic fitness improved in the intervention group compared with controls. There was no difference in weight gain, quality of life, pregnancy outcomes, or postnatal maternal body composition between groups (Seneviratne et al. 2016). In a systematic study, the authors reviewed the benefits and harms of an exercise intervention for pregnant women who are overweight or obese. The studies included were randomized controlled trials comparing supervised antenatal exercise intervention with routine standard antenatal care in women who were overweight or obese during pregnancy. The primary outcome was maternal GWG. Six randomized controlled trials and one quasirandomized trial were identified and included, involving a total of 276 women who were overweight or obese during pregnancy. The findings were that a supervised antenatal exercise intervention was associated with lower gestational weight when compared with standard antenatal care. So, monitored physical activity intervention appears to be successful in limiting GWG; however, the effect on maternal and infant health is less certain (Sui et al. 2012). In the pilot BAMBINO study, the authors investigated if exercise in obese pregnant women could reduce GWG and improve maternal circulating lipid profile, as well as alter leptin, interleukin-8 (IL-8), and monocyte chemoattractant protein-1 (MCP-1) levels. Obese pregnant women were recruited at 12 weeks of gestation and equally randomized to an exercise intervention or standard obstetric care until delivery. Women in the exercise intervention group received an individualized exercise plan based on personal preferences and ability, monthly face-to-face exercise advice by physiotherapists, and paper-based diaries for self-monitoring of activity. Blood samples, exercise diary, and pedometer data were obtained at 12, 20, 28, and 36 weeks of gestation. Cord blood was obtained at delivery. The low level of physical activity achieved in obese women in the exercise intervention group was insufficient to alter GWG, leptin, MCP-1, IL-8, or circulating lipid levels (Dekker Nitert et al. 2015). The cardiorespiratory responses and work efficiency of graded treadmill exercise in healthy nonpregnant, normal weight, and obese pregnant women were compared, to assess the effects of obesity on pregnant women at 16–20 weeks of gestation while exercising. The results showed that exercise duration and peak treadmill speed were lower in normal weight pregnant women than in nonpregnant women and were further reduced in pregnant obese women, which indicates a limitation to performing exercise. Resting heart rate and work rate were not significantly different between groups. The ventilatory response at both rest and exercise were more augmented in obese pregnant women. Thus, healthy obese pregnant women have the aerobic capacity to undertake structured walking activities (Mottola 2013). In a randomized controlled trial, a supervised exercise-based intervention to prevent excessive GWG was effective in normal weight women. However, there were no significant treatment effects in overweight or obese women (Ruiz et al. 2013). There are contradictory studies about the effects of physical activity during pregnancy in women who are overweight or obese. In a systematic review and meta-analysis of randomized controlled trials show that physical activity interventions were effective for overweight or obese pregnant, as well as postpartum women. Pregnant women in the intervention groups gained less weight and lost more body weight postpartum (Choi et al. 2013). On the other hand, insulin resistance and hyperglycemia are the main pathophysiological factors leading to gestational diabetes mellitus type 2 diabetes in pregnant women. Physical activity can help to prevent gestational diabetes mellitus by improving insulin sensitivity and excessive GWG, which, in turn, may help to prevent offspring postnatal complications, including childhood obesity and diabetes in adult life (Cid and Gonzalez 2016) (Figure 21.2).

21.5.2 Animal Studies

Physical exercise is recommended not only to assist weight loss and maintenance during the treatment of obesity but also to enhance whole-body insulin sensitivity and to improve the overall metabolic profile (Goularte et al. 2012). In experimental models, exercise has attenuated weight gain in rats fed a high-fat diet by reducing food intake (Wang et al. 2008). In a study conducted in female rats (aged 3 weeks), they were divided for the following treatments: rats were fed with cafeteria diet over 34 weeks or rats ate cafeteria diet plus physical exercise (starting at week 26 for 8 weeks). Physical exercise was able to improve insulin sensitivity even if obese rats were resistant to insulin and were eating the cafeteria diet (Goularte et al. 2012). Another study reported that exercise in pregnant mice fed a high-fat diet significantly reduced weight gain and fat mass and improved glucose tolerance and significantly increased insulin-stimulated phosphorylated Akt expression in adipose tissue. Voluntary exercise improves glucose homeostasis and body composition in pregnant female mice and points out the need of future studies to investigate the potential long-term health benefits in offspring born to obese exercising dams (Carter et al. 2015). In our group, we have recently reported the effects of an exercise intervention in obese rats before and during pregnancy on mothers. Exercise did not change maternal weight, but did completely prevent the rise in maternal triglycerides and partially the increases in glucose, insulin, cholesterol, leptin, fat, and oxidative stress. Exercise also recovered in female rats the decreased fertility induced by obesity (Vega et al. 2015) (Figure 21.4). Other studies in mice fed with a high-fat diet also demonstrated that maternal exercise before and during pregnancy has beneficial effects on the offspring metabolism and endocrine function (Laker et al. 2014).

However, if interventions cannot be applied in obese pregnant women, it is necessary to determine whether interventions in offspring are beneficial. One study aimed to investigate the effects of postweaning exercise in male offspring born from obese mothers and found that exercise reduced both adiposity and plasma leptin. In addition, the intracerebroventricular injection of leptin in the male pups suppressed food intake with a higher leptin-induced phospho-signal transducer and activator of transcription 3 (STAT3) level in the arcuate nucleus. Therefore, the authors concluded that although postweaning exercise provided no protection against gaining weight, it reduced adipose depots in the offspring born from obese mothers, which may have a relationship with improved central leptin sensitivity and changed hypothalamic neuropeptide expression (Sun et al. 2013). In our group, we have shown that maternal obesity in the rat increases both testicular and sperm oxidative stress, reduces sperm quality, and decreases fertility rate in rat offspring (Rodriguez-Gonzalez et al. 2015) and that physical voluntary exercise even in old male offspring of obese mothers has beneficial effects on adiposity index, gonadal fat, oxidative stress markers, sperm quality, and fertility. Thus, regular physical exercise in male offspring from obese mothers recuperates key male reproductive functions even at advanced age. The encouraging feature of these data is the indication that it is never too late for exercise to be beneficial (Santos et al. 2015).

21.6 CONCLUSION

Pregnancy seems to be a critical stage for the prevention of noncommunicable disease in future generations. Therefore, specific interventions during pregnancy provide a window of opportunity to promote the health not only of the mother but also of the child.

REFERENCES

Armitage J. A., Khan I. Y., Taylor P. D., Nathanielsz P. W., Poston L. Developmental programming of the metabolic syndrome by maternal nutritional imbalance: How strong is the evidence from experimental models in mammals?. *J Physiol* 561 Pt 2 (2004): 355–377.

Armitage J. A., Poston L., Taylor P. D. Developmental origins of obesity and the metabolic syndrome: The role of maternal obesity. *Front Horm Res* 36 (2008): 73–84.

Armitage J. A., Taylor P. D., Poston L. Experimental models of developmental programming: Consequences of exposure to an energy rich diet during development. *J Physiol* 565 Pt 1 (2005): 3–8.

Bispham J., Gopalakrishnan G. S., Dandrea J. et al. Maternal endocrine adaptation throughout pregnancy to nutritional manipulation: Consequences for maternal plasma leptin and cortisol and the programming of fetal adipose tissue development. *Endocrinology* 144 no. 8 (2003): 3575–3585.

Bodnar L. M., Catov J. M., Roberts J. M., Simhan H. N. Prepregnancy obesity predicts poor vitamin D status in mothers and their neonates. *J Nutr* 137 no. 11 (2007): 2437–2442.

Bondesson M., Hao R., Lin C. Y., Williams C., Gustafsson J. A. Estrogen receptor signaling during vertebrate development. *Biochim Biophys Acta* 1849 no. 2 (2015): 142–151.

Carruth B. R., Skinner J. D. Practitioners beware: Regional differences in beliefs about nutrition during pregnancy. *J Am Diet Assoc* 91 no. 4 (1991): 435–440.

Carter L. G., Ngo Tenlep S. Y., Woollett L. A., Pearson K. J. Exercise Improves glucose disposal and insulin signaling in pregnant mice fed a high fat diet. *J Diabetes Metab* 6 no. 12 (2015): pii: 634.

Caspersen C. J., Powell K. E., Christenson G. M. Physical activity, exercise, and physical fitness: Definitions and distinctions for health-related research. *Public Health Rep* 100 no. 2 (1985): 126–131.

Catalano P. M., Ehrenberg H. M. The short- and long-term implications of maternal obesity on the mother and her offspring. *BJOG* 113 no. 10 (2006): 1126–1133.

Choi J., Fukuoka Y., Lee J. H. The effects of physical activity and physical activity plus diet interventions on body weight in overweight or obese women who are pregnant or in postpartum: A systematic review and meta-analysis of randomized controlled trials. *Prev Med* 56 no. 6 (2013): 351–364.

Cid M., Gonzalez M. Potential benefits of physical activity during pregnancy for the reduction of gestational diabetes prevalence and oxidative stress. *Early Hum Dev* 94 no. (2016): 57–62.

Clapp J. F., 3rd. The effects of maternal exercise on fetal oxygenation and feto-placental growth. *Eur J Obstet Gynecol Reprod Biol* 110 no. Suppl 1 (2003): S80–85.

Clapp J. F., 3rd, Capeless E. L. Neonatal morphometrics after endurance exercise during pregnancy. *Am J Obstet Gynecol* 163 no. 6 Pt 1 (1990): 1805–1811.

Clapp J. F., 3rd, Little K. D., Appleby-Wineberg S. K., Widness J. A. The effect of regular maternal exercise on erythropoietin in cord blood and amniotic fluid. *Am J Obstet Gynecol* 172 no. 5 (1995): 1445–1451.

Clapp J. F., 3rd, Simonian S., Lopez B., Appleby-Wineberg S., Harcar-Sevcik R. The one-year morphometric and neurodevelopmental outcome of the offspring of women who continued to exercise regularly throughout pregnancy. *Am J Obstet Gynecol* 178 no. 3 (1998): 594–599.

Clapp J. F., 3rd, Stepanchak W., Tomaselli J., Kortan M., Faneslow S. Portal vein blood flow-effects of pregnancy, gravity, and exercise. *Am J Obstet Gynecol* 183 no. 1 (2000): 167–172.

Clark M., Ogden J. The impact of pregnancy on eating behaviour and aspects of weight concern. *Int J Obes Relat Metab Disord* 23 no. 1 (1999): 18–24.

de Ferranti S., Mozaffarian D. The perfect storm: Obesity, adipocyte dysfunction, and metabolic consequences. *Clin Chem* 54 no. 6 (2008): 945–955.

Dekker Nitert M., Barrett H. L., Denny K. J. et al. Exercise in pregnancy does not alter gestational weight gain, MCP-1 or leptin in obese women. *Aust N Z J Obstet Gynaecol* 55 no. 1 (2015): 27–33.

Dodd J. M., Grivell R. M., Crowther C. A., Robinson J. S. Antenatal interventions for overweight or obese pregnant women: A systematic review of randomised trials. *BJOG* 117 no. 11 (2010): 1316–1326.

Dodd J. M., McPhee A. J., Turnbull D. et al. The effects of antenatal dietary and lifestyle advice for women who are overweight or obese on neonatal health outcomes: The LIMIT randomised trial. *BMC Med* 12 (2014): 163.

Dodd J. M., Turnbull D., McPhee A. J. et al. Antenatal lifestyle advice for women who are overweight or obese: LIMIT randomised trial. *BMJ* 348 (2014): g1285.

Donnelly J. M., Walsh J. M., Byrne J., Molloy E. J., McAuliffe F. M. Impact of maternal diet on neonatal anthropometry: A randomized controlled trial. *Pediatr Obes* 10 no. 1 (2015): 52–56.

Faust I. M., Johnson P. R., Stern J. S., Hirsch J. Diet-induced adipocyte number increase in adult rats: A new model of obesity. *Am J Physiol* 235 no. 3 (1978): E279–286.

Forhead A. J., Fowden A. L. The hungry fetus? Role of leptin as a nutritional signal before birth. *J Physiol* 587 Pt 6 (2009): 1145–1152.

Garcia-Mantrana I., Collado M. C. Obesity and overweight: Impact on maternal and milk microbiome and their role for infant health and nutrition. *Mol Nutr Food Res* 60 no. 8 (2016): 1865–1875. doi:10.1002/mnfr.201501018.

Goularte J. F., Ferreira M. B., Sanvitto G. L. Effects of food pattern change and physical exercise on cafeteria diet-induced obesity in female rats. *Br J Nutr* 108 no. 8 (2012): 1511–1518.

Hedderson M. M., Gunderson E. P., Ferrara A. Gestational weight gain and risk of gestational diabetes mellitus. *Obstet Gynecol* 115 no. 3 (2010): 597–604.

Helland I. B., Smith L., Blomen B. et al. Effect of supplementing pregnant and lactating mothers with n-3 very-long-chain fatty acids on children's IQ and body mass index at 7 years of age. *Pediatrics* 122 no. 2 (2008): e472–479.

Hiort O. The differential role of androgens in early human sex development. *BMC Med* 11 (2013): 152.

Holick M. F. Vitamin D deficiency. *N Engl J Med* 357 no. 3 (2007): 266–281.

Huang T., Brown F. M., Curran A., James-Todd T. Association of pre-pregnancy BMI and post-partum weight retention with postpartum HbA1c among women with Type 1 diabetes. *Diabet Med* 32 no. 2 (2015): 181–188.

Institute of Medicine of National Academies. *Weight Gain During Pregnancy: Reexamining the Guidelines*, 2009. Washington, DC: The National Academies Press.

Isolauri E., Rautava S., Collado M. C., Salminen S. Role of probiotics in reducing the risk of gestational diabetes. *Diabetes Obes Metab* 17 no. 8 (2015): 713–719.

Kennelly M. M., McCaffrey N., McLoughlin P., Lyons S., McKenna P. Fetal heart rate response to strenuous maternal exercise: Not a predictor of fetal distress. *Am J Obstet Gynecol* 187 no. 3 (2002): 811–816.

Laker R. C., Lillard T. S., Okutsu M. et al. Exercise prevents maternal high-fat diet-induced hypermethylation of the Pgc-1alpha gene and age-dependent metabolic dysfunction in the offspring. *Diabetes* 63 no. 5 (2014): 1605–1611.

Lane R. H. Fetal programming, epigenetics, and adult onset disease. *Clin Perinatol* 41 no. 4 (2014): 815–831.

Lapillonne A. Vitamin D deficiency during pregnancy may impair maternal and fetal outcomes. *Med Hypotheses* 74 no. 1 (2010): 71–75.

Lindsay K. L., Walsh C. A., Brennan L., McAuliffe F. M. Probiotics in pregnancy and maternal outcomes: A systematic review. *J Matern Fetal Neonatal Med* 26 no. 8 (2013): 772–778.

Luo Z. C., Fraser W. D., Julien P. et al. Tracing the origins of "fetal origins" of adult diseases: Programming by oxidative stress? *Med Hypotheses* 66 no. 1 (2006): 38–44.

May L. E., Glaros A., Yeh H. W., Clapp J. F., 3rd, Gustafson K. M. Aerobic exercise during pregnancy influences fetal cardiac autonomic control of heart rate and heart rate variability. *Early Hum Dev* 86 no. 4 (2010): 213–217.

May L. E., Scholtz S. A., Suminski R., Gustafson K. M. Aerobic exercise during pregnancy influences infant heart rate variability at one month of age. *Early Hum Dev* 90 no. 1 (2014): 33–38.

May L. E., Suminski R. R., Langaker M. D., Yeh H. W., Gustafson K. M. Regular maternal exercise dose and fetal heart outcome. *Med Sci Sports Exerc* 44 no. 7 (2012): 1252–1258.

McGowan C. A., McAuliffe F. M. The influence of maternal glycaemia and dietary glycaemic index on pregnancy outcome in healthy mothers. *Br J Nutr* 104 no. 2 (2010): 153–159.

McGowan C. A., Walsh J. M., Byrne J., Curran S., McAuliffe F. M. The influence of a low glycemic index dietary intervention on maternal dietary intake, glycemic index and gestational weight gain during pregnancy: A randomized controlled trial. *Nutr J* 12 no. 1 (2013): 140.

Mottola M. F. Physical activity and maternal obesity: Cardiovascular adaptations, exercise recommendations, and pregnancy outcomes. *Nutr Rev* 71 no. Suppl 1 (2013): S31–36.

Nakae J., Kido Y., Accili D. Distinct and overlapping functions of insulin and IGF-I receptors. *Endocr Rev* 22 no. 6 (2001): 818–835.

Nathanielsz P. W., Ford S. P., Long N. M. et al. Interventions to prevent adverse fetal programming due to maternal obesity during pregnancy. *Nutr Rev* 71 no. Suppl 1 (2013): S78–87.

Organization World Health. *2008–2013 Action Plan for the Global Strategy for the Prevention and Control of Noncommunicable Diseases: Prevent and Control Cardiovascular Diseases, Cancers, Chronic Respiratory Diseases and Diabetes*, 2008. Geneva: WHO.

Ozcan U., Cao Q., Yilmaz E. et al. Endoplasmic reticulum stress links obesity, insulin action, and type 2 diabetes. *Science* 306 no. 5695 (2004): 457–461.

Perera F., Herbstman J. Prenatal environmental exposures, epigenetics, and disease. *Reprod Toxicol* 31 no. 3 (2011): 363–373.

Poston L. Maternal obesity, gestational weight gain and diet as determinants of offspring long term health. *Best Pract Res Clin Endocrinol Metab* 26 no. 5 (2012): 627–639.

Roberts V. H., Pound L. D., Thorn S. R. et al. Beneficial and cautionary outcomes of resveratrol supplementation in pregnant nonhuman primates. *FASEB J* 28 no. 6 (2014): 2466–2477.

Rodriguez J. S., Rodriguez-Gonzalez G. L., Reyes-Castro L. A. et al. Maternal obesity in the rat programs male offspring exploratory, learning and motivation behavior: Prevention by dietary intervention pre-gestation or in gestation. *Int J Dev Neurosci* 30 no. 2 (2012): 75–81.

Rodriguez-Gonzalez G. L., Vega C. C., Boeck L. et al. Maternal obesity and overnutrition increase oxidative stress in male rat offspring reproductive system and decrease fertility. *Int J Obes* 39 no. 4 (2015): 549–556.

Rooney B. L., Mathiason M. A., Schauberger C. W. Predictors of obesity in childhood, adolescence, and adulthood in a birth cohort. *Matern Child Health J* 15 no. 8 (2011): 1166–1175.

Rooney B. L., Schauberger C. W., Mathiason M. A. Impact of perinatal weight change on long-term obesity and obesity-related illnesses. *Obstet Gynecol* 106 no. 6 (2005): 1349–1356.

Ruiz J. R., Perales M., Pelaez M. et al. Supervised exercise-based intervention to prevent excessive gestational weight gain: A randomized controlled trial. *Mayo Clin Proc* 88 no. 12 (2013): 1388–1397.

Santos M., Rodriguez-Gonzalez G. L., Ibanez C. et al. Adult exercise effects on oxidative stress and reproductive programming in male offspring of obese rats. *Am J Physiol Regul Integr Comp Physiol* 308 no. 3 (2015): R219–225.

Schack-Nielsen L., Michaelsen K. F., Gamborg M., Mortensen E. L., Sorensen T. I. Gestational weight gain in relation to offspring body mass index and obesity from infancy through adulthood. *Int J Obes* 34 no. 1 (2010): 67–74.

Segovia S. A., Vickers M. H., Gray C., Reynolds C. M. Maternal obesity, inflammation, and developmental programming. *Biomed Res Int* 2014 no. (2014): 418975.

Seneviratne S. N., Jiang Y., Derraik J. et al. Effects of antenatal exercise in overweight and obese pregnant women on maternal and perinatal outcomes: A randomised controlled trial. *BJOG* 123 no. 4 (2016): 588–597.

Seneviratne S. N., McCowan L. M., Cutfield W. S., Derraik J. G., Hofman P. L. Exercise in pregnancies complicated by obesity: Achieving benefits and overcoming barriers. *Am J Obstet Gynecol* 212 no. 4 (2015): 442–449.

Shah B. R., Retnakaran R., Booth G. L. Increased risk of cardiovascular disease in young women following gestational diabetes mellitus. *Diabetes Care* 31 no. 8 (2008): 1668–1669.

Simopoulos A. P. Importance of the ratio of omega-6/omega-3 essential fatty acids: Evolutionary aspects. *World Rev Nutr Diet* 92 no. (2003): 1–22.

Skouteris H., Hartley-Clark L., McCabe M. et al. Preventing excessive gestational weight gain: A systematic review of interventions. *Obes Rev* 11 no. 11 (2010): 757–768.

Sui Z., Grivell R. M., Dodd J. M. Antenatal exercise to improve outcomes in overweight or obese women: A systematic review. *Acta Obstet Gynecol Scand* 91 no. 5 (2012): 538–545.

Sun B., Liang N. C., Ewald E. R. et al. Early postweaning exercise improves central leptin sensitivity in offspring of rat dams fed high-fat diet during pregnancy and lactation. *Am J Physiol Regul Integr Comp Physiol* 305 no. 9 (2013): R1076–1084.

Thangaratinam S., Rogozinska E., Jolly K. et al. Effects of interventions in pregnancy on maternal weight and obstetric outcomes: Meta-analysis of randomised evidence. *BMJ* 344 (2012a): e2088.

Thangaratinam S., Rogozinska E., Jolly K. et al. Interventions to reduce or prevent obesity in pregnant women: A systematic review. *Health Technol Assess* 16 no. 31 (2012b): iii–iv, 1–191.

Tuersunjiang N., Odhiambo J. F., Long N. M. et al. Diet reduction to requirements in obese/overfed ewes from early gestation prevents glucose/insulin dysregulation and returns fetal adiposity and organ development to control levels. *Am J Physiol Endocrinol Metab* 305 no. 7 (2013): E868–878.

Vega C. C., Reyes-Castro L. A., Bautista C. J. et al. Exercise in obese female rats has beneficial effects on maternal and male and female offspring metabolism. *Int J Obes* 39 no. 4 (2015): 712–719.

Vega C. C., Reyes-Castro L. A., Rodriguez-Gonzalez G. L. et al. Resveratrol partially prevents oxidative stress and metabolic dysfunction in pregnant rats fed a low protein diet and their offspring. *J Physiol* 594 no. 5 (2016): 1483–1499.

Walsh J. M., Mahony R., Byrne J., Foley M., McAuliffe F. M. The association of maternal and fetal glucose homeostasis with fetal adiposity and birthweight. *Eur J Obstet Gynecol Reprod Biol* 159 no. 2 (2011): 338–341.

Wang J., Chen C., Wang R. Y. Influence of short- and long-term treadmill exercises on levels of ghrelin, obestatin and NPY in plasma and brain extraction of obese rats. *Endocrine* 33 no. 1 (2008): 77–83.

Wrotniak B. H., Shults J., Butts S., Stettler N. Gestational weight gain and risk of overweight in the offspring at age 7 y in a multicenter, multiethnic cohort study. *Am J Clin Nutr* 87 no. 6 (2008): 1818–1824.

Zambrano E., Ibanez C., Martinez-Samayoa P. M. et al. Maternal obesity: Lifelong metabolic outcomes for offspring from poor developmental trajectories during the perinatal period. *Arch Med Res* 47 no. 1 (2016): 1–12.

Zambrano E., Martinez-Samayoa P. M., Rodriguez-Gonzalez G. L., Nathanielsz P. W. Dietary intervention prior to pregnancy reverses metabolic programming in male offspring of obese rats. *J Physiol* 588 Pt 10 (2010): 1791–1799.

Zambrano E., Nathanielsz P. W. Mechanisms by which maternal obesity programs offspring for obesity: Evidence from animal studies. *Nutr Rev* 71 Suppl 1 (2013): S42–54.

Index

Printed and bound by CPI Group (UK) Ltd, Croydon, CR0 4YY

24/10/2024

01778308-0013